MOOD DISORDERS IN WOMEN

MOOD DISORDERS IN WOMEN

Edited by

Meir Steiner MD, PhD, FRCPC

Professor of Psychiatry & Behavioural Neurosciences and Obstetrics and Gynaecology
McMaster University
Hamilton, Ontario, Canada

Kimberly A Yonkers MD

Associate Professor
Department of Psychiatry
Yale University School of Medicine
New Haven, CT, USA

Elias Eriksson MD

Associate Professor
Department of Pharmacology
Göteborg University
Göteborg, Sweden

MARTIN DUNITZ

© Martin Dunitz Ltd 2000

First published in the United Kingdom in 2000
Paperback edition published in the United Kingdom in 2001 by

Martin Dunitz Ltd
The Livery House
7–9 Pratt Street
London NW1 0AE

Tel: +44-(0)20-7482-2202
Fax: +44-(0)20-7267-0159
E-mail: info.dunitz@tandf.co.uk
Website: http://www.dunitz.co.uk

A CIP catalogue record for this book is available from the British Library

ISBN 1-85317-545-5 hardback edition
ISBN 1-84184-107-2 paperback edition

Distributed in the USA by
Fulfilment Center
Taylor & Francis
7625 Empire Drive
Florence, KY 41042, USA
Toll Free Tel: 1-800-634-7064
Email: cserve@routledge ny.com

Distributed in Canada by
Taylor & Francis
74 Rolark Drive
Scarborough
Ontario M1R 4G2, Canada
Toll Free Tel: 1-877-266-2237
Email: tal fran@istar.ca

Distributed in the rest of the world by
ITPS Limited
Cheriton House
North Way, Andover
Hampshire SP10 5BE, UK
Tel: +44 (0) 1264 332424
Email: reception@itps.co.uk

Cover illustration: Trotula of Salerno, 11th century female physician, lithograph. Reproduced courtesy of the Museum of the Medical School of Salerno.

Composition by Wearset, Boldon, Tyne and Wear.
Printed and bound in Spain by Grafos S.A. Arte sobre papel

CONTENTS

List of Contributors

Beth Alder PhD
Department of Epidemiology and Public
Health
University of Dundee
Ninewells Hospital and Medical School
Dundee
Scotland

Torbjörn Bäckström MD
Department of Obstetrics and Gynaecology
Umeå University
SE 901 85 Umeå
Sweden

Leslie Born MSc
Women's Health Concerns Clinic
St Joseph's Hospital
Hamilton, Ontario
Canada L8N 4A6

Karen D Bradshaw MD
5959 Harry Hines Boulevard
Dallas, TX 75235
USA

Olga Brawman-Mintzer MD
Associate Professor of Psychiatry
Department of Psychiatry
Medical University of South Carolina
Charleston, SC 29425
USA

Yulia Chentsova-Dutton BA
Department of Psychiatry
University of California, San Diego
La Jolla, CA 92093
USA

John T Condon MB, BS, MD, Dipl Psychother
Associate Professor of Psychiatry
Flinders University of South Australia
Flinders Medical Centre
Bedford Park
South Australia 5042
Australia

Koen Demyttenaere MD, PhD
University Hospital Gasthuisberg
Department of Psychiatry
Leuven University Fertility Centre, and
Institute of Family and Sexological Sciences
3000 Leuven
Belgium

Edward J Dunn PhD
Associate Professor
Pathology and Molecular Medicine
McMaster University, and
Department of Laboratory Medicine
St Joseph's Hospital
Hamilton, Ontario
Canada L8N 4A6

Lisa Ekselius MD, PhD
Associate Professor in Psychiatry
Department of Neuroscience, Psychiatry
Uppsala University
SE 751 85 Uppsala
Sweden

Elias Eriksson MD
Associate Professor
Department of Pharmacology
Göteborg University
SE 405 30 Göteborg
Sweden

Carl-Gerhard Gottfries MD
Department of Psychiatry and Neurochemistry
Sahlgrenska University Hospital/Mölndal
SE 431 80 Mölndal
Sweden

Uriel Halbreich MD
BioBehavioral Program
State University of New York at Buffalo
Buffalo, NY 14215
USA

Katherine A Halmi MD
Professor of Psychology in Psychiatry
Director Cornell Eating Disorders Program
Weill Medical College at Cornell
The New York Presbyterian Hospital
Westchester Division
White Plains, NY 10605
USA

Shirley Y Hill PhD
Department of Psychiatry
University of Pittsburgh Medical Center
Pittsburgh, PA 15213
USA

Amy Hostetter BA
Department of Psychiatry and Behavioral
Sciences
Emory University School of Medicine
Atlanta, GA 30322
USA

Linda S Kahn PhD
Biobehavioral Program
State University of New York at Buffalo
Buffalo, NY 14215
USA

Siegfried Kasper MD
Department of General Psychiatry
University of Vienna
1090 Vienna
Austria

Ronald C Kessler PhD
Department of Health Care Policy
Harvard Medical School
Boston, MA 02115-5899
USA

Lars von Knorring MD, PhD
Professor in Psychiatry
Department of Neuroscience, Psychiatry
Uppsala University
SE 751 85 Uppsala
Sweden

Mikael Landén MD, PhD
Department of Psychiatry and Neurochemistry
Göteborg University
Göteborg
Sahlgrenska University Hospital/Mölndal
SE 431 80 Mölndal
Sweden

Ellen Leibenluft MD
Chief, Unit on Affective Disorders
Pediatric and Developmental Neuropsychiatry
Branch
Bethesda, MD 20892
USA

Alexis Llewellyn BA
Department of Psychiatry and Behavioral
Sciences
Emory University School of Medicine
Atlanta, GA 30322
USA

Peter Marton PhD
Psychologist
101 Queensway W, Suite 105
Mississauga, Ontario
Canada

Margaret M McCarthy PhD
Department of Physiology
University of Maryland
Baltimore, MD 21201
USA

Michael T McGuire MD
Department of Psychiatry/Biobehavioral
Sciences
Brain Research Institute
School of Medicine
University of California at Los Angeles
Los Angeles, CA 90095
USA

Marta Meana PhD
Assistant Professor
Department of Psychology
University of Nevada, Las Vegas
Las Vegas, NV 89154
USA

Kathleen R Merikangas PhD
Professor of Epidemiology, Psychiatry, and
Psychology
Yale University School of Medicine
Genetic Epidemiology Research Unit
New Haven, CT 06510
USA

Charles B Nemeroff MD, PhD
Ruenette W Harris Professor and Chairman
Department of Psychiatry and Behavioral
Sciences
Emory University School of Medicine
Atlanta, GA 30322
USA

Alexander Neumeister MD
Department of General Psychiatry
University of Vienna
1090 Vienna
Austria

Michael W O'Hara PhD
Department of Psychology
University of Iowa
Iowa City, IA 52242
USA

Veronica O'Keane PhD, MB, MRCPsych,
MRCPI
Department of Psychiatry
Beaumont Hospital
Dublin 9
Republic of Ireland

Kelley Phillips MD, MPH, FRCPS(C), FAPA
President
American College of Women's Health
Physicians
Foundation for Women's Health
Washington, DC 20007
USA

Natalie L Rasgon MD
Department of Psychiatry/Biobehavioral
Sciences
School of Medicine
University of California at Los Angeles
Los Angeles, CA 90024
USA

Malcolm P Rogers MD
Associate Clinical Professor of Psychiatry
Department of Psychiatry
Harvard Medical School
Boston, MA 02115
USA

Stephen R Shuchter MD
Professor of Psychiatry
Department of Psychiatry
University of California, San Diego
La Jolla, CA 92093
USA

Deborah Sichel MD
Hestia Institute
Wellesley, MA 02481
USA

Micah J Sickel MS
Department of Physiology
University of Maryland
Baltimore, MD 21201
USA

Meir Steiner MD, PhD, FRCPC
Professor of Psychiatry & Behavioural
Neurosciences and Obstetrics and Gynaecology
McMaster University, and
Director of Research
Department of Psychiatry
St Joseph's Hospital
Hamilton, Ontario
Canada L8N 4A6

Donna E Stewart MD, FRCP(C)
Lillian Love Chair in Women's Health
University Health Network
Toronto General Hospital
University of Toronto
Toronto, Ontario
Canada M5G 2C4

Zachary N Stowe MD
Associate Professor
Department of Psychiatry and Behavioral
Sciences
Emory University School of Medicine
Atlanta, GA 30322
USA

Scott Stuart MD
Department of Psychiatry
University of Iowa
Iowa City, IA 52242
USA

Suzanne R Sunday PhD
Assistant Professor of Psychology in Psychiatry
Weill Medical College at Cornell
The New York Presbyterian Hospital
White Plains, NY 10605
USA

Charlotta Sundblad MD
Department of Pharmacology
Göteborg University
SE 405 30 Göteborg
Sweden

Eva M Szigethy MD, PhD
Assistant Professor
Department of Psychiatry
Boston Children's Hospital
Boston, MA 02115
USA

Alfonso Troisi MD
University of Rome 'La Sapienza'
Tor Vergata
Rome
Italy

Claire V Wiseman PhD
Assistant Professor of Psychology in
Psychiatry
Weill Medical College at Cornell
The New York Presbyterian Hospital
White Plains, NY 10605
USA

Katherine L Wisner MD, MS
Director, Women's Services
Department of Psychiatry
Case Western Reserve University School of
Medicine
Cleveland, OH 44106
USA

Judith J Wurtman PhD
Department of Brain and Cognitive Science
Massachusetts Institute of Technology
Cambridge, MA 02139
USA

Kimberly A Yonkers MD
Associate Professor
Department of Psychiatry
Yale University School of Medicine
New Haven, CT 06520
USA

Sidney Zisook MD
Professor of Psychiatry
University of California, San Diego
Department of Psychiatry
La Jolla, CA 92093
USA

Introduction

Evaluating physical, social and mental impacts of disease, and using the disability-adjusted life-year formula, depression was the fourth leading cause on the Global Burden of Illness list in 1990 and is predicted to be the first leading cause by the year 2020. The morbidity associated with depression in women is even greater. Not only do at least twice as many women suffer from the disorder when compared to men, but they also have a higher rate of depression-associated comorbid conditions (both physical and mental). From the age of menarche until well after menopause, women suffer from specific mood disorders, including premenstrual and perimenopausal dysphoria, depression associated with pregnancy and the postpartum period, as well as mood disorders associated with infertility and pregnancy loss. Untreated depression in elderly women is associated with an almost four-fold increase in mortality rates when compared to non-depressed, age-matched women.

Women also suffer more from eating disorders and autoimmune disease, are less tolerant to alcohol use and have a higher prevalence of pain disorders. They are influenced to a greater degree by seasonality, suffer more from jet lag and from shift-work and, last but not least, metabolize drugs differently than men. Some of this information is very new. In fact, most of it has been accumulated in the last 25 years, but some of it has been known since antiquity.

Trotula of Salerno, an eleventh century female gynaecologist (shown on the cover of this book), described, in her book, premenstrual symptoms ('There are young women who are relieved when the menses are called

forth'), postpartum blues ('If the womb is too moist the brain is filled with water & the moisture running over to the eyes compels them involuntarily to shed tears'), as well as disorders associated with the menopause ('There are also older women who give forth blood matter especially as the menopause approaches them').

In the seventeenth century, hysteria and melancholia were described as female-specific disorders in terms such as 'a disease called the suffocation of the mother' (Jordan, 1603); and 'maids', nuns' and widows' melancholy' (Burton, 1640). The notion that the origin of these disorders was in the uterus or in the gall-bladder was soon abandoned, and an abundance of theories about the mind–body relationship flourished in the eighteenth and nineteenth centuries. Some of these led to the evolution of both the psychoanalytical movement and the rediscovery of sexuality, as well as to the more medically oriented psychosomatic concepts.

The evolutionary perspective suggests that possible male–female asymmetries in preference for certain types of relationships, a differential investment in reproduction and offspring, as well as social options (or their lack), all contribute to the fact that women are more vulnerable to mood and other disorders than are men. While it is widely recognized that mood disorders are more common in women, it is still the case that depression is underdiagnosed and undertreated.

It is imperative that we learn about sex and gender differences in the aetiology, presentation, prevention and treatment of mood disorders. The failure to recognize depression in women is not due to the fact that they present less frequently to health care providers. Until very recently, women were systematically discriminated against in medical research in the USA and elsewhere. In 1977, the FDA issued a guideline for the clinical evaluation of drugs that mandated the exclusion of women with childbearing potential. These guidelines were revised in 1993; however, pharmaceutical companies and funding agencies have been slow in adopting the new recommendations. Reports on sex differences in drug pharmacokinetics, pharmacodynamics and response in both animals and humans should, by now, have convinced everybody of the importance of including women in all phases of clinical trials. The NIH, which has now created an Office for Research on Women's Health, is not only devoting its attention to the inclusion of women in clinical trials but has also become the watchdog to ensure that women's health research is an integral part of the scientific fabric.

The American Psychiatric Association, the World Health Organization and many of the major pharmaceutical companies now have Women's Offices. The American College of Obstetrics and Gynecologists has recently pledged to focus its attention on depression in women, and the American Board of Internal Medicine, in 1997, approved specific recommendations on required core competencies in women's health for internists.

Yet very little is known about the reasons for the differences in prevalence rates of depression, nor do we know much about sex differences in antidepressant effectiveness, tolerability and safety and in particular about the efficacy and safety of these agents during pregnancy and postpartum.

It is estimated that 7 million US women suffer from major depressive disorder at any given time, and the prevalence worldwide is much the same. This is the single most serious mental health problem for women. For many women, the only physician they will ever see is an obstetrician–gynaecologist or a general practitioner. This puts us psychiatrists in a very unique domain within academic medicine.

It is the purpose of this book to draw the attention of as many healthcare professionals as possible to the present state of knowledge of mood disorders in women, from bench to bedside. We hope that the information provided here will not only improve the care of women but will also be an incentive to study further those areas where our knowledge is still incomplete.

Meir Steiner
Kimberly Yonkers
Elias Eriksson

Acknowledgements

A book of this kind ultimately represents the efforts of many individuals. We would like to acknowledge the expertise and professionalism of our editors, Ian Mellor, Tanya Wiedeking, Julie Gorman and Alison Campbell, and the staff at Martin Dunitz Publishers for their hard work and dedication and for their confidence in us despite our many missed deadlines. Most of all we owe tremendous gratitude to Janice Rogers, Leslie Born, Carol Ballantyne and Annette Wilkins from the Women's Health Concerns Clinic at St Joseph's Hospital, McMaster University, Hamilton, Ontario, Canada for all their help and hard work in 'orchestrating' 31 chapters into one volume; and to Denise Landers from the University of Texas Southwestern Medical Center, who coordinated the work on many chapters in conjunction with Dr Yonkers.

And finally each of us would also like to thank our loved ones: MS to Jutta, Juwal, Inbal, Ronni and Jasmin; KY to Charles, Ethan, Arielle and Justin; and EE to Agneta, Jakob, Arvid and Agnes.

1

Epidemiology of mood disorders in women

Kathleen R Merikangas

Overview of evidence for sex differences in the prevalence of mood disorders

A substantial increase in the risk of mood disorders among women compared to men has been consistently observed in clinical and epidemiological samples. There is abundant literature describing possible explanations for the female preponderance of depression, and several reviews of this topic are available.[1-4] The goals of this chapter are: (1) to review the epidemiological evidence regarding sex differences in depression; (2) to evaluate possible explanations for the female preponderance of depression; and (3) to illustrate the application of genetic epidemiological studies to investigate sources of sex differences in depression.

Epidemiological data provide an important source of information on both artefactual and real explanations for sex differences, because they provide the most accurate representation of the expression of disorders in the general population. The major advantages of the epidemiological approach over the use of strictly clinical samples include: (1) increased generalizability of findings through the use of representative samples that reflect the various strata of the general population; (2) larger sample sizes that allow for the ability to control for multiple confounding factors associated with differential base frequencies of disorders; (3) greater statistical power and therefore enhanced ability to examine subtypes of disorders; and (4) elimination of bias associated with treatment-seeking behaviours (e.g. Berkson's bias).[5]

Although most reviews have concluded that the sex difference in depression is real, it is still necessary to evaluate systematically possible artefactual explanations for the female preponderance of depression. These include: sampling bias (i.e. increased detection of females in clinical samples); definition or detection bias (i.e. the thresholds for depression biased towards women, greater tendency to detect or report depression); and confounding with another correlate of depression (i.e. comorbidity with anxiety, anxiety which increases the risk for depression, or alcoholism as a *formes fruste* of depression in women). After exclusion of possible artefactual explanations for the female excess of mood disorders, numerous classes of explanations have been considered. These include: genetics (e.g. females have increased genetic loading for mood disorders); neurobiological factors (e.g. fluctuation of reproductive hormones, increased stress reactivity in women); greater exposure to environmental stressors (e.g. role stress, life events); increased prevalence of premorbid risk factors for depression in women (e.g. temperamental factors); or, more likely, a combination of the aforementioned explanations.

Sex differences in mood disorders in community surveys

Increased representation of females in clinical settings as an explanation for the sex difference in depression has become implausible with the increased availability of large-scale epidemiological data that confirm the preponderance of women with depression in the community. The results of two major community-based surveys of psychiatric disorders that have been conducted in the USA, the Epidemiological Catchment Area study (ECA) and the National Comorbidity Study (NCS), confirm the sex difference in mood disorders that has been reported in earlier epidemiological studies across the world over the last several decades.[2,6–14] The ECA consisted of a large-scale study that included a probability sample of adults across five sites in the USA. Diagnostic information necessary for ascertaining the DSM-III criteria for the major psychiatric disorders was collected via a structured diagnostic instrument, the Diagnostic Interview Survey (DIS),[15] which was adminis-

tered by lay interviewers. The NCS was based on a nationally stratified multi-stage area probability sample of non-institutionalized adults. The Composite International Diagnostic Interview (CIDI),[16] a structured diagnostic instrument, was used to collect the diagnostic information. The major differences between these two large-scale studies, which were conducted a decade apart, include: (1) a national sampling frame of the NCS compared to the five-site design in the ECA; (2) the use of DSM-III-R; and (3) different diagnostic instruments in the NCS rather than the DSM-III criteria used in the ECA.

Table 1.1 presents the sex-specific lifetime rates and sex ratios for the major subtypes of mood disorders assessed in the ECA and NCS. Although the magnitude of the rates of mood disorders varies substantially between the two studies, the sex ratio is consistently greater for women, with a 1.6–2-fold elevation in lifetime rates of major depression and dysthymia. Thus, data from large-scale epidemiological studies in the USA nearly a decade apart reveal that a greater proportion of females than males report all of the subtypes of non-bipolar mood disturbances. In contrast, the sex ratio for bipolar disorder in community samples is approximately equal.

Not only is there a consistent sex difference in mood disorders in the USA, but there is also international evidence that women have greater rates of depression. In a recent summary of the lifetime prevalence rates of depression in 10 countries, Weissman et al[17] found a greater proportion of females with depression across all studies. However, there was a wide difference in the magnitude of the sex differences, with the lowest sex ratio in Taiwan and the greatest in Italy and West Germany.

The strength of evidence from community surveys excludes the explanation that the female preponderance of depression is related

Table 1.1 Sex-specific lifetime prevalence rates of mood disorders in community surveys in the USA.

Affective disorders	Epidemiological Catchment Area Study (ECA)[17]			National Comorbidity Survey (NCS)[24]		
	Males	Females	Sex ratio (F/M)	Males	Females	Sex ratio (F/M)
All affective disorders	5.2	10.2	2.0	14.7	23.9	1.6
Major depression	2.6	7.0	2.7	11.0	18.6	1.7
Dysthymia	2.2	4.1	1.9	4.8	8.0	1.7
Manic episode	1.1	1.4	1.3	0.4	0.5	1.2

to an increased tendency for women to seek treatment. Nevertheless, data from community samples do confirm the increased representation of women in clinical settings. For example, data from the prospective epidemiological study of young adults in Zurich, Switzerland demonstrated that depressed females are more likely to seek treatment than are males.[18] Table 1.2 presents the sex-specific rates of treatment by affective subtype among participants in the Zurich Cohort Study of Young Adults. These data reveal a three-fold increase in treatment rates among women compared to men.

Studies of sex differences in treatment settings generally find a significantly greater proportion of females with depression. A recent study of depressive and anxiety disorders in primary care settings in 15 centres from four continents revealed a preponderance of females with current depression.[19] However, the magnitude and consistency of the sex differences were less pronounced than those observed in the epidemiological studies shown in Table 1.1. Table 1.3 shows the sex-specific rates and sex ratio of current depression in the World Health

Table 1.2 Zurich Cohort Study: sex differences in proportion of patients treated by depressive subtypes.[18]

Depression subtype	Male	Female	Sex ratio (F/M)
Major depression	2.8	10.8	3.9
Dysthymia	0.7	1.7	2.4
Recurrent brief	2.8	11.1	3.9
Minor depression	0.6	3.4	5.7
All depression	5.7	17.5	3.1

Organization Study of Psychologic Problems in General Health Care.[19] Statistical analysis of the sex ratio across centres revealed an odds ratio of 1.6 for a physician-identified current episode of major depression in females versus males, with no sex by centre interaction. The authors concluded that the consistency of the sex difference across such a large and culturally diverse sample implicates biological factors or non-specific psychosocial factors that transcend cultural barriers in the aetiology of depression. Moreover, there is some suggestive evidence that physicians are more likely to diagnose and treat depression in women than in men.

Explanations for sex differences in mood disorders

Since the sex difference in depression does not appear to be an artefact of the sampling source, other possible methodological explanations for the female excess of depression must be consid-

Table 1.3 Sex-specific prevalence and sex ratio of current depressive episode in primary care.[19]			
Centre	Men	Women	Sex ratio (F/M)
Ankara, Turkey	9.8	12.5	1.3
Athens, Greece	6.5	6.4	1.0
Bangalore, India	4.8	13.3	2.8
Berlin, Germany	3.7	7.7	2.1
Groningen, The Netherlands	13.0	17.9	1.4
Ibadan, Nigeria	5.3	3.8	0.7
Mainz, Germany	9.8	12.3	1.3
Manchester, UK	13.9	18.3	1.3
Nagasaki, Japan	2.3	2.8	1.2
Paris, France	9.3	18.7	2.0
Rio de Janiero, Brazil	5.8	19.6	3.4
Santiago, Chile	11.2	36.8	3.3
Seattle, USA	6.0	6.5	1.1
Shanghai, China	3.3	4.4	1.3
Verona, Italy	3.2	5.5	1.7
Total	7.1	12.5	1.8

ered. In the following section, sex differences in reporting, the components of the definition of depression, age at onset and course and comorbidity are reviewed.

Sex differences in reporting of depression

In a longitudinal study of an epidemiological sample, Angst and Dobler-Mikola[20] found that males were more likely to forget the occurrence of depressive symptoms over time than were females. Moreover, Briscoe[21] showed that women more readily report minor psychiatric disturbances to their physicians, possibly due to a greater awareness of symptoms and/or a lower threshold of discomfort before symptom recognition. In their comprehensive review of sex differences in definitional and reporting biases, Ernst and Angst[4] concluded that, despite the tendency for females to report more accurately the components of depression, such artefactual explanations are unlikely sources of the consistent sex difference in depression.

In assessing possible explanations for sex differences in depression and anxiety among adolescents, Lewinsohn et al[22] concluded that the sex difference could not be attributed to reporting bias, because there was no gender difference in measures of social desirability. However, this still did not rule out possible gender differences in reporting of depressive symptoms because of other reasons, such as differential awareness or cognitive interpretation between males and females.

Some of the major impediments of assessing depression in young children include the lack of stability of reporting symptoms, insufficient cognitive development to judge the meaning of physical symptoms and signs, and the significance of fears and worries. The use of a maternal report to provide the context for symptoms in children has helped to determine the significance of self-reported symptoms of depression in children. Among adolescents, Compas et al[23] found that the sex difference in depression among adolescents was less pronounced by maternal report than by self-report of the adolescent. Thus, it is unlikely that reporting bias can explain the large differences in prevalence of depression among females; however, there is some suggestive evidence that males tend to underreport symptoms during direct interviews, which may lead to an increase in the magnitude of the sex ratio for mood states.

Sex differences in the clinical components and correlates of depression

One of the first systematic reviews of sex differences in the components of depression was conducted by Angst and Dobler-Mikola,[20] who reported that the sex ratio was strongly associated with the definition of depression. As the number of symptoms increased, the discrepancy in the rates between males and females became greater. The female preponderance of depression is also found for depressive symptoms, subthreshold definitions of depression, and several components of the diagnostic categories of mood disorders, including severity, recurrence, impairment and course.

Data from both the ECA and NCS likewise illustrate a direct relationship between the number of symptoms of depression and the sex ratio.[17,24] The sex-specific rates of depressive symptoms with a 2-week duration reported in the ECA study revealed greater rates of all symptoms among women.[17] Likewise, Kessler et al[24] found that women reported far more symptoms of depression than did men; the sex ratio increased with increasing numbers of criterial symptoms of depression. Data from both the

ECA and NCS as well as other community surveys also revealed that the female preponderance of depression was observed across all prevalence periods, increasingly strict definitions of depression, and all ages throughout adulthood. More recently, evaluation of the sex differences in subthreshold manifestation of depression revealed a direct relationship between the magnitude of the sex ratio and the severity of depression.[18]

Inspection of the sex differences in the components of depression in children and adolescents have the advantage of minimizing potential recall bias. The Oregon Adolescent Depression Project (OADP) provides some of the most significant evidence regarding the sex difference of depression in adolescents.[25] The OADP is a prospective longitudinal study of adolescents aged 14–18 from the general community in which sex differences in the prevalence, course, risk factors, onset and comorbidity of mood disorders were examined.[25] Figure 1.1 shows the sex difference in depression by the various time periods of assessment, ranging from lifetime to current as well as recurrence of previous cases. As compared to males, females had greater rates of both major depression and dysthymia across all time periods (Figure 1.1).

Other epidemiological surveys of adolescents have yielded similar findings. For example, Compas et al[23] found significant sex differences for all definitions of depression, ranging from depressed mood to depression/anxiety syndrome, as well as an analogue rating of DSM-IV major depression. In contrast, the results of a recent large-scale twin survey revealed that although females reported more depressive symptoms, the sex difference in depression was minimal when the criteria for depression included impairment.[26]

Similar reviews of artefactual explanations for the sex difference in depression have also concluded that females truly manifest increased

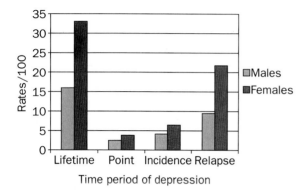

Figure 1.1 Sex ratio of depression in adolescents. Lifetime: current and past episodes. Point: current episodes. Incidence: new onset. Relapse: new episodes in previous cases.

rates of depression, irrespective of the sampling, definition of depression and methods of assessment.[2]

Sex differences in onset and course

Although cross-sectional epidemiological data demonstrate consistently increased prevalence rates of depression among women, inspection of the evolution of the sex difference over time is critical to identifying risk factors associated with depression in women. Retrospective data from the NCS indicate that females have greater rates of major depression across the lifespan, with the exception of the ages 35–39, when new onsets among males temporarily exceed those of females. Thereafter, the female predominance re-emerges, with an increase in prevalence after age 45.[24]

Epidemiological studies of mood disorders in childhood and adolescence may also provide clues regarding possible explanations for the sex difference in depression by examining the

age at which the discrepancy becomes apparent as well as the changes in risk factors and correlates of depression across the progression of the period of risk for onset of the depression. Although the results of these studies reveal that females have greater rates of depression than males, the most informative data are those derived from prospective longitudinal data that examine the course of males and females across the period at which the female excess begins to emerge.

In light of the compelling evidence for the increased prevalence of mood disorders among women, one of the key explanations of the gender difference may be provided by the age at which the sex difference emerges. The sex-specific rates of mood disorders in several large-scale community and school-based surveys of children and adolescents[25–28] demonstrate that the sex difference in females first emerges in late childhood and early adolescence. Whereas an equivalent proportion of males and females have depression in childhood, increasing proportions of females as compared to males tend to develop depression during the early teen years.[29–42] For example, Offord et al[43] reported that the sex ratio for emotional disorders was 1.1 at ages 4–11 years, whereas it was 2.7 at ages 12–16. Thereafter, the female preponderance remains elevated across the lifespan.

Increasing evidence of the evolution of sex differences in depression exists among community samples of children and adolescents. The results of prospective studies of children and adolescents reveal that the female excess of depression tends to emerge around the age of 13.[30,31,34,44,45] Lewinsohn et al reported that the incidence rates of depression were greater among females than males across all ages between mid-to-late adolescence.[25] However, the findings did not indicate that the sex difference between males and females became greater with increasing age, since there was no sex by age interaction during the mid-teen years.

Two prospective longitudinal follow-up studies of children and adolescents have shown a greater stability of internalizing disorders in girls compared to boys.[40,44,46] Likewise, the results of other studies suggest a sex difference in the continuity of emotional problems. Bolognini et al[47] found that girls without emotional problems in childhood who developed new-onset emotional problems in adolescence tended to have persistent problems into adulthood, whereas boys with emotional disorders in childhood tended to remit in adulthood. Likewise, Lewinsohn et al[25] reported that females had greater relapse rates than males when evaluated prospectively.

Finally, evidence from studies of clinical samples of both children and adults have been inconsistent in their conclusions regarding sex differences in the treatment outcome and course of depression among patients with mood disorders. Some investigators reported few significant sex differences in the course of depression in terms of time to recovery, the overall time to first recurrence, or the number or severity of recurrences of major depressive episodes in clinical samples followed prospectively;[48,49] epidemiological studies tend to show that females do experience greater duration, recurrence, chronicity and global manifestations of depression than males throughout early to middle adulthood.[4] However, in general, the epidemiological and clinical data converge in demonstrating a more severe and chronic course among women.[50,51]

Comorbidity as an explanation for sex difference

Comorbidity between mood disorders and other psychiatric disorders may provide one explanation for the sex difference in depression. Breslau et al[52] reported that the higher rates of anxiety among females early in life may in part explain the sex difference in depression among adult females. However, since there was no interaction between primary anxiety and depression and sex, the observed gender difference in depression cannot be wholly attributable to the anxiety–depression link.

Sex differences in the patterns of comorbidity between depression and specific subtypes of anxiety states were also assessed in the Zurich Cohort Study.[4] Whereas comorbidity between depression and panic or generalized anxiety was independent of sex, comorbidity of phobic states and depression (called 'sex-dependent comorbidity' by the authors) was limited to females. Family and twin studies also show common underlying aetiological factors for the broad diagnostic categories of anxiety and depression, but longitudinal studies of comorbidity tend to reveal that anxiety disorders, particularly phobic disorders, tend to have far more stability over time than depression.[53]

Likewise, there is fairly compelling evidence that comorbidity between depression and substance disorders does not explain the increased rates of depression among females. This explanation posits that the higher rate of substance disorders in males results from the male tendency to use alcohol or drugs to self-medicate underlying mood disorders. However, the results of several epidemiological studies have found that comorbidity between depressive disorders and either alcohol or drug dependence tends to be either more common in females[53,54] or equal across gender.[55] This suggests that the sex difference in mood disorders cannot be explained by the increased frequency of substance disorders in males resulting from masked expression of underlying mood states, since females are even more likely to exhibit both depression and substance disorders despite their lower rates of substance abuse and dependence.

Evidence from family study data also tends to rule out comorbidity between substance and mood disorders as an artefactual explanation for the lower rates of depression in males. Despite the widely held belief that alcoholism represents the male form of expression of depression, family studies have provided rather consistent evidence for specificity of familial aggregation of alcoholism among both males and females. Many family and twin studies have failed to provide evidence for sex-specific cross-aggregation of depression and alcoholism.[56-58]

Comorbidity between mood disorders and other DSM-III-R or -IV disorders is even more common in adolescents than in adults.[59] Epidemiological studies of children and adolescents reveal that depression is associated with all of the other major classes of disorders, including anxiety disorders, disruptive behaviours, eating disorders, and substance use (e.g. Lewinsohn et al[25]). In the Virginia Twin Study of Adolescent Behavioral Development (VTSABD), depression was significantly associated with all other disorders except attention deficit hyperactivity disorder. Among the depression cases with impairment, 77% of the cases were comorbid with at least one other emotional disorder, and 27% with two or more other disorders.[26] In a review of the literature on comorbidity of anxiety and depression in youth, Brady and Kendall[60] suggested that anxiety and depression may be part of a developmental sequence in which anxiety is expressed earlier in life than depression. Thus, because comorbidity between anxiety and both depression and substance problems is quite common in children and adolescents of both genders, it is unlikely to provide an explanation for the sex difference in depression.

Risk factors for depression among women

Although the specific domains of risk which potentially explain the female preponderance of depression are reviewed in depth in the remainder of this book (see Chapters 4, 5 and 13), epidemiological data may provide insights regarding possible aetiological risk factors for depression in women. Striking evidence for the role of endocrine factors in the onset of depression in girls was reported recently by Angold et al.[61] Based on prospective evaluation of a community sample, it was found that the increase in depressive symptoms in girls relative to boys was attributable to pubertal stage (i.e. Tanner stage III) rather than to age. Moreover, this developmental transition was rather sharply demarcated.

Prospective epidemiological studies have also provided numerous clues regarding risk factors that underlie the female preponderance of depression.[62] These include: pre-existing anxiety disorders, increased vulnerability to environmental stress such as familial discord, life events and physical illness, decreased coping skills, and lack of social support. The increased sensitivity to life events among girls confirms the results of a prospective longitudinal study of youth that revealed that parental death evoked depression in female but not male offspring.[63] Perhaps more compelling are explanations that invoke multiple domains of risk which may either mediate or moderate expression of depression in susceptible individuals. For example, Davies and Windle[64] concluded that there were gender-specific pathways to depression through marital discord and maternal depression, with girls having greater vulnerability to familial disruption than boys. Future studies will need to examine simultaneously the overlap between genetic, biological and environmental factors in order to enhance our understanding of sex-specific pathways to depression.

Explanations for sex differences using family study designs

The familial aggregation of all of the major subtypes of depression has been well established.[65] The results of twin studies of depressive symptoms and disorders reveal that familial clustering of depression can be attributed largely to genetic factors.[66–69] Several studies have investigated sex differences in the genetic factors underlying the components of depression. The findings confirm that the same genetic factors underlie depression in both males and females. For example, Madden et al[70] reported no difference in the genetic factors underlying seasonal depression in men and women.

In addition to providing evidence regarding the possible role of transmissible genetic factors, family studies may be employed to investigate sources of a sex difference in the prevalence of a particular disorder. The sex effect can be treated as a differential threshold, with the less commonly affected sex having the higher threshold.[71] Accumulation of more genetic and/or environmental factors is required for the disorder to become manifest at the higher threshold. Because such individuals have increased genetic and/or environmental loading for the trait, they have more factors to transmit or share with their relatives. Therefore, the relatives of probands with the more deviant threshold are more likely to be affected by the disorder.[72]

With respect to depression, relatives of males would be expected to exhibit greater rates of depression than relatives of females if the sex difference in depression can be attributed to genetic factors. If one applies this principle to major depression, males should have a higher threshold than females; this requires the accumulation of more risk factors in males in order for depression to manifest itself. Relatives of male probands would then be expected to have greater risk for depression than relatives of female probands if the sex difference for major depression were genetic. The results of a familial aggregation study by Merikangas et al[2] demonstrated that despite an increased prevalence of depression in female relatives compared with male relatives, this excess was not attributable to increased genetic loading for depression in women. Several subsequent investigations of sex differences in familial transmission of affective disorders have yielded inconsistent conclusions. These differences in the conclusions may be attributed to the subtypes of affective disorder (i.e. bipolar versus unipolar) and generational composition of the family study sample.[73]

In a compilation of existing family study data on bipolar disorder, Baron et al[74] reported that the patterns of familial aggregation were consistent with X-linked transmission based on the low frequency of male-to-male transmission and excess risk among female relatives. Other models of sex differences in familial transmission, including sex-linked transmission and autosomal transmission with non-familial effects, have been summarized by Faraone et al,[75] who also concluded that the sex difference in affective disorders could not be attributed to genetic factors. Recent analyses of a large-scale controlled family study revealed an increased risk of major depression among relatives of female probands, the opposite pattern to that predicted by the above-cited expectations of genetic-based sex differences in depression.[57] Therefore, current evidence does not support genetic explanations for the preponderance of females with depression.

Summary and conclusions

In summary, there is consistent evidence that women have higher rates of mood disorders and symptoms than men across the age span. Systematic review of possible artefactual explanations, including sampling or methodological factors, cannot explain the large female preponderance of depression. However, there is some evidence that males are less likely to report depressive symptoms, to recall depressive episodes and to suffer from the same magnitude of impairment and distress as women. In a review of the multiple possible explanations for the higher rates of depression in women, the most compelling explanation is that, given the same degree of genetic vulnerability for depression, women are more likely to have higher levels of somatic symptoms, rumination, feelings of worthlessness and guilt than are men.

There is now abundant evidence from epidemiological studies that the sex difference in depression emerges in early adolescence and remains fairly stable across life. Prospective epidemiological studies have also provided numerous clues regarding risk factors that underlie the sex difference in depression. These include: pre-existing anxiety disorders, pubertal hormones, increased vulnerability to environmental stress such as familial discord, life events and physical illness, decreased coping skills, lack of social support, increased severity and expressivity of depression, and greater levels of expression of underlying vulnerability for depression, as well as increased severity and frequency of depressive symptoms among ongoing cases.

There are several areas in need of additional research. Future studies should address the following issues:

- Studies designed to develop more accurate and developmentally sensitive methods of assessment of the components of depression, including mood regulation, cognitive development, neurovegetative signs and stress reactivity with a focus on developing objective measures of the components of depression

- Follow-up studies of community-based samples of individuals with depression to examine the longitudinal stability of depression, the overlap between the mood disorders and other types of psychiatric and medical disorders, and risk factors and correlates associated with chronicity and remission

- Additional research on the role of comorbidity of anxiety and depression in the sex differences for emotional disorders

- Following up the intriguing evidence that the onset of depression is associated with specific stages of pubertal development, further research attention to hormonally mediated neurobiological function is needed in order to understand gender differences predisposing women to experience decreased resilience to extrinsic and intrinsic stress

- Systematic study of the role of sex-specific transmission in family, twin and high-risk studies of mood disorders and their overlap with anxiety disorders in order to identify the extent to which genetic and environmental factors contribute to the aetiology of depression

- Simultaneous investigation of the overlap between genetic, biological and environmental factors in order to enhance our understanding of sex-specific pathways to depression

In addition to research implications of this work, there are several clinical issues of relevance to mood disorders in women. First, the sheer magnitude of affective states, affecting up to one-third of women across the lifespan, warrants intensive focus on increased education and treatment of depression in the general population. Second, the focus on links between depression and the female reproductive cycle has failed to consider the importance of anxiety symptoms and disorders that may even overshadow those of depression, particularly in younger women. Third, the importance of early intervention in mood disorders is highlighted by the evidence of its temperamental underpinnings and chronicity across the lifespan. The dramatic increase in rates of onset of mood disorders during the early stages of adolescence provides an important target for prevention of the crystallization of these disorders and subsequent impairment in the accomplishment of both education and social life goals. The over-

whelming focus on disruptive behaviour problems in youth should be balanced by new initiatives to identify those who suffer quietly from depression and anxiety, thereby minimizing opportunities for application of the intervention and treatment strategies that have been well developed for depression in clinical settings.

Acknowledgments

This research is supported in part by grants AA07080, DA05348, AA09978, DA09055, and MH36197, and a Research Scientist Development Award K02 from Alcohol, Drug Abuse, and Mental Health Administration of the United States Public Health Service.

References

1. Weissman MM, Klerman GL, Sex differences and the epidemiology of depression, *Arch Gen Psychiatry* 1977; **34**:98–111.
2. Merikangas KR, Weissman MM, Pauls DL, Genetic factors in the sex ratio of major depression, *Psychol Med* 1985; **15**:63–9.
3. Nolen-Hoeksema S, Sex differences in unipolar depression: evidence and theory, *Psychol Bull* 1987; **101**:259–82.
4. Ernst C, Angst J, The Zurich Study: XII. Sex difference in depression. Evidence from longitudinal epidemiological data, *Eur Arch Psychiatry Clin Neurosci* 1992; **241**:222–30.
5. Berkson J, Limitation of the application of the 4-fold table analysis to hospital data, *Biometrics* 1946; **2**:47–53.
6. Canino GJ, Bird HR, Shrout PE et al, The prevalence of specific psychiatric disorders in Puerto Rico, *Arch Gen Psychiatry* 1987; **44**:727–35.
7. Bland RC, Orn H, Newman SC, Lifetime prevalence of psychiatric disorders in Edmonton, *Acta Psychiatr Scand Suppl* 1988; **338**:24–32.
8. Faravelli C, Guerrini Degl'Innocenti B, Giardnelli L, Epidemiology of anxiety disorders

in Florence, *Acta Psychiatr Scand* 1989; **79**:308–12.
9. Wells JE, Bushnell JA, Hornblow AR et al, Christchurch psychiatric epidemiology study: methodology and lifetime prevalence for specific psychiatric disorders, *Aust NZ J Psychiatry* 1989; **23**:315–26.
10. Angst J, Comorbidity of anxiety, phobia, compulsions, and depression, *Int Clin Psychopharmacol* 1993; **8**(suppl 1):21–5.
11. Lee CK, Kwak YS, Yamamototo J et al, Psychiatric epidemiology in Korea: Part 1. Gender and age differences in Seoul, *J Nerv Ment Dis* 1990; **178**:242–6.
12. Wacker H, Mullejans R, Klein K et al, Identification of cases of anxiety disorders and affective disorders in the community according to the ICD-10 and DSM-III-R by using the Composite International Diagnostic Interview (CIDI), *Int J Methods Psychiatr Res* 1992; **2**:91–100.
13. Lepine JP, Pariente P, Boulenger JP et al, Anxiety disorders in a French general psychiatric outpatient sample. Comparison between

DSM-III and DSM-III-R criteria, *Soc Psychiatry Psychiatr Epidemiol* 1989; **24**:301–8.

14. Wittchen HU, Essau CA, von Zerssen D et al, Lifetime and six-month prevalence of mental disorders in the Munich Follow-Up Study, *Eur Arch Psychiatry Clin Neurosci* 1992; **241**: 247–58.

15. Robins LN, Helzer JE, Croughan J et al, The National Institute of Mental Health Diagnostic Interview Schedule: its history, characteristics, and validity, *Arch Gen Psychiatry* 1981; **38**:381–9.

16. Robins LN, Wing J, Wittchen HU et al, The Composite International Diagnostic Interview, *Arch Gen Psychiatry* 1988; **45**:1069–77.

17. Weissman MM, Bland R, Joyce PR et al, Sex differences in rates of depression: cross national perspectives, *J Affect Disord* 1993; **29**:77–84.

18. Angst J, Merikangas KR, Preisig M, Subthreshold syndromes of depression and anxiety in the community, *J Clin Psychiatry* 1997; **58**(suppl 8):6–10.

19. Gater R, Tansella M, Korten A et al, Sex differences in the prevalence and detection of depressive and anxiety disorder in general health care settings, *Arch Gen Psychiatry* 1998; **55**:405–13.

20. Angst J, Dobler-Mikola A, Binder J, The Zurich Study: a prospective epidemiologic study of depressive, neurotic and psychosomatic syndromes. I. Problems methodology, *Eur Arch Psych Clin NeuroSci* 1984; **234**:13–20.

21. M, Sex differences in psychological well-being, *Psychol Med* 1982; **1**(suppl):1–46.

22. Lewinsohn PM, Gotlib IH, Lewinsohn M et al, Gender differences in anxiety disorders and anxiety symptoms in adolescents, *J Abnorm Psychol* 1998; **107**:109–17.

23. Compas BE, Oppedisano G, Connor JK et al, Gender differences in depressive symptoms in adolescence: comparison of national samples of clinically referred and nonreferred youths, *J Consult Clin Psychol* 1997; **65**:617–26.

24. Kessler RC, McGonagle KA, Swartz M et al, Sex and depression in the National Comorbidity Survey I: Lifetime prevalence, chronicity and recurrence, *J Affect Disord* 1993; **29**:85–96.

25. Lewinsohn PM, Hops H, Roberts RE et al, Adolescent psychopathology: I. Prevalence and incidence of depression and other DSM-III-R disorders in high school students, *J Abnorm Psychol* 1993; **102**:133–44.

26. Simonoff E, Pickles A, Meyer JM et al, The Virginia twin study of adolescent behavioral development: influences of age, sex, and impairment on rates of disorders, *Arch Gen Psychiatry* 1997; **54**:801–8.

27. Costello EJ, Angold A, Burns B et al, The Great Smoky Mountains Study of Youths: goals, design, methods, and the prevalence of DSM-III-R disorders, *Arch Gen Psychiatry* 1996; **53**:1129–36.

28. Wittchen HU, Nelson CB, Lachner G, Prevalence of mental disorders and psychosocial impairments in adolescents and young adults, *Psychol Med* 1998; **28**:109–26.

29. Rutter M, Graham P, Chadwick OF et al, Adolescent turmoil: fact or fiction? *J Child Psychol Psychiatry* 1976; **17**:35–56.

30. Anderson JC, Williams S, McGee R et al, DSM-III disorders in preadolescent children: prevalence in a large sample from the general population, *Arch Gen Psychiatry* 1987; **44**:69–76.

31. Cohen P, Brook J, Family factors related to the persistence of psychopathology in childhood and adolescence: 2. Persistence of disorders, *J Child Psychol Psychiatry* 1987; **34**:869–77.

32. Kashani JH, Beck NC, Hoeper EW et al, Psychiatric disorders in a community sample of adolescents, *Am J Psychiatry* 1987; **144**:584–9.

33. Kashani JH, Orvaschel H, Rosenberg TK et al, Psychopathology in a community sample of children and adolescents: a developmental perspective, *J Am Acad Child Adolesc Psychiatry* 1989; **28**:701–6.

34. Velez CN, Johnson J, Cohen P, A longitudinal analysis of selected risk factors for childhood psychopathology, *J Am Acad Child Adolesc Psychiatry* 1989; **28**:861–4.

35. Fleming JE, Offord DR, Epidemiology of childhood depressive disorders: a critical review, *J Am Acad Child Adolesc Psychiatry* 1990; **29**:571–80.

36. McGee R, Feehan M, Williams S et al, DSM-III disorders in a large sample of adolescents, *J Am Acad Child Adolesc Psychiatry* 1990; **29**:611–19.

37. Reinherz HZ, Giaconia RM, Pakiz B et al, Psychosocial risks for major depression in late adolescence: a longitudinal community study, *J Am Acad Child Adolesc Psychiatry* 1993; **32**:1155–63.

38. Lewinsohn PM, Gotlib IH, Seeley JR, Adolescent psychopathology: IV. Specificity of psychosocial risk factors for depression and substance abuse in older adolescents, *J Am Acad Child Adolesc Psychiatry* 1995; **34**: 1221–9.

39. Whitaker A, Johnson J, Shaffer D et al, Uncommon troubles in young people: prevalence estimates of selected psychiatric disorders in a nonreferred population, *Arch Gen Psychiatry* 1990; **47**:487–96.

40. Feehan M, McGee R, Williams SM, Mental health disorders from age 15 to 18 years, *J Am Acad Child Adolescent Psychiatry* 1993; **32**: 1118–26.

41. Fergusson DM, Horwood LJ, Lynskey MT, Prevalence and comorbidity of DSM-III-R diagnoses in a birth cohort of 15 year olds, *J Am Acad Child Adolesc Psychiatry* 1993; **32**: 1127–34.

42. Verhulst FC, van der Ende J, Ferdinand RF et al, The prevalence of DSM-III-R diagnoses in a national sample of Dutch adolescents, *Arch Gen Psychiatry* 1997; **54**:329–36.

43. Fleming J, Offord D, Boyle M, Prevalence of childhood and adolescent depression in the community, Ontario Child Health Study, *Br J Psychiatry* 1989; **155**:647–54.

44. McGee R, Feehan M, Williams S et al, DSM-III disorders from age 11 to age 15 years, *J Am Acad Child Adolesc Psychiatry* 1992; **31**:50–9.

45. Cohen P, Cohen J, Kasen S et al, An epidemiological study of disorders in late childhood and adolescence—I. Age and gender-specific prevalence, *J Child Psychol Psychiatry* 1993; **34**:851–67.

46. Ferdinand RF, Verhulst FC, Psychopathology from adolescence into young adulthood: an 8-year follow-up study, *Am J Psychiatry* 1996; **152**:1586–94.

47. Bolognini M, Bettschart W, Plancherel B et al, From the child to the young adult: sex differences in the antecedents of psychological problems. A retrospective study over ten years, *Soc Psychiatry Psychiatr Epidemiol* 1989; **24**:179–86.

48. Keller MO, Lavori PW, Rice J et al, The persistent risk of chronicity in recurrent episodes of nonbipolar major depressive disorder: a prospective follow-up, *Am J Psychiatry* 1986; **143**:24–8.

49. Simpson HB, Nee JC, Endicott J, First-episode major depression, *Arch Gen Psychiatry* 1997; **54**:633–9.

50. Aneshensel CS, Huba GJ, Depression, alcohol use, and smoking over one year: a four-wave longitudinal causal model, *J Abnorm Psychol* 1983; **92**:134–50.

51. Sargeant JK, Bruce MV, Florio L et al, Factors associated with 1-year outcome of major depression in the community, *Arch Gen Psychiatry* 1990; **47**:519–26.

52. Breslau N, Schultz L, Peterson E, Sex differences in depression: a role for pre-existing anxiety, *Psychiatry Res* 1995; **58**:1–12.

53. Angst J, Vollrath M, Merikangas K et al, Comorbidity of anxiety and depression in the Zurich Cohort Study of young adults. In: Maser J, Cloninger C, eds, *Comorbidity of Mood and Anxiety Disorders* (American Psychiatric Press: Washington, DC, 1990) 123–37.

54. Kessler R, The National Comorbidity Survey: preliminary results and future directions, *Int J Methods Psychiatr Res* 1995; **5**:139–51.

55. Schneier FR, Johnson J, Hornig CD et al, Social phobia: comorbidity and morbidity in an epidemiologic sample, *Arch Gen Psychiatry* 1992; **49**:282–8.

56. Merikangas KR, Gelernter CS, Co-morbidity for alcoholism and depression, *Psychiatr Clin North Am* 1990; **13**:613–32.

57. Merikangas K, Stevens D, Fenton B et al, Comorbidity and familial aggregation of alcoholism and anxiety disorders, *Psychol Med* 1998; **28**:773–88.

58. McGue M, Genes, environment, and the etiology of alcoholism. In: Zucker R, Boyd G, Howard J, eds, *The Development of Alcohol Problems: Exploring the Biopsychosocial Matrix*, Research monograph no. 26 (US Department of Health and Human Services, Public Health Service, National Institutes of Health, National Institute on Alcohol Abuse and Alcoholism: Rockville, MD, 1994) 1–39.

59. Rhode P, Lewinsohn PM, Seeley JR, Comparability of telephone and face-to-face interviews in assessing axis I and II disorders, *Am J Psychiatry* 1997; **154**:1593–8.

60. Brady EU, Kendall PC, Comorbidity of anxiety and depression in children and adolescents, *Psychol Bull* 1992; **111**:244–55.

61. Angold A, Costello EJ, Worthman CM, Puberty and depression: the roles of age, pubertal status and pubertal timing, *Psychol Med* 1998; 28:51–61.

62. Lewinsohn PM, Roberts RE, Seeley JR et al, Adolescent psychopathology: II. Psychosocial risk factors for depression, *J Abnorm Psychol* 1994; **103**:302–15.

63. Reinherz HZ, Stewart-Berghauer G, Pakiz B et al, The relationship of early risk and current mediators to depressive symptomatology in adolescence, *J Am Acad Child Adolesc Psychiatry* 1989; 28:942–7.

64. Davies PT, Windle M, Gender-specific pathways between maternal depressive symptoms, family discord, and adolescent adjustment, *Dev Psychol* 1997; 33:657–68.

65. Merikangas KR, Swendsen JD, Genetic epidemiology of psychiatric disorders, *Epidemiol Rev* 1997; **19**:144–55.

66. Kendler KS, Heath AC, Martin NG et al, Symptoms of anxiety and symptoms of depression: same genes, different environments? *Arch Gen Psychiatry* 1987; 44:451–7.

67. Kendler KS, Neale MC, Kessler RC et al, A population-based twin study of major depression in women: the impact of varying definitions of illness, *Arch Gen Psychiatry* 1992; 49:257–66.

68. Kendler KS, Neale MC, Kessler RC et al, Major depression and phobias: the genetic and environmental sources of comorbidity, *Psychol Med* 1993; 23:361–71.

69. Kendler KS, Walters EE, Neale MC et al, The structure of the genetic and environmental risk factors for six major psychiatric disorders in women: phobia, generalized anxiety disorder, panic disorder, bulimia, major depression, and alcoholism, *Arch Gen Psychiatry* 1995; **52**: 374–83.

70. Madden PA, Heath AC, Rosenthal NE et al, Seasonal changes in mood and behavior: the role of genetic factors, *Arch Gen Psychiatry* 1996; 53:47–55.

71. Kidd K, Spence M, Genetic analyses of pyloric stenosis suggesting a specific maternal effect, *J Med Genet* 1976; **13**:290–4.

72. Carter C, Genetics of common disorders, *Br Med Bull* 1969; **25**:52–7.

73. Rice J, Reich T, Andreasen N et al, Sex-related differences in depression: familial evidence, *J Affect Disord* 1984; **71**:199–210.

74. Baron M, Rainer J, Risch N, X-linkage in bipolar affective illness: perspectives on genetic heterogeneity, pedigree analysis and the X-chromosome map, *J Affect Disord* 1981; **3**: 141–57.

75. Faraone S, Lyons M, Tsyang M, Sex differences in affective disorder: genetic transmission, *Genet Epidemiol* 1987; **4**:331–43.

2

Gender differences in the prevalence and correlates of mood disorders in the general population

Ronald C Kessler

This chapter reviews recent research on the general population epidemiology of mood disorders among women and men, with an emphasis on findings regarding prevalence, course, consequences, and patterns of help-seeking. The main results are fairly easy to summarize. Women have consistently been found in community epidemiological surveys to have a higher rate of depression than men, while no evidence has been found for a gender difference in the prevalence of mania. The course of mood disorders has not been found to differ by gender. Mood disorders have a wide variety of adverse consequences, some of which are gender-specific, but all have very high personal and societal costs for women and men alike. Women have a higher probability than men of seeking professional help for mood disorders.

Beyond these basics, there is a great deal of subtlety in our current knowledge about gender differences in the epidemiology of mood disorders. For example, a variety of issues have been studied involving the possibility of gender-linked methodological biases in report-ing mood disorders. A number of interesting epidemiological studies have been done to study substantive determinants of gender differences in mood disorders. Recent studies of the social consequences of depression have documented gender-specific effects of great importance both to the current debate on health reform and to social policy concerns about the global burden of disease. Finally, new research has studied the factors that account for gender differences in patterns of help-seeking for mood disorders. All these issues are reviewed in this chapter.

Gender differences in the lifetime prevalences of depression and mania

One of the most widely documented findings in psychiatric epidemiology is that women have higher rates of major depressive episodes than men. This has been found throughout the world using a variety of diagnostic schemes and interview methods.[1–16] The prevalence of major depression among women in these studies has typically been between one and a half and three times that of men. Despite this consistency, there has been enormous variation in the estimated total population prevalence of major depression, with lifetime prevalence estimates ranging between 6%[17] and 17%.[18]

A substantial number of epidemiological studies have also examined gender differences in dysthymia.[2–4,9,19–21] These studies have consistently found that dysthymia is more prevalent among women than among men, with female/male (F/M) prevalence ratios generally around 2 : 1. Total population lifetime prevalence estimates of dysthymia are typically in the range of 6–8% when diagnostic hierarchy rules are not made. However, when the definition of dysthymia excludes respondents with a concurrent major depressive episode over a 2-year period, the total population lifetime prevalence estimate of dysthymia drops to less than 3%.[19]

Smaller numbers of epidemiological studies have examined gender differences in minor depression[22] or brief recurrent depression,[23] and have consistently found that these types of subthreshold depression are more prevalent among women than among men. Epidemiological studies have not found meaningful gender differences, in comparison, in the prevalence of mania.[24,25] It is important to note that the evaluation of mania has low validity in community epidemiological surveys.[26,27] This low validity, in conjunction with the low total population prevalence of true mania (1–2% lifetime prevalence), introduces considerable uncertainty into the evaluation of gender differences. However, treatment studies have also failed to find a gender difference in mania,[24] adding support to this finding in general population surveys.

Differential validity

Before turning to substantive issues, it is useful to consider the possibility that societal norms and sex role socialization experiences make it easier for women than for men to admit depression in epidemiological surveys.[28,29] If this is so, then the higher reported prevalences of depression among women in such surveys might be due to nothing more than differential reporting bias. However, the available evidence is inconsistent with this hypothesis in two important ways.

First, a number of methodological studies have been carried out on this type of response bias in community surveys of non-specific psychological distress.[30–32] These studies used standard psychometric methods to assess potential biasing factors such as social desirability, expressivity, lying, and yeasaying/naysaying. No evidence was found in any of these studies that the significantly higher levels of self-reported distress found among women than among men was due to these biasing factors.

Second, a more indirect, but in some ways more revealing, evaluation of the impact of response bias on the gender difference in major depression was carried out by Young et al.[29] They hypothesized that lower reluctance to admit depression should lead women to be more likely than men to admit ever having a period lasting 2 weeks or longer of being sad, blue, or depressed, but should not affect reports of the less stigmatizing symptoms that cluster with depressed mood to make up a major depressive episode, such as sleep disturbance, eating disturbance, and lack of energy. Yet the opposite was found by Young et al in an analysis of a representative sample of non-patient relatives of depressed probands. The F/M ratio of a 2-week period of depressed mood or anhedonia (1.3) was much smaller than the ratio of less stigmatizing associated

Table 2.1 Female/male prevalence ratios of lifetime DSM-III-R major depressive episodes in the National Comorbidity Survey by varying diagnostic criteria.

Diagnostic criteria	Lifetime prevalence		
	Female (%)	Male (%)	Female/Male
Stem	57.6	45.7	1.30
Stem plus 1 or more symptoms	35.9	25.2	1.40
Stem plus 2 or more symptoms	32.0	20.9	1.50
Stem plus 3 or more symptoms	26.9	16.6	1.60
Stem plus 4 or more symptoms	21.3	12.7	1.70
Stem plus 5 or more symptoms	16.6	8.5	2.0
Stem plus 6 or more symptoms	11.0	5.7	1.9
Stem plus 7 or more symptoms	6.1	3.3	1.8
Stem plus all 8 symptoms	3.0	1.2	2.5

Reprinted from Kessler et al[33] with kind permission from Elsevier Science. © 1993.

symptoms (1.7). As shown in Table 2.1, we found very similar results in the nationally representative general population data collected in the US National Comorbidity Survey (NCS).[33] The F/M odds ration (OR) for the lifetime prevalence of DSM-III-R[34] major depression in the NCS increased steadily from 1.3 for endorsement of the major depression diagnostic stem question to 2.5 for endorsement of the stem question plus all eight of the other A Criteria stipulated in DSM-III-R. It is implausible that a pattern of this sort would be due to greater reluctance to admit depression on the part of men than women.

Before concluding that this pattern argues against a differential reporting bias, it is important to recognize that this is exactly what one would expect from invalidity due to differential forgetting. The notion here is that men might remember the vague outlines of past depressive episodes as well as women but are more likely

than women to minimize in memory the impairment and constellation of symptoms associated with these episodes. Angst and Dobler-Mikola[35] reported a pattern of this sort in a longitudinal study of young adults. Prospective data in their study showed no gender difference in the period prevalence of depression even though retrospective data over the same recall period suggested that women had higher rates than men.

Wilhelm and Parker[36] subsequently reported a similar result regarding male underreporting in a separate sample and added the important finding that women were more likely to over-report depression than were men (i.e. retrospectively to report a previously reported subclinical episode as having met full criteria). These results argue persuasively that the gender difference in reported lifetime depression is, at least in part, due to a gender difference in accuracy of retrospective reporting.

As noted by Ernst and Angst,[23] it is unlikely that this differential retrospective reporting bias completely explains the gender difference in reported depression. The most important evidence in this regard comes from studies of current or recent prevalence, where recall becomes unimportant. Women consistently have higher rates of current depression than do men in these studies.[17,18] This finding, of course, is not definitive. It could be that a higher proportion of depressed men than women consistently refuse to admit their depression to survey interviewers. However, this possibility is inconsistent with the fact that a higher prevalence of current depression among women than among men is found not only in studies that rely on self-report but also in those that use informant reports.[37]

Another methodological possibility is that men are as likely to be depressed as women, but that some sort of recognition bias (as opposed to bias due to differential recall failure or differential willingness to report) leads to more underreporting among men than among women. This would come about if men were more likely than women to mask their depression so completely that neither they nor those close to them are aware of it. It would also come about if depression among men was more likely than depression among women to manifest itself as irritability rather than dysphoria or anhedonia. Current diagnostic systems allow for this possibility among children and adolescents, but not adults. It would be informative to explore this possibility in future epidemiological studies.

The evaluation of irritability also raises questions about the accuracy of the assessment of mania. In community epidemiological surveys that use fully structured diagnostic interviews, the majority of respondents who are classified as manic meet criteria by reporting periods of irritability with four or more associated symptoms, but deny ever having euphoria. This is very different from the typical symptom profile seen clinically, where a lifetime history of episodes with euphoria is characteristic of the vast majority of manics.[24] Research exploring the validity of diagnostic assessment in community surveys shows that respondents with irritability but not euphoria are very often incorrectly diagnosed as manics.[38] As these people are more likely to be men than women, a more rigorous assessment of mania in the general population, which would exclude these false positives, might find that women have a higher prevalence of true mania than men.

Age of onset distributions

A question can be raised as to whether lifetime F/M prevalence differences are the same regardless of the age of respondents. This question derives from the possibility suggested in recent research that women and men might have been getting more similar in their rates of depression in recent years.[39,40] We are aware of only one direct examination of this possibility.[41] This study made use of NCS respondent retrospective reports of the age when they first experienced their depression. By comparing these reports across subsamples of respondents who differed in age at the time of interview but focusing on the same recalled ages (e.g. comparing respondents who are currently in their twenties, thirties, forties and fifties but all having had their first onset of depression prior to the age of 20), it was possible to generate synthetic age of onset curves for each sample cohort to see whether there had been a change over time.

These curves are presented in Figures 2.1 and 2.2 for the cumulative lifetime prevalence of ever having a major depressive episode. Separate curves are presented for each of four NCS 10-year birth cohorts, beginning with the

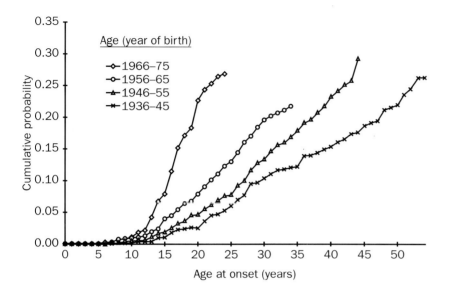

Figure 2.1 Cohort differences in the cumulative lifetime prevalence of DSM-III-R major depressive episodes among women in the National Comorbidity Survey. Reprinted from Kessler et al[41] with kind permission from Elsevier Science. © 1994.

oldest respondents, who were born in the decade before the end of World War II (1936–45), and ending with the youngest respondents, who were born during the decade spanning the second half of the 1960s and the first half of the 1970s (1966–75). The first of the two figures shows the estimated cumulative lifetime prevalence of depression among women in these four cohorts, while the second shows parallel results for men. There is a consistent trend for lifetime prevalence to be higher at all ages in successively younger cohorts in both figures. This means that lifetime major depression is becoming more common in recent cohorts. Similar results are found for most other disorders considered in the survey.

But is this increase associated with a change in the F/M lifetime prevalence ratio? The answer is presented in Table 2.2, where we see cohort-specific cumulative ratios of this sort by 5-year age intervals. An elevated female ratio can be observed by age 14 in the youngest

cohort and by age 9 in the next two older cohorts, but not until age 24 in the oldest cohort. This much later emergence of the gender difference in the oldest cohort could be due to a true cohort effect or to less accurate recall of early-onset depression in the oldest cohort. We would not expect this cohort effect to exist if biological factors were largely responsible for the gender difference in depression (e.g. if onset of puberty played a powerful part in causing the emergence of depression among girls). Therefore, if this cohort effect is genuine and not a result of bias, it must be due to environmental rather than biological risk factors.

Despite this cohort difference in the age at which the gender difference first emerges, the F/M ratio does not differ greatly across cohorts by age 24, the oldest age at which we can compare all four NCS cohorts. The ratio is 1.9 in the youngest cohort and decreases monotonically to 1.6 in the oldest cohort, a difference that is not statistically significant in this sample. Past the age of 24, the ratio tends to be

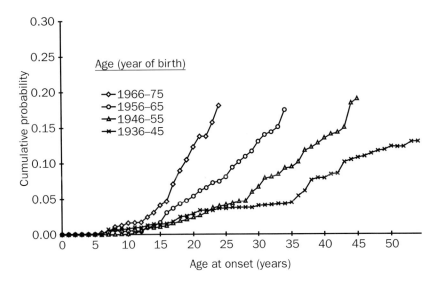

Figure 2.2 Cohort differences in the cumulative lifetime prevalence of DSM-III-R major depressive episodes among men in the National Comorbidity Survey. Reprinted from Kessler et al[41] with kind permission from Elsevier Science. © 1994.

larger in successively older cohorts, suggesting that the gender difference in the onset of depression during the middle years of life has become smaller in more recent cohorts. However, only one of the 14 possible pairwise inter-cohort comparisons in Table 2.2 beginning at age 24 is statistically significant—the difference between the 1.5 ratio at age 34 in the 1956–65 cohort and the 2.8 ratio at the same age in the 1936–45 cohort ($z = 2.2$, $P = 0.026$). The general similarity of the ratios across cohorts beginning at age 24 is much more impressive than this one significant difference, with the average of the ratios being equal to 1.8 and the range between 1.5 and 2.8. This similarity across cohorts is particularly striking in light of the finding shown in Figures 2.1 and 2.2 that there is a roughly five-fold increase in the lifetime prevalence of major depression across these cohorts.

The effects of prior psychopathology

Breslau[42] proposed the existence of an interesting specification: that the gender difference in depression is partly due to a difference in prior anxiety. She supported this claim by showing that the OR of gender predicting major depression substantially attenuates when controls are introduced for the prior existence of anxiety. A similar result was recently reported by Wilhelm et al.[43] This finding is indirectly consistent with the finding, reported above, that the cohort effect for major depression is largely confined to secondary depression. However, this finding is limited in the same way as is the result regarding sexual trauma, in that it focuses on a predictor that is characteristic of women (i.e. anxiety) while ignoring other comparable predictors that are more characteristic of men (e.g. alcohol/drug abuse, conduct disorder, antisocial personality disorder).

Table 2.2 Cumulative F/M rate ratios for lifetime DSM-III-R major depressive episode in the National Comorbidity Survey by age and cohort.

Age	Cohort (year of birth)							
	1966–75		1956–65		1946–55		1936–45	
	OR	(95% CI)	OR	(95% CI)	OR	(95% CI)	OR	(95% CI)
9	0.7	(0.2, 1.9)	1.9	(0.4, 7.9)	1.7	LP	0.2	LP
14	2.0[a]	(1.0, 3.8)	2.4[a]	(1.3, 4.3)	1.5	(0.8, 3.2)	0.6	(0.1, 2.8)
19	2.0[a]	(1.3, 3.2)	1.6[a]	(1.2, 2.3)	1.5	(0.9, 2.6)	0.8	(0.3, 2.2)
24	1.9[a]	(1.3, 2.9)	1.8[a]	(1.4, 2.3)	1.6[a]	(1.1, 2.4)	1.6	(0.7, 3.4)
29			1.6[a]	(1.3, 2.1)	1.7[a]	(1.2, 2.4)	2.6[a]	(1.5, 4.5)
34			1.5[a]	(1.2, 2.0)	1.9[a]	(1.4, 2.5)	2.8[a]	(1.7, 4.5)
39					1.8[a]	(1.4, 2.3)	2.0[a]	(1.3, 3.0)
44					1.7[a]	(1.4, 2.2)	1.8[a]	(1.2, 2.7)
49							1.9[a]	(1.2, 2.8)
54							2.0[a]	(1.3, 3.0)

[a] Significant at the 0.05 level (two-tailed test).
LP, low precision; OR, odds ratio; CI, confidence interval.
The results are based on a series of discrete-time survival models in which gender and age (person-year) were used to predict onset of major depressive episodes using retrospective age of onset reports in subsamples defined by the cross-classification of age (person-year) and cohort. The ORs are gender effects.
Reprinted from Kessler et al[41] with kind permission from Elsevier Science. © 1994.

In an effort to investigate this issue, Breslau's result was replicated in the NCS by estimating a pair of survival models to predict first onset of major depression.[44] The only predictor in the first model was gender. The F/M OR in this model was 1.9. The second model introduced a series of controls for prior anxiety disorders (panic, simple phobia, social phobia, agoraphobia, generalized anxiety disorder, post-traumatic stress disorder). Consistent with Breslau, the introduction of these controls was found to reduce the F/M OR to 1.6.

However, a third model was also estimated that controlled for prior substance use disorders and conduct disorder rather than prior anxiety disorders. The F/M OR in this third model increased to 2.4. This means that the higher risk of depression among women than among men would be even greater than it is were it not for the fact that men are more likely than women to have prior substance and conduct problems.

Finally, a model was estimated that controlled simultaneously for prior anxiety disorders, substance use disorders and conduct disorder. The F/M OR in this final model was

1.9—exactly what it was in the model that had no controls. Furthermore, in the subsample of respondents with no history of any of these prior disorders, the F/M OR was 2.2. These results show clearly, contrary to Breslau's conclusion, that history of prior psychiatric disorders does not play an important part in explaining the observed gender difference in onset risk of major depression.

Gender differences in the course of depression and mania

There are some theories about the reasons for gender differences in depression that emphasize the importance of differential persistence. For example, sex role theories suggest that the chronic stresses and lack of access to effective coping resources associated with traditional female roles lead to the higher prevalence of depression found among women than among men,[45,46] while rumination theory suggests that women are more likely than men to dwell on problems and, because of this, to let transient symptoms of dysphoria grow into clinically significant episodes of depression.[12] Both of these perspectives imply that the higher point prevalence of clinically significant depression among women is due, at least in part, to a higher persistence than among men.

There is some evidence from retrospective studies that women do, in fact, have a more chronic course of depression than do men.[23] However, the differential recall bias discussed in the previous section appears to explain this effect. Indeed, Ernst and Angst[23] found that evidence for a higher recurrence risk of major depression among women than among men disappears entirely when adjustments are made for differential recall bias. Furthermore, in the

NCS, where special procedures were used to stimulate active memory search,[27] no gender difference in recurrence risk was found.[41] The NCS also failed to find evidence of a gender difference in either speed of episode recovery or chronicity. Furthermore, a recent report from the NIMH Collaborative Program on the Psychobiology of Depression reported prospective data that showed no gender difference in the subsequent course of respondents who were followed over time after their first episode of depression.[47]

Additional information about gender differences in the course of mood disorders comes from the same epidemiological studies that documented a higher lifetime prevalence of major depression among women than among men. These studies also show that women are more likely than men to have had a recent episode of depression. Between one-third and more than half of the respondents in these surveys who were estimated to ever experience depression are classified in these studies as having had an episode of depression during the year prior to the interview, while up to 80% of those with a prior history of mania are estimated to have had a past-year episode of either mania or depression. However, although no explicit investigations of course were carried out in most of these studies, inspection of the prevalence estimates shows that the ratios of current to lifetime prevalence, a rough indicator of persistence, do not differ consistently by gender.

These indirect results are not definitive, as they fail to adjust for the possibility of gender differences in either age of onset or time since onset. A more formal analysis of persistence with cross-sectional data is possible by controlling for age of onset and years since onset. Results of such an analysis carried out in the NCS[48] are presented in Table 2.3. The coefficients presented in this table are the F/M ORs

Table 2.3 Gender differences (F/M ratios) in the persistence of DSM-III-R mood disorders in the National Comorbidity Survey.

	OR	(95% CI)
Major depression episode	1.0	(0.7–1.4)
Manic episode	0.5	(0.2–1.3)
Dysthymia	0.8	(0.5–1.3)

[a]None of the three odds ratios is significant at the 0.05 level (two-tailed test).
OR, odds ratio; CI, confidence interval.
Persistence is defined as 12-month prevalence among respondents with a lifetime history of the disorder and age of onset more than 1 year prior to the time of interview. The ORs are the effects of gender (female/male) in a multivariate logistic regression equation controlling for age of onset and number of years since onset.
Reprinted from an earlier NCS report[48] with kind permission from the American Medical Women's Association. © 1998.

of 12-month prevalence among people with a lifetime disorder, controlling for age of onset and years since onset of that disorder. Results are shown for major depressive episode, dysthymia, and mania. There is no evidence in Table 2.3 for a gender difference in the course of mood disorders.

One exception to this general pattern is the finding in many clinical studies that women with bipolar disorder have a higher proportion of depressive than manic episodes compared with men with bipolar disorder.[49–51] I am aware of only one attempt to verify this pattern in a general population sample.[38] No evidence was found in this one study of a gender difference in the ratio of manic to depressive episodes among people with bipolar disorder.

Gender differences in current depression

The finding of a gender difference in lifetime prevalence in conjunction with the absence of a gender difference in course implies that there should be a gender difference in current depression equivalent to the gender difference in lifetime prevalence. This is, in fact, what is generally found in epidemiological studies. However, the fact that the gender difference in current depression is entirely due to a difference in lifetime history often goes unrecognized in more analytical studies of the determinants of current depression.

This lack of recognition is particularly evident in research on the effects of sex roles on the gender difference in depression. It has been known for nearly two decades, since the early empirical studies of the relationship between sex roles and mental illness,[52,53] that the gender difference in depressed mood is stronger for married people than for the unmarried. The same is true for current major depression. But, contrary to the interpretation of sex role theorists, this pattern is not due to a greater protective effect of marriage on men than on women. As noted above, the gender difference in risk of first onset of major depression is the same among the married as among the never married or previously married. Instead, there are two other processes at work that lead to a stronger gender difference in depression among married than among unmarried people.

First, as documented below, depression has different consequences for men and women, including different effects on educational attainment, teen childbearing, marital timing, and marital stability. Second, although there is no gender difference in the chronicity or recurrence of major depression, the environmental experiences that are associated with chronicity and recurrence are different for men and women. For example, financial pressures are more depressogenic for men than for women, while family problems are more depressogenic for women than for men.[54] Together, these two processes create variation in the relationship between gender and current depression across sectors of the population defined in terms of roles. It is a mistake to get confused into thinking that these specifications give us insights into the causes of the gender differences in depression.

An important example of this confusion can be found in the recent work of Nazroo et al[55] on the differential effects of life events on men and women. Nazroo et al argued that the gender difference in risk of past-year episodes of major depression is due in large part to a greater vulnerability to the effects of stressful life events and difficulties among women than among men. However, given that the vast majority of past-year episodes of major depression in the adult general population are recurrences rather than first onsets, this line of thinking is attempting to explain something that does not exist: a gender difference in recurrence risk of depression.

How is it that Nazroo et al were able to find a gender difference in their analysis if no such difference exists? The answer is this. By failing to distinguish first onsets from recurrences in

the analysis of past-year episode onset, Nazroo et al confounded three separable processes: the gender difference in risk of first onset in the subsample of respondents who had never been depressed prior to the past year (a difference that is statistically significant); the gender difference in recurrence risk in the subsample of respondents who were asymptomatic at the beginning of the past year but who had a subsequent recurrence of major depression (a difference that is not significant); and the gender difference in the proportion of respondents who have an elevated risk of episode recurrence because they have a history of depression (a difference that is significant).

Furthermore, exposure to stressful life experiences is higher among people with a history of depression than among those without such a history.[56] In addition, the impact of stress on the onset of depressive episodes is stronger among people with a history of depression than among those without such a history. Given that women are more likely than men to have a history of depression, these differences in exposure and impact will create the impression that the higher rate of past-year episode onset among women than among men is due to a combination of differential exposure and differential reactivity to stress, when, in fact, it is largely due to a higher proportion of women than men having a history of depression and this history being associated with risk of subsequent episode onset.

To illustrate, the F/M OR for past-year episode onset of major depression in the total NCS is a statistically significant 2.2. This OR is reduced by controls for past-year stressful events and difficulties. However, when we disaggregate the data into the subsample of respondents with a history of depression, the OR becomes 1.0 with or without controls for past-year stress. The OR is 2.6, in comparison, in the subsample of respondents with no prior history of depression before controlling for stress. This OR decreases to 2.3 after controlling for stress. There is no significant interaction between gender and stress in predicting past-year first onset of major depression.

Our work with the NCS has shown that a number of putative predictors of the gender difference in depression work in exactly the same way. One of the most important of these is personality. There has been considerable discussion of the possibility that personality differences account for the higher prevalence of depression among women than among men. Low self-esteem, interpersonal dependency, pessimistic attributional style, low perceived control, expressiveness and instrumentality have all been implicated in this way.[12,57–62] However, few of the empirical studies that have documented these effects controlled for prior history of depression, and those that did failed to find powerful effects of personality on the gender difference in depression.[63,64] When we carried out similar analyses in the NCS, we found that personality differences appeared to explain part of the association between gender and current depression in the total sample when we did not control for prior history of depression. When we controlled for history of depression, however, all such significant associations disappeared.

The consequences of mood disorders

The past decade has seen a growing interest in the social consequences of psychiatric disorders. This work has documented that psychiatric disorders often have substantial personal and social costs[65] and that the impairments associated with these disorders are as great as those associated with serious chronic physical illnesses.[9] Psychiatric disorders are associated with overall reduced quality of life[66] and impaired work role functioning.[67] The analysis of gender differences has not played a prominent role in these investigations, although there is reason to believe that the implications of psychiatric disorders could be quite different for women than for men because of the greater importance of interpersonal competence in the roles typically occupied by women.

One of the ways in which psychiatric disorders can be consequential is by affecting important life-course transitions. A series of investigations of such effects were carried out as part of the NCS. The basic logic of these analyses was to use retrospectively reported age of onset data to classify respondents according to the existence of psychiatric disorders prior to the age of the relevant transition and then to use discrete-time survival analysis in a logistic regression framework with the disorders treated as time-varying covariates to determine whether these disorders significantly predicted the transitions.

The first of these analyses focused on educational attainment and documented that early-onset psychiatric disorders are powerful predictors of failure to graduate from high school, failure to go on to college after high school graduation, and failure to complete college after college entry.[68] Mood disorders were shown to be especially important in a third of these transitions. However, no significant overall pattern of gender differences in these effects was found.

A second set of analyses focused on teenage childbearing (for women) and fathering (for men). Early-onset psychiatric disorders were found to be significant predictors of these outcomes.[69] Mood disorders were among the significant predictors, with ORs that did not differ by gender.

A third set of analyses studied marital timing

and marital stability.[70] We began by estimating separate prediction equations for early marriage (prior to age 18), on-time marriage (18–25), and later marriage (26+). The ORs associated with prior disorders, mood disorders included, were consistently greater than 1.0 in predicting early marriage, which means that adolescents with a history of these disorders are more likely than others to marry by age 18. In comparison, the majority of the coefficients were less than 1.0 for later marriages, which can most reasonably be interpreted as suggesting that psychiatric disorders are a handicap in the marriage market among people who do not marry by the age of 18. The strongest effects of this sort were found for mood disorders. As in analyses of other role transitions, no consistent pattern of gender differences in the ORs was found.

We also studied the effects of psychiatric disorders on employment.[48] However, as no data on lifetime employment history were obtained in the NCS, we focused on current employment. In order to avoid the possibility of interpretational confusion due to reciprocal effects between current disorders and current employment status, we estimated the effects of psychiatric disorders as of the age of completing school on current employment status, controlling for amount of education and time since completion of education, and number and ages of children at home, and looking separately at married and unmarried NCS respondents who were not students.

We found that a history of mood disorders is associated with an elevated chance of being employed in the subsample of married women (OR = 1.7) but not in any of the other subsamples. Further analysis showed that this pattern of results is a consequence of the fact that women with a history of mood disorders are more likely than other women to be married to men who are either unemployed or who have

low earnings, increasing the necessity for the wives to be employed. This result confirms our earlier speculation that mood disorders create disadvantages for women in the marriage market.

We also looked at the association between past-month mood disorders and workplace functioning in the subsample of NCS respondents who were employed at the time of interview.[67] A significantly higher proportion of women (5.9%) than men (4.0%) reported past-month mood disorders. Respondents with these mood disorders reported 40 more work-loss days per 100 worker-months and 270 more work-cutback days per 100 worker-months than workers without mood disorders. There were no significant gender differences in these impairments.

Use of services for mood disorders

Prior to the NCS, the most recent general population data in the USA regarding gender differences in use of services for psychiatric disorders came from the Epidemiologic Catchment Area (ECA) Study.[71] The ECA was a survey of over 20 000 persons in five US communities carried out between 1980 and 1985 that estimated the prevalences of specific DSM-III disorders and past-year use of services for these disorders in different sectors of the de facto mental and addictive disorders service system. The ECA data suggested that women with a recent psychiatric disorder were significantly more likely than comparable men to obtain treatment.[72]

This result is consistent with virtually all previous US evidence on gender differences in mental health service use.[73,74] It is not plausible to argue that this gender difference in seeking help is due to women having more psychiatric problems than men, as the ECA investigators and others before them found that the difference in use persists after adjusting for differential need for services. Nor is it plausible to argue that women have more ready access to services than men, as available evidence is clear in showing that both financial[75] and non-financial[76] barriers to seeking care are greater for women than for men.

The more recent data from the NCS are reported in Table 2.4. As shown in the first two rows of the table, women with a 12-month mood disorder were significantly more likely than their male counterparts to seek help from the general medical sector (14.5% versus 8.6%). Because of slightly higher rates of ser-

vices use in the mental health specialty and self-help sectors among men, though, there was no gender difference in the overall proportion of respondents who sought some type of service for a mood disorder (36.8% versus 35.6%). We also looked at the average number of visits in each service sector among respondents undergoing treatment for a mood disorder and found no significant gender difference.

The third and fourth rows of Table 2.4 show that, unlike the situation for mood disorders, women with any NCS/DSM-III-R disorder (including anxiety disorders, mood disorders, substance use disorders, and non-affective psychosis) were significantly more likely than comparable men to seek some type of service for a psychiatric problem (27.7% versus 21.1%).

Table 2.4 Gender-specific probabilities of 12-month service use for mood disorders in separate service sectors by 12-month DSM-III-R disorders in the National Comorbidity Survey.

Disorder	Service use for psychiatric problems during the past 12 months											
	MHS		GM		HCS		HS		SH		ANY	
	%	(se)	%	(se)	%	(se)	%	(se)	%	(se)	%	(se)
1. Any mood disorder												
Female	19.8	(2.2)	14.5[a]	(2.2)	29.0	(2.7)	14.4	(1.5)	7.5	(1.0)	36.8	(2.8)
Male	23.2	(3.2)	8.6	(2.3)	26.0	(3.5)	12.8	(2.6)	10.1	(2.0)	35.6	(4.0)
2. Any 12-month NCS disorder												
Female	13.4	(1.2)	10.7[a]	(1.5)	20.3[a]	(1.8)	10.5[a]	(0.9)	6.4	(0.7)	27.7[a]	(1.7)
Male	11.2	(1.4)	4.5	(1.0)	13.7	(1.6)	6.9	(1.0)	8.6	(1.2)	21.1	(1.9)
3. No 12-month NCS disorder												
Female	4.2[a]	(1.0)	2.2	(0.5)	5.5	(1.0)	4.3	(1.1)	1.7	(0.5)	9.8[a]	(1.4)
Male	1.5	(0.4)	2.0	(1.0)	3.5	(1.1)	2.5	(0.7)	1.0	(0.2)	6.5	(1.1)

[a] Significant gender difference at the 0.05 level (two-tailed test).
MHS, mental health specialty; GM, general medical; HCS, health care system (either MHS or GM); HS, human services; SH, self-help; ANY, any services.
Reprinted from an earlier NCS report[48] with kind permission from the American Medical Women's Association. © 1998.

The last two rows, finally, show that women without any NCS/DSM-III-R disorders were significantly more likely than comparable men to seek some type of service for a psychiatric problem (9.8% versus 6.5%). Why the situation is different for mood disorders is unclear.

Previous research has suggested that the gender difference in rates of seeking treatment for psychiatric problems might be due to women being more likely than men to perceive themselves as needing help even when they have the same level of measured need as men. We were able to investigate this issue in the NCS by creating a 'perceived need' score that combined (1) the people who reportedly sought treatment because of perceived need as opposed to involuntarily seeking treatment under pressure from a loved one or legal authorities with (2) the people who reportedly felt that they needed help at some time during the past year but did not get it.

A strong monotonic relationship was found between objective measures of need (e.g. number of disorders, how recent, impairments) and this measure of perceived need among both women and men.[48] However, we also found that women have a significantly higher level of perceived need than do men, controlling for objective measures of need. Furthermore, we found that there is no significant gender difference in the proportions of women and men who seek help for psychiatric problems after controlling for perceived need. This means that the higher perception of need among women than among men plays a critical role in the higher rate of help-seeking for psychiatric problems among women than among men.

Discussion

While methodological limitations could lead to some distortion in the epidemiological evidence regarding prevalence and course of mood disorders, the most reasonable conclusion based on the available evidence is that women have much higher lifetime prevalences of non-bipolar mood disorders than men, but do not differ from men either in the lifetime prevalence of bipolar depression or in the course of either depression or mania. There appears to have been little change in these F/M ratios over the past few decades. The fact that significant cohort effects were documented for most of these disorders separately among women and men strongly suggests that environmental factors play a strong part in bringing them about and presumably in accounting for the gender differences. We also know from twin and adoption studies, though, that there are powerful genetic effects on mood disorders,[77,78] suggesting that some combination of environmental and genetic influences is at work. It is quite possible that these include genetic influences on sensitivity to environmental effects.

The results regarding social consequences suggest that mood disorders significantly influence a variety of important life-course role transitions as well as role functioning. We know that some of these processes affect women more powerfully than they do men. This is certainly the case with both teenage childbearing, which leads to more financial adversity for women than for men. Furthermore, there is good reason to think that these adverse effects are on the rise because of an increase in the prevalence of early-onset psychiatric disorders. These results have important implications for the policy debate on national health-care insurance, a large part of which involves evaluation of the various costs and benefits associated with providing universal access to health care. The findings reported here add to the growing body of evidence that early-onset mood disorders have important societal costs. An accounting scheme that includes these costs may well lead to the conclusion that we cannot afford to forego the opportunity to develop early interventions and treatments to prevent these costly consequences for society and some of its most vulnerable citizens.

The NCS data on help-seeking show that women are significantly more likely than men to seek professional help for most types of psychiatric problem, but not for mood disorders. This is true despite the fact that women are disadvantaged relative to men in access to health insurance. An important factor appears to be that women with these problems are more aware than men that they need help. As reported elsewhere,[48] this difference was found to be especially pronounced at the lower levels of need, suggesting that there is a lower threshold for seeking help among women than among men. A similar gender difference in threshold for help-seeking has been documented for physical illness.[79,80]

There are at least two plausible explanations for this difference. One is that women might be more sensitive than men to bodily symptoms and thereby more likely to recognize and seek help for a symptom.[81] However, the empirical data on this possibility fail to show a strong difference of this sort.[80] A second possibility is that women are socialized in such a way as to more readily adopt the sick role than men. Numerous beliefs and attitudes have been cited

as instances of such a gender difference.[82,83] Furthermore, a great deal of inferential evidence consistent with this hypothesis has been found in health surveys, such as the finding that women report a greater tendency to consult a physician for hypothetical physical health problems than do men[84] and are more likely than men to believe in the efficacy of medical intervention.[85] Although we are not aware of any direct evidence in support of these suggestions, this is likely to be a fruitful area of future research, addressing the problem of unmet need for treatment that is found among women and men alike.

Acknowledgments

Preparation of this chapter was partially supported by grants R01 MH41135, R01 MH46376, R01 MH49098 and K05 MH00507 from the US National Institute of Mental Health with supplemental support from the National Institute of Drug Abuse (through a supplement to MH46376) and the WT Grant Foundations (Grant 90135190). Portions of this chapter previously appeared in the *Journal of Affective Disorders* (**30**:15–26) and the *Journal of the American Medical Women's Association* (**53**:148–58), and are reproduced here with permission of the publishers.

References

1. Bebbington P, Hurry J, Tennant C et al, The epidemiology of mental disorders in Camberwell, *Psychol Med* 1981; **11**:561–79.
2. Bland RC, Newman SC, Orn H, Period prevalence of psychiatric disorders in Edmonton, *Acta Psychiatr Scand* 1988; **338**:33–42.
3. Bland RC, Orn H, Newman SC, Lifetime prevalence of psychiatric disorders in Edmonton, *Acta Psychiatr Scand* 1988; **338**:24–32.
4. Canino GJ, Bird HR, Shrout PE et al, The prevalence of specific psychiatric disorders in Puerto Rico, *Arch Gen Psychiatry* 1987; **44**:727–35.
5. Cheng TA, Sex difference in prevalence of

minor psychiatric morbidity: a social epidemiological study in Taiwan, *Acta Psychiatr Scand* 1989; 80:395–407.

6. Hwu HG, Yeh EK, Chang LY, Prevalence of psychiatric disorders in Taiwan defined by the Chinese Diagnostic Interview Schedule, *Acta Psychiatr Scand* 1989; 79:136–47.

7. Lee CK, Han JH, Choi JO, The epidemiological study of mental disorders in Korea (IX): alcoholism, anxiety and depression, *Seoul J Psychiatry* 1987; 12:183–91.

8. Weissman MM, Myers JK, Affective disorders in a US urban community: the use of research diagnostic criteria in an epidemiologic survey, *Arch Gen Psychiatry* 1978; 35:1304–11.

9. Wells JE, Bushnell JA, Hornblow AR et al, Christchurch Psychiatric Epidemiology Study, Part I: Methodology and lifetime prevalence for specific psychiatric disorders, *Aust NZ J Psychiatry* 1989; 23:315–26.

10. Wittchen H-U, Essau CA, von Zerssen D et al, Lifetime and six-month prevalence of mental disorders in the Munich follow-up study, *Eur Arch Psychiatry Clin Neurosci* 1992; 241:247–58.

11. Bebbington PE, The social epidemiology of clinical depression. In: Henderson AS, Burrows GD, eds, *Handbook of Social Psychiatry* (Elsevier: Amsterdam, 1988) 87–102.

12. Nolen-Hoeksema S, Sex differences in unipolar depression: evidence and theory, *Psychol Bull* 1987; 101:259–82.

13. Weissman MM, Klerman GL, Sex differences and the epidemiology of depression, *Arch Gen Psychiatry* 1977; 34:98–111.

14. Weissman MM, Klerman JK, Gender and depression, *Trends Neurosci* 1985; 8:416–20.

15. Weissman MM, Klerman GL, Depression: current understanding and changing trends, *Annu Rev Public Health* 1992; 13:319–39.

16. Weissman MM, Leaf PJ, Holzer CE III et al, The epidemiology of depression. An update on sex differences in rates, *J Affect Disord* 1984; 7:179–88.

17. Weissman MM, Bruce ML, Leaf PJ et al, Affective disorders. In: Robins LN, Regier DA, eds, *Psychiatric Disorders in America: The Epidemiologic Catchment Area Study* (Free Press: New York, 1991) 53–80.

18. Blazer DG, Kessler RC, McGonagle KA, Swartz MS, The prevalence and distribution of major depression in a national community sample: The National Comorbidity Survey, *Am J Psychiatry* 1994; 151:979–86.

19. Kessler RC, McGonagle KA, Nelson CB et al, Sex and depression in the National Comorbidity Survey. II: Cohort effects, *J Affect Disord* 1994; 30:15–26.

20. Lee CK, Kwak YS, Yamamoto J et al, Psychiatric epidemiology in Korea: Part 1. Gender and age differences in Seoul, *J Nerv Ment Dis* 1990; 178:242–6.

21. Weissman MM, Leaf PJ, Bruce ML, Florio L, The epidemiology of dysthymia in five communities: rates, risks, comorbidity, and treatment, *Am J Psychiatry* 1988; 145:815–19.

22. Kessler RC, Zhao S, Blazer DG, Swartz M, Prevalence, correlates and course of minor depression and major depression in the National Comorbidity Survey, *J Affect Disord* 1997; 45:19–30.

23. Ernst C, Angst J, The Zurich study XII. Sex differences in depression. Evidence from longitudinal epidemiological data, *Eur Arch Psychiatry Clin Neurosci* 1992; 241:222–30.

24. Goodwin FK, Jamison KJ, *Manic-Depressive Illness* (Oxford University Press: New York, 1990).

25. Kessler RC, Nelson CB, McGonagle KA et al, Comorbidity of DSM-III-R major depressive disorder in the general population: results from the US National Comorbidity Survey, *Br J Psychiatry* 1996; 168(suppl 30):17–30.

26. Wittchen H-U, Reliability and validity studies of the WHO-Composite International Diagnostic Interview (CIDI): a critical review, *J Psychiatr Res* 1994; 28:57–84.

27. Kessler RC, Wittchen H-U, Abelson JM et al, Methodological studies of the Composite International Diagnostic Interview (CIDI) in the US National Comorbidity Survey, *Int J Methods Psychiatr Res* 1998; 7:33–55.

28. Phillips DL, Segal BE, Sexual status and psychiatric symptoms, *Am Sociol Rev* 1969; 34:58–72.

29. Young MA, Fogg LF, Scheftner WA et al, Sex differences in the lifetime prevalence of depression: does varying the diagnostic criteria reduce the female/male ratio? *J Affect Disord* 1990; 18:187–92.

30. Clancy K, Gove W, Sex differences in mental illness: an analysis of response bias in self-reports, *Am J Clin Hypnosis* 1972; **14**:205–16.

31. Gove WR, Geerken MR, Response bias in surveys of mental health: an empirical investigation, *Am J Sociol* 1977; **82**:1289–317.

32. Gove WR, Sex differences in mental illness among adult men and women: an evaluation of four questions raised regarding the evidence on the higher rates of women, *Soc Sci Med* 1978; **12**:187–98.

33. Kessler RC, McGonagle KA, Swartz M et al, Sex and depression in the National Comorbidity Survey I: lifetime prevalence, chronicity and recurrence, *J Affect Disord* 1993; **29**:85–96.

34. American Psychiatric Association, *Diagnostic and Statistical Manual of Mental Disorders*, 3rd edn revised (American Psychiatric Association: Washington DC, 1987).

35. Angst J, Dobler-Mikola A, Do the diagnostic criteria determine the sex ratio in depression? *J Affect Disord* 1984; **7**:189–98.

36. Wilhelm K, Parker G, Sex differences in lifetime depression rates: fact or artefact? *Psychol Med* 1994; **24**:97–111.

37. Kendler KS, Davis CG, Kessler RC, The familial aggregation of common psychiatric and substance use disorders in the National Comorbidity Survey: a family history study, *Br J Psychiatry* 1997; **170**:541–8.

38. Kessler RC, Rubinow DR, Holmes C et al, The epidemiology of DMS-III-R bipolar I disorder in a general population survey, *Psychol Med* 1997; **27**:1079–89.

39. Kessler RC, McRae JA Jr, Trends in the relationship between sex and psychological distress: 1957–1976, *Am Sociol Rev* 1981; **46**:443–52.

40. Murphy JM, Trends in depression and anxiety: men and women, *Acta Psychiatr Scand* 1986; **73**:113–27.

41. Kessler RC, McGonagle KA, Nelson CB et al, Sex and depression in the National Comorbidity Survey II: cohort effects, *J Affect Disord* 1994; **30**:15–26.

42. Breslau N, Schultz L, Peterson E, Sex differences in depression: a role for preexisting anxiety, *Psychiatry Res* 1995; **58**:1–12.

43. Wilhelm K, Parker G, Hadzi-Pavlovic D, Fifteen years on: evolving ideas in researching sex differences in depression, *Psychol Med* 1997; **27**:875–83.

44. Kessler RC, Gender differences in major depression: epidemiologic findings. In: Frank E, ed., *Gender and its Effects on Psychopathology* (American Psychiatric Press: Washington, DC, 2000) 61–84.

45. Barnett RC, Baruch GK, Social roles, gender and psychological distress. In: Barnett RC, Biener L, Baruch GK, eds, *Gender and Stress* (The Free Press: New York, 1987) 122–43.

46. Mirowsky J, Ross CE, *Social Causes of Psychological Distress* (Aldine De Gruyter: New York, 1989).

47. Simpson HB, Nee JC, Endicott J, First-episode major depression. Few sex differences in course, *Arch Gen Psychiatry* 1997; **54**:633–9.

48. Kessler RC, Gender differences in DSM-III-R psychiatric disorders in the United States: results from the National Comorbidity Survey, *J Am Med Wom Assoc* 1998; **53**:148–58.

49. Dunner DL, Hall KS, Social adjustment and psychological precipitants in mania. In: Belmaker RH, van Praag HM, eds, *Mania: An Evolving Concept* (Spectrum Publications: Jamaica NY, 1980) 337–47.

50. Taylor MA, Abrams R, Gender differences in bipolar affective disorder, *J Affect Disord* 1981; **3**:261–71.

51. Roy-Byrne P, Post RM, Uhde TW et al, The longitudinal course of recurrent affective illness: life chart data from research patients at the NIMH, *Acta Psychiatr Scand* 1985; **317**:1–34.

52. Gove WR, The relationship between sex roles, marital status, and mental illness, *Social Forces* 1972; **51**:34–44.

53. Gove WR, Tudor JF, Adult sex roles and mental illness, *Am J Sociol* 1973; **78**:812–35.

54. Kessler RC, McLeod JD, Sex differences in vulnerability to undesirable life events, *Am Sociol Rev* 1984; **49**:620–31.

55. Nazroo JY, Edwards AC, Brown GW, Gender differences in the onset of depression following a shared life event: a study of couples, *Psychol Med* 1997; **27**:9–19.

56. Kessler RC, Magee WJ, Childhood adversities and adult depression: basic patterns of association in a US National Survey, *Psychol Med* 1993; **23**:679–90.

57. Abrahams B, Feldman S, Nash SC, Sex-role self concept and sex-role attitudes: enduring personality characteristics or adaptations to changing life situations? *Dev Psychol* 1978; **14**:393–400.

58. Abramson LY, Andrews DE, Cognitive models of depression: implications for sex differences in vulnerability to depression, *Int J Mental Health* 1982; **11**:77–94.

59. Bassoff ES, Glass GV, The relationship between sex roles and mental health: a meta-analysis of twenty-six studies, *The Counseling Psychologist* 1982; **10**:105–12.

60. Baucom DH, Danker-Brown P, Sex role identity and sex-stereotyped tasks in the development of learned helplessness in women, *J Pers Soc Psychol* 1984; **46**:422–30.

61. Klerman GL, Hirshfeld RMA, Personality as a vulnerability factor: with special attention to clinical depression. In: Henderson AS, Burrows GD, eds, *Handbook of Social Psychiatry* (Elsevier: New York, 1988) 41–53.

62. Whiteley BE Jr, Sex role orientation and psychological well-being: two meta-analyses, *Sex Roles* 1985; **12**:207–25.

63. Hirschfeld RMA, Klerman GL, Clayton PJ et al, Assessing personality: effects of the depressive state on trait measurement, *Am J Psychiatry* 1983; **140**:695–9.

64. Hirschfeld RMA, Klerman GL, Clayton PJ et al, Personality and gender-related differences in depression, *J Affect Disord* 1984; **7**:211–21.

65. Kouzis AC, Eaton WW, Emotional disability days: prevalence and predictors, *Am J Public Health* 1994; **84**:1304–7.

66. Wohlfarth TD, van den Brink W, Ormel J et al, The relationship between social dysfunctioning and psychopathology among primary care attenders, *Br J Psychiatry* 1993; **163**:37–44.

67. Kessler RC, Frank RG, The impact of psychiatric disorders on work loss days, *Psychol Med* 1997; **27**:861–73.

68. Kessler RC, Sonnega A, Bromet E et al, Posttraumatic stress disorder in the National Comorbidity Survey, *Arch Gen Psychiatry* 1995; **52**:1048–60.

69. Kessler RC, Berglund PA, Foster CL et al, Social consequences of psychiatric disorders: II. Teenage parenthood. *Am J Psychiatry* 1997; **154**:1405–11.

70. Kessler RC, Forthofer MS, The effects of psychiatric disorders on family formation and stability. In: Cox MJ, Brooks-Gunn J, eds, *Conflict and Cohesion in Families: Causes and Consequences* (Cambridge University Press: New York, 1999).

71. Robins LN, Regier DA, eds, *Psychiatric Disorders in America: The Epidemiologic Catchment Area Study* (Free Press: New York, 1991).

72. Robins LN, Locke BZ, Regier DA, An overview of psychiatric disorders in America. In: Robins LN, Regier DA, eds, *Psychiatric Disorders in America: The Epidemiologic Catchment Area Study* (Free Press: New York, 1991) 328–66.

73. Kessler RC, Brown RL, Broman CL, Sex differences in psychiatric help-seeking: evidence from four large-scale surveys, *J Health Soc Behav* 1981; **22**:49–64.

74. Leaf PJ, Bruce ML, Gender differences in the use of mental health-related services: a re-examination, *J Health Soc Behav* 1987; **28**:171–83.

75. Wilensky GR, Cafferata GL, Women and the use of health services, *Women Health* 1983; **73**:128–33.

76. Gove WR, Gender differences in mental and physical illness: the effects of fixed roles and nurturant roles, *Soc Sci Med* 1984; **19**:77–91.

77. Kendler KS, Neale MC, Kessler RC et al, A population based twin study of major depression in women: the impact of varying definitions of illness, *Arch Gen Psychiatry* 1992; **49**:257–66.

78. Cadoret RJ, *Adoption Studies in Psychosocial Epidemiology* (Rutgers University Press: New Brunswick NJ, 1991).

79. Davis MA, Sex differences in reporting osteoarthritic symptoms: a sociomedical approach, *J Health Soc Behav* 1981; **22**:298–310.

80. Kessler RC, Sex differences in the use of health services. In: McHugh S, Vallis TM, eds, *Illness Behavior: A Multidisciplinary Model* (Plenum: New York, 1986) 135–48.

81. Mechanic D, Correlates of physician utilization: why do major multivariate studies of physician utilization find trivial psychosocial and organizational effects? *J Health Soc Behav* 1979; **20**:387–96.

82. Mechanic D, Sex, illness, illness behaviour, and the use of health services, *J Human Stress* 1976; **2**:29–40.

83. Nathanson CA, Sex, illness, and medical care: a review of data, theory, and method, *Soc Sci Med* 1977; **11**:13–25.

84. Cleary PD, Mechanic D, Greenley JR, Sex differences in medical care utilization: an empirical investigation, *J Health Soc Behav* 1982; **23**:106–19.

85. Depner CE, *Predictor Variables. Health in Detroit Study*, Technical Report No. 2 (Institute for Social Research, The University of Michigan: Ann Arbor MI, 1981).

3

Evolutionary concepts of gender differences in depressive disorders

Natalie L Rasgon, Michael T McGuire and Alfonso Troisi

Introduction

In both medicine and psychiatry, males and females differ in their predispositions to certain illnesses. Women are particularly vulnerable to somatic pathologies such as thyroid disorders, rheumatological spectrum disorders (e.g. rheumatoid arthritis, fibrositis, systemic lupus erythematosus, polymyalgia rheumatica), and the migrainous disorders.[1,2] Men are at greater risk of developing disorders of the cardiovascular system and alcoholism. Women also have greater lifetime risks for eating disorders and depression.[3–5] Sex differences in the onset and prevalence of depressive disorders begin to appear after puberty and are maintained throughout the reproductive years. Compared to men, women are more often diagnosed with unipolar depression, the depressive subtype of bipolar depression, and cyclical forms of affective illness such as rapid-cycling manic-depressive illness, dysthymia, and seasonal affective disorder.[5–7] Psychosocial, biomedical and evolutionary factors have been implicated in prevalence differences in depression. This chap-

ter begins with a selected review of psychosocial and biomedical explanations of prevalence differences. It then turns to evolutionary explanations.

Psychosocial explanations of male–female prevalence differences

Numerous studies have focused on interactions between psychosocial factors and depression in women. Rate increases in depression often correlate with periods of rapid social change, and current epidemiological findings are consistent with the view that the USA is experiencing a period of rate increase.[4,5] Schwab and Bell[8] have pointed to possible historical parallels with the current era and late Elizabethan and early 17th-century England, when depression reached epidemic proportions. Rosen,[9] discussing late 18th-century England, quotes Edgar Shepherd, who, in the year 1773, attributed the rise in mental illness to the wear and tear of civilization and speculated on the causes for male–female prevalence differences in mental disorders. Rising expectations, access to new opportunities and efforts to redress traditional social inequalities of women have been suggested as reasons for the increase in depression among women.[10] New role expectations may have unexpected outcomes, such as creating personal conflicts, particularly for women involved in traditional family tasks who also desire employment and recognition outside the family.[10]

Most psychosocial theories of depression either assume or postulate that women are either more vulnerable to depression or have greater difficulty in recovering from depression.[11] Women are thought to derive the majority of their self-esteem from social relationships rather than from the mastery of the physical environment. They are also thought to be more dependent and less able to take control of their lives. And they are thought to be more likely to internalize stress and develop self-blame.[12] The influence of social factors on the course and treatment of depression in women may also be important. For example, there is evidence that what is frequently viewed as the typical female psychological structure cannot be separated easily from gender-specific socialization and that these factors may influence the clinical course of mental disorders.[13] Women's roles in most societies are defined in terms of caring for others and engaging in specific tasks, neither of which may be assigned high status or correlate with social influence; for example, on average women get lower wages than men. Other studies[14] suggest that more women live in poverty and that they have higher rates of victimization compared to males. The relationship between poverty and depression has been well described for both men and women, yet it appears to be a particularly critical factor among women who are depressed.[14] A number of studies have described both high rates of victimization in women who are depressed and high rates of depression in women who have been victimized.[15,16] Greater victimization among women compared to men may be a contributing factor to prevalence differences.

Despite their intuitive appeal, the degree to which psychosocial explanations are compelling remains problematic. Studies designed to test psychosocial hypotheses have often failed to yield consistent results.[12] There are good reasons why this is so. Taken as a whole, psychosocial explanations postulate multiple psychological and social contributing factors. Moreover, each factor may have its own disorder-contributing threshold. Further, the form and intensity of factors across any two-study situations will vary despite investigators' attempts to minimize variance. The implication of these points is that, short of extreme situations (e.g. solitary confinement), replication studies are likely to yield inconsistent results. Granting these points, what does emerge from these studies is that psychosocial explanations are in agreement with the idea that females are more vulnerable to the negative effects of social events than are males and that these differences appear to influence prevalence rates.

Biomedical explanations of male–female prevalence differences in depression

Biomedical explanations for the female preponderance in mood disorders build on a number of not mutually exclusive ideas ranging from hormonal status, to entrainment, to kindling.

Hormones are partial determinants of behaviours and interact with psychological, social and physiological factors. Throughout both the menstrual cycle and the life cycle, women are subject to hormonal fluctuations. Hormonal fluctuations often correlate with rates of depression. Examples include depression associated with premenstrual dysphoric disorder,[17-19] postpartum depression,[6,7] menopause[7,20,21] and oral contraceptives.[7,21] One biological theory suggests that the menstrual cycle modulates mood and behavioural disturbances and thereby modifies the severity of appearance of certain mental illnesses.[22] In turn, modifications may trigger the recrudescence of previously experienced mental illnesses.[6,21] The hormonal status explanation is consistent with several surveys that have demonstrated increased psychiatric admissions during the para-menstrual phases of the menstrual cycle (4–5 days before onset and during the menses[23,24])—that is, when compared to the mid-follicular and early-to-mid-luteal phases of the menstrual cycle, the late luteal and menstrual phase of the cycle are associated with significantly higher rates of admissions to psychiatric facilities. Other research reports provide supportive findings. For example, in one study, 46% of 276 emergency psychiatric admissions occurred during the para-menstrual phases;[23] Jacobs and Charles[25] and Abramowitz et al[26] have reported, respectively, 47% and 47.8% psychiatric admission rates during the para-menstrual interval. These findings invite the hypothesis that premenstrual biological change in individuals who are vulnerable to mental disorders may be sufficient to trigger mental illness and lead to hospitalization.[27]

A related theory focuses on the menstrual cycle itself, which may be powerful enough to entrain a variety of episodic disorders by serving as a *zeitgeber* (synchronizer) of disorder expression.[6,22] During the reproductive years, premenstrual worsening of depressed and/or dysphoric mood has been described.[28,29] In a retrospective study of 70 women with primary recurrent depression,[30] approximately 30% experienced their first depressive episode during the period of reproductive hormonal change, whether premenstrually or at menopause. That recurrent changes in depressive mood can be linked to the menstrual cycle suggests a possible relationship between depressive illness and menstrual cyclicity.[22] A link is also suggested by the finding that some women with prospectively diagnosed premenstrual dysphoric disorder (PMDD) show characteristic postmenstrual periods of euphoria which are analogous to the mood state changes observed in bipolar illness.[22] Further, some women with PMS may experience a menstrual cycle-entrained cyclic mood disorder that has become linked with, although not necessarily caused by, the menstrual cycle.[19,22]

Pregnancy has been considered as another example of the influence of reproductive hormonal milieu on mood changes across the life cycle.[7] The relatively low rate of mental disorders during pregnancy is associated with elevated levels of steroid hormones, although recently the view of pregnancy as a 'psychiatric oasis' is undergoing revision.[7] During the postpartum period, abrupt shifts in hormonal levels may predispose women to an increased risk of developing a major psychiatric illness, such as mood disorder or psychosis.[7] This view is consistent with the hypothesis that ovarian failure and subsequent disintegration of the menstrual cyclicity observed in menopause is one of the factors in the development of menopause-related mood and behaviour disorders.[21]

Research into the neurobiology of mood disorders during the last decade has led to the development of hypotheses of kindling and behavioural sensitization.[31-33] Kindling hypotheses focus on the spatial–temporal effects of neurobiological development that are thought to be linked with the progression of mood disorders.[32] In kindling, one observes an increased behavioural responsiveness to the same stimulus over time, with progression to spontaneity following sufficient numbers of triggered kindled events (e.g. seizures).[34] Applying this hypothesis to changes in a mood state, if, for example, repeated separations or losses are associated with dysphoric reactions, the anticipation of such experiences may become associated with dysphoric states. Initial stresses may be insufficient to precipitate full-blown episodes of mood disorders. However, with the repetition of stressors or stimuli of sufficient magnitude, neurobiological alterations associated with full-blown episodes of affective disorder may be induced.[33]

The influence of ovarian sex steroids on various brain functions could be exerted at several levels, for example receptors, converting enzymes, and interactions among neurotransmitter systems.[6,7] Glucocorticoids have also been implicated in the mediation of depression, and changes in glucocorticoid function may explain why an extrinsic stress may result in certain features of depressive disorders.[35] The neuroendocrine response to stress involves a cascade of secretory events that are initiated by the hypothalamic neuropeptides, corticotrophin-releasing hormone and arginine–vasopressin. This cascade culminates in the release of glucocorticoids from the adrenal cortex. Release elicits a host of biological effects that allow the organism to meet the requirements imposed by stressful challenges. Circulating glucocorticoids regulate the hypothalamic–pituitary–adrenal (HPA) axis through feedback effects on the synthesis and secretion of hypothalamic and pituitary hormones, thus 'resetting' the activity of the system to basal levels. The neuroendocrine response to stress displays significant male–female differences that are thought to be associated with the presence of sex-specific gonadal steroids.[36] This view is consistent with findings showing sex differences in treatment responses to antidepressants (tricyclic antidepressants)—males are more responsive than females, despite similar plasma levels of drugs.[37] Further, women often experience premenstrual exacerbation of an underlying psychiatric disorder, which may be a result of the reproductive hormonal influence on the pharmacokinetics of psychotropic medications.

Although we have reviewed only a part of the literature and thus only a subset of the psychosocial and biomedical explanations that have been offered for depression, several points are suggested by the review. First, there are consistently detectable differences in the prevalence rates of depression among males and females. Second, there are also consistently detectable differences in the clinical course of depression. Third, age of onset of first episodes does not appear to differ among males and females. Fourth, biological factors particular to females, such as reproduction-related hormonal changes and cycling, possibly entrainment and kindling, are implicated in prevalence differences. For details see also Chapters 5 and 13.

Evolutionary approaches to male–female prevalence differences in depression

There are a number of evolutionary explanations of depression, many of which are reviewed elsewhere.[38,39] Here, examples are discussed with the aim of illustrating how evolutionary ideas can be applied to the analysis of male–female prevalence differences.

But first, a few comments point out evolutionary explanations as they apply to mental disorders. In one sense, these explanations are not so much alternative explanations as they are explanations that introduce an evolutionary framework for explaining and integrating findings from psychiatry's many subdisciplines (e.g. psychosocial, biomedical). In an evolutionary context, explanations like those discussed in the first half of this chapter are proximate explanations. They focus on the immediate effects of social contexts, psychological states, physiological states, and the influence of genetic information. The primary limitation of proximate explanations is that they overlook the possible contributions of function (the purpose of behaviour) and strategies as contributing factors to disorder phenotypes, that is that disorders themselves or, better, features of what are normally called disorders, have evolved (selected for in the Darwinian sense) and that these features have or had adaptive functions. Evolutionary explanations are as much at home with proximate explanations as they are with explanations that take function and adaptive possibilities into account,[38,39] but a comprehensive explanation requires the integration of proximate with functional and adaptive explanations.

There is yet another factor that differentiates evolutionary explanations of mental disorders from current approaches. From an evolutionary perspective, it is questionable if disorders qua disorders actually exist.[39] Put another way, it is questionable if the current emphasis on diagnoses has explanatory utility. Why might one argue this way? There are several reasons. First, clinical profiles of depression in two otherwise comparable individuals (e.g. monozygotic twins raised together) are never quite the same. This clinical fact not only suggests the obvious point that individuals differ despite genetic and upbringing similarity, but also that the expression of depression may have explanations other than those that are normally put forth in the biomedical model (e.g. dysregulated physiological state) or in most psychosocial models (e.g. some combination of adverse upbringing and/or current stressful circumstances). Second, there is no reason to assume that somewhat similar clinical manifestations in males and females have the same causal origins. Much of evolution is about sex differences and the different selection pressures that contributed to genetic, hormonal, behavioural and psychological differences between the two sexes. Clearly, males and females are different in multiple ways. Equally clearly, the same symptom or sign may have different causal origins and social meaning across the sexes. Third, variation is a cardinal principle of evolutionary theory and research. Each creation of a new human being is somewhat similar to a dice throw with respect to the combination of resulting genes. Some human beings can run fast while others cannot, and some have perfect pitch or photographic memory while others cannot detect a discordant note or remember. We usually take these attribute variations as part of human nature until we come to the concept of disorders, when we seem to forget that variation is just as likely to be present in moments of distress as it is during less stressful moments. Fourth, different causal variables may result in similar phenotypes.

The upshot of the four above points is that it should be helpful to look at depression from a different perspective. Evolutionary theory introduces such a perspective. What follows are examples of this perspective. The implications are clear: collect different data than the ones usually collected in psychiatric studies and offer alternative interpretations for the data. We begin with a discussion of sex-related differences in the clinical presentations of mood disorders.

Sex-related differences in symptoms

Available epidemiological data on sex differences in depressive symptomatology among non-patient samples (e.g. community-based populations, college students) show that depressed women report a greater number of symptoms than depressed men.[40] In these studies, women also experienced more neurovegetative symptoms (e.g. appetite, sleep changes) and feelings of worthlessness or guilt. Other studies show that non-patient depressed males do not endorse crying, social withdrawal, feelings of failure or somatic complaints, whereas non-patient depressed women are more likely to report self-dislike and indecisiveness.[41]

In clinical populations, male–female differences are also evident in symptom presentations. Women more frequently report an increase in food intake, written expressions of feelings, difficulty in making decisions, sleep disturbances, diminished appetite, and worry about their health and verbal hostility.[42] Compared to women, depressed men are more likely to exhibit both trait and state hostility,[43] which suggests that men may be at greater risk than women for developing patterns of aggressive behaviour during depressive episodes. Conversely, among both non-clinical subjects and depressed patients, crying behaviour is significantly more frequent in women than in men.[44,45] The evolutionary hypothesis that social manipulation is an important functional aspect of depression may explain in part these sex-related differences.[46] When confronted with situations in which the costs of behaviour exceed the benefits, women may adopt those behaviours that are likely to elicit the support of significant others.[39] Crying behaviour is very powerful in humans as a means of eliciting caring behaviour from others.[44] In contrast, men tend to experience hostility and to employ aggression to change a situation that is characterized by an unfavourable cost/benefit ratio.

Why depression is triggered by different events in women and men

Reproduction is more important for women than for men. The evolutionary reasons for this difference are related to paternity uncertainty (males are uncertain if they are the biological father of their offspring) and maternal certainty. Further, to assess the adaptiveness of their social behaviour, women monitor social support and reproductive success while men monitor resource access and control and sexual success.[39] There is a large body of evidence pointing to the relationship between reproduction and depression in women. Among parents who have lost a child through sudden infant death syndrome, neonatal death or stillbirth, 25–30% of mothers have high levels of depression. The results for fathers are 4–10%.[47] Infertile women show higher distress compared to their partners on both a global measure of psychiatric symptoms and subclass of depression.[48] Furthermore, despite the stresses associated with pregnancy and impending childbirth, pregnant women have a significantly lower risk of suicide than women of childbearing age who are not pregnant.[49]

Postpartum depression

The other side of reproduction in women is that the majority of reproductions are timed to take into account such factors as number and age of live offspring, resource predictability for the foreseeable future, and available social support systems. It follows that the frequency of postpartum depression should increase in situations in which these factors are absent. Available evidence supports this view. Postpartum depression is more frequent at the extremes of reproductive age, with undesired pregnancies, with being unmarried, with feeling unloved by one's husband, with reduced emotional support, with economic pressures, and with the birth of a high-risk or premature infant.[50] These factors indicate that the reproductive event is at risk and they predict reduced fitness payoffs. Under these conditions, depression might either elicit more help from others or favour maternal divestment of offspring.

Psychosocial factors

Gender differences in depression do not appear to be constant, but rather to vary over time. Prevalence differences (women > men) are higher among generations of males and females who reached adolescence when women had greater opportunities than their mothers for academic or professional achievement compared to those persons who reached adolescence when women had equal or less opportunity than their mothers for academic or professional achievement.[46] From an evolutionary perspective, these findings are not surprising. Trying to emancipate oneself from traditional social roles, which usually means taking on a new social role, may have negative psychological consequences, for example conflicts between academic or professional achievement and reproduction.

The social competition hypothesis of depression

The social competition hypothesis is the work of Price et al[51] and is perhaps the most well-known evolutionary hypothesis of depression. A central idea of this hypothesis is that human beings share with their more primitive ancestors an evolutionary mechanism for yielding in competitive situations. This 'involuntary subordinate strategy' has three main functions: (1)

an executive function which prevents the individual from attempting to make a 'comeback' by inhibiting aggressive behaviour toward rivals and superiors (but not dependents) and by creating a subjective sense of incapacity; (2) a communicative function that signals 'no threat' to rivals and 'out of action' to any kin who might wish to put an individual back into the area of fight on their behalf; and (3) a facultative function that puts the individual into a 'giving-up' state of mind that encourages acceptance of the outcome of competition and promotes behaviour that expresses voluntary yielding.[51]

Two ideas implicit in the social competition hypothesis are worth noting, male–female asymmetry and the physiological effects of social interactions. Among males and females, asymmetries are present in who determines sexual access (females control sexual access while males seek sexual access), predispositions to engage in rank (males > females) and coalition (females > males) relationships, social options (males generally have a greater number of social options than females), the importance of reproduction, and relationship exit costs. Considering rank and coalition relationships first, there is compelling evidence that males are more inclined than females to engage in overt competitive contests and hierarchy-related behaviour,[52–54] while females are more inclined to engage in coalition relationships. These differences influence male–female relationships in specific ways. For example, males are more inclined to have specific expectations and responses that are influenced by hierarchical considerations (e.g. sex-specific expectations, more direct and threatening communications), while females are more inclined to negotiate and engage in coercive communications.

Relationship exit costs are also a factor. Costs are likely to be greater for females than for males. There are both practical and psychological reasons for these differences. For females, practical reasons include disruptions of offspring upbringing and established social support networks, reduced access to resources, and priority changes. Psychological reasons include social isolation, shame (possibly), and reduced self-esteem (e.g. 'I couldn't manage the relationship'). For males, financial compromise and reduced access to offspring are usually the highest cost features. Of course, degree and type of asymmetry will differ in any given male–female relationship. However, asymmetries may occur with enough consistency to influence prevalence rates, and the most likely influence is that females more than males will be disadvantaged more frequently as a result of asymmetries.

There is an extensive literature (reviewed in McGuire and Troisi[39]) that addresses the influence of neutral, negative or absent social information on psychological and neurochemical states, mood, and behaviour. This literature is relevant to prevalence differences in depression in at least two ways. First, neutral or non-responsive behaviour by others in contexts where positive social interactions are expected can trigger central nervous system physiological changes and increase risk for depression. The central nervous system and triggering effects are even more striking when negative information such as criticisms, threats or rejections are frequent. To the degree that females are more involved and responsive in both male–female and female–female relationships than are males, the greater is their vulnerability to neutral and negative information and the greater is the likelihood that disorder might be triggered. Differences in the response to antidepressant drugs may be relevant here. Such differences introduce the possibility that sex-related physiological differences may contribute to prevalence differences.

Adaptive interpretations

Turning to the adaptive interpretations of depression, at first glance it may seem counter-intuitive to argue that depression can be adaptive or have adaptive features. However, the fact that depression occurs with such a high frequency and with such great predictability in certain situations (e.g. loss, defeat) suggests that depression may have been selected and that it can confer an adaptive advantage. Adaptive hypotheses of depression build from the idea that depression is in part a response to situations in which the existing costs of social interactions or activities (e.g. achieving goals) exceed the benefits. (Depression differs from anxiety in that anxiety is viewed as a response to the anticipation that the costs of activities or social interactions will exceed the benefits.) Examples of high-cost/low-benefit situations include loss of a significant other, loss of a job, failure at an activity in which one has invested a great deal of time and effort (e.g. failure to find a publisher for a novel), loss of physical capacities, and loss in competition.

Many of the research findings from studies of depression are consistent with the cost/benefit view. Behavioural change, social withdrawal and signalling are examples.

Behavioural changes refer to the reduction in interest and libido and initiated activities that often accompanies depression as well as the inability to concentrate, remember, and think creatively. These features result in a 'slowing down' of behaviour which may be mirrored physiologically and which is postulated to result in the preservation of energy and the avoidance of new, possibly costly or disappointing, activities or interactions. In effect, the possibility that a person will incur further costs is reduced. This hypothesis also addresses the fact that further benefits are unlikely following behavioural changes. However, the absence of benefits is one of the contributing factors to depression, so in the short term the loss of potential benefits is less relevant than the avoidance of further losses.

Social withdrawal has analogous consequences to behavioural change. Withdrawal reduces the frequency of social interactions, which in turn reduces the need to attend to others, to listen to what they say, and to interact. One has more time to ruminate and to be concerned about oneself. Although rumination and self-concern are often viewed as symptoms of depression, they may have adaptive features in that, like behavioural changes, they reduce the probability of engaging in new and possibly costly interactions.

Considering signalling, in most instances the signs and symptoms of depression are accurately signalled to known others, and known others are likely to recognize these signals. Those who recognize signals usually change their behaviour. They offer help, reduce social expectations, and take on new responsibilities. Furthermore, these behaviours usually occur without expectations of paybacks, a factor which, from a social interaction perspective, reduces the cost to depressed persons of accepting them.

There are, of course, qualifications to the view that depression may be adaptive. The points above are consistent with time-limited, non-severe, forms of depression. They are less consistent with depression associated with severe weight loss, extreme social withdrawal, and suicide. Extreme cases of depression may represent instances in which adaptive responses are unable to offset other compromised capacities.

Conclusion

There can be little doubt that depression is a common human affliction. There is also little doubt about the pervasiveness of the sex differences in the course, manifestations and biological underpinnings of depression. Our review suggests that there is a variety of reasons (e.g. biological, psychosocial) to suspect that females are more vulnerable to depression than are males. These suspicions are informed by evolutionary analysis, which suggests that evolved male–female asymmetries in preference for certain types of relationships, investment in reproduction and offspring, physiology and social options contribute to this vulnerability. The effects of negative or neutral information that often occur in competitive situations can be viewed as one of several depression-triggering mechanisms.

References

1. Sullivan J, The sex difference in ischemic heart disease, *Perspect Biol Med* 1983; **26**:657–71.
2. Robins LN, Helzer JE, Weismann MM et al, Lifetime prevalence of specific psychiatric disorders in three sites, *Arch Gen Psychiatry* 1984; **41**:949–58.
3. Kendell RE, Hall DJ, Hailey A et al, The epidemiology of anorexia nervosa, *Psychol Med* 1973; **3**:200–3.
4. Merikangas KR, Weissman MM, Pauls DJ, Genetic factors in the sex ratio of major depres-

sion, *Psychol Med* 1985; **15**:63–9.
5. Kessler RC, Nelson CB, Gonagle MC et al, Comorbidity of DSM-III-R major depressive disorder in the general population: results from the US National Comorbidity Survey, *Br J Pyschiatry* 1996; **168**(suppl):17–30.
6. Steiner M, Female-specific mood disorders, *Clin Obstet Gynecol* 1992; **35**:599–611.
7. Parry BL, Reproductive factors affecting the course of affective illness in women, *Psych Clin North Am* 1989; **12**:207–20.

8. Schwab JJ, Bell RA, *Social Order and Mental Health* (Brunner/Mazel: New York, NY, 1979).

9. Rosen G, Social stress and mental disease from the 18th century to the present: some origins of social psychiatry, *Milbank Mem Fund Q* 1989; 37:5–3ND.

10. Weissman MM, Klerman GL, Sex differences and the epidemiology of depression, *Arch Gen Psychiatry* 1977; **34**:98–111.

11. Pajer K, New strategies in the treatment of depression in women, *J Clin Psychiatry* 1995; **56** (suppl 2):30–7.

12. Whitley BE, Sex role orientation and psychological well-being: two meta-analyses, *Sex Roles* 1985; **12**:207–25.

13. Schwartz S, Women and depression: a Durkheimian perspective, *Soc Sci Med* 1991; **32**:127–40.

14. Sorenson SB, Golding JM, Depressive sequelae of recent criminal victimization, *J Traum Stress* 1990; **3**:337–50.

15. Carmen EH, Riecker PP, Mills T, Victims of violence and psychiatric illness, *Am J Psychiatry* 1984; **141**:378–83.

16. Roth S, Leibowitz L, The experience of sexual trauma, *J Traum Stress* 1988; **1**:79–107.

17. Rubinow DR, Hoban MC, Grover GN et al, Changes in plasma hormones across the menstrual cycle in patients with menstrually related mood disorder and in control subjects, *Am J Obstet Gynecol* 1988; **158**:5–11.

18. Veeninga AT, Westenberg HG, Serotonergic function and late luteal phase dysphoric disorders, *Psychopharmacology* 1992; **108**:153–8.

19. Rubinow DR, Roy-Byrne PP, Hoban MC et al, Prospective assessment of menstrually related mood disorders, *Am J Psychiatry* 1984; **141**:684–6.

20. Paykel ES, Depression in women, *Br J Psychiatry* 1991; **158**(suppl 10):22–9.

21. Schmidt PJ, Rubinow DR, Menopause-related affective disorders: a justification for further study, *Am J Psychiatry* 1991; **148**:844–52.

22. Rubinow DR, Psychiatric disorders of the luteal phase. In: *Psychopharmacology in Practice: Clinical and Research Update* (Foundation for Advanced Education in the Sciences: Bethesda, MD, 1995) 155–84.

23. Dalton K, Menstruation and acute psychiatric illness, *Br Med J* 1959; **5115**:148–9.

24. Rubinow DR, Roy-Byrne PP, Premenstrual syndromes: overview from a methodologic perspective, *Am J Psychiatry* 1984; **141**:163–72.

25. Jacobs TJ, Charles E, Correlation of psychiatric symptomatology and the menstrual cycle in an outpatient population, *Am J Psychiatry* 1970; **126**:1504–8.

26. Abramowitz ES, Baker AH, Fleisher SF, Onset of depressive psychiatric crises and the menstrual cycle, *Am J Psychiatry* 1982; **139**:475–8.

27. Zola P, Meyerson AT, Reznikoff JM et al, Menstrual symptomatology and psychiatric admission, *J Psychosom Res* 1979; **23**:241–5.

28. Warner P, Bancroft J, Factors related to self-reporting of the premenstrual syndrome, *Br J Psychiatry* 1990; **157**:249–60.

29. Halbreich U, Endicott J, Relationship of dysphoric premenstrual changes to depressive disorders, *Acta Psychiatr Scand* 1985; **71**:331–8.

30. Kolakowska T, The clinical course of primary recurrent depression in pharmacologically treated female patients, *Br J Psychiatry* 1975; **126**:336–45.

31. Post RM, Kopanda RT, Cocaine, kindling, and psychosis, *Am J Psychiatry* 1976; **133**:627–34.

32. Post RM, Therapies of rapid-cycling and ultra-rapid cycling bipolar illness. In: *Psychopharmacology in Practice: Clinical and Research Update* (Foundation for Advanced Education in the Sciences: Bethesda, MD, 1995) 315–83.

33. Post RM, Rubinow DR, Ballenger JC, Conditioning and sensitization in the longitudinal course of affective illness, *Br J Psychiatry* 1986; **149**:191–201.

34. Racine R, Kindling: the first decade, *Neurosurgery* 1978; **3**:234–52.

35. Dinan TG, Glucocorticoids and the genesis of depressive illness: a psychobiological model, *Br J Psychiatry* 1994; **164**:365–71.

36. Kant GJ, Lenox RH, Bunnel BN et al, Comparison of stress response in male and female rats: pituitary cyclic AMP and plasma prolactin, growth hormone and corticosterone, *Psychoneuroendocrinology* 1983; **8**:421–8.

37. Aneshensel CS, The natural history of depressive symptoms, *Res Commun Ment Health* 1985; **5**:45–74.

38. McGuire MT, Troisi A, Raleigh MJ, Depression in evolutionary context. In: Baron-Cohen S, ed.,

The Maladapted Mind: Classic Readings in Evolutionary Psychopathology (Erlbaum: London, 1997) 255–82.

39. McGuire MT Troisi A, *Darwinian Psychiatry* (Oxford University Press: New York, 1998).

40. Angst J, Dobler-Mikola A, Do the diagnostic criteria determine the sex ratio in depression, *J Affect Disord* 1984; 7:189–98.

41. Nolan R, Willson VL, Gender and depression in an undergraduate population, *Psychol Rep* 1994; 75:1327–30.

42. Frank E, Carpenter AB, Kupfer DJ, Sex differences in recurrent depression: are there any that are significant? *Am J Psychiatry* 1988 145:41–5.

43. Fava M, Nolan S, Kradin R, Rosenbaum J, Gender differences in hostility among depressed and medical outpatients, *J Nerv Ment Disord* 1995; 183:10–14.

44. Williams DG, Weeping by adults: personality correlates and sex differences, *J Psychol* 1982; 110:217–26.

45. Davis D, Lamberti J, Ajans AZ, Crying in depression, *Br J Psychiatry* 1969; 115:597–8.

46. Silverstein B Perlick D, Gender differences in depression: historical changes, *Acta Psychiatr Scand* 1991; 84:327–31.

47. Vance JC, Foster WJ, Najman JM et al, Early parental responses to sudden infant death, stillbirth or neonatal death, *Med J Australia* 1991; 155:292–7.

48. Wright J, Duchesne C, Sabourin S et al, Psychosocial distress and infertility: men and women respond differently, *Fert Sterility* 1991; 55:100–8.

49. Marzuk PM, Tardiff K, Leon AC et al, Lower risk of suicide during pregnancy, *Am J Psychiatry* 1997; 154:122–3.

50. Hopkins J, Marcus M, Campbell SB, Postpartum depression: a critical review, *Psychol Bulletin* 1984; 95:498–515.

51. Price J, Sloman L, Gardner R Jr et al, The social competition hypothesis of depression, *Br J Psychiatry* 1994; 164:309–15.

52. Barkow JH, Darwin, sex, and status. In: *Biological Approaches to Mind and Culture* (University of Toronto Press: Toronto, 1989).

53. Salter FK, Emotions in command. In: *A Naturalistic Study of Institutional Dominance* (Oxford University Press: New York, 1995).

54. Savin Williams RC, *Adolescence. An Ethological Perspective* (Springer-Verlag: New York, 1987).

4

Neuroanatomical sex differences

Micah J Sickel and Margaret M McCarthy

Introduction

The frequent conflict between the viewpoints of biomedical science and cultural politics is perhaps no better illustrated than by the topic of sex differences in the human brain. While few will argue that men and women on average *behave* differently, the putative source of this difference is markedly influenced by personal opinion, anecdote or even, perhaps, a hidden agenda. Frequent reports of conflicting data or failure of replication have contributed to a feeling that this research field lacks objectivity and rigour. However, rather than being the result of some nefarious agenda by dishonest scientists, the more likely source of data discrepancies can be found in the very nature of the neuroanatomical sex differences themselves; they are small, subtle and only apparent on a group level. For the most part, the neuroanatomy is far more similar in males and females than it is different. But small differences can have large impacts on neuronal functioning, and it will be the goal of this review to highlight those areas in which the data are

unequivocal and to identify those in which future research may be required.

Historical perspective

The original reports of neuroanatomical sex differences in the mammalian brain involved the detection of small differences in the shape and size of neurons in the preoptic area,[1,2] and received relatively little notice, since the effects were, as expected, small. It was generally considered that the obvious sex differences in behaviour were the result of other regulatory factors such as dimorphisms in gonadal steroids (oestrogens and androgens), or perhaps the distribution and quantity of their cognate receptors. The notion that there were no real structural differences in male and female brains was widely accepted, and at times championed. The catalyst that changed this view came from an unlikely and unanticipated source, bird brains. By their own admission, neither investigator was looking for a sex difference. In 1976, Nottebohm and Arnold[3] reported that brain nuclei associated with the production of song in two species of birds were substantially larger in males than in females. In fact, they were so much larger as to be readily visible to the naked eye. Even more importantly, these brain nuclei were clearly tied to the sexually dimorphic behaviour of singing. Following on the heels of this report was an equally startling discovery of a sex difference in the mammalian brain, now known as the sexually dimorphic nucleus of the preoptic area, or SDN-POA.[4] From that point forward, sex differences in the brain were no longer considered trivial or so small as to be of little significance. In fact, the list of neuroanatomical sex differences seems to grow at such a rate that it raises questions of whether any neuroanatomical structure is completely identical in males and females.

In recent years, investigation of sex differences in the human brain has garnered wide attention. Many of these data are controversial and some remain inconclusive in the absence of replication. This situation is no doubt due in large part to the particular difficulties and limitations inherent in working with human tissue of variable sources, origins and qualities. In this chapter, we include both the human neuroanatomical data and functional data, such as those concerning cognitive ability tests, lateralization of function, and glucose metabolism. In the last section, we attempt to bring all of this work together and propose ideas which can link the neuroanatomical data to particular illnesses. This last part is composed of a discussion about the links between oestrogen, neuroanatomy and affective (depression and manic-depression) and anxiety disorders.

Guiding principles

An informed discussion on neuroanatomical sex differences requires the elucidation of certain generalities. First and foremost is the fact that the brain is a heterogeneous organ composed of complex interconnections, circuits and relays. Neuroanatomical sex differences in a discrete brain region cannot be interpreted in the absence of understanding the relation that area has to the rest of the brain. Perhaps because of this, in the majority of instances the functional significance of neuroanatomical sex differences is largely unknown.

A second essential guiding principle regarding neuroanatomical sex differences is the importance of gonadal and adrenal steroid hormones in both the developing and adult brains. Of particular importance is the concept of sexual differentiation of the brain. A developing fetus possesses a bipotential or 'indifferent' gonadal system. The activation of a gene on the Y chromosome, called SRY (sex-determining region of the Y chromosome), induces a cascade of events that results in the differentiation of the male gonadal system. The absence of this gene, as in the case of two X chromosomes, is a prerequisite for the development of a female gonadal and ductal system. Like the gonadal system, the developing brain is also bipotential. However, rather than responding to the presence or absence of a single gene, the brain is differentiated by the steroid hormone milieu which is produced by the differentiated gonads. Early experience, such as pre- or postnatal stress, can also result in steroid hormone release which influences the developing brain. For these reasons, we do not think of sexual differentiation of the brain as being strictly the result of a genetic process; rather, it is a hormonal process dictated by genes and a heterogeneous distribution of functional hormone receptors. In a very simplified view, a hormone molecule enters a cell and binds its cognate receptor, and the complex then binds the DNA and alters transcription. The majority of neurons containing steroid receptors are found in the hypothalamus and limbic system, although recent evidence suggests that the developing cortex also consists of a substantial number of oestrogen receptor-containing neurons.[5] In order to have a better understanding of neuro-anatomical sex differences, it is best to start with a brief overview of the basic neuro-anatomy.

Basic neuroanatomy of the hypothalamus and limbic system

The nervous system is divided into a central component, consisting of the brain and spinal cord, and a peripheral component, consisting of the nerves which project to the body and send information regarding sensory and proprioceptive stimuli back to the central nervous system. The brain can be divided into the forebrain, midbrain and hindbrain. These divisions are useful for delineating brain functions on a simplistic level. In general, the forebrain and midbrain are most importantly involved in regulation of behaviour, whereas the hindbrain is important for regulation of vegetative functions such as control of heart rate and respiration. Understanding the role of the brain in regulation of behaviour requires thinking in terms of functional systems. For instance, the perception of light involves the 'visual system', an inter-connected series of discrete brain regions which act together in a coordinated fashion so that light hitting the retinae is ultimately perceived as a blue sky or your grandmother's face. Information flows from the retinae into the brain along a specified pathway, with different way stations along the route integrating and refining the information. Similarly, there are also discrete pathways for the formation and retrieval of memories, in the reward system, to control appetite and feeding and so on. Some

systems or pathways are more discretely defined than others, and some involve the simultaneous recruitment and/or exclusion of other pathways. For example, the expression of rage involves activation of the peripheral nervous system in a 'fight or flight' response, but it also suppresses systems involved in feeding, perception of pain and sexual behaviour.

The concept that emotional responses in humans could have a discrete anatomical localization was somewhat slow to develop. The prevailing notion was that emotionality was a product of activity within the entire brain, a so-called emergent property. It is now clear that very specific emotional responses can be elicited by stimulating specific parts of the brain in experimental animals and humans. In addition, certain neurological disorders manifested as changes in emotionality have been associated with specific neuroanatomical defects. For example, damage to a specific region of the right temporal cortex (Wernicke's area) leads to disturbances in the comprehension of the emotional aspects of language. Conversely, damage to a closely related but distinct cortical area (Broca's area) results in difficulty in expressing the emotional aspect of language. Further demonstrations of the localization of affect in the human brain are found in patients with chronic temporal lobe epilepsy, who exhibit characteristic emotional changes, and from patients with panic attack disorder, who show abnormal bloodflow in a circumscribed region of the temporal lobe.[6] However, while the cortex is importantly involved in the regulation of human behaviour, it is certainly not the only brain region modulating affective behaviour, and it is often just one component of a functional system. Many neuroanatomical sex differences are found in the hypothalamus and components of the limbic system, and reports of differences in cortical regions and fibre tracts are increasing annually.

Hypothalamus

The hypothalamus is located within the ventro-medial portion of the diencephalon. This heterogeneous brain region is critical for the control of many bodily functions, including fluid regulation/thirst, thermoregulation, food intake, various aspects of reproduction, sympathetic and parasympathetic function, and circadian rhythms. Many of these actions are related to hypothalamic control of anterior and posterior pituitary functioning.

The hypothalamus is composed of many distinct nuclei and regions (Table 4.1, Figure 4.1) (a nucleus refers to an aggregation of neuronal cell bodies, or somata). The major nuclei in a rostral-to-caudal gradient would be the preoptic area (POA), suprachiasmatic nucleus (SCN), supraoptic nucleus (SON), paraventricular nucleus (PVN), ventromedial nucleus (VMN),

and arcuate nucleus (ARC). Each of these is involved in specialized functions. For instance, the PVN produces the hypothalamic hypophysiotropic hormones which are released into the portal vessel system. These peptides are transported into the anterior pituitary, or adenohypophysis, where they either stimulate or inhibit the release of yet other hormones. For instance, thyrotrophin-releasing hormone (TRH) and corticotrophin-releasing hormone (CRH), are made in the PVN parvocellular neurosecretory cells and released into the anterior pituitary, where they cause the respective release of thyroid-stimulating hormone (TSH) and adrenocorticotrophic hormone (ACTH). These latter hormones then act on their respective effector organs, in this case the thyroid, which then releases thyroid hormone, and the adrenal gland, which releases corticosteroids. In both cases there is a negative feedback loop in that

---

Table 4.1 List of major hypothalamic nuclei.

Preoptic area	Located rostral to the optic chiasm, this grouping of many nuclei is integrally involved in sexual behavior.
Paraventricular nucleus	Contains magnocellular neurosecretory cells which synthesize vasopressin and oxytocin to be released into the bloodstream via the posterior pituitary. This nucleus also plays a key role in hypothalamic-pituitary-adrenal (HPA) axis function, known as the stress axis.
Supraoptic nucleus	Located just above the optic chiasm, this nucleus, like the PVN, also contains magnocellular neurosecretory cells which synthesize and secrete vasopressin and oxytocin into the bloodstream via the posterior pituitary.
Suprachiasmatic nucleus	Known as the circadian rhythm generator, it is located just rostral to the arcuate nucleus.
Ventromedial nucleus	Involved in sexual and feeding behaviour in rats, the ventrolateral portion has many oestrogen receptor-containing cells.
Arcuate nucleus	Located just ventral and medial to the VMN, it may play a role in pulsatile LHRH secretion.

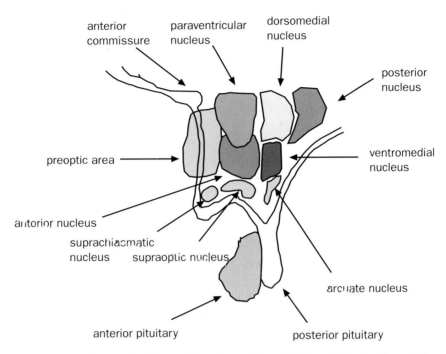

Figure 4.1 Sagittal view of the major hypothalamic nuclei and their relation to the pituitary gland. From rostral to caudal, they are: POA, preoptic area; SCN, suprachiasmatic nucleus; SON, supraoptic nucleus; PVN, paraventricular nucleus; ANT, anterior nucleus; DMN, dorsomedial nucleus; VMN, ventromedial nucleus; ARC, arcuate nucleus.

the hormones produced (glucocorticoids or thyroid hormone) move from the circulation into the brain, where they turn off the stimulus for their initial release. In this way the hypothalamus functions as a thermostat to control circulating hormone levels, and hormones in turn act on the brain to modulate behaviour. All of these functional systems serve to coordinate peripheral physiological events with appropriate behavioural responses. An example of this is the coordination of ovulation, a peripheral event, with the central control of sexual receptivity in order for reproduction to be achieved.

The PVN and SON contain magnocellular neurosecretory cells which send their axons into the posterior pituitary, or neurohypophysis, where they release the peptide hormones vasopressin (antidiuretic hormone) and oxytocin, directly into the bloodstream. Vasopressin causes vasoconstriction and water retention, thus affecting blood pressure and maintenance of a constant blood osmolality. Oxytocin, on the other hand, causes milk letdown during lactation as well as uterine contractions during childbirth. However, both of these neurohypophyseal hormones also act in the brain to modulate neuronal activity and exert profound influences on behaviour. For example, oxytocin has anxiolytic properties and it is this property which may allow for increased social interactions.[7,8]

The POA plays a critical role in sexual behaviour. Lesioning this brain region will result in a loss of sexual activity in male rodents, but will actually increase sexual receptivity in females. The POA, along with the SCN, which is the circadian rhythm generator, work together to produce a cyclical release of gonadotrophin-releasing hormone (GnRH). GnRH is therefore important in maintaining the cyclicity inherent in female reproduction. (GnRH stimulates the release of gonadotrophins luteinizing hormone (LH) and follicle-stimulating hormone (FSH), both of which act on the testes and ovaries). Conversely, males have a constant low level of GnRH release beginning at puberty which stimulates both spermatogenesis (via FSH) as well as the release of yet another hormone, testosterone (via LH). The ARC is also important in the regulation of gonadotrophin and prolactin release by the anterior pituitary. Thus it is apparent that through its control of pituitary functioning, the hypothalamus can regulate a wide range of physiological responses.

Limbic system

The limbic system is a functionally organized group of brain regions involved in many affective behaviours. This collection of brain structures, along with those regulating olfactory input, is considered to be phylogenetically ancient. The limbic system includes the hippocampus, which is integral to learning and memory, the amygdala, which is central to the perception of fear and expressions of anxiety, and some primitive portions of the cortex. The amygdala receives olfactory information, often relaying it to the hippocampus, thus providing the neural underpinnings of a phenomenon known to everyone, the sudden evoking of an old memory by a familiar smell. Not far from the amygdala is found the nucleus accumbens, a brain area that has been dubbed 'the reward centre' because of its crucial involvement in numerous addictive and affiliative behaviours.

An additional and important site for integration of varying and often conflicting input from the forebrain is found in the midbrain. Alternatively referred to as the periaqueductal grey (PAG) or midbrain central grey (MCG), this brain area is a major relay station for the regulation of responses as diverse as aggression, anxiety, pain perception and sexual behaviour.[9]

Organizational–activational hypothesis of steroid hormones action in the brain

Central to understanding the aetiology of sex differences in the brain is the concept of an initial organizing effect of steroid hormones early in development, followed by the activation of this organized neural circuit in adulthood. The organizational hypothesis, first proposed by Phoenix et al in 1959,[10] holds that neural circuits are permanently laid down or organized by the actions of steroid hormones during early life. The developmental window during which the neural substrate can be organized by steroids is referred to as the 'sensitive' or 'critical' period. Sex differences in the organization of neural circuits arise from sex differences in exposure to steroids, and this is in turn the result of sex differences in gonadal activation. In rodents, on embryonic day 18, the testes begin to release copious quantities of testosterone into the bloodstream, a portion of which gains access to the brain and permanently alters its development. There is an additional surge of testosterone production by the testes on the day of birth (embryonic day 22), further differentiating the developing brain, after which steroid levels fall and remain close to undetectable until puberty. As a result of this perinatal steroid exposure, the brain is considered 'masculinized'. In the developing female rodent the gonads remain relatively quiescent and there are no surges in steroid hormones, and subsequently the female brain remains undifferentiated or 'feminized'. There are human counterparts to these surges of testosterone. They take place during the first half of gestation, the perinatal period, and puberty. For instance, during the period from 34 to 41 weeks of gestation, male fetuses have a level of testosterone that is 10-fold higher than female levels.[11] It is fair to assume that these surges have analogous effects on the human brain in terms of sexual differentiation. Evidence in support of this comes from documented changes in the psychosexual differentiation of girls prenatally exposed to high levels of androgens because of a defect in adrenal steroid-metabolizing enzymes, referred to as congenital adrenal hyperplasia.[12] Additionally, boys prenatally exposed to high levels of diethylstilboestrol (DES), a potent oestrogen, showed higher incidences of major depressive disorder, which is more common in women, compared to their unexposed siblings.[13]

There still remains substantial controversy as to whether the development of the female brain is an entirely passive process or whether feminization is the result of an active differentiation via mechanisms that are not yet well understood. Nonetheless, at the end of the sensitive period, the brain is either masculinized or feminized. This does not mean that the brain cannot be influenced by steroids later in life, but rather that it can only be modified within the framework of what was laid down during the neonatal period.

In the current context, activation is the modification or 'activation' of a particular neural circuit by steroid hormones. Because of the foundation laid down during the neonatal period, a neural circuit will be modified in a way which is different from the modification that would have taken place within the same hormonal environment had the brain been organized differently. A dramatic example of this is the ability of the brain to regulate gonadal function. Ovulation requires a surge of LH from the anterior pituitary, and this surge is in turn dependent on neuronal signals from the hypothalamus. These neuronal signals are under the regulation of oestrogen, and in most mammalian species the male brain is insensitive to this effect of oestrogen. If a newborn female is exposed to exogenous testosterone during the sensitive period for sexual differentiation of the brain, she will permanently lose the ability to respond to oestrogen in a manner that will support ovulation, because of the organizing effects of this steroid exposure. Although not so definitive, there is a myriad of additional behavioural and physiological responses that are altered by this neonatal exposure to testosterone and its metabolites.

Neuroanatomical sex differences in the rodent brain

Volumetric differences in specific brain nuclei

The organization of neurons into specific nuclei, particularly in the hypothalamus, allows for relatively easy volumetric analysis at the macroscopic level. The original discovery of the SDN-POA precipitated similar analyses of other hypothalamic and limbic nuclei, and although many other volumetric sex differences have been found, none have compared in magnitude to that of the SDN-POA. First described by Gorski in 1978, this intensely staining area located in the medial preoptic nucleus is four to eight times larger in volume in the male and can be used as a marker for sexual differentiation of the brain because its volume is hormone dependent.[4] Hormonal manipulation of adult animals does not produce changes in the volume of the SDN-POA. However, if males are gonadectomized on the day of birth, the size of the SDN-POA is significantly reduced compared to males gonadectomized at the time of weaning, ie at about days 20–22 of life.[4] Similarly, newborn females treated with testosterone developed larger SDN-POA volumes than control females.[4]

Additional studies demonstrated that males gonadectomized and treated with a single injection of testosterone on days 2–5 of life had increased SDN-POA volumes compared to gonadectomized males that did not receive testosterone replacement and to males that did not receive the testosterone injection until days 6–8 of postnatal life.[14] Similarly, females treated with testosterone on days 2–5 showed a significant increase in SDN-POA volume compared to females that did not receive a testosterone injection until days 6–8 of life.[14] These findings illustrate the principle of a 'sensitive period' by demonstrating a loss of sensitivity to the differentiating effect of testosterone as development progresses.

Recent studies have taken the opposite approach; that is, instead of adding gonadal steroids, the gonads are removed at different time points postnatally. Males that had a gonadectomy delayed until postnatal day 4, 5, 6 or 7 had significantly reduced SDN-POA volumes compared to gonadally intact males, but none of them was significantly different from males gonadectomized on the day of birth.[15] However, males that had their gonads removed on the day of birth showed more female-typical sexual behaviour as adults than did males that

were gonadectomized on postnatal day 4, 5, 6 or 7.[15] These data indicate that the SDN-POA is not the only structure regulating sexual behaviours, since males with similar SDN-POA volumes displayed very dissimilar levels of sexual receptivity and/or there are non-volumetric differences present in the SDN-POA.

A second important concept that emerged from studies of the SDN-POA is that the hormonally mediated effects are actually due to the action of a testosterone metabolite, oestrogen (testosterone is aromatized to oestrogen by the P450 enzyme aromatase). Administration of the oestrogen antagonist tamoxifen to males on the day of birth reduces the volume of the SDN-POA.[16] A similar finding is observed following administration directly into the neonatal hypothalamus of antisense oligonucleotides to oestrogen receptor mRNA, confirming that oestrogen is acting at the oestrogen receptor.[17]

In general, most volumetric measurements of nuclei indicate a larger structure in males. However, the anteroventral periventricular nucleus (AVPv) is a notable exception to the rule, because of its greater size in females.[18,19] It is thought to be a regulator of gonadotrophin release, a sexually dimorphic process whereby females have an LH surge followed by ovulation. The AVPv is also the origin of a sexually dimorphic projection to the ARC; there are eight times as many neurons projecting from the female AVPv to the ARC compared to that of the male, and this is believed to be the neuroanatomical basis for its regulation of gonadotrophin release (review: Gu and Simerly[20]). An additional component of sexual dimorphism in the AVPv is the three-fold greater number of dopaminergic neurons in the female brain.[19] These findings illustrate the important principle of a sexually dimorphic circuit and its neurochemical underpinnings.

One complex grouping of nuclei in the preoptic area is known collectively as the bed nucleus of the stria terminalis (BNST). The posteromedial portion of the nucleus is 2.5 times larger in the male,[11] and as with the SDN-POA, this is the result of gonadal steroid hormone exposure. On the other hand, the female medioanterior portion of this nucleus is greater in volume. Females also have more cells within the medioanterior region and in the lateral region of the nucleus. These differences in the lateral division can be reversed with neonatal gonadectomy of males and testosterone treatment of females (review: Guillamon and Segovia[21]). Similarly, in the limbic system, the subdivisions of the amygdaloid complex are steroid sensitive during development. Males and females treated with oestrogen for the first 30 days of life both have a larger medial amygdaloid nucleus, while the lateral amygdaloid nucleus is the same volume in males and females.[22] The presence of oestrogen receptors within the medial amygdaloid nucleus and their absence within the lateral amygdaloid nucleus is a likely source of this divergence. Thus gonadal steroids can have highly localized effects.

It is apparent from this cataloging of sexually dimorphic brain nuclei that the preoptic area is a brain region where these dimorphisms are particularly prevalent. Nuclei in the caudal hypothalamus, such as the PVN, VMN, dorsomedial nucleus (DMN) and ARC, do not appear to vary much in volume between the sexes. However, there are profound sex differences in these nuclei at the neurochemical and microneuroanatomical levels.

Fibre tracts and neuronal projections

Fibre tracts are bundles of axons that connect one area with another so that the two areas can communicate. As was mentioned before, the AVPv is the source of a highly sexually dimorphic projection to the ARC. The corpus callo-sum (CC) is the structure which lies between the two hemispheres of the brain, and it contains a majority of the fibres which cross between the hemispheres. In rats, sex differences have been found in the ratio of unmyelinated to myelinated axons in the anterior region of the CC known as the genu (female > male),[23] in the number of total axons in another region known as the splenium (female > male),[24] and in the number of myelinated axons in the splenium (males > females).[24] By affecting the myelination of fibres, gonadal steroids could thereby affect neural conduction, with a consequence being a change in summation of signals and thus modulation of higher-order functions. Alternatively, myelinated and unmyelinated neurons may originate from different regions, and differences in their numbers may reflect differences in regional nuclear volumetric differences.

Synaptic patterning

A synapse is a point at which one neuron makes contact with another at either the neuronal cell body, dendrite, or axon (Figure 4.2). A neuron transmits information via release of a neurochemical that is either a neurotransmitter or neuropeptide. The neurochemical is released from the presynaptic terminal to the postsynaptic terminal membrane, where it binds its cognate receptor. Synapses onto dendrites are either on the dendritic shaft or the dendritic spine.[25] These dendritic spines look like little knobs or appendages poking out from the dendrites and they are thought to be the sites of excitatory synaptic contact (typically glutamatergic) between two neurons. This is in contrast to other types of synapses, which are usually inhibitory. While volumetric and fibre tract differences are intriguing, it is the patterns of connectivity between neurons and their variable firing rates that ultimately dictate behavioural responses.

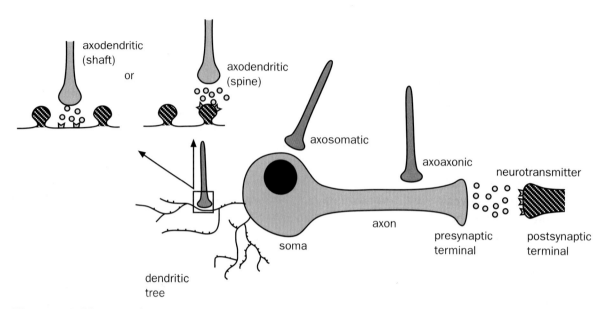

Figure 4.2 Diagram of a neuron demonstrating four different types of synapses: axodendritic (shaft), axodendritic (spine), axosomatic, and axoaxonic. The stereotyped postsynaptic terminal can be the dendritic shaft or spine, cell soma, or axon shaft. Synapses can also be formed on the presynaptic terminal, also called the terminal bouton.

Techniques developed in the 1800s allowed for the visualization of individual neurons in post-mortem tissue by impregnating them with heavy metals. Microscopic analysis allows for the discrimination of minute neuronal structures, including dendritic spines. These spines are now generally accepted as hallmarks of a synapse. When the levels of oestrogen and progesterone fluctuate over the oestrous cycle, so too do the number and types of spines found throughout many neuronal populations. For example, within the VMN there is an increase and subsequent decrease in the number of dendritic spines over the course of the oestrous cycle.[26] The use of electron microscopy allows for an even finer analysis, as well as for the distinction between synapses on dendritic spines, dendritic shafts, and neuronal somata. For example, in the ventrolateral portion of the

VMN, an area with a high concentration of oestrogen receptors, male rats have more dendritic shaft and spine synapses than do females.[25] These differences are not seen in the dorsomedial portion of the VMN, an area with relatively few oestrogen receptor-containing neurons.

Although a direct functional relationship cannot currently be found between patterns of synaptic connectivity and behaviour, it is likely that the expression of sex-typical behaviour in rodents is at least in part due to sex differences in neuronal 'wiring'. Sex differences in the pattern of synaptic connectivity are widespread and include the ARC, POA, amygdala (AMYG) and hippocampus, in addition to the VMN. The best evidence for the functional significance of these changes in synaptic connections is found in the hippocampus. As in the

VMN, the number of dendritic spines fluctuates during the oestrous cycle within the CA1 region of the hippocampus,[26] and the change is specific to a type of synaptic structure known as the multiple-synapse bouton. As the name implies, a multiple-synapse bouton is a neuronal ending (bouton) that makes contact with multiple postsynaptic cells, thus differentiating it from a single-synapse bouton, which makes contact with only a single postsynaptic cell. When oestrogen is given to an ovariectomized female rat, there are increases in both the percentage of presynaptic terminals forming multiple synaptic contacts and the number of synapses formed by the presynaptic terminals.[27]

Oestrogen has been shown to enhance the formation of long-term potentiation (LTP),[28] a cellular process believed to be related to learning and memory. Not only has LTP been produced at the same type of synapses which fluctuate during the oestrous cycle, but the degree of LTP induction within the stratum radiatum of the hippocampus is greatest during the time of the cycle when synapse numbers within that region are highest.[28] Also, a correlation has been found between oestrogen-induced increases in dendritic spines and the increased excitability of hippocampal neurons.[29] These data point to a modulation in hippocampal function by oestrogen and possibly other hormones, and this could in turn produce differences in learning strategies and emotionality of male and female rats. Other sex differences in the hippocampus have been found in the mossy fibre system, which connects the dentate gyrus with areas CA2, CA3 and CA4 of the hippocampus. It has been shown that female rats have a lower volume of mossy fibres and the number of varicosities per unit length of mossy fibre is also lower in females.[30] Varicosities are thought to be points of synaptic contact. However, the density of synapses between mossy fibres and CA3 neurons is greater in

females.[30] So, although females have less volume of these fibres, their synapses are more dense, probably making up for the lack of volume.

In the ARC the sex differences in synaptic patterning are particularly dramatic. Females have twice as many dendritic spine synapses as males, but half the number of somatic synapses.[25] This difference is no doubt functionally related to the pivotal importance of the ARC in the control of gonadotrophin secretion from the anterior pituitary, a process which is highly sexually dimorphic. Similar to the case in the ARC, normal males and neonatally androgenized females have greater numbers of dendritic shaft synapses in the medial amygdaloid nucleus than do normal females and neonatally castrated males.[25] These changes show the organizational effects that oestrogen has on synaptic morphology. The functional significance of these hormonally mediated sex differences in the amygdala is currently unknown.

An additional mechanism by which synaptic patterns can be changed involves steroid modulation of the non-neuronal glial cells. There are a variety of glial cell types and they serve a host of different functions. Generally, these functions have been considered in the context of a supportive role for neurons, but it has recently become clear that glia can be major effectors of synaptic transmission. This is in large part due to their ability to dramatically alter their morphology and thereby physically ensheath and block a synapse on a temporary basis. A common method to assess glial morphology is by immunocytochemical visualization of a glial-specific intermediate filament protein, known as glial fibrillary acidic protein (GFAP). Neonatal testosterone and/or oestrogen treatment dramatically and permanently alters glial morphology. Castration of males on the day of birth, or testosterone treatment of females, results in decreased GFAP levels within the hippocampus and ventromedial part of the ARC when brains are examined at 3 months of age.[31] Similar changes are seen during neonatal life.[32] Arcuate and hippocampal glia remain responsive to steroids in adulthood and will alter their content of GFAP, and hence their morphology, in response to gonadectomy and hormone replacement, and across the oestrous cycle.[33,34] Although confirming these effects in humans is not an option, these findings are of great importance, as it is likely that these same principles apply to the physiology of the human brain.

Cortical layer thickness

Differences in cortical thickness have been found on a global level as well as on a more local level. Globally, the male cortex appears to be longer as well as wider than in females, with the exception of the temporal cortex, where these differences are not found.[35] On a more local level, a great deal of work has been done to examine sex differences in the visual cortex. The male visual cortex has both a greater volume and a greater number of cells, and layers within one of its subfields are thicker in the male.[36] Differences have also been found in total dendritic length within subregions of the visual cortex.[37] Sex differences in cortical areas would seem to indicate sex differences in higher-order neural processing, such as retrieval of memories, learning, and perception of what one sees.

Neurochemistry

While morphological sex differences in neurons and glia are of obvious importance to understanding the sexual dimorphism of neural functioning, of equal importance are both the amount and distribution of neurochemicals in the brain. These neurochemicals include the neurotransmitters and neuropeptides which directly alter synaptic functioning, as discussed previously, as well as the enzymes which synthesize and degrade them. Of equal importance, of course, are the receptors, including receptors for steroid hormones. Substantial research effort has been directed towards mapping and quantifying all aspects of neurotransmitter systems and steroid hormone receptors and related enzymes in the brain. Reviewing all of these would quickly prove exhausting and largely uninformative. Therefore, we will focus on those systems that we think are particularly relevant to the neuroanatomical basis of mood disorders and sex differences therein.

Some obvious candidates for a sex dimorphism in neurochemistry are the steroid receptors and the critical metabolizing enzymes involved in the synthesis of the major gonadal steroids: androgens, oestrogens, and progestogens. Sex differences in the quantities of oestrogen, progesterone and androgen receptors have been reported, although none quite as dramatic as those in a recent report by Wagner et al.[38] They reported that male rats have significantly more progesterone receptor (PR) than females at embryonic days 20 and 21 and day of birth. These differences were found specifically within the POA, and are most likely a result of the testosterone surge that occurs around embryonic day 19 (E19). Steroid hormones exert their effect on the brain by inducing gene expression, and there are some sex differences in the magnitude of induction of particular genes in response to oestrogen treatment.[39] But again, these differences are relatively small and are not likely in and of themselves to be accountable for the dramatic differences in neuronal responsiveness of male and female brains.

Variation in neurotransmission is tantamount to variance in neural functioning. The number of identified neurotransmitters and neuropeptides in the brain is of the order of 30, and virtually every system has been reported to be influenced by gonadal steroids during development, adulthood or both. Three neurotransmitters are of particular interest to the current discussion. They are the dopaminergic system, which is important in reward and affect, the serotonergic system, which is implicated in major depression, and the GABAergic system, which influences a variety of behavioural responses related to mood and anxiety.

The release of dopamine into the nucleus accumbens, the so-called 'reward centre' of the brain, is enhanced by oestrogen and progesterone.[40] There are also sex differences in the production of dopamine receptors in this brain area.[41] Since increased dopamine release in this brain structure is correlated with increasing pleasure or reward properties of a stimulus, it is clear that hormones would be an important source of variability in these responses, and this has in fact been found to be the case. The rewarding properties of brain stimulation were found to be greatest at the time in the oestrous cycle when both oestrogen and progesterone levels were high.[42] Monoamine oxidase (MAO) is an enzyme involved in the breakdown of various monoamines, including dopamine, noradrenaline and serotonin and is the enzyme inhibited by the class of antidepressants known as the monoamine oxidase inhibitors (MAOIs). Oestrogen has been shown to regulate the levels of MAO within key reproduction-related nuclei. Oestradiol delivered to male rats can reduce MAO activity by 30–50% within the ventrolateral VMN (vlVMN), ARC, and median eminence.[43] In contrast, oestradiol actually increased MAO activity within the female vlVMN and midbrain central grey.[44] When oestrogen was administered to ovariectomized rats, there was a resultant 30% decrease in MAO-A activity in the basomedial

hypothalamus and in the corticomedial amygdala, with no effect on MAO-B activity.[45] Also, there are changes in MAO-A activity over the course of the oestrous cycle.[46] These data reveal oestrogen modulation of MAO-A activity within prescribed areas of the brain.

GABA (γ-aminobutyric acid) is the major inhibitory neurotransmitter in the brain, although early in development it is excitatory and thought to play a key role in the sexual differentiation of synaptic patterning.[47] One way to regulate GABA levels is through altering levels of its synthesizing rate-limiting enzyme glutamic acid decarboxylase (GAD). GAD levels are sexually dimorphic prior to 2 weeks of life, at which time the critical period for sexual differentiation of the brain closes.[48] In adult rats, GABA levels are also modulated by gonadal steroids, in particular oestrogen. During early pro-oestrus, a time when oestrogen levels are high, GABA levels are high in the VMN and low in the POA. During late pro-oestrus, when oestrogen levels are at their lowest, GABA levels are decreased in the VMN and increased in the POA.[49] These cyclic changes play a role in the sexual receptivity of the female. In addition to modulating GABA levels, steroids also modulate the expression of the postsynaptic GABA receptor subunits.[50] Thus gonadal steroids play a role in GABAergic system modulation, at both the neurochemical level and neuroreceptor levels, and at both the organizational and activational levels.

Benzodiazepines, a group of anxiolytic drugs, work at the GABA$_A$ receptor. When diazepam (valium) is injected into the midbrain central grey of a female rat, the rat demonstrates increased exploratory behaviour, and hence lower anxiety levels, as well as an increased lordosis quotient, that is, a greater degree of sexual receptivity.[51] Furthermore, oestrogen has been found to enhance the anxiolytic action of diazepam,[51] and this has been found to be true of other benzodiazepines as well. Allopregnanolone, a metabolite of progesterone and neuromodulator at the $GABA_A$ receptor, has also been shown to have anxiolytic properties in animal models.[52] Others have found that levels of allopregnanolone are inversely correlated with levels of energy, wellbeing and cheerfulness, and levels of 5α-pregnane-3,20-dione (5α-DHP), an intermediate metabolite of progesterone, are inversely related with levels of fatigue and depression (see Chapter 12).[53] These types of data may shed light on the relationship between depression and anxiety, which are often comorbidly expressed.

Serotonin is a neurotransmitter familiar to many as the target of the selective serotonin reuptake inhibitors (SSRIs), a class of drugs frequently used in the treatment of major depression. In the brain, serotonin (5-hydroxytryptamine (5-HT)) receptor levels fluctuate within the basal forebrain of the cycling female rat, with lower levels occurring on pro-oestrus and oestrus.[46] During development, there are sex differences in levels of serotonin, and these differences can be modulated with hormone treatment as well as by removal of the gonads.[54] An agonist of the serotonin somatodendritic $5-HT_{1A}$ autoreceptor, 8-hydroxy-2-(di-n-propylamino)tetralin (8-OH-DPAT), has been shown to inhibit lordosis in females and also causes hyperphagia, and both of these effects are attenuated by oestradiol.[55,56] Oestradiol's attenuation of the 8-OH-DPAT inhibitory effects on lordosis may be through its action in the midbrain central grey or through the VMN.[55]

If the above findings are taken together, it is apparent that oestrogen exerts potent effects on the dopaminergic, serotonergic and GABAergic neurotransmitter systems. While it is tempting to infer functional relationships between these effects (i.e. attenuation of serotonin and simultaneous enhancement of GABA), a coordinated analysis of oestrogen's effects on neurotransmission within one animal species is lacking. Thus one of the great challenges remaining to neuroendocrinologists is the development of a coherent picture of how oestrogen influences neurotransmission and ultimately how it alters behaviour.

Functional significance of neuroanatomical sex differences in rodent brain

Over the oestrous cycle there are both structural changes in synaptic and glial morphology within the hippocampus and functional changes with regard to the induction of LTP. The relationship between the structural changes and functional changes is not entirely clear, but evidence is converging in support of a critical role for structural changes in altering neural activity. Other examples of ultrastructural differences and functional significance have been discussed above; however, we have yet to address any functional significances of volumetric differences. Since the greatest volumetric differences have been found in the SDN-POA, it has naturally been the target of the majority of investigations into functional significance of volumetric differences. Bilateral lesions of the SDN-POA in the male rat caused an attenuation in the rise of plasma LH and FSH subsequent to immediate gonadectomy or even when gonadectomy took place at 7 and 14 days post-lesioning.[57] It also caused a decrease in plasma prolactin levels when compared to gonadectomized controls and pre-lesioned levels.[57] This hints at a role of the SDN-POA in regulation of LH, FSH and prolactin secretion, which are sexually dimorphic responses. However, the POA is also the major brain region regulating male sexual behaviour. Attempts to unambiguously implicate only the SDN subdivision of the POA in male sex behaviour have generally failed. Nonetheless, it is clear that the dimorphic nature of the entire POA region contributes to differences in neuronal activity and that these differences in turn are important to the regulation of sex-typical reproductive behaviour.[58]

Neuroanatomical sex differences in the primate brain

Although not nearly as voluminous as the non-primate literature, the human and non-human primate literature on sex differences in neuroanatomy increases annually. Since the SDN-POA is probably the most recognizable neuroanatomical sex difference in the non-primate literature, we will begin with what is thought to be the correlate in humans, the interstitial nucleus of the anterior hypothalamus 1, or INAH-1 (Figure 4.3).

Comparison to the findings in rodents

Volumetric differences in specific brain nuclei

The human INAH-1 possesses interesting similarities to the rat SDN-POA. Both in humans and in rats, this nucleus possesses galanin- and TRH-containing neurons. Equally compelling is the fact that the male INAH-1 has twice as many cells as that of the female and is twice the volume.[11] Swaab and Hofman found that the size of the INAH-1 increases until about 2–4 years of age, when the sex difference becomes apparent. While the number of cells in the female INAH-1 begins to decrease after around the fourth year of life, the number remains con-

stant in the male nucleus until around the fiftieth year of life, when it, too, begins to decline (Figure 4.4). Others have not found this sex difference in the volume of the INAH-1, but have found a sex difference in INAH-2 and INAH-3, or in INAH-3 but not INAH-1 or INAH-2.[59,60] These conflicting findings make it difficult to come to a definitive conclusion; however, it is likely that the conflict results from variation in fixation procedures, staining techniques, and other inter-laboratory differences. There is a good possibility that real sex differences do exist in these hypothalamic nuclei, but we do not yet know which ones they are.

An additional volumetric difference in humans has been reported for the SCN. The shape of the SCN differs between men and women. In women, it appears to be more elongated, while in men it is more spherical.[11] Also, the vasoactive intestinal polypeptide(VIP)-containing subnucleus of the male SCN contains twice as many cells as that in the female and is twice as large in males aged 10–30.[11] The latter two differences disappear with increasing age. Because there is no clear connection between the SCN and any sexually dimorphic response, this reported sex difference has received less attention than it probably should have.

Fibre tracts and/or neuronal projections

The largest fibre tract in the brain is the CC, which connects the two hemispheres. As with most findings in the field of sexual differentiation of the brain, there is considerable controversy concerning the sex differences in the CC. Some groups have found that the total size of the CC and the sizes of certain regions within it, particularly the genu and the splenium, are smaller in females, while others have not found these differences (review: Bishop and Wahlsten[61]). While debates as to the size and shape of the CC will continue, there does

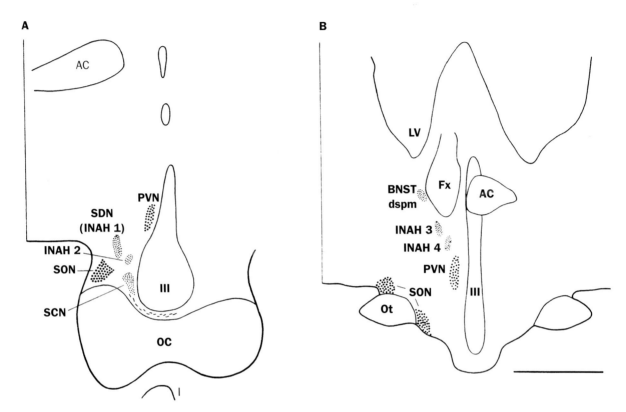

Figure 4.3 Topography of the sexually dimorphic structures in the human hypothalamus. **A** is a more rostral view than **B**. III, third ventricle; AC, anterior commissure; BNST-dspm, darkly staining posteriomedial component of the bed nucleus of the stria terminalis; Fx, fornix; I, infundibulum; INAH1-4, interstitial nucleus of the anterior hypothalamus 1-4; LV, lateral ventricle; OC, optic chiasm; Ot, optic tract; PVN, paraventricular nucleus; SCN, suprachiasmatic nucleus; SDN, sexually dimorphic nucleus of the preoptic area; SON, supraoptic nucleus. Scale bar, 5 mm. Reprinted from Swaab et al[11] with kind permission from Elsevier Science. © 1995.

appear to be a difference in the number of myelinated and unmyelinated axons within different regions of it. As people age, it seems that the number of medium and large fibres increases, and this increase is significantly greater in females.[62] Also, as they age, males and females have increases in different areas of the CC. Development appears to follow a different time course in the sexes within three delineated regions (the CC is divided into seven different regions in this study[63]). These three areas in the male attain maximum width at 20 years of age and then decrease in size, while the female counterpart does not achieve maximum width until 41–50 years of age.[63] Thus there are many reports of differences in CC size, development, and fibre composition, and these differences may reflect the many neural sex differences found throughout the brain. An obvious question is whether size difference in fibre tracts is due to gonadal steroid influence. Part of this answer lies in the rat model, where oestradiol and progesterone both increase myelination[64,65] and 5-α-reductase (the enzyme

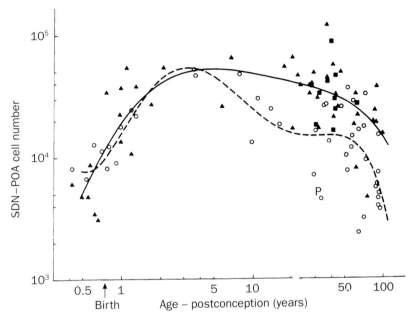

Figure 4.4 Development and sexual differentiation of the human sexually dimorphic nucleus of the preoptic area (SDN-POA) of the hypothalamus. Log–log scale. Note that, at the moment of birth, the SDN-POA is equally small in boys (▲) and girls (○) and contains only about 20% of the cell number found at 2–4 years of age. Cell numbers reach a peak value around 2–4 years postnatally, after which a sexual differentiation occurs in the SDN-POA as a result of a decrease in cell number in the SDN-POA of women, whereas the cell number in men remains approximately unchanged up to the age of 50. The SDN-POA cell number in homosexual men (■) does not differ from that in the male reference group. The curves are quintic polynomial functions that are fitted to the original data for males (solid line) and females (broken line). P, progesterone. Reprinted from Swaab et al[11] with kind permission from Elsevier Science. © 1995.

that converts testosterone to dihydrotestosterone, which only acts at androgen receptors) levels are inversely related with levels of myelination.[66]

The anterior commissure is a fibre tract that connects the two temporal neocortices, and it is 12% larger in females. The massa intermedia (MI) is a fibre tract which connects the two thalami; it is present in only 78% of females and 68% of males, and, when present, is about 53% larger in females.[67] In animal models the MI seems to be involved in dopamine release. If

the MI is missing in 20–30% of all people, one wonders if it has a critical function or is just a vestige of days past, like a neural appendix.

Cortical layer thickness
While differences in something as gross as brain size are still controversial (some say the male brain is larger, while others say that when body size is factored in, the difference disappears), a recent report show that the male brain contains about 16% or 3.5 billion more neocortical neurons (19.5 billion versus 22.8

billion) than the female brain.[68] They also found a greater neocortical surface area, volume and thickness in the male brain. As an example of the heterogeneity of the brain, other data show that the female brain has 11% more neurons per unit volume within the temporal cortex.[35] This difference was attributed to differences specifically in layers II and IV, which are part of the granular system, an input component of the cortex; the granular system, as it turns out, contains mostly GABAergic neurons. As many point out, the female brain is not just a miniature version of the male brain, but rather a differently organized brain which is also differently activated.

Functional significance of neuroanatomical sex differences in primate brain

Glucose utilization

The use of PET scans to examine brain glucose metabolism indicates that right–left metabolic asymmetry in the frontal lobe is significantly less in women.[69] As women age, they have significantly greater decline in hippocampal and thalamic glucose metabolism. Interestingly, until the twenty-fourth year of age, women have significantly higher thalamic metabolism, and at the seventieth year, women's hippocampal glucose metabolism becomes significantly less than that of men.[69] At rest, men have relatively higher glucose metabolism in temporolimbic regions and in the cerebellum and lower glucose metabolism in cingulate regions.[70] Thus it appears that men and women have different levels of glucose metabolism in their brains, and changes in glucose metabolism with age are also different between the sexes. Since glucose metabolism is indicative of neural activity, these data show that men and women have different basal activity levels, and

this may be indicative of differences which would manifest themselves during a specific task.

Lateralization of language

While men tend to perform better on some spatial and motor tasks, women do better on some verbal tasks (reviewed by Collaer and Hines[71]). However, conflicts frequently arise in research which looks at the lateralization of verbal function and sex differences therein. While it appears that all studies do not find a sex difference, when a difference is found it is males who are more lateralized in verbal ability. Also, when a brain injury is sustained, it is the males who develop verbal deficits after left-hemisphere damage and non-verbal damage deficits after right-hemisphere damage, while in women the functional deficit is not specific to the hemisphere which was damaged.[72,73] Employing functional magnetic resonance imaging (MRI), sex differences were found in the functional organization of the brain such that during phonological (rhyme) tasks, male brain activation was significantly more lateralized to the left inferior frontal gyrus region, while females showed a more dispersed activation pattern which included both left and right frontal gyri.[74]

Potential impact of neuroanatomical sex differences on mood and anxiety disorders

Although there seems to be a vast sea of sex differences in the brain, from the organ level, to the nuclear and fibre tract level, all the way down to the neurochemical and microanatomical level, it would be unwise at this moment to jump from a single data point or even a collection of data points to a direct correlation with a complex mental illness. With any mental illness, there is likely to be a host of factors, genetic and otherwise.

When the statistics for the disorders to be discussed here are examined, the question arises of whether there is some link between hormones, neuroanatomy, and the particular mental illness. Over a lifetime, depression will afflict an estimated 8–20% of the population, with women being closer to 20%,[75] and the female/male ratio is 2 : 1 (see Chapters 1 and 2).[76] The aetiology of depression is constantly debated. For our purposes, the idea of depression as a result of menopause is relevant; however, a direct correlation between menopause and depression is difficult to make. This difficulty is due to other factors, such as life stressors related to the menopause, as opposed to hormonal changes which result directly from the menopause, both of which may contribute to depression.[77] It is unclear from studies on hormone replacement therapy (HRT) whether replacing oestrogen really ameliorates depression. A meta-analysis study looked at hormone replacement and depression and came to the conclusion that HRT reduced depressed mood or other mild depressive symptoms in women, but that because studies involving severe depression were few and far between, no conclusion could be drawn about HRT and amelioration of severe depression (see Chapters 13 and 22).[78]

An excellent model of the interactions between oestrogen and mental illness is the postpartum onset of depression and anxiety. Postpartum depression occurs in about 10% of women within the first few months after childbirth, and has a relapse rate in subsequent pregnancies of about 25–40% (see Chapter 18).[79,80] Postpartum oestrogen treatment has been found to be effective in this population of women. Ten of eleven women who presented with postpartum depression were successfully treated during the period immediately following delivery and for the first postpartum year during which they were observed.[80] The authors caution that their particular regimen of treatment is specific for those women who do not experience a depressive disorder outside of the context of their pregnancy; that is, they do not normally experience a non-puerperal depression. The simultaneous appearance of a mental disorder with the period just after delivery, or even the lesser symptoms that typically appear during the menstrual cycle, may relate to circulating oestrogen levels. During a normal menstrual cycle, oestrogen levels go from a low of around 20–50 pg/ml up to a high of about 200 pg/ml around the time of the LH surge (Figure 4.5). During pregnancy, there is a gradual rise of oestrogen, with a peak of about 18 ng/ml occurring at the time of the delivery.[81] But the absolute levels of oestradiol are probably not the key here; rather, it is the precipitous drop in oestradiol levels that occurs just after delivery. Within 48 h of delivery, oestrogen levels are back down to follicular phase levels,[80] around 20–50 pg/ml, an almost 400–1000-fold drop. Thus the term that has been coined for this event is 'oestrogen withdrawal',[80] and it is possible that a susceptible subpopulation of women experiences a mental disorder as a result. This withdrawal of oestrogen not only precipitates depressive disorder, but has also been shown to precipitate anxiety and panic disorders, as well as obsessive-compulsive disorder.[82,83] One of the critical points here is that these women usually do not have a previous history of a mental illness, although some may have had previous postpartum-onset mental illness. While many of these studies remain unreplicated, it seems plausible that fluctuating hormone levels, particularly fluctuating oestrogen and progesterone, could precipitate a depressive episode. However, this may or may not explain why

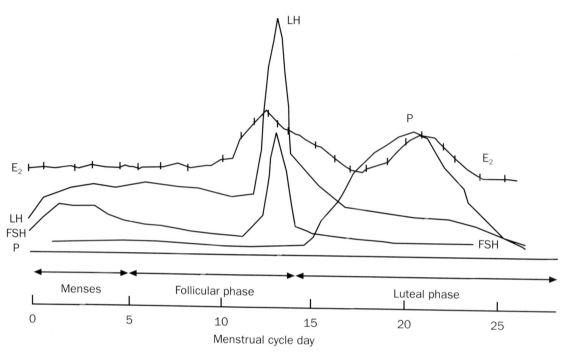

Figure 4.5 Hormonal changes during the human menstrual cycle. Peak hormone levels are as follows: oestradiol (E_2) = 200 pg/ml; progesterone (P) = 10 ng/ml; follicle-stimulating hormone (FSH) = 25 mIU/ml; luteinizing hormone (LH) = 60 mIU/ml. Ovulation occurs subsequent to the rise in LH, known as the LH surge, while menses begins with the withdrawal of oestrogen and progesterone. (Adapted from Thorneycroft et al.[85])

10% of pregnant women in the USA experience a major depression over the course of their pregnancy (see Chapter 17).[84] And, as was stated above, hormones will not be the only factors precipitating the depression; rather, it is a combination of fluctuating hormone levels and the impending responsibilities that go along with the birth of a child.

The prevalence of anxiety disorders is also sexually dimorphic. While 2–3% of women have anxiety disorders, only 0.5–1.5% of men have them. There is clearly a heritable component to these disorders, since monozygotic twins are five times more likely to have an anxiety disorder than are dizygotic twins.[75] Also, as stated above, anxiety disorder can be precip-

itated during the postpartum period. In this case, patients have been successfully treated with SSRIs.[82]

Bipolar disorder has a prevalence of about 0.5–1%, with a female/male ratio of 3 : 2.[75] It is characterized by highs and/or lows; the type which afflicts women tends to be more of the depressive type (type II). Twin studies have shown that genetic factors play a very large role in the mood disorders, but these same studies also show that genes are not the only variables, since there is not a 100% concordance among monozygotic twins.

There is an abundance of evidence for sex differences in mood and anxiety disorders as well as in the relevant neuroanatomy and neurochemistry. Is the relationship between these neuroanatomical/neurochemical differences and mental illness correlative or causative? While this is as yet unknown, it is clear that there is a complex interplay between genes and environment. Neuroanatomical sex differences are the results of this gene–environment interaction. Future research is required to further elucidate the intricacies of this relationship and its importance to neural functioning.

References

1. Raisman G, Field PM, Sexual dimorphism in the preoptic area of the rat, *Science* 1971; **173**:731–3.
2. Pfaff DW, Morphological changes in the brains of adult male rats after neonatal castration, *J Endocrinol* 1966; **36**:415–16.
3. Nottebohm F, Arnold AP, Sexual dimorphism in vocal control areas of the songbird brain, *Science* 1976; **194**:211–13.
4. Gorski RA, Gordon JH, Shryne JE, Southam AM, Evidence for a morphological sex difference within the medial preoptic area of the rat brain, *Brain Res* 1978; **148**:333–46.
5. Toran-Allerand CD, Miranda RC, Hochberg RB, MacLusky NJ, Cellular variations in estrogen receptor mRNA translation in the developing brain: evidence from combined [I-125]estrogen autoradiography and non-isotopic in situ hybridization histochemistry, *Brain Res* 1992; **576**:25–41.
6. Kandel ER, Schwartz JH, *Principles of Neural Science*, 2nd edn (Elsevier Science Publishing Co, Inc.: New York, 1985) 5–17.
7. McCarthy MM, McDonald CH, Brooks PJ, Goldman D, An anxiolytic action of oxytocin is enhanced by estrogen in the mouse, *Physiol Behav* 1996; **60**:1209–15.
8. Elands J, de Kloet ER, de Wied D, Neurohypophyseal hormone receptors: relation to behavior. In: Ermisch A, Landgraf R, Ruhle H-J, eds, *Progress in Brain Research*, Vol. 91 (Elsevier: New York, 1992) 459–64.
9. Bandler R, Shipley MT, Columnar organization in the midbrain periaqueductal gray: modules for emotional expression? *Trends Neurosci* 1994; **17**:379–89.
10. Phoenix CH, Goy RW, Gerall AA, Young WC, Organizing action of prenatally administered testosterone propionate on the tissues mediating mating behavior in the female guinea pig, *Endocrinology* 1959; **65**:369–82.
11. Swaab DF, Hofman MA, Sexual differentiation of the human hypothalamus in relation to gender and sexual orientation, *Trends Neurosci* 1995; **18**:264–70.
12. Zucker KJ, Bardley SJ, Oliver G et al, Psychosexual development of women with congenital adrenal hyperplasia, *Horm Behav* 1996; **30**:300–18.
13. Pillard RC, Rosen LR, Meyer-Bahlburg H et al, Psychopathology and social functioning in men prenatally exposed to diethylstilbestrol (DES), *Psychosom Med* 1993; **55**:485–91.
14. Rhees RW, Shryne JE, Gorski RA, Termination of the hormone-sensitive period for differentiation of the sexually dimorphic nucleus of the preoptic area in male and female rats, *Brain Res* 1990; **52**:17–23.
15. Davis EC, Shryne JE, Gorski RA, A revised critical period for the sexual differentiation of the sexually dimorphic nucleus of the preoptic area in the rat, *Neuroendocrinology* 1995; **62**:579–85.
16. Dohler KD, Srivastava SS, Shryne JE et al, Differentiation of the sexually dimorphic nucleus in the preoptic area of the rat brain is inhibited by postnatal treatment with an estrogen antagonist, *Neuroendocrinology* 1984; **38**:297–301.
17. McCarthy MM, Schlenker E, Pfaff DW, Enduring consequences of neonatal treatment with antisense oligonucleotides to estrogen receptor messenger ribonucleic acid on sexual differentiation of rat brain, *Endocrinology* 1993; **133**:433–9.
18. Byne W, Bleier R, Medial preoptic sexual dimorphisms in the guinea pig. I. An investigation of their hormonal dependence, *J Neurosci* 1987; **7**:2688–96.

19. Bloch GJ, Gorski RA, Estrogen/progesterone treatment in adulthood affects the size of several components of the medial preoptic area in the male rat, *J Comp Neurol* 1988; **275:** 613–22.

20. Gu G, Simerly RB, Hormonal regulation of opioid peptide neurons in the anteroventral periventricular nucleus, *Horm Behav* 1994: **28:**503–11.

21. Guillamon A, Segovia S, Sexual dimorphism in the CNS and role of steroids. In: Stowe TW, ed., *CNS Neurotransmitters and Neuromodulators* (CRC Press: Boca Raton, FL, 1996) 127–52.

22. Mizukami S, Nishizuka M, Arai Y, Sexual difference in nuclear volume and its ontogeny in the rat amygdala, *Exp Neurol* 1983; **79:**569–75.

23. Mack CM, Boehm GW, Berrebi AS, Denenberg VH, Sex differences in the distribution of axon types within the genu of the rat corpus callosum, *Brain Res* 1995; **697:**152–60.

24. Kim JHY, Ellman A, Juraska JM, A reexamination of sex differences in axon density and number in the splenium of the rat corpus callosum, *Brain Res* 1996; **740:**47–56.

25. Matsumoto A, Synaptogenic action of sex steroids in developing and adult neuroendocrine brain, *Psychoneuroendocrinology* 1991; **16:** 25–40.

26. McEwen BS, Woolley CS, Estradiol and progesterone regulate neuronal structure and synaptic connectivity in adults as well as developing brain, *Exp Gerontol* 1994; **29:**431–6.

27. Woolley CS, Wenzel HJ, Schwartzkroin PA, Estradiol increases the frequency of multiple synapse boutons in the hippocampal CA1 region of the adult female rat, *J Comp Neurol* 1996; **373:**108–17.

28. Warren SG, Humphreys AG, Juraska JM, Greenough WT, LTP varies across the estrous cycle: enhanced synaptic plasticity in proestrus rats, *Brain Res* 1995; **703:**26–30.

29. Woolley CS, Weiland NG, McEwen BS, Schwartzkroin PA, Estradiol increases the sensitivity of hippocampal CA1 pyramidal cell to NMDA receptor-mediated synaptic input: correlation with dendritic spine density, *J Neurosci* 1997; **17:**1848–59.

30. Madeira MD, Sousa N, Paula-Barbosa MM, Sexual dimorphism in the mossy fiber synapses of the rat hippocampus, *Exp Brain Res* 1991; **87:**537–45.

31. Garcia-Segura LM, Suarez I, Segovia S et al, The distribution of glial fibrillary acidic protein in the adult rat brain is influenced by the neonatal levels of sex steroids, *Brain Res* 1988; **456:**357–63.

32. Mong JA, Kurzweil RL, Davis AM et al, Evidence for sexual differentiation of glia in rat brain, *Horm Behav* 1996; **30:**553–62.

33. Day JR, Laping NJ, Lampert-Etchells M et al, Gonadal steroids regulate the expression of glial fibrillary acidic protein in the adult male rat hippocampus, *Neuroscience* 1993; **55:**435–43.

34. Garcia-Segura LM, Luquin S, Parducz A, Naftolin F, Gonadal hormone regulation of glial fibrillary acidic protein immunoreactivity and glial ultrastructure in the rat neuroendocrine hypothalamus, *Glia* 1994; **10:**59–69.

35. Witelson SF, Glezer II, Kigar DL, Women have greater density of neurons in posterior temporal cortex, *J Neurosci* 1995; **15:**3418–28.

36. Reid SN, Juraska JM, Sex differences in the number of synaptic junctions in the binocular area of the rat visual cortex, *J Comp Neurol* 1995; **352:**560–6.

37. Seymoure P, Juraska JM, Sex differences in cortical thickness and the dendritic tree in the monocular and binocular subfields of the rat visual cortex at weaning age, *Brain Res* 1992; **69:**185–9.

38. Wagner CK, Nakayama AY, De Vries GJ, Potential role of maternal progesterone in the sexual differentiation of the brain, *Endocrinology* 1998; **139:**3658–61.

39. Lauber AH, Pfaff D, Estrogen regulation of mRNAs in the brain and relationship to lordosis behaviour, *Curr Top Neuroendocrinol* 1990; **10:**115–47.

40. Saigusa T, Takada K, Baker SC et al, Dopamine efflux in the nucleus accumbens evoked by dopamine receptor stimulation in the entorhinal cortex is modulated by oestradiol and progesterone, *Synapse* 1997; **25:**37–43.

41. Andersen SL, Rutstein M, Benzo JM et al, Sex differences in dopamine receptor overproduction and elimination, *Neuroreport* 1997; **8:** 1495–8.

42. Bless EP, McGinnis KA, Mitchell AL et al, The effects of gonadal steroids on brain stimulation

reward in female rats, *Behav Brain Res* 1997; 82:235–44.

43. Luine VN, Rhodes JC, Gonadal hormone regulation of MAO and other enzymes in hypothalamic areas, *Neuroendocrinology* 1983; 36: 235–41.

44. Luine VN, Hearns M, Relationship of gonadal hormone administration, sex, reproductive status and age to monoamine oxidase activity within the hypothalamus, *J Neuroendocrinol* 1990; 2:423–8.

45. Luine VN, McEwen BS, Effect of oestradiol on turnover of type A monoamine oxidase in brain, *J Neurochem* 1977; 28:1221–7.

46. Biegon A, Bercovitz H, Samuel D, Serotonin receptor concentration during the estrous cycle of the rat, *Brain Res* 1980; 187:221–5.

47. McCarthy MM, Davis AM, Mong JA, Excitatory neurotransmission and sexual differentiation of the brain, *Brain Res Bull* 1997; 44:487–95.

48. Davis AM, Grattan DR, Selmanoff M, McCarthy MM, Sex differences in glutamic acid decarboxylase mRNA in neonatal rat brain: implications for sexual differentiation, *Horm Behav* 1996; 30:538–52.

49. McCarthy MM, Masters DB, Fiber JM et al, GABAergic control of receptivity in the female rat, *Neuroendocrinology* 1991; 53:473–9.

50. O'Connor LH, Nock B, McEwen BS, Regional specificity of gamma-aminobutyric acid receptor regulation by estradiol, *Neuroendocrinology* 1988; 47:473–81.

51. McCarthy MM, Felzenberg E, Robbins A et al, Infusions of diazepam and allopregnanolone into the midbrain central gray facilitate open-field behavior and sexual receptivity in female rats, *Horm Behav* 1995; 29:279–95.

52. Baulieu EE, Steroid hormones in the brain: several mechanisms? In: Fuxe K, Gustafsson JA, Wetterberg L, eds, *Steroid Hormone Regulation of the Brain* (Pergamon Press: Oxford, 1981) 3–14.

53. Wang M, Seippel L, Purdy RH, Backstrom T, Relationship between symptom severity and steroid variation in women with premenstrual syndrome: study on serum pregnenolone, pregnenolone sulfate, 5α-pregnane-3,20-dione and 3α-hydroxy-5α-pregnan-20-one, *J Clin Endocrinol Metab* 1996; 81:1076–82.

54. Giulian D, Pohorecky LA, McEwen BS, Effects of gonadal steroids upon brain 5-hydroxytryptamine levels in the neonatal rat, *Endocrinology* 1973; 93:1329–35.

55. Jackson A, Uphouse L, Prior treatment with estrogen attenuates the effects of the 5-HT1A agonist, 8-OH-DPAT, on lordosis behavior, *Horm Behav* 1996; 30:145–52.

56. Salamanca S, Uphouse L, Estradiol modulation of the hyperphagia induced by the 5-HT1A agonist, 8-OH-DPAT, *Pharmacol Biochem Behav* 1992; 43:953–5.

57. Preslock JP, McCann SM, Lesions of the sexually dimorphic nucleus of the preoptic area: effects upon LH, FSH, and prolactin in rats, *Brain Res Bull* 1987; 18:127–34.

58. Kartha KN, Ramakrishna T, The role of sexually dimorphic medial preoptic area of the hypothalamus in the sexual behaviour of male and female rats, *Physiol Res* 1996; 45:459–66.

59. LeVay S, A difference in hypothalamic structure between heterosexual and homosexual men, *Science* 1991; 253:1034–7.

60. Allen LS, Hines M, Shryne JE, Gorski RA, Two sexually dimorphic cell groups in the human brain, *J Neurosci* 1989; 9:497–506.

61. Bishop KM, Wahlsten D, Sex differences in the human corpus callosum: myth or reality? *Neurosci Biobehav Rev* 1997; 21:581–601.

62. Aboitiz F, Rodriguez E, Olivares R, Zaidel E, Age-related changes in fibre composition of the human corpus callosum: sex differences, *Neuroreport* 1996; 7:1761–4.

63. Cowell PE, Allen LS, Zalatimo NS, Denenberg VH, A developmental study of sex and age interactions in the human corpus callosum, *Brain Res* 1992; 66:187–92.

64. Curry JJ, Heim LM, Brain myelination after neonatal administration of oestradiol, *Nature* 1966; 209:915–16.

65. Koenig HL, Schumacher M, Ferzaz B et al, Progesterone synthesis and myelin formation by Schwann cells, *Science* 1995; 268:1500–3.

66. Celotti F, Melcangi RC, Negri-Cesi P et al, Differential distribution of the 5-alpha-reductase in the central nervous system of the rat and the mouse: are the white matter structures of the brain target tissue for testosterone action? *J Steroid Biochem* 1987; 26:125–9.

67. Allen LS, Gorski RA, Sexual dimorphism of the

anterior commissure and massa intermedia of the human brain, *J Comp Neurol* 1991; **312**:97–104.

68. Pakkenberg B, Gundersen HJ, Neocortical neuron number in humans: effect of sex and age, *J Comp Neurol* 1997; **384**:312–20.

69. Murphy DG, DeCarli C, McIntosh AR et al, Sex differences in human brain morphometry and metabolism: an in vivo quantitative magnetic resonance imaging and positron emission tomography study on the effect of aging, *Arch Gen Psychiatry* 1996; **53**:585–94.

70. Gur RC, Mozley LH, Mozley PD et al, Sex differences in regional cerebral glucose metabolism during a resting state, *Science* 1995; **267**: 528–31.

71. Collaer ML, Hines M, Human behavioral sex differences: a role for gonadal hormones during early development? *Psychol Bull* 1995; **118**: 55–107.

72. Inglis J, Lawson JS, Sex differences in the effects of unilateral brain damage on intelligence, *Science* 1981; **212**:693–5.

73. Inglis J, Ruckman M, Lawson JS, MacLean AW, Monga TN, Sex differences in the cognitive effects of unilateral brain damage, *Cortex* 1982; **18**:257–76.

74. Shaywitz BA, Shywitz SE, Pugh KR et al, Sex differences in the functional organization of the brain for language, *Nature* 1995; **373**:607–9

75. Leibenluft E, Women with bipolar illness: clinical and research issues, *Am J Psychiatry* 1996; **153**:163–73.

76. Andreasen NC, Black DW, *Introductory Textbook of Psychiatry*, 2nd edn (WB Saunders: Washington, DC, 1995) 247–320.

77. Coope J, Hormonal and non-hormonal interventions for menopausal symptoms, *Maturitas* 1996; **23**:159–68.

78. Zweifel JE, O'Brien WH, A meta-analysis of the effect of hormone replacement therapy upon depressed mood, *Psychoneuroendocrinology* 1997; **22**:189–212.

79. Gregoire AJ, Kumar R, Everitt B et al, Transdermal oestrogen for treatment of severe postnatal depression, *Lancet* 1996; **347**:930–3.

80. Sichel DA, Cohen LS, Robertson LM et al, Prophylactic estrogen in recurrent postpartum affective disorder, *Biol Psychiatry* 1995; **38**: 814–18.

81. Wilson JD, Foster DW, *Williams Textbook of Endocrinology*, 7th edn (WB Saunders: Philadelphia, PA, 1985) 438–51.

82. Sichel DA, Cohen LS, Dimmock JA, Rosenbaum JF, Postpartum obsessive compulsive disorder: a case series, *J Clin Psychiatry* 1993; **54**:156–9.

83. Metz A, Sichel DA, Goff DC, Postpartum panic disorder, *J Clin Psychiatry* 1988; **49**:278–9.

84. Wobie K, Eyler FD, Behnke M, Conlon M, Symbolic expression of feelings and depressive symptoms in high-risk pregnant women, *J Fla Med Assoc* 1997; **84**:384–90.

85. Thorneycroft IH, Mishell DR, Stone SC et al, The relation of serum 17-hydroxyprogesterone and estradiol-17-beta levels during the human menstrual cycle, *Am J Obstet Gynecol* 1971; **111**:947–51.

5

The functional neurochemistry of mood disorders in women

Edward J Dunn and Meir Steiner

Introduction

The lifetime prevalence of mood disorders (major depression, dysthymia and anxiety disorders) in women is approximately twice that of men (see also Chapters 1 and 2). This higher incidence of depression in women is primarily seen from puberty on and is less marked in the years after menopause.[1] The underlying causality of this gender difference in mood-related disorders is not clear at this time. As outlined elsewhere in this book, the aetiology is multifactorial and depends on genetic, environmental, neuroanatomical and biochemical factors (see Chapters 4, 8, 12 and 13). Since mood disorders occur in both men and women, it is assumed that a unified basis for the development of these diseases exists. The principal constituent of this unified theory is believed to be related to genetic predisposition. Multiple environmental stressful events cause biochemical changes in a host of neuroendocrine systems and neuroanatomical areas. The genetic predisposition, which is multifocal, determines how stressful life events are interpreted and predicts the response, which can

lead to the development of mood disorders. The higher prevalence of mood disorders in women could be related to either an increased genetic predisposition, an increased vulnerability/exposure to stressful life events, modulation of the neuroendocrine system by fluctuating gonadal hormones, or a combination of any or all of these factors.

We have previously proposed a biological susceptibility hypothesis to account for gender differences in the prevalence of mood disorders, based on the idea that there is a disturbance in the interaction between the hypothalamic–pituitary–gonadal (HPG) axis and other neuromodulators in women.[2] According to this hypothesis, the neuroendocrine rhythmicity related to female reproduction is vulnerable to change and is sensitive to psychosocial, environmental and physiological factors. Thus, premenstrual dysphoric disorder (PMDD), depression with postpartum onset (PPD) and mood disorders associated with the use of oral contraceptives or with menopause are related to hormone-modulated changes in neurotransmitter function.

The challenge now is to identify genetic markers and understand the neuroendocrine changes involved in the development of mood disorders. This will not be easy, since changes in one system often produce a cascade effect, leading to changes in other systems. Understanding the interactions of hormones and neurotransmitter systems will not only elucidate the pathophysiology of these diseases, but also provide better tools for diagnosis and treatment. This chapter will present examples from both animal and clinical studies, illustrating some of the potential neurochemical mechanisms that may be of importance in the aetiology of female-specific mood disorders.

Effects of steroid hormones on neurotransmitter systems

Control of mood and behaviour involves many different neurotransmitter systems, including glutamate, γ-aminobutyric acid (GABA), acetylcholine (ACh), serotonin (5-HT), dopamine, noradrenaline/adrenaline and neuropeptides. Given the observation that prevalence and symptomatology of mood disorders are often different between males and females, it is presumed that gonadal steroid hormones are somehow involved. For example, declining levels of oestrogen in women have been associated with postnatal depression and postmenopausal depression, and the cyclical variations of oestrogens and progesterone are probably the trigger for premenstrual complaints in women with premenstrual syndrome (PMS).[3,4] The interaction between neurotransmitters and steroid hormones is extremely complex and delicately balanced. Each system appears to have a modulatory function on the other, and changes in one system may have dramatic effects on the other systems.

Glucocorticoid and gonadal steroid receptors are abundant in different areas of the brain. Gonadal steroid receptors are found in the amygdala, hippocampus, basal forebrain, cortex, cerebellum, locus ceruleus (LC), midbrain raphe nuclei, pituitary gland and hypothalamus.[5] Oestrogen receptors are located in the preoptic area and amygdala[6] and the ventromedial nucleus and arcuate nucleus of the hypothalamus.[7]

Activation of cholinergic, dopaminergic or adrenergic neurotransmitter systems can alter concentrations of cytosolic hypothalamic oestrogen receptors. Muscarinic agonists and antagonists can increase oestrogen-binding sites in the female rat hypothalamus.[8,9] Oestrogen, progesterone and glucocorticoid receptors can also be activated by insulin-like growth factor 1 (IGF-1), epidermal growth factor (EGF), transforming growth factor alpha (TGF-α), cyclic AMP, protein kinase activators and various neurotransmitters.[10] Thus activation of neurotransmitter systems can have a direct modulatory effect on the binding of gonadal hormones in the central nervous system (CNS).

Conversely, steroid hormones can modulate neuronal transmission by a variety of mechanisms. They may affect the synthesis and/or release of neurotransmitters, as well as the expression of receptors, membrane plasticity and permeability. It has been suggested that steroid hormone receptors function as general transcription factors to achieve integration of neural information in the CNS.[11] Steroids are believed to act primarily by classical genomic mechanisms through intracellular receptors to modulate transcription and protein synthesis. This mechanism involves the binding of the steroid to a cytoplasmic or nuclear receptor. The hormone–receptor complex then binds to DNA to trigger RNA-dependent protein synthesis. The response time for this mechanism is of the order of several minutes, hours or days.

Recently, however, it has been shown that steroids can also produce rapid effects on electrical excitability and synaptic function through direct membrane mechanisms, such as ligand-gated ion channels, G-proteins and neurotransmitter transporters.[12] These short-term (seconds to minutes) effects of steroids may occur through binding to the cell membrane, binding to membrane receptors, modulation of ion channels, direct activation of second-messenger systems,[13] or activation of receptors by factors such as cytokines and dopamine.[14] Topical application of oestrogen or progesterone to nervous tissue has been shown to result in a rapid change in membrane potential, and sex steroids can affect membrane fluidity, thereby modifying ion transport or receptor function.[15]

The following are specific examples of how gonadal and adrenal steroids can influence the different neurotransmitter systems interacting with them.

The glutamate system

Neurosteroids can also act as modulators of N-methyl-D-aspartate (NMDA), a subtype of the glutamate receptor.[16] Androgens can modulate NMDA-mediated depolarization in CA1 hippocampal pyramidal cells.[17] Oestradiol increases the number of NMDA agonist binding sites in the CA1 region of the hippocampus, increasing the sensitivity of the hippocampus to stimulation by glutamate.[18] This increased sensitivity may in turn mediate some of the effects of oestrogen on cognitive function and epileptic seizure activity.[18]

The binding of sex steroids to NMDA and sigma receptors may provide yet another mechanism by which these steroids can confer neuroprotective effects. The risk and severity of dementia are decreased in women receiving oestrogen therapy. Weaver et al suggest that this may occur by direct inhibition of the NMDA receptor, protecting against NMDA-induced neuronal death.[19]

The GABA system

Progesterone is converted to neuroactive steroids (5α-pregnane steroids) in the brains of males and females. Neuroactive steroids can interact with progesterone receptors, induce DNA binding and activate transcription of the progesterone receptor.[20,21] Neuroactive steroids have anxiolytic properties resulting from their allosteric interaction with the GABA-A/benzodiazepine receptor complex. Withdrawal of progesterone increases seizure susceptibility and insensitivity to benzodiazepine sedatives, presumably through an effect on gene transcription.[22] Ovarian steroids are also suggested to play a role in modifying the stress response of the benzodiazepine receptor.[23] A decline in circulating levels of progesterone will lead to a decrease in 3α-OH-5α-pregnan-20-one (3α,5α-THP) production. This reduction in the level of 3α,5α-THP enhances transcription of the α4 subunit of the GABA-A receptor. The increased production of GABA-A receptors may then lead to increased anxiety and seizure susceptibility.[22]

The GABA system can also be modulated by modification of the neurosteroids. Pregnenolone is a potent positive allosteric modulator of the GABA-A receptor, whereas pregnenolone sulphate is a potent negative modulator.[24] Allopregnanolone and tetrahydrodeoxycorticosterone enhance GABA-mediated chloride currents, whereas pregnenolone sulphate and dehydroepiandrosterone sulphate (DHEA-S) are GABA-A receptor antagonists.[22] Regulation of steroid sulphation may therefore have important behavioural and morphological effects on the CNS.[24] Neurosteroids can attenuate exaggerated responsiveness to glucocorticoid feedback, and they can alter the transcription of the corticotrophin-releasing hormone (CRH) gene in the hypothalamus and the glucocorticoid receptor (GR) in the hippocampus.[25] Neurosteroids, corticosteroids and gonadal steroids have also been shown to contribute to the modulation of GABA-A receptor binding in the brains of male and female mice.[26]

Recent studies indicate that dysfunction in the GABA-A/neurosteroid system may play a significant role in the aetiology of mood disorders. Romeo et al have found that patients experiencing a major depressive episode have low levels of $3\alpha,5\alpha$-THP and $3\alpha,5\beta$-THP, which are positive allosteric modulators of GABA-A, as well as a concomitant increase in $3\beta,5\alpha$-THP. Treatment with antidepressants corrects this dysequilibrium of neuroactive steroids.[27] Symptoms of PMS, anxiety and seizure susceptibility may be associated with sharp declines in progesterone and consequently decreased levels of $3\alpha,5\alpha$-THP.[22,28] PMS symptoms may also be due, in part, to alterations in GABA-A receptor subunit expression, as a result of progesterone withdrawal.[22] Dysregulated sensitivity of GABA-A receptor has also been suggested in patients with PMS[29] (see also Chapter 12).

The serotonergic (5-HT) system

Serotonergic dysfunction has been implicated in the aetiology of many psychiatric disorders, including depression, anxiety, somatization and eating disorders.[30] Serotonergic dysfunction has also been implicated in PMDD, PPD and perimenopausal mood disorders.[31] The exact role that 5-HT plays in these disorders is unclear; however, it is likely that there is a generalized decrease in activity of the serotonergic system, which increases vulnerability to depression. This decreased activity may result from any or all of the following: decreased synthesis of 5-HT; increased turnover; or decreased sensitivity of 5-HT receptors. There are huge methodological difficulties in assessing properly the serotonergic activity in different brain regions of humans, but some studies suggest tentatively that major depression is associated with an increased number of postsynaptic 5-HT_2 receptors, decreased or desensitized postsynaptic 5-HT_{1A} receptors and decreased or desensitized presynaptic 5-HT transporter (5-HTT).[32]

Gonadal and adrenal steroid hormones are involved in regulating the expression of 5-HT receptors. Oestrogen administered alone or in combination with progesterone reduces 5-HTT mRNA in female ovariectomized rhesus macaque monkeys.[33] However, oestrogen stimulates an increase in density of 5-HT_{2A} in the anterior frontal, cingulate and primary olfactory cortex and also in the nucleus accumbens in rats.[3] Long-term treatment with imipramine causes a decrease in concentration of 5-HT_2 receptors in rat brain frontal cortex, which appears to be dependent on the presence of testosterone. Castration abolishes this decline, whereas the addition of testosterone reverses the effect.[34] Conversely, castration in male rats decreases 5-HT_{1A} receptor density.[35] These results suggest that testosterone may influence depressed mood as well as the effect of antidepressant treatment by interacting with brain 5-HT neurotransmission (see also Chapter 14).

It is evident that the gonadal hormones affect the production of 5-HT receptors at the transcriptional level. The altered distribution or function of 5-HT receptor subtypes brought on by changes in the hormonal milieu, such as at puberty, menopause or during the menstrual cycle, may increase vulnerability to mood disorders.

Adrenal steroids also affect 5-HT receptors. Expression of 5-HT_{1A} and 5-HT_7 mRNA is increased in the hippocampus of adrenalectomized animals, whereas hippocampal 5-HT_{1C} and D1 dopamine receptors are not altered.[36] This effect is negated by administration of corticosterone at the time of adrenalectomy, suggesting a negative regulatory effect of corticosterone on the production of mRNA coding for certain 5-HT receptors.[21] Consistently elevated adrenocortical activity along the hypothalamic–pituitary–adrenal (HPA) axis has been found in many patients with major depression[37,38] (see also Chapter 8). Chronically elevated cortisol or repeated stressful life events may produce genomic events that alter the number and distribution of 5-HT receptor subtypes, leading to dysfunction or altered sensitivity in the 5-HT system.[39]

The dopamine system

Dopamine has been shown to influence reproductive behaviour through D5 dopamine receptor-mediated modulation of the progesterone receptor in rat CNS.[40] The oestrogen receptor can similarly be activated by dopamine[41] with dopamine agonists.[42] Dopamine can also regulate the biological effect of oestradiol in the anterior pituitary by decreasing its binding to the oestrogen receptor.[43] Dopamine can activate progesterone receptor in a ligand-independent manner[44] and can cause the translocation of the progesterone receptor from the cytoplasm to the nucleus.[45]

The dopamine system is, in turn, modulated by gonadal steroids. These steroids display short-term non-genomic effects, as well as long-term genomic effects on the dopaminergic processes.[46] The responsiveness of tubero-infundibular dopaminergic (TIDA) neurons has been shown to be regulated by gonadal steroids,[47] and oestrogen stimulates a significant increase in D2 dopamine receptors in the striatum.[3] Steroids can also modulate receptor expression by pre- and post-translational modifications. There are two forms of rat D2 dopamine receptors generated by alternate splicing of the pre-messenger RNA. The long isoform of the receptor is found primarily in the pituitary and striatum, and the short form in the hypothalamus and substantia nigra. Changes in circulating sex hormones affect the splicing without changing the total amount of receptor mRNA. Castration of male rats increases the ratio of long to short isoforms. Testosterone and 17β-oestradiol reverse this effect.[48]

The effect of circulating sex steroids on dopamine receptor expression and modification may be implicated in the gender differences observed in schizophrenia and Parkinson's disease. Women tend to have a later age of onset of schizophrenia (2–10 years), more severe positive symptoms and less severe negative symptoms than men,[49] whereas neurotoxic agents such as methamphetamine induce greater neurotoxicity in male rats than in female rats.[50] Evidence suggests that oestrogen is protective against the onset of schizophrenia and that oestrogen interacts with the dopamine system in a manner similar to neuroleptics.[49] Evidence that oestrogen may have neuroprotective effects lies in the fact that the incidence of Parkinson's disease is greater in men than in women (3 : 2) and that Alzheimer's disease progresses more slowly in women receiving hormone replacement therapy (HRT) (see also Chapter 22).

The adrenergic system

Noradrenergic regulation of oestrogen receptor levels has been demonstrated in the hypothalamus of female guinea pigs.[51] Oestradiol and progesterone also seem to modulate hypothalamic noradrenaline release in the ventromedial hypothalamus (VMH);[52] however, the effect of steroid hormones on the regulation of adrenergic receptors is not clear. Changes in plasma concentrations of gonadal steroids during the oestrus cycle seem to influence the density of β-adrenergic receptors in the cerebral cortex, hypothalamus and anterior pituitary involved in the control and release of anterior pituitary gonadotrophins.[53] Similarly, an increase in oestradiol and progesterone in females during the luteal phase is accompanied by an increase in the number of lymphocyte $β_2$-adrenoceptors,[54] and exogenous progesterone given to healthy females in the follicular phase also increases the number of lymphocyte $β_2$-adrenoceptors.[55]

In contrast, Wilkinson et al have shown that the affinity, but not maximum binding, of hypothalamic β-adrenergic binding sites is reduced in rats treated with oestrogen for 3 months.[56] Similarly, oestradiol and progesterone given to healthy males did not have any significant effect on lymphocyte $β_2$-adrenoceptors.[57]

The effect of oestrogen on central $α_2$-adrenergic receptors is not clear. Oestrogen was shown to have no effect on $α_2$-adrenergic receptors in guinea pigs[51] and on the expression of mRNA for noradrenaline transporter in non-human primates.[58] However, $α_2$-adrenergic receptor density in male rabbit urethral smooth muscle is increased with oestrogen administration.[59]

The inconsistent effect of steroids on the expression of adrenergic receptors may be due to methodological differences or may relate to the presence or absence of steroid receptors on the particular cell type being studied. The effect of oestrogen on $β_2$-adrenoceptors may, however, play an important role in PMDD. Gurguis et al have shown that follicular $β_2$-adrenergic receptor density is higher in patients with PMDD than in controls and that receptor binding measures correlated with luteal symptom severity.[60] Lack of cyclical control of $β_2$-adrenoceptor regulation or abnormal coupling of the receptors to the second-messenger system require further investigation to help define their contribution to PMDD.

The cholinergic system

Gibbs has hypothesized that the increased risk for Alzheimer's-related dementia in postmenopausal women is due, in part, to the loss of ovarian function and to the effects that decreased levels of ovarian hormones have on basal forebrain cholinergic function.[61] Decreased levels of choline acetyltransferase (ChAT) were found in the medial septum (MS) and nucleus basalis magnocellularis (NBM) of female rats following ovariectomy relative to age-matched, gonadally intact controls. Short-term oestrogen replacement, initiated 6 months following ovariectomy and administered for 3 days prior to sacrifice, partially restored ChAT mRNA levels. This suggests that long-term loss of ovarian function produces a decrease in the functional status of basal forebrain cholinergic neurons projecting to the hippocampus and cortex.[61]

The non-steroidal anti-oestrogen, tamoxifen, has been shown to inhibit cationic currents of adult-type human muscle nicotinic ACh receptors expressed in *Xenopus* oocytes.[62] Progesterone has been shown to inhibit the neuronal nicotinic ACh receptor,[63] and the steroid, promegestone, is a non-competitive antagonist of the *Torpedo* nicotinic ACh receptor.[64] The direct effects of gonadal hormones on the expression of the nicotinic ACh receptor are unclear at this time.

The opiate system

Endogenous opioid peptides control the release of luteinizing hormone (LH) by inhibiting the activity of hypothalamic neurons that release gonadotrophin-releasing hormone (GnRH). Administration of naloxone to fertile females increases LH levels in the luteal phase but not in the follicular phase. In postmenopausal females, naloxone has no effect on LH release, but HRT increases LH response.[65] Clearly, the release of LH is modulated by the sex steroid hormonal milieu.

The density of μ-opioid receptors in the medial preoptic area (MPOA) of the rat hypothalamus is cyclical and sexually dimorphic. MPOA μ-opioid receptor density increases and decreases in parallel with the oestrus cycle,[66] with a dense concentration of μ-opioid receptors located in MPOA during oestrus and dioestrus in female rats but not in pro-oestrus or in male rats.[67] Similarly, μ- and δ-opioid receptor density changes are observed in the hypothalamus of normal cycling ewes; however, no differences in κ-type receptors were observed across the cycle.[68] It has similarly been shown that administration of gonadal steroid hormones to rats upregulates μ-opioid receptors in the hypothalamus[56] and the MPOA.[69] Oestrogen and stress also increase levels of κ-opioid receptor mRNA in the paraventricular nucleus (PVN) of the hypothalamus of castrated male rats.[70]

Oestrogens (diethylstilboestrol, 17-α-oestradiol, 17-α-ethinyloestradiol, oestriol, oestrone and 17-β-oestradiol) have been shown to interact with rat brain δ, μ and κ opioid receptors.[71] 17-α-Oestradiol has antagonist/agonist activity, whereas 17-α-dihydroequilin and 17-α-dihydroequilenin are pure antagonists.[72] These steroids can influence intrinsic excitability and sensitivity to neurotransmitters in opiodergic neurons,[73] suggesting that oestrogens may also produce non-genomic effects at target neuronal cell membranes.[71]

These observations suggest that oestrogens can directly affect the number and function of opioid receptors and may directly stimulate these receptors. It has also been shown that cyclical administration of oestrogen–progestin to menopausal women significantly increases serum levels of β-endorphin.[74] The observed beneficial effects of HRT on behaviour and mood may therefore also relate to changes in circulating opioid levels.

The vasopressin system

Fink et al have demonstrated that oestrogen stimulates expression of arginine vasopressin (AVP) in the bed nucleus of the stria terminalis,[3] indeed castration of golden hamsters results in decreased vasopressin receptor binding in the ventrolateral hypothalamus.[75] Symptomatic women with PMS have lower AVP levels throughout the menstrual cycle than asymptomatic or normal women.[76] These observations suggest that oestrogen and testosterone may modulate the expression of AVP and vasopressin receptors in the hypothalamus, which results in the expression of certain symptoms or behaviours. Again, these studies illustrate that sex steroids can interact with multiple systems, producing either an increased vulnerability or a psychoprotectant effect.

Conclusions

The complex integration of the neurotransmitter and steroid hormone systems implies that

Table 5.1 Effect of steroid hormones on some of the major neurotransmitter systems.

	5-HTT	5-HT$_2$	5-HT$_{1a}$	β-Adrenergic	D2	GABA-A	Opioid	NMDA	AVP
Oestrogen	↓	↑		↑	↑		↑	↑	
Progesterone				↑		↓			
Testosterone		↓	↑						↑
Cortisol		↓					↑		

circulating steroid hormones from peripheral endocrine glands can directly regulate brain function and modulate behaviour. Regulation occurs, for example, through direct interaction with or upregulation of specific receptors on neuronal cells. Thus, the hormonal milieu surrounding a neuronal cell will, in part, determine the response of that cell to various stimuli.

Adrenal and gonadal steroids regulate the transcription of serotonin, dopamine, adrenaline, GABA, glutamate, AVP and sigma receptors at the genomic level. These effects are summarized in Table 5.1.

Steroid hormones also have direct effects on neuronal cell function by non-genomic mechanisms, influencing the sensitivity and responsiveness of the neurons.

Levels of oestrogen and progesterone vary significantly across the female lifespan. At puberty, there is an increase in oestrogen and initiation of cyclic and diurnal variation in oestrogen production. The sudden appearance of higher levels of oestrogen in puberty alters the sensitivity of the neurotransmitter systems. Behaviours such as moodiness, irritability and conflicts with parents around this time may, in part, reflect this increased sensitivity (see Chapter 15). The constant flux of oestrogen and progesterone levels continues throughout the reproductive years. The neurotransmitter systems are thus constantly being attenuated or amplified. PMS and PMDD may be the result of an altered activity

(or sensitivity) of certain neurotransmitter systems (e.g. 5-HT) (see Chapter 16). Pregnancy and delivery produce dramatic changes in oestrogen and progesterone levels, possibly increasing vulnerability to depression (see Chapters 17 and 18). Finally, at menopause, oestrogen levels decline while pituitary LH and follicle-stimulating hormone (FSH) levels increase. The loss of the modulating effects of oestrogen and progesterone may underlie the development of perimenopausal mood disorders in vulnerable women (see Chapter 22).

Since these hormonal changes occur in all women, it seems safe to speculate that the development of mood disorders requires more than just fluctuating levels of hormones, but also a genetic predisposition. These genetic as yet unidentified 'defects' probably relate to subtle alterations in number and function of various receptors and enzymes and to subtle structural and anatomical differences in the CNS. These subtle differences caused by genetic polymorphism, combined with the flux in the hormonal milieu, determine how the system reacts to multiple environmental stresses and predicts the development of mood disorders. Further research into this complex system is needed to be able to identify specific 'genetic markers', which might help us better understand how the balance between oestrogen, progesterone, testosterone and other steroid hormones affects neurotransmitter function.

References

1. Weissman MM, Olfson M, Depression in women: implications for health care research, *Science* 1995; **269**:799–801.
2. Steiner M, Female-specific mood disorders, *Clin Obstet Gynecol* 1992; **35**:599–611.
3. Fink G, Sumner BE, Rosie R et al, Estrogen control of central neurotransmission: effect on mood, mental state, and memory, *Cell Mol Neurobiol* 1996; **16**:325–44.
4. Sumner BE, Fink G, The density of 5-hydroxy-tryptamine$_{2A}$ receptors in forebrain is increased at pro-oestrus in intact female rats, *Neurosci Lett* 1997; **234**:7–10.
5. Stomati M, Genazzani AD, Petraglia F, Genazzani AR, Contraception as prevention and therapy: sex steroids and the brain, *Eur J Contracept Reprod Health Care* 1998; **3**:21–8.
6. McEwen BS, Genomic regulation of sexual behavior, *J Steroid Biochem* 1988; **30**:179–83.
7. Herbison AE, Horvath TL, Naftolin F, Leranth C, Distribution of estrogen receptor-immunoreactive cells in monkey hypothalamus: relationship to neurones containing luteinizing hormone-releasing hormone and tyrosine hydroxylase, *Neuroendocrinology* 1995; **61**:1–10.
8. Lauber AH, Whalen RE, Muscarinic cholinergic modulation of hypothalamic estrogen binding sites, *Brain Res* 1988; **443**:21–6.
9. Lauber AH, Bethanechol-induced increase in hypothalamic estrogen receptor binding in female rats is related to capacity for estrogen-dependent reproductive behavior, *Brain Res* 1988; **456**:177–82.
10. Culig Z, Hobisch A, Cronauer MV et al, Activation of the androgen receptor by polypeptide growth factors and cellular regulators, *World J Urol* 1995; **13**:285–9.
11. Mani SK, Blaustein JD, O'Malley BW, Progesterone receptor function from a behavioral perspective, *Horm Behav* 1997; **31**:244–55.
12. Wong M, Thompson TL, Moss RL, Nongenomic actions of estrogen in the brain: physiological significance and cellular mechanisms, *Crit Rev Neurobiol* 1996; **10**:189–203.
13. Moss RL, Gu Q, Wong M, Estrogen: nontranscriptional signaling pathway, *Recent Prog Horm Res* 1997; **52**:33–68; discussion 68–9.
14. Brann DW, Hendry LB, Mahesh VB, Emerging diversities in the mechanism of action of steroid hormones, *J Steroid Biochem Mol Biol* 1995; **52**:113–33.
15. Maggi A, Perez J, Role of female gonadal hormones in the CNS: clinical and experimental aspects, *Life Sci* 1985; **37**:893–906.
16. Baulieu EE, Neurosteroids: of the nervous system, by the nervous system, for the nervous system, *Recent Prog Horm Res* 1997; **52**:1–32.
17. Pouliot WA, Handa RJ, Beck SG, Androgen modulates N-methyl-D-aspartate-mediated depolarization in CA1 hippocampal pyramidal cells, *Synapse* 1996; **23**:10–19.
18. Weiland NG, Estradiol selectively regulates agonist binding sites on the N-methyl-D-aspartate receptor complex in the CA1 region of the hippocampus, *Endocrinology* 1992; **131**:662–8.
19. Weaver CE Jr, Park Chung M, Gibbs TT, Farb DH, 17beta-Estradiol protects against NMDA-induced excitotoxicity by direct inhibition of NMDA receptors, *Brain Res* 1997; **761**:338–41.
20. Rupprecht R, Hauser CA, Trapp T, Holsboer F, Neurosteroids: molecular mechanisms of action and psychopharmacological significance, *J Steroid Biochem Mol Biol* 1996; **56**:163–8.
21. Rupprecht R, The neuropsychopharmacological potential of neuroactive steroids, *J Psychiatr Res* 1997; **31**:297–314.
22. Smith SS, Gong QH, Hsu FC et al, GABA(A) receptor alpha4 subunit suppression prevents withdrawal properties of an endogenous steroid, *Nature* 1998; **392**:926–30.
23. Bitran D, Dowd JA, Ovarian steroids modify the behavioral and neurochemical responses of the central benzodiazepine receptor, *Psychopharmacology (Berl)* 1996; **125**:65–73.
24. Compagnone NA, Salido E, Shapiro LJ, Mellon SH. Expression of steroid sulfatase during embryogenesis, *Endocrinology* 1997; **138**:4768–73.
25. Patchev VK, Montkowski A, Rouskova D et al, Neonatal treatment of rats with the neuroactive steroid tetrahydrodeoxycorticosterone (THDOC) abolishes the behavioral and neuroendocrine consequences of adverse early life events, *J Clin Invest* 1997; **99**:962–6.

26. Akinci MK, Johnston GA, Sex differences in the effects of gonadectomy and acute swim stress on GABA-A receptor binding in mouse forebrain membranes, *Neurochem Int* 1997; **31**:1–10.

27. Romeo E, Ströhle A, Spalletta G et al, Effects of antidepressant treatment on neuroactive steroids in major depression, *Am J Psychiatry* 1998; **155**:910–3.

28. Rapkin AJ, Morgan M, Goldman L et al, Progesterone metabolite allopregnanolone in women with premenstrual syndrome, *Obstet Gynecol* 1997; **90**:709–14.

29. Sundström I, Ashbrook D, Bäckström T, Reduced benzodiazepine sensitivity in patients with premenstrual syndrome: a pilot study, *Psychoneuroendocrinology* 1997; **22**:25–38.

30. Eriksson E, Humble M, Serotonin in psychiatric pathophysiology. In: Pohl R, Gershon S, eds, *The Biological Basis of Psychiatric Treatment* (Karger: Basel, 1990) 66–119.

31. Steiner M, Dunn EJ, The psychobiology of female-specific mood disorders, *Infertil Reprod Med Clin North Am* 1996; **7**:297–313.

32. Maes M, Meltzer HY, The serotonin hypothesis of major depression. In: Bloom FE, Kupfer DJ, eds, *Psychopharmacology: the Fourth Generation of Progress* (Raven Press: New York, 1994) 933–44.

33. Pecins Thompson M, Brown NA, Bethea CL, Regulation of serotonin re-uptake transporter mRNA expression by ovarian steroids in rhesus macaques, *Brain Res Mol Brain Res* 1998; **53**:120–9.

34. Kendall DA, Stancel GM, Enna SJ, The influence of sex hormones on antidepressant-induced alterations in neurotransmitter receptor binding, *J Neurosci* 1982; **2**:354–60.

35. Frankfurt M, McKittrick CR, Mendelson SD, McEwen BS, Effect of 5,7-dihydroxytryptamine, ovariectomy and gonadal steroids on serotonin receptor binding in rat brain, *Neuroendocrinology* 1994; **59**:245–50.

36. Chalmers DT, Kwak SP, Mansour A et al, Corticosteroids regulate brain hippocampal 5-HT$_{1A}$ receptor mRNA expression, *J Neurosci* 1993; **13**:914–23.

37. Sapolsky RM, Plotsky PM, Hypercortisolism and its possible neural bases, *Biol Psychiatry* 1990; **27**:937–52.

38. Carroll BJ, Feinberg M, Greden JF et al, A specific laboratory test for the diagnosis of melancholia. Standardization, validation, and clinical utility, *Arch Gen Psychiatry* 1981; **38**:15–22.

39. Mann JJ, Malone KM, Diehl DJ et al, Demonstration in vivo of reduced serotonin responsivity in the brain of untreated depressed patients, *Am J Psychiatry* 1996; **153**:174–82.

40. Apostolakis EM, Garai J, Fox C et al, Dopaminergic regulation of progesterone receptors: brain D5 dopamine receptors mediate induction of lordosis by D1-like agonists in rats, *J Neurosci* 1996; **16**:4823–34.

41. Smith CL, Conneely OM, O'Malley BW, Modulation of the ligand-independent activation of the human estrogen receptor by hormone and antihormone, *Proc Natl Acad Sci USA* 1993; **90**:6120–4.

42. Gangolli EA, Conneely OM, O'Malley BW, Neurotransmitters activate the human estrogen receptor in a neuroblastoma cell line, *J Steroid Biochem Mol Biol* 1997; **61**:1–9.

43. Szijan I, Burdman JA, Alonso GE, Effect of dopamine agonists and antagonists on the binding of [3H]estradiol to its receptors in the anterior pituitary gland of male rats, *Endocrinology* 1985; **117**:1742–8.

44. Mani SK, Allen JM, Clark JH et al, Convergent pathways for steroid hormone- and neurotransmitter-induced rat sexual behavior, *Science* 1994; **265**:1246–9.

45. Power RF, Mani SK, Codina J et al, Dopaminergic and ligand-independent activation of steroid hormone receptors, *Science* 1991; **254**:1636–9.

46. Di Paolo T, Modulation of brain dopamine transmission by sex steroids, *Rev Neurosci* 1994; **5**:27–41.

47. Manzanares J, Wagner EJ, LaVigne SD et al, Sexual differences in kappa opioid receptor-mediated regulation of tuberoinfundibular dopaminergic neurons, *Neuroendocrinology* 1992; **55**:301–7.

48. Guivarch D, Vernier P, Vincent JD, Sex steroid hormones change the differential distribution of the isoforms of the D2 dopamine receptor messenger RNA in the rat brain, *Neuroscience* 1995; **69**:159–66.

49. Lindamer LA, Lohr JB, Harris MJ, Jeste DV, Gender, estrogen, and schizophrenia,

Psychopharmacol Bull 1997; **33**:221–8.

50. Miller DB, Ali SF, O'Callaghan JP, Laws SC, The impact of gender and estrogen on striatal dopaminergic neurotoxicity, *Ann NY Acad Sci* 1998; **844**:153–65.

51. Tetel MJ, Blaustein JD, Immunocytochemical evidence for noradrenergic regulation of estrogen receptor concentrations in the guinea pig hypothalamus, *Brain Res* 1991; **565**:321–9.

52. Etgen AM, Karkanias GB, Estrogen regulation of noradrenergic signaling in the hypothalamus, *Psychoneuroendocrinology* 1994; **19**:603–10.

53. Petrovic SL, McDonald JK, De Castro JC et al, Regulation of anterior pituitary and brain beta-adrenergic receptors by ovarian steroids, *Life Sci* 1985; **37**:1563–70.

54. Wheeldon NM, Newnham DM, Coutie WJ et al, Influence of sex-steroid hormones on the regulation of lymphocyte beta 2-adrenoceptors during the menstrual cycle, *Br J Clin Pharmacol* 1994; **37**:583–8.

55. Tan KS, McFarlane LC, Coutie WJ, Lipworth BJ, Effects of exogenous female sex-steroid hormones on lymphocyte beta 2-adrenoceptors in normal females, *Br J Clin Pharmacol* 1996; **41**:414–6.

56. Wilkinson M, Bhanot R, Wilkinson DA, Brawer JR, Prolonged estrogen treatment induces changes in opiate, benzodiazepine and beta-adrenergic binding sites in female rat hypothalamus, *Brain Res Bull* 1983; **11**:279–81.

57. Tan KS, McFarlane LC, Lipworth BJ, Effect of exogenous female sex-steroid hormones on beta 2-adrenoceptors in healthy males, *Eur J Clin Pharmacol* 1997; **52**:281–3.

58. Schutzer WE, Bethea CL, Lack of ovarian steroid hormone regulation of norepinephrine transporter mRNA expression in the non-human primate locus coeruleus, *Psychoneuroendocrinology* 1997; **22**:325–36.

59. Morita T, Tsuchiya N, Tsujii T, Kondo S, Changes of the autonomic receptors following castration and estrogen administration in male rabbit urethral smooth muscle, *Tohoku J Exper Med* 1992; **166**:403–5.

60. Gurguis GN, Yonkers KA, Blakeley JE et al, Adrenergic receptors in premenstrual dysphoric disorder. II. Neutrophil beta2-adrenergic receptors: Gs protein coupling, phase of menstrual cycle and prediction of luteal phase symptom

severity, *Psychiatry Res* 1998; **79**:31–42.

61. Gibbs RB, Impairment of basal forebrain cholinergic neurons associated with aging and long-term loss of ovarian function, *Exper Neurol* 1998; **151**:289–302.

62. Allen MC, Newland C, Valverde MA, Hardy SP, Inhibition of ligand-gated cation-selective channels by tamoxifen, *Eur J Pharmacol* 1998; **354**:261–9.

63. Baulieu EE, Schumacher M, Neurosteroids, with special reference to the effect of progesterone on myelination in peripheral nerves, *Mult Scler* 1997; **3**:105–12.

64. Blanton MP, Xie Y, Dangott LJ, Cohen JB, The steroid promegestone is a noncompetitive antagonist of the Torpedo nicotinic acetylcholine receptor that interacts with the lipid–protein interface, *Mol Pharmacol* 1999; **55**:269–78.

65. Genazzani AR, Gastaldi M, Bidzinska B et al, The brain as a target organ of gonadal steroids, *Psychoneuroendocrinology* 1992; **17**:385–90.

66. Mateo AR, Hijazi M, Hammer RP Jr, Dynamic patterns of medial preoptic mu-opiate receptor regulation by gonadal steroid hormones, *Neuroendocrinology* 1992; **55**:51–8.

67. Hammer RP Jr, Mu-opiate receptor binding in the medial preoptic area is cyclical and sexually dimorphic, *Brain Res* 1990; **515**:187–92.

68. Thom B, Canny BJ, Cowley M et al, Changes in the binding characteristics of the mu, delta and kappa subtypes of the opioid receptor in the hypothalamus of the normal cyclic ewe and in the ovariectomised ewe following treatment with ovarian steroids, *J Endocrinol* 1996; **149**:509–18.

69. Zhou L, Hammer RP Jr, Gonadal steroid hormones upregulate medial preoptic mu-opioid receptors in the rat, *Eur J Pharmacol* 1995; **278**:271–4.

70. Yukhananov RY, Handa RJ, Alterations in kappa opioid receptor mRNA levels in the paraventricular nucleus of the hypothalamus by stress and sex steroids, *Neuroreport* 1996; **7**:1690–4.

71. Schwarz S, Pohl P, Steroids and opioid receptors, *J Steroid Biochem Mol Biol* 1994; **48**:391–402.

72. LaBella FS, Opiate receptor activity of 17-alpha-estradiol and related steroids, *Prog Clin*

Biol Res 1985; **192**:323–8.

73. Zakon HH, The effects of steroid hormones on electrical activity of excitable cells, *Trends Neurosci* 1998; **21**:202–7.

74. Ortega E, Cuadros JL, Gonzalez AR, Ruiz E, Effects of estrogen–progestin replacement therapy on plasma beta-endorphin levels in menopausal women, *Biochem Mol Biol Int* 1993; **29**:831–6.

75. Delville Y, Mansour KM, Ferris CF, Testosterone facilitates aggression by modulating vasopressin receptors in the hypothalamus, *Physiol Behav* 1996; **60**:25–9.

76. Rosenstein DL, Kalogeras KT, Kalafut M et al, Peripheral measures of arginine vasopressin, atrial natriuretic peptide and adrenocorticotropic hormone in premenstrual syndrome, *Psychoneuroendocrinology* 1996; **21**:347–59.

6

Grief and bereavement in women
Sidney Zisook, Yulia Chentsova-Dutton and Stephen R Shuchter

The death of a loved one is a disruptive, traumatic and tragic experience with profound consequences. Cross-culturally, people react to it with overwhelming sadness and longing, and each culture has recognized the distress of grief, and developed mourning rituals to assist people in dealing with their loss. Throughout the ages, the image of a woman in grief has served as a powerful symbol of the agony of loss. In the myth of Venus and Adonis, Venus hurries to her lover's side only to find him dead:

She alighted and bending over his lifeless body beat her breast and tore her hair. Reproaching the Fates, she said, 'Yet theirs shall be a partial triumph; memorials of my grief shall endure, and the spectacle of your death, my Adonis, and of my lamentation shall be annually renewed. Your blood shall change into a flower; that consolation none can envy me.[1]

This short quote embodies the pain of bereavement and the strength of surviving a tragic loss. Annual rituals to commemorate her loved one's death and turning his blood, the very symbol of his death, into something alive and beautiful helped the widowed Venus to withstand her grief.

This chapter will examine the bereavement of women, first by outlining the dimensions of distress among widows, then by discussing the gender differences and risk factors in bereavement, and finally by reviewing the course and outcome of bereavement adjustment and examining the treatment options.

Women experience losses and tragedies throughout their lives. Relatives and friends die, couples separate and divorce, and children leave the home, causing the painful 'empty nest' syndrome. There is the anguish of miscarriage and excruciating pain of seeing a child die. All of these experiences can trigger grief. The only life stressor that seems to be more harmful to a woman's psychological and physical health than the loss of a husband is the loss of a child. It disrupts family life, has detrimental effects on surviving children, and provokes an intense psychological reaction of guilt, depression and anxiety in the bereaved mother.

Leahy[2] compared the levels of depression in women following the loss of a child, a parent and a husband, and demonstrated that bereaved mothers were more depressed than widows, whereas both groups were far more depressed than bereaved adult daughters. In this chapter we will focus on the best studied form of bereavement—spousal bereavement.

Women tend to live longer than men, and the number of widows far outweighs the number of widowers. According to the *Statistical Abstract of the United States 1996*, the ratio of bereaved women to men is about 5 : 1. In 1995 there were 11.1 million widowed women in the USA alone. The risk of losing a husband is much higher for older women, and 47.3% of women in the USA who are 65 and over are widowed.[3]

The loss of a spouse has been defined as a prototypical severe life stressor.[4] It creates a powerful disruption in a woman's life. This tragic and traumatic event affects her health, mood, and social and spiritual life, deprives her of companionship and often depletes her financial resources and forces her to alter her established lifestyle. Often, it is losing one's best friend, lover, companion and source of support all in one. Given the enormity of such a loss, grief pervades all aspects of one's being. Thus, Shuchter and Zisook have formulated a multidimensional way of evaluating spousal bereavement.[5] Their model emphasizes the following six dimensions of grief: emotional and cognitive experiences, coping, the continuing relationship with the deceased, functioning, relationships and identity. We will illustrate our discussion of these dimensions by including quotes and data collected from 350 widows and widowers who participated in the longitudinal San Diego Widowhood Project. Subjects in this study were contacted and interviewed 2 months after the deaths of their spouses. Follow-up questionnaires were completed by participants at 7, 13, 19 and 25 months. A full description of the population is available elsewhere.[6]

Dimension 1: Emotional and cognitive experiences

The feelings inflicted by a loved one's death encompass shock and disbelief, numbness and a sense of loss, anguish and despair, fear and anxiety, as well as anger and depression. The emotional pain of loss is intense and unrelenting. Often coming in waves of anguish and longing, the so-called pangs of grief, the distress can be relatively constant initially, only later becoming episodic, resurfacing with reminders of the lost loved one. Loneliness truly becomes a daily reminder of one's grief, and the widow must face the trial of everyday life without the support and companionship of her deceased husband. In addition to seriously affecting a widow's mood, bereavement also diminishes her ability to concentrate and think clearly. Mental disorganization due to the trauma of loss often causes widows to complain of forgetfulness, inability to concentrate and distractibility. In the early weeks and months, the widow often feels in a fog, dissociated from the world around her, and perhaps even estranged from her own family. This anguish may be accompanied by deteriorating health and developing substance use problems. One of the participants of the San Diego Widowhood Project describes her life 2 months after her husband's death: 'My life had no meaning. I could not, nor could anyone, help to alleviate my depression, fear, anger, emptiness, hopelessness. Certainly not God ... I would have welcomed death ... My health was not good before I was widowed and rapidly grew worse over that time. I could not eat or sleep, but I could drink and work and drink some more.'

As illustrated by the data from the San Diego Widowhood Project presented in Table 6.1, the most prevalent emotional responses experienced by widows soon after the death of their spouses include difficulties in believing in the death or talking about the deceased spouse without crying, yearning for the spouse, being overwhelmed and feeling lonely. Some feelings tended to persist over the first 2 years of widowhood. For example, emotional responses such as difficulty in talking about her spouse without crying, fear of death and being overwhelmed did not substantially diminish over time. Other feelings, such as apathy, were more common at 2 months, but became less so after the initial months of bereavement.

Early in the bereavement, somatic symptoms such as loss of appetite, palpitations, chest pain, nausea, gastrointestinal problems, dizziness and others can cause considerable discomfort. About 44% of new widows complain of pronounced sleep disturbances.[7] Intrusive images of the spouse's death and recurrent vivid memories of him are common in widows. Unfortunately, all too often these psychological and somatic upheavals are not merely transient, time-limited phenomena, but, for many widows, may last for years, often indefinitely.[8,9] Stages of grief do not merely pass; there is an ebb and flow of emotion, with some feelings greatly diminishing over time, but others persisting as sources of pain and distress for years if not lifetimes. Grief does not end, but it does become more tolerable.

Full-blown major depressive disorders and anxiety disorders can be precipitated and/or worsened by the stress of bereavement. Several studies show that the onset or exacerbation of depressive and anxiety disorders are common and often long-lasting among both bereaved men and women.[10-15] Almost half (49.6%) of the widows in one study[2] suffered from moderate to severe depression.

Research shows that 19–58%[8,16,17] of widows are depressed at 1 month after bereavement as compared with 7% of married controls. Approximately 26% of widows are still depressed at 6 months after the loss.[18] After a year, about 17%[16] remain depressed, and this number is reduced to about 14% by 2 years.[17] While the number of depressed widows diminishes over time, as a group widows continue to be more depressed than married controls even at 2 years after their husbands' deaths.[9,18] For many widows, this depression tends to be persistent and debilitating. In fact, bereavement is established to be associated with depression to such an extent that bereavement is included in the DSM-IV as the only environmental stressor which can negate the diagnosis of major depression. Thus, a diagnostic code for 'bereavement' is provided in the DSM-IV to account for depressive symptoms experienced by those in grief. However, even when termed 'bereavement' rather than major depression, the syndrome can be associated with severe and debilitating symptoms such as overwhelming sadness, fatigue and difficulty in concentrating, feelings of hopelessness and helplessness, and inability to enjoy life.[19] Furthermore, the depressive episodes associated with bereavement are every bit as debilitating as any other form of depression. Compared with bereaved individuals who do not meet criteria for major depression, those widows with depression have more difficulties in adjusting to the loss, getting along with children, other relatives and friends, and in their workplace; they experience more problems with physical health, and are less likely to develop new relationships. They are more likely to remain depressed over much of the immediate future. In short, they have 'real' major depression.

Several cases of mania associated with bereavement have been reported.[20] However, no larger studies have examined the prevalence

Table 6.1 Emotional and cognitive responses to the death of a spouse and coping.

	% Endorsing each item		
	At 2 months	At 13 months	At 25 months
Emotional and cognititve responses			
Emotional pain of grief/loss			
I can't talk about him without crying	62	64	78
Yearning for spouse	75	59	45
Anger at self	11	7	5
Guilt	12	7	4
Anxiety and fearfulness			
Nervous when left alone	11	7	4
Fearful of death	10	11	8
Overwhelmed			
More demands than I can handle	37	34	32
Loneliness	56	41	29
Apathy	18	15	9
Coping			
Disbelief			
It's hard to believe	75	53	38
Emotional control			
Numbness	13	4	3
I push my feelings away	48	50	42
Rationalization			
Spouse's death was for the better	58	45	43
Faith			
Prayer has helped me with my feelings	74	71	70
Avoidance			
I avoid looking at pictures or belongings	19	15	15
Being busy/active distraction			
I've been so busy I haven't had time to grieve	26	29	26
Involvement with others			
I've become involved in trying to help others	53	61	65
Expression			
I talk with people a lot about my loss	58	37	29
I express my feelings whenever possible	71	65	65

of manic symptoms among bereaved individuals, and the lower prevalence of mania than depression in the general population would suggest that those with pre-existing bipolar disorder are at some risk for this development.

Bereaved women also commonly experience heightened anxiety and anxiety-spectrum problems such as somatic distress, interpersonal sensitivity, obsessions and compulsions, panic attacks and phobias, as well as post-traumatic stress disorder (PTSD)-like syndromes.[6] Bereavement-related anxiety is more prevalent and chronic than is often assumed. The loss of a husband triggers a psychological regression characterized by excessive worrying and feelings of insecurity and fear. The sense of security that was once reinforced by the presence of a spouse vanishes, creating an eruption of fears and worries about the widow's own safety. Tasks that were once routine can become frightening. Bereaved women report having fears of being alone, becoming more hesitant to go out by themselves, and developing anxiety-related symptoms, such as palpitations and dizziness, in the first 2 years following their husbands' deaths. Research has demonstrated that the prevalence rates of panic disorder, generalized anxiety disorder (GAD) and hypervigilance among bereaved men and women were higher than community prevalence rates, and one study found that over 40% of widows and widowers report at least one anxiety disorder.[21] We have found that widows are more likely to experience anxiety symptoms than widowers.[22] A study focusing on bereavement-related anxiety in widows has demonstrated that over 50% of bereaved women report increased worrying, panic and fear since bereavement.[23] Lindstrom[24] has found that the level of anxiety among widows 4–6 weeks after their husbands' deaths was comparable to that of medical, surgical and neuropsychiatric patients. Anxiety-related symptoms last through-

out the first year of bereavement, may not subside at the same rate as depression, and often become chronic.[21] Horowitz et al[25] have also described PTSD-like syndromes associated with bereavement. As a consequence of the intense and unrelenting anxiety, many widows turn to anti-anxiety medications. We found that the number of bereaved women taking anti-anxiety medications after their spouses' deaths is higher than before death, but does tail off after the first several months.[6]

Dimension 2: Coping

In an attempt to defend themselves against the onslaught of the symptoms described above, widows turn to a variety of coping mechanisms. These strategies include suppression of emotions with numbing and disbelief, avoidance of reminders, intellectualization and humour. While some may seek out reminders of the deceased, others avoid all possible reminders and may distract themselves in either passive (e.g. watching television) or active (e.g. charity work) ways. Many widows find solace in activity, be it work, remodelling the house or helping others in need. 'I find that caring about others is one of the greatest helps. So many need our love and friendship, and when you are busy with others and see their needs, there is no time to pity yourself,' testifies one widow months after her loss. Some widows turn to faith for consolation, while developing new friendships and new romantic relationships helps others. Some coping strategies are less adaptive than others. Unfortunately, some widows attempt to deal with their loss by overindulging in potentially self-destructive activities, such as promiscuity, uncontrollable overeating or substance abuse. Usually, such behaviours are exacerbations of old problems rather than newly developed disturbances.

As demonstrated in Table 6.1, widows in our

study made use of a variety of coping strategies 2 months after their losses. More than a half of all widows found it hard to believe the fact of their husband's death, rationalized that their spouse's death was for the better, turned to their faith, became involved in helping others and expressed their feelings as much as possible. It was less often that widows engaged in avoidance or used active distraction when faced with intense thoughts and/or feelings related to the loss. As would be expected, inability to accept the loss became less common as time went on. On the other hand, other coping strategies continued to be useful throughout the first 2 years of widowhood.

Dimension 3: The continuing relationship with the deceased

Perhaps the most powerful means of mitigating the pain of losing a loved one is to maintain strong ties with that person. While a harsh external reality demands acceptance of the loss, an equally compelling psychological reality implores that the relationship be maintained. This tug of war between accepting the fact of death and maintaining an attachment to the deceased goes on for years, if not lifetimes, in many widows. The relationship may be maintained in several ways, for example localizing the husband in a special place, such as heaven, the grave site or urn, or believing in the oneness of nature, introjecting certain traits, mannerisms, symptoms or illnesses and thereby keeping a piece of him with the bereaved wife, focusing on deeds, living legacies, and 'seeing him' in surviving children or grandchildren, sensing his presence, actual visions and hearing his voice, and finally experiencing memories and dreams. All of these are quite common in perfectly normal widows and other bereaved individuals, and may be comforting and sustaining.

Table 6.2 shows that an overwhelming majority of widows in our study found it comforting to know that their spouse was in heaven and were interested in carrying out his wishes throughout the first 2 years after the loss. A large proportion of widows (30–50%) maintained their relationship with their husbands by talking with them, keeping one of their belongings nearby, identifying with them and dreaming about them.

The physical absence of the spouse seems in contradiction to the continuing thoughts, emotions and behaviours related to the relationship. It is not unusual for a widow to live in anticipation that her husband will walk into the house or call her name. Hearing the voice of a spouse or his footsteps, or noticing his silhouette in a crowd, are also within the context of normal grieving. One of the widows in the San Diego Widowhood Project has shared her experiences: 'Recently my husband's presence has seemed very close. I actually received communications ... I really enjoy when these infrequent experiences occur. Usually they are about things we did and enjoyed together.' Many widows and widowers continue to maintain aspects of their relationships by talking to their late spouses, seeing them in their dreams and keeping their clothes, letters and photographs. 'The well-meaning ladies here said it would be better if I put away all photos of my spouse. I did for a week, but put them up again and they are still up and I feel real good about it, too,' writes another participant. Annual rituals, daily memories and visits to the grave often continue as the most enduring means of reconnecting to the past with a deceased spouse.

Dimension 4: Functioning

Loss of a spouse can impact on one's functioning by affecting finances, health, work performance and social functioning. Financially, widows are

Table 6.2 The continuing relationship with the dead spouse and changes in relationships.

	% Endorsing each item		
	At 2 months	At 13 months	At 25 months
Continuing relationship with dead spouse			
Location			
Comforted that spouse is in heaven	84	74	75
Continuing contact with the deceased			
Look for spouse in crowd	19	13	12
Feel spouse is with me at times	73	66	62
Talk with spouse regularly	41	34	25
Symbolic representation			
Keep one of his/her belongings near me	50	43	39
Living legacies			
I seem to be more like my spouse	40	44	38
I find myself doing things like my spouse	51	49	47
I'm interested in carrying out his/her wishes	78	66	58
Dreams			
I see my spouse in dreams	34	40	43
Old relationships			
Children			
Better (than before death)	55	49	46
Worse	4	7	5
Parents			
Better (than before death)	24	28	40
Worse	9	12	2
Friends			
Better (than before death)	40	42	39
Worse	1	5	3
New relationships			
Dating			
It's difficult to think about dating	77	60	53
I feel guilty about dating	29	27	21
Romantic relationships			
I'm fearful of getting romantic with another person	40	47	51
I'm only interested in developing friendships	85	71	70
I will be able to love someone else	42	54	56
I'm involved in a new romantic relationship	3	18	19
Remarriage			
I have positive thoughts about remarriage	24	40	46
Sexuality			
I have less than usual interest in sex	46	40	38
General			
New relationships have been hard to develop	46	62	58
My feelings are easily hurt	16	12	8

less equipped to survive the loss than widowers. Women, more than men, experience a dramatic decline in family income as a result of spousal bereavement. Not only are widows more likely to have economic problems than married women, but they also do not have partners to rely on for assistance in solving these problems. Older bereaved women living alone or with non-relatives are four times more likely to be living in poverty than are widowed men.[26] Many women take time off from their jobs to raise families and, as a consequence, have less work experience, and may find it particularly difficult to find jobs after their husbands' deaths. Compared with widowers, it is also harder for widows to find new relationships that can provide them with new sources of companionship, closeness and support.

The loss of a spouse disrupts a woman's life, forcing her to realign her roles and responsibilities. Adjustments that need to be made range from everyday tasks like balancing a cheque-book to more serious and overwhelming problems such as the task of raising a family with a diminished income. Incompetence in these novel areas can become long-lasting. A bereaved woman may require assistance during this critical time in her life in order to be able to adjust to life without a spouse.

As demonstrated by the data from the San Diego Widowhood Project presented in Table 6.3, psychological, social, occupational and physical functioning are all impacted by the loss of a husband. About a quarter of all widows meet criteria for major depressive syndrome at 2 months. Thirty-four per cent of widows report having fewer social activities outside of their homes since their husbands' deaths. Social functioning does not return to the pre-bereavement levels for one-third of the widows even after 2 years. Lack of satisfaction with work performance reflects difficulties in occupational functioning; a feeling of dissatis-

faction and the tendency to make mistakes at work do not diminish over time.

The detrimental effects of bereavement on health are reflected in widows' estimates of their health 2 months after the loss of a husband, as well as in their increased use of alcohol. Twenty-eight per cent report that their health is poor or fair at 2 months after death, decreasing to 22% at 2 years after death. This decrease is noticeable because the health of widows in this age range would be expected to worsen, whereas this group's estimate of their health actually improves as they recover from the trauma of bereavement. It is alarming that a large number of widows report increased frequency and quantity of alcohol consumption. Unfortunately, this tendency does not diminish with time. In fact, the elevated quantity of alcohol consumption increases from 7% at 2 months after the loss to 32% 2 years after the loss.

Research shows that conjugal bereavement puts a survivor at risk for general medical health problems.[26,27] The number of medical consultations following bereavement increases among widows of all ages.[28] This trend is even more pronounced among younger widows. Studies examining mortality rates among bereaved individuals demonstrate that death rates are higher for both widows and widowers than for married men and women.[29–33] Increased mortality rates may be more pronounced for bereaved men than they are for women.[34] However, widowed women are also at somewhat higher risk than their married counterparts.[35] For widows, the excessive risk is more significant when their husbands' deaths are preceded by chronic medical conditions.[36] Wives of patients with chronic medical illnesses often assume a role of a primary caregiver, so the added stress of caregiving may account for this trend. When death rates from suicide are examined, several studies show that widowers

Table 6.3 Changes in functioning and identity.

	% Endorsing each item		
	At 2 months	At 13 months	At 25 months
Functioning			
Overall psychological adjustment	36	28	21
Depression			
Downhearted, sad, blue	30	17	13
Feeling hopeless about future	15	10	8
Major depressive syndrome	24	18	15
Anxiety			
Spells of terror or panic	6	4	2
So restless I couldn't keep still	14	9	3
Social functioning			
Decreased number of social days/month	34	36	30
Occupational functioning			
Not satisfied with work performance	28	28	33
More mistakes than usual	11	13	8
Health			
Poor–fair physical health	28	25	22
Alcohol – increased frequency of consumption	16	24	29
Identity			
Self-perceptions			
Feel self-sufficient	76	74	81
Feel useful and needed	68	59	66
Self-esteem			
I feel good about myself	82	80	87
Unlovable	13	17	14
Surprise myself by new tasks I have mastered	61	71	77
Philosophy/worldview			
My life is pretty full	66	59	71
I try to get the most out of every day	88	87	90
Direction/purpose			
I don't know where my life is headed	61	65	61
I look forward to tomorrow	78	83	85
I enjoy the freedom of being on my own	39	56	16
I like making decisions just for me	53	64	66

have a greater suicide risk than married men. On the other hand, most studies have not found widows to differ in suicide rates from their married counterparts.[37,38]

Findings conflict regarding the time of highest risk of mortality for widows. Jones[39] and Mellstrom and Kaprio (as outlined in Stroebe and Stroebe[35]) have identified the first 6 months after bereavement as the time of highest risk of mortality; McNeill[30] and Cox and Ford (as outlined in Stroebe and Stroebe[35]) have found a morbidity peak for older widows during the second year after their husbands' deaths. It appears that mortality risk peaks immediately after the loss and continues to be excessive into the second year.

Dimension 5: Relationships

Relationships with family members and friends often change for a woman after her spouse passes away; some ties may become closer, while others may weaken. A death of a family member can repair strained relationships, but the turmoil of loss can also tear a family apart. A widow may have to alter a role she plays in the family and learn how to be a single woman again. Some widows seek social opportunities and confide in their friends to ease their loneliness. Others react to pain with withdrawal, like a widow in our study who commented: 'I have been going through a long spell where I don't want to go out anywhere, for any reason.'

Widows in our study reported (Table 6.2) that their relationships with relatives and friends became better after the loss. This support diminished somewhat over time but continued to be substantial. Widows' answers revealed feelings of insecurity and ambivalence about developing new romantic relationships, but a majority reported that they are interested in developing new friendships. The capacity to

form new romantic relationships is one of the measures of post-bereavement adjustment. Those widows who go on to develop new romantic relationships report experiencing fewer symptoms of depression and anxiety. Remarriage is associated with better adjustment to widowhood. Here is a testimonial from one of the participants of the San Diego Widowhood Project concerning the power of new romance: 'When I look back on my spouse's death, I feel total blackness, total hopelessness and total loneliness. Since I have remarried I am extremely happy, hopeful and fulfilled. I hope others may know that life can be wonderful again, that life can go on and that it is possible to feel well and complete again.'

Our study demonstrated that widowers remarry or form new romantic relationships more often than do widows.[40] Two months after their spouses' deaths, 12% of men become involved in a new romantic relationship, whereas only 3% of widows do so. This difference is just as pronounced 25 months after the spouses' deaths, when 61% of men and only 19% of women report a new romantic involvement. Women report having difficulty in thinking about a new romance and developing a new relationship, they feel more guilty about dating than do men, and are more fearful of getting romantic.

This contrast between widows and widowers in dating and remarriage after widowhood can be partially accounted for by demographic factors. Men tend to die younger than women, thus leaving fewer available men in the widows' age group. In addition, widowers may be socialized to pursue new relationships more aggressively than widows.

Dimension 6: Identity

Bereavement may lead to profound changes in a woman's identity. The feminist theorist Gilligan[41] argues that women, more than men, define their sense of self through their relationships with others. For a married woman, the relationship with her husband represents a core part of who she is. The loss of a husband disrupts this identity, forcing her to realign her likes and dislikes, roles and relationships, and to establish a life independent of her deceased spouse; this trauma can also affect a woman's sense of self in a positive way, allowing her to feel stronger and more in control of her life.

Table 6.3 shows that among widows in the San Diego Widowhood Project, sense of identity was very stable throughout the first 2 years of widowhood. As time went on, widows reported feeling slightly better about themselves. Independence brought some rewarding feelings. By the end of the second year after the loss, more widows reported being pleased by new tasks that they had mastered, looking forward to tomorrow and enjoying the opportunity to make their own decisions. While more than half of the widows reported enjoying the freedom of being on their own 1 year after the loss, this number decreased to 16% after the second year. Perhaps freedom had lost its novelty, and the price that came with it had become more apparent by the second year.

Widowhood can become a time for women to develop new skills and interests. One of the widows in the San Diego Widowhood Project has shared her joy of rediscovering her life after the initial shock of losing her husband: 'I am travelling a great deal, having driven across country several times alone. Hopefully, I'll be able to go to Europe in the fall . . . I truly enjoy being alone, and being my own boss. At times I miss my husband dreadfully, but I am doing things he wouldn't do. I am enjoying life: I look forward to each day.'

Risk factors

Given the complexity and variability of bereavement-associated difficulties, it is important to identify individuals at risk for poor adjustment. Multiple risk factors for poor psychological and physical adaptation following conjugal bereavement have been identified.[42,43] These risk factors include: characteristics of the person (demographics, early experiences, health history, depression history, resiliency etc.), characteristics of the relationship with the deceased (was it close or ambivalent?), the characteristics of death (was it sudden or expected?) and post-bereavement factors (availability of social support, use of coping mechanisms, financial security).

The person

Some of the demographic factors known to play a role in bereavement adaptation are gender, age and socio-economic status. Differences between patterns of adjustment to conjugal bereavement among men and women have been a focus of numerous studies. However, the role of gender in post-bereavement adjustment is not well understood. In interpreting the results of these studies it is important to keep in mind that females report more depressive symptoms, higher distress and more health complaints than do males in the general population.[44] Our data (Table 6.4) show gender differences on many individual items.

One set of studies suggests that females experience more distress than males after their spouses' deaths. Women report higher levels of depression[10,45–49] and more symptoms of psychopathology such as anxiety, phobic anxiety, somatization and obsessive-compulsive symptoms[10,22,48,50] than men. However, this pattern does not differ significantly from non-bereaved samples. Women report more distress than do

Table 6.4 Gender differences at 2, 13 and 25 months.

	Significant gender differences ($P < 0.01$)		
	At 2 months	At 13 months	At 25 months
Affects			
Fearful	F > M	F = M	F = M
Nervous when left alone	F > M	F = M	F = M
Helpless	F = M	F > M	F = M
Difficulty in making decisions	F > M	F > M	F = M
Coping			
It's hard to believe	F > M	F = M	F = M
Prayer has helped me with my feelings	F = M	F > M	F = M
I talk with people a lot about my loss	F > M	F = M	F = M
I express my feelings whenever possible	F > M	F > M	F > M
Crying spells	F > M	F > M	F > M
Continued relationships			
I seem to be more like my spouse	F = M	F > M	F = M
I've had physical symptoms like my spouse	F = M	F > M	F = M
Functioning			
I eat as much as usual	F > M	F = M	F = M
Trouble in falling asleep	F > M	F > M	F = M
Trouble in sleeping through the night	F = M	F > M	F = M
Tense or keyed up	F > M	F > M	F = M
Spells of terror or panic	F > M	F > M	F = M
Relationships			
I'm not sure how a single person acts these days	F = M	F > M	F > M
It's difficult to think about dating	F > M	F > M	F = M
I'm only interested in friendships	F > M	F > M	F > M
I will be able to love someone else	F < M	F < M	F < M
I'm involved in a new romantic relationship	F < M	F < M	F < M
My feelings are easily hurt	F < M	F = M	F = M
Feel inferior to others	F = M	F > M	F > M
Identity			
I continue to surprise myself by new tasks I have mastered	F > M	F > M	F > M
I don't know where my life is headed	F = M	F > M	F = M

F, females; M, males.

men regardless of bereavement status. We have found that widows tend to experience a greater degree of helplessness,[5] lower levels of self-efficacy[46] and more hopelessness than do men. Their ability to plan for the future and complete plans is also impaired as compared to widowers. Nolen-Hoeksema et al[45] provide data that allow us to account for this gender discrepancy. They demonstrate that bereaved women, as do women in general, utilize more ruminative coping strategies. After their spouses' deaths, women tend to passively ruminate on their feelings of sadness and loneliness, which may facilitate more severe and prolonged symptoms of distress.

On the other hand, another set of data asserts that males are at higher risk for poor adaptation after bereavement than are women. They have been found to experience more distress[51] and depression,[18] at least in the first several months after the loss. Bereaved men are at greater risk for mortality and suicide than are women.[31–33,37]

Other studies suggest that bereavement among women and men is more similar than it is different. No difference was found between the two genders on measures of physical and psychosocial health dysfunction,[52] depression, self-rated mental health, anxiety, somatization and general malaise.[11,17,50,53,54] While widows report higher levels of depression at the moderate levels, the two genders do not differ at severe levels of distress.[11] Finally, men and women do not differ greatly in their expressions of grief.[10,50] It has been hypothesized that expressions of grief are consistent with both male and female gender roles, whereas expressions of sadness and despair are traditionally associated with a female gender role.[10] Thus, widows and widowers may report different levels of depression, while grieving in a similar way.

In addition to gender, other demographic factors have been shown to play roles in the bereavement reaction. In particular, the age of a widow can help us to account for her adaptation to bereavement. Younger widows are more likely to develop prolonged and severe symptoms than are older widows. Widows under 65 are at higher mortality risk than those who are older, and that trend is even more pronounced for the youngest group of widows.[33] The mortality rate of widows under 35 is higher than the mortality rate of older widows.[29] Younger widows report more symptoms overall, higher anxiety and more restlessness than their older counterparts and experience a higher intensity of grief.[6,7,55] This trend can be explained if we take into account that losing one's spouse relatively early in life is an unanticipated trauma, and younger women are not prepared to assume the role of a widow.

A history of other stressors can contribute to the severity of the bereavement reaction in widows. A widow's adjustment to her loss may be related to her experiences with losses as a child. Bowlby[56] developed a theory of anxious attachment, stating that children who are frequently separated from their care-takers develop anxious attachment styles and often carry this vulnerability to loss into adulthood when they show more distress after experiencing a loss, especially when the loss is as fundamental as the loss of a spouse.[23] Stoll[57] provided empirical support for this hypothesis, demonstrating that a higher number of actual childhood separations and threats of childhood separations from primary caregivers was related to severity of depression and psychosomatic symptoms during bereavement.

Prior mental health is also a factor in post-bereavement adjustment. Widows with a history of psychological problems tended to have higher levels of psychosocial dysfunction[52] and depression.[58] In particular, past depression has been linked to post-bereavement depression, anxiety,[22] and even substance abuse.[59] Poor early adaptation can be predictive of long-term difficulties. Several groups have found that intense symptoms of distress early in bereavement are predictive of higher levels of depression and anxiety later on.[6,55,60,61] Linking early adjustment with other risk factors, Parkes and Weiss[60] describe a subgroup of widows whose early intense yearning for their husbands expressed not only a sense of continued connection to their husbands, but also a sense of inability to manage alone. These widows were dependent on their spouses during marriage and their grieving was unlikely to be resolved.

Relationship with the deceased

Pre-bereavement marital adjustment also plays a role in bereavement adaptation. Freud postulated that the loss of an ambivalently loved object (person) is the principal basis for melancholia. However, the recent literature has not always validated his theory. Indeed, in one study of both bereaved men and women, high ratings of marital adjustment were associated with higher levels of depression; relying on subjects' retrospective ratings in this study makes it difficult to interpret these results.[48] While it is possible that happily married individuals experience more distress after losing their spouse, it is also possible that depressed widows and widowers idealize their lost relationship with their spouse. Parkes and Weiss[60] also have found that widows and widowers whose marriages were conflict-laden, marked by ambivalence and anger, show less emotional stress early in bereavement compared to those whose marriages were happy. The follow-up interviews, however, revealed that a year after the loss most of the widows and widowers with marriages low in conflict returned to normal functioning, while those with high-conflict marriages were less likely to recover from their grief, experienc-

ing more problems with social, emotional and psychological functioning in the long run. They seemed ready to move on early after their loss, but found it hard to accept the loss later on, yearning for their spouses and feeling guilty and angry. While ambivalent feelings may interfere with normal grieving and take longer to resolve,[60] it is also possible that insecure attachments can complicate adjustment to the loss of a high-conflict relationship.

The death

Another factor related to bereavement outcome was death expectancy. Some investigators have found that widows who did not anticipate their husbands' deaths had more intense grief reactions[7] and higher levels of anxiety[6] than those who knew that their husbands were terminally ill. On the other hand, other studies show no relationship between death expectancy and subsequent adjustment.[62] As discussed earlier, one study reports that mortality rates are greater among widows whose husbands died after chronic illness.[36]

Post-bereavement factors

Deterioration in socio-economic status often follows the loss of a spouse and is especially dramatic for widows. Women are more likely to experience a decline in family income after their spouses' deaths than are men, and widows of lower socio-economic status are more likely to experience bereavement-associated depression[57] and anxiety[6] than are their wealthier counterparts. One study demonstrated that the absence of resources (material as well as psychological and social) is related to lower levels of physical and psychosocial function.[52]

Other recent losses[52] and stressful life changes[57,63] also emerge as risk factors for women following spousal bereavement. Widows who experienced additional simultaneous losses had more physical and psychosocial dysfunction and succumbed to the effects of multiple stressors. Along the same lines, women experiencing stressful changes in their lives after their husbands' deaths were more likely to report depressive and psychosomatic symptoms.

The quality and availability of social support is important for a widow's adjustment to bereavement. Widows with more friends, well-developed social networks and close relationships with their children reported requiring less help for emotional problems.[64] The level of interpersonal support is inversely related to the levels of depression. Employment history also plays a role. Widows who worked outside the home prior to bereavement (and thus developed a network of friends and colleagues) experienced less distress after their husbands' deaths.[58] Finally, post-bereavement physical and mental health are strongly associated with outcome. While bereavement can affect health, it also is true that health affects one's ability to cope with widowhood. We have found that a widow's or widower's medical health at the time of the loss is one of the most powerful predictors of depression 2 years after the loss.[9]

Course and outcome of bereavement

Stages of grief

Bereavement is a complex phenomenon, and people experience it in a variety of ways. There is no single course that a widow ought to take on her way to adaptation. Research attests that the bereaved population shows a high degree of individual variability in their courses of adjustment to loss.[65,66] A number of individual characteristics, including the risk factors outlined

above as well as cultural and gender differences, may account for these differences. Variability in adjusting to loss exists not only between different individuals, but also among the different spheres of functioning within single individuals. Thus, the 'stage' theories of grief should be viewed as flexible guidelines rather than prerequisites for 'normal' adjustment. The stages may overlap rather than follow one another in a linear fashion. Some symptoms subside over time, whereas other complaints persist for years and may never fully disappear. Therefore, attempting to outline a typical or 'normal' course of bereavement is a very complex task.

Numerous stage theories, outlining the 'typical progression' through the ordeal of bereavement, have been proposed.[12,67-69] According to most of these models, a bereaved woman passes from an initial period of shock, denial, numbness and confusion into a period of acute grief and mourning, when the widow experiences intense feelings of despair and anger, and withdraws socially. During this phase, she is overwhelmed by yearning and preoccupied with thoughts of her deceased husband. These disruptive initial stages of acute separation distress are followed by months of mourning, characterized by episodes of depressed mood and anxiety, pangs of nostalgia and loneliness, and insomnia and loss of interest in things that were once enjoyable. A bereaved woman progresses towards recovery by gradually adjusting to widowhood, reconstructing her identity and returning to normal functioning. Grief becomes submerged and less troubling with time, but it never fully resolves, as particular symptoms may continue to re-emerge years later.

The duration of grief

There is little agreement about the duration of symptoms of distress associated with bereavement. Some symptoms are most intense immediately after the loss and diminish in intensity over the first year of bereavement. However, even though the intensity of distress may lessen within months, widows do not return to normal functioning for a much longer period of time. We have found that affective and symptomatic distress following the loss significantly lessen but do not disappear within months in most widows and widowers.[70] Several studies show that, while improving significantly in the first 6 months, mental health and levels of depression of the bereaved do not return to the level of the non-bereaved population until after a year or two.[8,50,71] The greatest improvement occurs in the first 6 months, with a slight increase in the second and third years.[50]

A more chronic distress is not uncommon. For some individuals, depression and anxiety persist and become long-lasting. 'I did believe that time heals all things. I don't anymore. Two years have gone by since the death of my husband, and I feel I miss him more,' writes one widow. Even at the end of the fourth year, 13% of widows and widowers in our study continued to experience significant depressive symptoms and 8% continued to feel angry.[70]

While some symptoms of distress diminish over the first year of bereavement, others appear to be more pervasive and long-lasting. Certain indications of depression in widows, such as feelings of hopelessness, worthlessness and thoughts of suicide, tend to continue throughout the first year.[72] The intensity of grief can decline slightly or remain stable during the course of the first $3\frac{1}{2}$ years after loss.[50,71] Anxiety among widows typically persists over the first 3 years.[23] Bereaved men and women report more health problems than their non-bereaved counterparts; this discrepancy does not disappear over the period of $3\frac{1}{2}$ years after loss.[71] Impairment in some areas of functioning following the loss of a spouse may be more chronic than in others, and some aspects of grieving may never end for otherwise well-adjusted bereaved individuals.

Complications in the course of grief

Complicated grief reactions such as atypical,[33] morbid,[73] pathological,[74,75] neurotic[76] or unresolved grief,[77] have been described. These syndromes refer to either absent, delayed, intensified or prolonged reaction to loss. Inhibited grief is characterized by the absence of a grief reaction and it is more common in young children and in elderly individuals.[78] Initial absence of grief followed by a typical or chronic reaction is often referred to as delayed grief. As we have discussed earlier, delayed grief is more likely to occur when the relationship between the bereaved and the deceased spouse was conflicted or ambivalent. Defining overly intense grief poses a challenge, because it is hard to judge how much intensity is too much. When pangs of longing and preoccupation with the deceased become so intense that they interfere with functioning, and when they do not lessen after the first few months, it is possible that the bereavement is complicated by a disorder such as major depression, anxiety disorder or post-traumatic stress disorder. Chronic grief is more intense and lasts longer than would be expected; it is marked not so much by the number of days, weeks or months it lasts, but rather by the extent to which unrelenting preoccupation with the deceased interferes with the drive to move forward. The most common pattern of 'atypical' grief is by far the chronic one.

Treatment options

Most widows grieve without turning to professional help. However, treatment options have been developed for those widows who do turn to counsellors or support groups for help. A variety of treatment interventions are aimed at supporting widows, providing them with an empathic environment, identifying those at risk and treating depression and anxiety. Grief counselling and self-help sessions led by professional counsellors or trained volunteers incorporate elements of supportive psychotherapy, attachment theory, dynamic perspectives and behavioural and cognitive approaches, to name a few. The goal of these preventive interventions and grief counselling programmes is to provide supportive environments for those recently bereaved and to facilitate the healthy passage from mourning to normal life. A number of programmes, such as the one developed at Boston State Hospital,[79] that facilitate one-on-one and group widow-to-widow contact have been developed in the past few decades. These programmes offer the widowed a crisis telephone line, home visits, social gatherings, and seminars on bereavement. Group and individual psychotherapy also represent excellent secondary preventive strategies. Therapeutic approaches aimed at helping widows to adjust to their losses include dynamic, interpersonal and cognitive-behavioural psychotherapies, as well as approaches such as 'guided mourning'[80] and re-grief work.[81] Typically, immediately after their loss, widows receive social support from their friends and family. Research shows that the typical widow is not ready to seek help outside her social network for the first few weeks after her husband's death (as outlined in Zisook et al[82]). However, as time goes on, the bereaved woman may find herself alienated, as it is often difficult for others to relate to her grief. A widow may isolate herself and avoid her acquaintances, for fear that interaction with them would bring up her pain and loneliness. One-on-one support from other widows or professional counsellors, support groups or a form of group therapy may prove beneficial for the bereaved, especially for those who are at risk for poor adaptation or do not have a close-knit social network.

These therapeutic measures offer education and acceptance of emotional reactions to the loss, focusing on alleviating separation distress and symptoms of depression and anxiety, and facilitating social adjustment. In most cases, therapeutic interventions are short term at the time of highest distress. They provide widows dealing with a complex process of grief with structures and therapeutic goals. Drawing from his work with widows and widowers, Shuchter proposes the following tasks to be addressed in bereavement therapy: learning to experience, express and integrate painful feelings; finding the most adaptive means of modulating painful feelings; integrating the continuing relationship with the dead spouse; maintaining health and continued functioning; adapting successfully to altered relationships; and developing an integrated, healthy self-concept and a stable worldview.[83] Along the same lines, Worden[84] outlines four essential therapeutic tasks: accepting the reality of the loss, working through the pain of separation, adjusting to an environment in which the deceased is missing, and emotionally relocating the deceased and moving on with one's life.

Bereaved individuals often experience grief counselling, therapy and self-help interventions as beneficial.[79,85] Despite these positive evaluations from widows and widowers, research shows no consistent findings regarding the effectiveness of various treatment formats. A set of studies comparing the effectiveness of crisis intervention support groups with controls shows no difference in reduction of grief, medical and psychiatric illnesses, or disturbed social functioning in treated bereaved individuals compared to controls.[85-87] Yet other studies do demonstrate the effectiveness of active treatments, including the usage of psychotropic medications, in the reduction of anxiety and depressive symptoms.[88-90] It has also been suggested that bereaved individuals who participate in widow-to-widow support programmes follow the same course of adaptation as those receiving no treatment, but reach the milestones of adaptation more quickly.[91]

Comparison of different treatment approaches yields few definitive differences between various forms of bereavement counselling. While some findings suggest that individual psychotherapy and support groups are about equally effective,[92] other studies[90] show that self-help groups are more effective than psychotherapy and vice versa. When the effectiveness of different treatments is evaluated for females, it appears that widows may benefit from a problem-focused approach more than from an emotion-focused treatment.[93] It has been suggested that females traditionally utilize emotion-focused rather than problem-focused coping, so problem-focused treatment aids widows in extending their coping faculties.

Special concerns arise for widows whose grief is complicated by the exacerbation or emergence of major depressive episodes. For most widows, acute grief following bereavement will gradually subside. Despite the severe stress of separation, they will be able to survive the loss, find new identity, realign their ties to the deceased spouse, assume new roles and take care of their daily needs while planning for the future. Their grief will not vanish completely, re-emerging on anniversaries, during holidays or when something reminds them of the deceased spouse. Despite these reminders of their loss, for most widows the time will come when their daily lives will no longer be characterized by a sense of longing, despair and anxiety. Their passage from mourning to normalcy will be unobstructed. However, bereavement makes some widows vulnerable to serious and long-lasting disorders. This concern is especially valid for those who fall into groups of highest risk, i.e. widows with a past personal or family history of mental illness. For those individuals, bereavement may instigate or exacerbate a major depressive disorder. Unfortunately, it is easy for a widow, her friends, relatives and healthcare providers to dismiss her symptoms as normal grief, not recognizing her passage from acute grief to a serious and deleterious illness. Thus, only about one-quarter of the bereaved with major depressive disorder receive any treatment for their symptoms.[94] Clinicians tend to dismiss depressive symptoms in bereaved patients, often assuming that such distress is normal. It is extremely important to recognize major depression and anxiety disorders behind the veil of mourning and provide active intervention as soon as possible. According to DSM-IV, the diagnosis of major depression should be made if the criteria for major depression are met 2 months after the loss. However, even if the symptoms are present within the first 2 months, a diagnosis of major depression should be considered if the symptoms began before the death, are particularly intense, do not subside with time, or appear to be independent of reminders of the deceased, or if a widow reports suicidal ideation. Depression associated with bereavement manifests itself with the same symptoms as any other depression and should be treated with the same clinical methods.

Unfortunately, evidence demonstrating the efficacy of therapeutic approaches to the treatment of bereavement-associated depression is limited to pilot studies and case reports. These show that treatment with antidepressants such as nortriptyline and desipramine is effective in alleviating symptoms of depression and insomnia as well as improving the general level of functioning.[95,96] These studies lack random assignment to treatment conditions and control subjects, so it is clear that further exploration of medication treatment in bereavement-associated depression is warranted.

Some literature also suggests that cognitive-behavioural therapy and interpersonal psychotherapy are useful for treatment of depressive symptoms associated with bereavement in widows.[97,98] Zisook et al have developed a treatment approach combining medication and a form of therapy emphasizing education and support.[82]

An ideal intervention for bereaved women would focus on assisting them in recognizing and expressing their feelings triggered by the loss, integrating their relationship with the deceased spouse into their lives, maintaining their health and functioning, and developing a new sense of identity. This intervention approach would be mindful of the religious and cultural background of the widows and would integrate their worldviews into the treatment. The treatment would be available to widows early in the course of their bereavement, with possible ongoing contact and/or availability, such as during anniversaries, at other life transitions, or when new stresses cause old trauma to resurface. Both short-term and long-term options would be available, providing continuous treatment for those in persistent distress. Finally, an ideal intervention would encompass various approaches to treat bereavement as a multidimensional syndrome. It would integrate therapeutic approaches such as psychodynamic, cognitive, behavioural, supportive and educational psychotherapies with medication.

Summary

Spousal bereavement is associated with tremendous distress and requires adjustments in many areas of a woman's life. It is associated with considerable psychological and medical morbidity. Bereavement is a process so complex that it can be fully understood only from a multidimensional perspective. A widow's thoughts and feelings, level of health and functioning, social environment and sense of self undergo powerful disruptions. Grief is a painful and disruptive process, but it can lead a widow to discover new resources and abilities within herself.

References

1. Bulfinch T, *Bulfinch's Mythology: The Greek and Roman Fables Illustrated* (Viking Press: New York, 1979).

2. Leahy JM, A comparison of depression in women bereaved of a spouse, child, or a parent, *Omega* 1992; **26**:207–17.

3. US Bureau of the Census, *Statistical Abstract of the United States 1996* (US Department of Commerce, Economics and Statistics Administration: Washington, DC, 1996).

4. Holmes TH, Rahe RH, The social readjustment rating scale, *J Psychosom Res* 1967; **11**:213–18.

5. Shuchter SR, Zisook S, The course of normal grief. In: Stroebe MS, Stroebe W, Hansson RO, eds, *Handbook of Bereavement* (Cambridge University Press: Cambridge, 1993) 175–95.

6. Zisook S, Mulvihill M, Shuchter SR, Widowhood and anxiety, *Psychiatr Med* 1990; **8**:99–116.

7. Ball JF, Widow's grief: the impact of age and mode of death, *Omega* 1977; **7**:307–33.

8. Harlow SD, Goldberg EL, Comstock GW, A longitudinal study of the prevalence of depressive symptomatology in elderly widowed and married women, *Arch Gen Psychiatry* 1991; **48**:1065–8.

9. Zisook S, Shuchter SR, Major depression associated with widowhood, *Am J Geriatr Psychiatry* 1993; **1**:316–26.

10. Thompson LW, Gallagher-Thompson D, Futterman A et al, The effects of late-life spousal bereavement over a 30-month interval, *Psychol Aging* 1991; **6**:434–41.

11. Feinson MC, Aging widows and widowers: are there mental health differences? *Int J Aging Human Dev* 1986; **23**:241–55.

12. Rubin SS, The resolution of bereavement: a clinical focus on the relationship to the deceased, *Psychotherapy* 1985; **22**:231–5.

13. Clayton PJ, Bereavement and depression, *J Clin Psychiatry* 1990; **51**:34–8.

14. Broadhead WE, Blazer DG, George LK et al, Depression, disability days, and days lost from work in a prospective epidemiologic survey, *JAMA* 1990; **264**:2524–8.

15. Breckenridge JN, Gallagher D, Thompson LW, Peterson J, Characteristic depressive symptoms of bereaved elders. *J Gerontol* 1986; **41**:163–8.

16. Bornstein PE, Clayton PJ, Halikas JA et al, The depression of widowhood after thirteen months, *Br J Psychiatry* 1973; **122**:561–6.

17. Lund DA, Caserta MS, Dimond MF, Gender differences through two years of bereavement among the elderly, *Gerontologist* 1986; **26**:314–20.

18. Richards JG, McCallum J, Bereavement in the elderly, *NZ Med J* 1979; **89**:201–4.

19. Zisook S, Shuchter SR, Depression through the first year after the death of a spouse, *Am J Psychiatry* 1991; **148**:1346–52.

20. Rickarby GA, Four cases of mania associated with bereavement, *J Nerv Ment Dis* 1977; **165**:255–62.

21. Jacobs S, Hansen F, Kasl S et al, Anxiety disorders during acute bereavement: risk and risk factors, *J Clin Psychol* 1990; **51**:269–74.

22. Zisook S, Shuchter SR, Lyons LE, Predictors of psychological reactions during the early stages of widowhood, *Psychiatr Clin North Am* 1987; **10**:355–68.

23. Sable P, Attachment, anxiety, and loss of a husband, *Am J Orthopsychiatry* 1989; **59**:550–6.

24. Lindstrom TC, Anxiety and adaptation in bereavement, *Anxiety Stress Coping* 1995; **8**:251–61.

25. Horowitz MJ, Stinson CH, Fridhandler B et al, Pathological grief: an intensive case study, *Psychiatry: Interpersonal Biol Process* 1993; **56**:356–74.

26. Arens DA, Widowhood and well-being: an examination of sex differences within a causal model, *Int J Aging Hum Dev* 1982; **15**:27–40.

27. Maddison D, Walker WL, Factors affecting the outcome of conjugal bereavement, *Br J Psychiatry* 1967; **113**:1057–67.

28. Parkes CM, The effects of bereavement on physical and mental health: a study of the case-records of widows, *Br Med J* 1964; **2**:274–9.

29. Kraus AS, Lilienfield AM, Some epidemiologic aspects of the high mortality rate in the young widowed group, *J Chronic Dis* 1959; **10**:207–17.

30. McNeill DN, Mortality among the widowed in Connecticut. Unpublished MPH essay (Yale University, 1973).

31. Jacobs S, Ostfeld A, An epidemiologic review of the mortality of bereavement, *Psychosom Med* 1977; **39**:344–57.

32. Stillon JM, Perspectives on the sex differential in death, *Death Educ* 1984; **8**:237–56.

33. Parkes CM, Brown RJ, Health after bereavement. A controlled study of young Boston widows and widowers, *Psychosom Med* 1972; **34**:449–61.

34. Stroebe W, Stroebe MS, *Bereavement and Health. The Psychological and Physical Consequences of Partner Loss* (Cambridge University Press: Cambridge, 1987).

35. Stroebe W, Stroebe MS, The mortality of bereavement: a review. In: Stroebe MS, Stroebe W, Hansson RO, eds, *Handbook of Bereavement* (Cambridge University Press: Cambridge, 1993) 175–95.

36. Smith KR, Zick CD, Risk of mortality following widowhood: age and sex differences by mode of death. *Soc Biol* 1996; **43**:59–71.

37. Li G, The interaction effect of bereavement and sex on the risk of suicide in the elderly: an historical cohort study, *Soc Sci Med* 1995; **40**:825–8.
38. Gove WR, The relationship between sex roles, marital roles and mental illness, *Soc Forces* 1972; **51**:33–44.
39. Jones DR, Heart disease mortality following widowhood: some results from the OPCS longitudinal study, *J Psychosom Res* 1987; **31**:325–33.
40. Schneider DS, Sledge PA, Shuchter SR, Zisook S, Dating and remarriage over the first two years of widowhood, *Ann Clin Psychiatry* 1996; **8**:51–7.
41. Gilligan C, *In a Different Voice* (Harvard University Press: Cambridge, 1982).
42. Sanders CM, Risk factors in bereavement outcome, *J Soc Issues* 1988; **44**:97–112.
43. Stroebe W, Stroebe MS, Determinants of adjustments to bereavement in younger widows and widowers. In: Stroebe MS, Stroebe W, Hansson RO, eds, *Handbook of Bereavement* (Cambridge University Press: Cambridge, 1993) 208–26.
44. Nolen-Hoeksema S, Sex differences in unipolar depression: evidence and theory, *Psychol Bull* 1987; **101**:259–82.
45. Nolen-Hoeksema S, Parker LE, Larson J, Ruminative coping with depressed mood following loss, *J Pers Soc Psychol* 1994; **67**:92–104.
46. Arbuckle NW, deVries B, The long-term effects of later life spousal and parental bereavement on personal functioning, *Gerontologist* 1995; **35**:637–47.
47. Bruce ML, Kim K, Leaf PJ et al, Depressive episodes and dysphoria resulting from conjugal bereavement in a prospective community sample, *Am J Psychiatry* 1990; **147**:608–11.
48. Futterman A, Gallagher D, Thompson LW et al, Retrospective assessment of marital adjustment and depression during the first two years of spousal bereavement, *Psychol Aging* 1990; **5**:277–83.
49. Jacobs S, Hansen F, Berkman L et al, Depression of bereavement, *Comp Psychiatry* 1989; **30**:218–24.
50. Farberow NL, Gallagher-Thompson D, Gilewski M, Thompson L, Changes in grief and mental health of bereaved spouses of older suicides, *J Gerontol* 1992; **47**:P357–66.
51. Stroebe MS, Stroebe W, Who suffers more? Sex differences in health risks of the widowed, *Psychol Bull* 1983; **93**:279–301.
52. Gass KA, Aged widows and widowers: similarities and differences in appraisal, coping, resources, type of death, and health dysfunction, *Arch Psychiatr Nurs* 1988; **2**:200–10.
53. McHorney CA, Mor V, Predictors of bereavement depression and its health services consequences, *Med Care* 1988; **26**:882–93.
54. Clayton PJ, Halikas JA, Maurice WL, The depression of widowhood, *Br J Psychiatry* 1972; **120**:71–7.
55. Zisook S, Shuchter SR, Sledge P, Bereavement, grief and anxiety, *Womens Psychiatr Health* 1992; **1**:3–5.
56. Bowlby J, *Attachment and Loss*, Vol. II, *Separation* (Hogarth: London, 1973).
57. Stoll M, Predictors of middle aged widows; psychological adjustment. In: Pottharst K, ed., *Research Explorations in Adult Attachment, American University Studies. Series 8: Psychology*, Vol. 14 (P. Lang Publishing: New York, 1990) 219–55.
58. Nuss WS, Zubenko GS, Correlates of persistent depressive symptoms in widows, *Am J Psychiatry* 1992; **149**:346–51.
59. Zisook S, Shuchter SR, Mulvihill M, Alcohol, cigarette, and medication use during the first year of widowhood, *Psychiatr Ann* 1990; **20**:318–26.
60. Parkes CM, Weiss RC, *Recovery From Bereavement* (Basic Books: New York, 1983).
61. Clayton PJ, Bereavement. In: Paykel ES, ed., *Handbook of Affective Disorders* (Churchill Livingstone: London, 1982) 403–15.
62. Hill CD, Thompson LW, Gallagher D, The role of anticipatory bereavement in older women's adjustment to widowhood, *Gerontologist* 1988; **28**:792–6.
63. Parkes CM, Determinants of outcome following bereavement, *Omega* 1975; **6**:303–23.
64. Goldberg EL, Comstock GW, Harlow SD, Emotional problems and widowhood, *J Gerontol* 1988; **43**:S206–8.
65. Zisook S, Shuchter SR, Sledge PA et al, The spectrum of depressive phenomena after spousal bereavement, *J Clin Psychiatry* 1994; **55**:29–36.

66. Levy LH, Martinkowski KS, Derby JF, Differences in patterns of adaptation in conjugal bereavement: their sources and potential significance, *Omega* 1994; **29**:71–87.

67. Schaie KW, Willis SL, *Adult Development and Aging*, 2nd edn (Little, Brown: Boston, 1986).

68. Jacobs S, *Pathologic Grief: Maladaptation to Loss* (APA Press: Washington DC, 1993).

69. Silverman PR, *Helping Each Other in Widowhood* (Health Sciences: New York, 1974).

70. Zisook S, Shuchter SR, The first four years of widowhood. *Psychiatr Ann* 1986; **6**:288–94.

71. Van Zandt S, Mou R, Abbott D, Mental and physical health of rural bereaved and non-bereaved elders: a longitudinal study. In: Lund DA, ed., *Older Bereaved Spouses* (Hemisphere Publishing Corporation: New York, 1989) 25–35.

72. Blanchard CG, Blanchard EB, Becker JV, The young widow: depressive symptomatology throughout the grief process, *Psychiatry* 1976; **39**:394–9.

73. Lindemenn E, Symptomatology and management of acute grief, *Am J Psychiatry* 1944; **101**:141–8.

74. Raphael B, The management of pathological grief, *Aust NZ J Psychiatry* 1975; **9**:173–80.

75. Volkan VD, The recognition and prevention of pathological grief, *Va Med Mon* 1972; **99**:535–40.

76. Wahl CW, The differential diagnosis of normal and neurotic grief following bereavement, *Psychosomatics* 1970; **11**:104–6.

77. Zisook S, DeVaul R, Unresolved grief, *Am J Psychoanal* 1985; **45**:370–9.

78. Parkes CM, Bereavement and mental illness, *Br J Med Psychol* 1965; **38**:13–26.

79. McCourt WF, Barnett RD, Brennen J, Becker A, We help each other: primary prevention for the widowed, *Am J Psychiatry* 1976; **133**:98–100.

80. Mawson D, Marks IM, Ramm L et al, Guided mourning for morbid grief: a controlled study, *Br J Psychiatry* 1981; **138**:185–93.

81. Volkan VD, Re-grief therapy. In: Schoenberg B, Gerber I, eds, *Bereavement: Its Psychological Aspects* (Columbia University Press: New York, 1975) 334–50.

82. Zisook S, Peterkin JJ, Shuchter SR, Bardone A, Death, dying, and bereavement. In: Nicassio PM, Smith TW, eds, *Managing Chronic Illness: A Biopsychosocial Perspective* (APA: Washington DC, 1995) 351–90.

83. Shuchter SR, *Dimensions of Grief* (Jossey-Bass Publishers: San Francisco, 1986).

84. Worden JW, *Grief Counseling and Grief Therapy*, 2nd edn (Springer: New York, 1991).

85. Sabatini L, Evaluating a treatment program for newly widowed people, *Omega* 1988; **19**:229–36.

86. Polak PR, Egan D, Vandenbergh R et al, Prevention in mental health: a controlled study, *Am J Psychiatry* 1975; **132**:146–9.

87. Videka-Sherman L, Lieberman M, The effects of self-help and psychotherapy intervention on child loss: the limits of recovery, *Am J Orthopsychiatry* 1985; **55**:70–82.

88. Constantino RE, Comparison of two group interventions for the bereaved, *Image J Nurse Sch* 1988; **20**:83–7.

89. Parkes CM, Evaluation of a bereavement service, *J Bereavement Service* 1981; **1**:179–88.

90. Lieberman MA, Videka-Sherman L, The impact of self-help groups on the mental health of widows and widowers, *Am J Orthopsychiatry* 1986; **56**:435–49.

91. Marmar CR, Horowitz MJ, Weiss DS et al, A controlled trial of brief psychotherapy and mutual-help group treatment of conjugal bereavement, *Am J Psychiatry* 1988; **145**:203–9.

92. Raphael B, Preventive intervention with the recently bereaved, *Arch Gen Psychiatry* 1977; **34**:1450–4.

93. Schut HA, Stroebe MS, van den Bout J et al, Intervention for the bereaved: gender differences in the efficacy of two counselling programmes, *Br J Clin Psychol* 1997; **36**:63–72.

94. Zisook S, Shuchter SR, Psychotherapy of the depressions in spousal bereavement, *In Session: Psychother Pract* 1996; **2**:31–45.

95. Jacobs SC, Nelson JC, Zisook S, Treating depressions of bereavement with antidepressants. A pilot study, *Psychiatr Clin North Am* 1987; **10**:501–10.

96. Pasternak RE, Reynolds CE, Schlernitzauer M et al, Acute open-trial nortriptyline therapy of bereavement-related depression in late life, *J Clin Psychiatry* 1991; **52**:307–10.

97. Miller MD, Frank E, Cornes C et al, Applying

interpersonal psychotherapy to bereavement-related depression following loss of a spouse in late life, *J Psychother Pract Res* 1994; **3**:149–62.

98. Florsheim MJ, Gallagher-Thompson D, Cognitive-behavioral treatment of atypical bereavement: a case study, *Clin Gerontologist* 1990; **10**:73–6.

7

Gender differences in dysthymia

Uriel Halbreich, Kimberly A Yonkers and Linda S Kahn

Introduction

Gender differences in the prevalence and treatment response are reported to exist in most affective disorders, especially major depressive disorder (MDD). The higher frequency of MDD in women has been amply documented.[1-4] Women also experience higher rates of 'atypical' depression, anxious depression,[5,6] and seasonal affective disorder (SAD).[7] Although women appear to be more prone to various affective disorders, there are other types, particularly bipolar disorder, which appear with equal frequency among men and women.[8] Only rapid cycling bipolar disorder is more prevalent among women.

Male–female differences in the nature and occurrence of affective disorders can be and probably are related to the combination of multiple processes attributed to several biological and social factors. The biological factors include genetic vulnerability, the effect of hormonal changes on neurotransmitter systems, and some biological variables putatively involved in the pathophysiology of depression.[9,10] Hormonal changes have been linked to a higher incidence of dysphoric states during key periods in women's life cycles, including puberty,[11,12] perimenstrual period,[13,14] postpartum[15] and surgically induced menopause.[16]

Psychological and socio-cultural factors also contribute to the higher reported incidence of chronic affective disorders among women. Women often balance several roles: worker, wife, mother, daughter. The combined pressures of making a living and confronting a second set of duties and responsibilities in the home can result in stress and affective disorders.[17] Women are also more inclined to seek treatment for affective disorders and depression. Certain types of stressors, including stressful events surrounding parenting and the home, are risk factors for depression in women.[18] Other risk factors include: less than a high school education,[19,20] being unemployed, particularly if educational attainment is low,[19,20] and young children at home.[21] As will be demonstrated in this chapter, in the context of other acute and chronic depressions, dysthymic disorder is no exception.

Dysthymic disorder: symptoms and diagnosis

Dysthymic disorder is a chronic depressive illness which affects 3–6% of the US adult population.[22,23] It is estimated that as many as 36% of patients who seek treatment at psychiatric outpatient clinics suffer from dysthymic disorder.[24] It is usually characterized by an insidious, often early onset and is distinct from unresolved or partially remitted major depression.[25,26] By definition, dysthymic disorder must not be the result of the continuance of a major depressive episode.

Because the symptoms of dysthymic disorder are less severe than those observed in patients with major depression, dysthymic disorder is often considered to be a dysphoric state of subsyndromal intensity.[27] Nevertheless, patients with this disorder experience considerable social dysfunction and disability,[28,29] including an increased likelihood of not completing high school or college.[30] Dysthymia patients are also more likely than the general population to use general health services, and they are more likely to take non-specific psychotropic drugs, such as minor tranquillizers and sedatives.[22]

Patients with dysthymic disorder are also at risk for comorbid illnesses: more than 75% of patients with dysthymic disorder have coexisting psychiatric disorders, including anxiety disorders and substance abuse.[22] Approximately 40% of patients with dysthymic disorder have coexisting major depression—a combination termed *double depression*.[22] Untreated dysthymic disorder rarely improves spontaneously over time,[31] and chronicity is one of the defining characteristics of the disorder.[22]

Dysthymic disorder has historically been underrecognized and undertreated.[32–34] One study of psychiatric outpatients who met the DSM-III criteria for dysthymic disorder found that a clinical diagnosis of dysthymic disorder had been considered in less than half of the patients who actually had it, and only 41% had received treatment with an adequate trial of antidepressant medication.[24]

Dysthymic disorder differs from MDD in severity and duration (Table 7.1). The DSM-IV criteria specify that a patient may be diagnosed with dysthymic disorder if they experience a depressed mood for most of the day, for more days than not, or for at least 2 years, and have two of the following symptoms during the depressed state: poor appetite or overeating, insomnia or hypersomnia, low energy or fatigue, low self-esteem, poor concentration or difficulty in making decisions, feelings of hopelessness.

The NIMH Task Force Report on Dysthymia[35] questioned the DSM-IV's inclusion of neurovegetative symptoms as criteria for diagnosing dysthymic disorder. Their criticism was based in part on the 1995 DSM-IV field trial results, which reported few patients presenting with these symptoms (i.e. changes in sleep or appetite). Among other recommendations, the Task Force agreed upon six essential core symptoms to be used in the diagnosis of dysthymia, and upheld the DSM-IV duration criteria (Table 7.2).

To accurately diagnose dysthymic disorder, other conditions and symptoms must be excluded. These include: manic, mixed or hypomanic episodes, chronic psychotic disorder (i.e. schizophrenia), reaction to a drug or medication, or general medical conditions.

Although MDD and dysthymic disorder share certain characteristics, in patients with MDD the depressive symptoms are usually more severe and sometimes cause a more marked change in the patient's functioning.[36]

Table 7.1 Comparison of DSM-IV diagnostic criteria of dysthymic disorder with those of chronic MDD, and double depression.

Dysthymic disorder	MDD	Double depression

Duration
  2 years
  Most of the day
  Most days
	2 years
	Continuously
	Most days
	Most of the day
		Continuously dysthymic
		
		MDD superimposed for at least 2 weeks

Specifiers
  Depression
  No MDD during first 2 years
  No mania or hypomania
  No cyclothymic disorder
	Depression	Depression
		
		No mania or hypomania
		No cyclothymic disorder

Two or more of:
  1. Poor appetite or overeating
  2. Insomnia or hypersomnia
  3. Low energy or fatigue
  4. Low self-esteem
  5. Poor concentration or difficulty in making decisions
  6. Feelings of hopelessness
	Four or more of:
	  1. Depressed mood most of the day, nearly every day
	  2. Markedly diminished interest or pleasure in almost all activities
	  3. Significant weight loss or weight gain
	  4. Insomnia or hypersomnia
	  5. Psychomotor agitation or retardation
	  6. Fatigue or low energy
	  7. Feelings of worthlessness or excessive or inappropriate guilt
	  8. Diminished ability to think or concentrate, or indecisiveness
	  9. Recurrent thoughts of death, recurrent suicidal ideation	

Table 7.2 Comparison of DSM-IV and NIMH core diagnostic criteria of dysthymic disorder.[35,36]

DSM-IV	NIMH Task Force
Two or more of:	Three or more of:
Poor appetite or overeating	Low self-esteem
Insomnia or hypersomnia	Pessimism, hopelessness
Low energy or fatigue	Social withdrawal
Low self-esteem	Irritability, excessive anger
Poor concentration or difficulty in making decisions	Concentration, thinking problems
Feelings of hopelessness	Low energy, low initiative

General treatment

Various studies have demonstrated the efficacy of antidepressants for the treatment of patients with dysthymic disorder.[37,38] In the first of these, Kocsis et al[39] studied 76 patients with DSM-III-defined dysthymic disorder in a 6-week, double-blind, placebo-controlled trial that compared imipramine and placebo. A favourable response was seen in 59% of the imipramine-treated patients and 13% of the placebo-treated patients. Nardi et al[40] compared the efficacy of imipramine and moclobemide in patients with either 'pure dysthymia' or double depression and reported that 54% of the moclobemide-treated patients and 49% of those who received imipramine no longer met the criteria for dysthymic disorder at the end of therapy, in contrast to 24% of the patients who received placebo.

The selective serotonin reuptake inhibitor (SSRI) fluoxetine has been found to be effective for the treatment of dysthymic disorder in several studies (review Yonkers et al[38]). For instance, Hellerstein et al compared fluoxetine and placebo in an 8-week trial that included 35 patients who met DSM-III-R criteria for dysthymic disorder.[41] A significantly higher percentage of the patients who received fluoxetine (62%) than those who received placebo (19%) responded.

Few studies have examined the efficacy of combining SRRIs and psychotherapy for treating dysthymia. Ravindran et al[42] compared the effectiveness of sertraline, placebo and group cognitive behavioural therapy alone and in combination. They found sertraline to be most effective in treating the clinical symptoms, while cognitive therapy alleviated functional impairments associated with dysthymia. Steiner et al[43] undertook a 2-year randomized clinical trial comparing the effects and expense of sertraline versus interpersonal psychotherapy (IPT) alone and in combination for treatment of dysthymia. They found sertraline alone and sertraline plus IPT were superior to IPT alone.

Data suggest that there may be differences in medication response among men and women with either MDD or dysthymic disorder. A meta-analysis of all imipramine treatment trials of MDD found that men have a more robust response to this tricyclic antidepressant (TCA) than do women.[44] This was reinforced by a large database analysis of men and women with MDD which found a preferential response to SSRIs, compared with TCAs.[45] A limited amount of research finds that such sex differences in treatment response may also exist in those with dysthymic disorder. In a small study of 20 patients treated with fluoxetine, more women than men had at least a 50% decrease in the Hamilton Rating Scale for Depression (HRS-D) score.[46] Although there is a possibility that sex differences in the clinical presentation and treatment response exist among those with dysthymic disorder, much less is published about the nature of these differences. Our group's experience with sertraline[37] suggests a better response of women with dysthymic disorder to SSRIs, while men respond somewhat better to TCAs.

Psychosocial effects

The Epidemiologic Catchment Area study estimated the lifetime prevalence of dysthymic disorder in the US population to be approximately 3%.[47] More recent results have indicated that the prevalence of dysthymic disorder is higher than previously thought and that most patients with this condition are undertreated.[48–50] It is relevant that more than one-half of the economic cost of depression in the USA is estimated to be derived from indirect costs due to absenteeism or impaired work functioning.[51]

Despite a generally milder level of depressive symptoms, the early onset and chronic course of dysthymic disorder may result in even greater impairments in both social and occupational functioning than those found with more episodic forms of major depression.[52–55] Cassano et al[55] used the Social Adjustment Scale to compare patients with acute or chronic depression and found greater social maladjust-

ment in the dysthymic patients. The Medical Outcomes Study[53] found that patients with dysthymic disorder (with and without concurrent major depression) had significantly lower functional status and wellbeing than patients with only depressive symptoms, as well as a high prevalence of poor general medical health and impaired physical functioning. A study of over 1000 primary care patients found that those with dysthymic disorder had substantial impairment in health-related quality of life and exhibited greater impairments in physical functioning, role functioning and social functioning than patients with major depression.[54]

Whereas studies of the efficacy of antidepressant therapy have traditionally concentrated primarily on symptom reduction and/or syndrome remission, more recent trials have recognized the importance of evaluating the effects of treatment on the psychosocial functioning and quality of life of patients with major depression.[56,57] Kocsis et al[58] analysed the effects of treatment with either sertraline or imipramine on both mood symptoms and psychosocial outcomes for a large group of patients with DSM-III-R-defined, early-onset primary dysthymic disorder (without concurrent major depression) and found that antidepressant treatment had a positive effect on their psychosocial and work functioning.

Gender differences

Dysthymic disorder is more frequently seen in women than in men. The National Comorbidity Survey reported that the lifetime prevalence of dysthymic disorder was 4.8% for men and 8.0% for women.[23] This gender difference with a higher prevalence among women is similar to that found for other chronic forms of depression. Weismann et al found that 5.4% of women and 2.6% of men suffered from an episode of dysthymic disorder.[59–61] One of the few studies to compare symptom profiles in males and females with dysthymic disorder was conducted in adolescents. Adolescent girls endorsed a non-significantly greater number of symptoms and had significantly more difficulty with self-esteem. Adolescent boys were more likely to have aggressive, externalized behaviours rather than poor self-esteem.[62]

Baseline characteristics of collaborative study

In our collaborative, multicentre study, we analysed data from a large sample of patients with dysthymic disorder to explore relationships between sex, clinical variables, and response to treatment.[63] The data set comprised 416 patients with DSM-III-R-defined early-onset dysthymic disorder who were enrolled in a 12-week, multicentre, randomized, double-blind trial comparing treatment with sertraline, imipramine, or placebo. Seventeen university-affiliated centres in the USA participated. Methodological details and outcome results of the study have been reported elsewhere[37] and have demonstrated that imipramine and sertraline were equivalent to each other and superior in efficacy to placebo.

In the intent-to-treat (ITT) sample, 144 men and 266 women were included. There were no significant differences between men and women in baseline scores for the psychiatric rating scales: the HRS-D, the Montgomery-Asberg Depression Rating Scale (MADRS), the Inventory of Depressive Symptomatology-Self Report (IDS-SR), or the Clinical Global Impression (CGI) scale. Similarly, there were no sex differences after controlling for treatment condition.[63]

Women were more likely than men to have had a history of MDD, although this was significant only at the trend level. When the numbers of episodes were compared, men and women were equally likely to have had more than one episode of MDD (25% of men and 27% of women), but women were more likely to have had only one previous episode of MDD. The other past psychiatric illness that differed by sex was alcohol abuse, with a higher incidence of previous episodes being found in men. Men were also more likely to meet criteria for passive-aggressive personality disorder, and histrionic personality disorder was more prevalent among men at a trend level (numbers of individuals in these groups were small, and, therefore, results should be cautiously interpreted).

Treatment response

A comparison of sertraline, imipramine and placebo (Yonkers et al, unpublished) showed that, overall, 40% of males and 40% of females had full remission. However, there was a gender difference in the rate of remission in response to each specific drug. Women responded better to sertraline (54% of women versus 40% of men), while the response rate to imipramine was almost similar (47% of men showed remission versus 40% of women).

The response rate seen in the placebo group was somewhat higher than expected (44%). All study participants made frequent and prolonged study visits to mental health professionals during a 3-month period to complete the many rating scales used to assess both depressive symptoms and psychosocial functioning. Thus, placebo treatment was not the equivalent of no treatment. While dysthymia is a chronic condition, the severity of depression in dysthymia patients waxes and wanes over time, and it is likely that patients will seek treatment when symptoms are most severe. The natural course of dysthymia would thus predict some amelioration of symptoms over the course of the trial in placebo-treated patients.[37]

When partial remission or response rates were considered (a 50% decrease in the HRS-D-17, 50% decrease in the IDS-SR, or a CGI improvement score of 1 or 2), there was a trend for women, compared with men, to respond at a higher rate to either active treatment (59% versus 48%) with the 50% decrease in HRS-D-17 definition. The gender differences became more apparent when the percentages of men and women responding in the sertraline group were compared (64% versus 42%).

While women were more likely to respond to sertraline than were men, men were slightly more likely to respond to imipramine when the CGI definition was used, although these differences were small and did not achieve statistical significance.

Subjects with the greatest symptom improvement also showed the greatest improvement in functional impairment and quality-of-life measures. In both domains measured by the Social Adjustment Scale-Self Report (SAS-SR) and the Quality of Life Enjoyment and Satisfaction Questionnaire (Q-LES-Q), there was a significant improvement among women but not among men.[63]

Women given active treatment experienced significantly greater improvement on all measures, compared to women given placebo. In men, placebo-active treatment differences were not found in symptom scales and were evident only in one measure of functioning, the SAS-SR. When both a loss of dysthymic disorder criteria and a 0 on the HRS-D depression item were used to define remission, women were more likely to remit, but this failed to achieve significance.

There were also sex differences in the two active-treatment cells. While the percentages of men and women remitting on imipramine were approximately equivalent, the largest remission rate, 53%, occurred among women treated with sertraline. This represents an increment of approximately 10% compared with the other treatment cells. Response, indicating improvement but not necessarily remission, was also evaluated. Women were more likely to be responders, particularly if they were assigned to sertraline. On the other hand, the rate of improvement for people who received imipramine was equivalent or slightly and nonsignificantly superior in men.

Suggestions that men may have a better response to TCAs have been reported.[44,64-66] These studies, however, have focused on MDD. In a 1974 paper, the results of two multicentre trials comparing responses of patients with MDD to treatment with chlorpromazine, imipramine and placebo were reanalysed by sex and age.[65] Younger women were found to have a less favourable response to imipramine than either men or older women. Davidson and Pelson[66] analysed treatment response by sex and atypicality in a group of 152 patients treated with either imipramine or a monoamine oxidase inhibitor (MAOI). They found that women, but not men, with atypical symptoms preferentially responded to an MAOI. In a third study, the numbers of men and women responding to imipramine did not differ, but 49% of male completers and only 32% of female completers experienced a 'normal response', defined as rapid and sustained recovery.[64] In a meta-analytic study of all published clinical trials $(N = 35)$ that reported imipramine response by sex, Hamilton et al[44] found a significantly greater likelihood that males would positively respond. The response rate was 67% in 342 men and 57% in 711 women. Finally, in a large pooled database of 717 men and women with MDD who were treated with imipramine, paroxetine or placebo, a greater response in the female group treated with the SSRI was found.[45] Thus, the majority of studies that have evaluated sex differences in MDD treatment response have found a higher rate of response to imipramine therapy for males, and some work suggests greater improvement for women if they are treated with an SSRI.

Our data are somewhat similar, although women had a slightly higher remission rate than men, even when taking imipramine. It is possible that the difference is more difficult to detect in their patient population, which had lower symptom severity than is usually seen in trials for MMD (mean HRS-D scores of 13.2 [4.0] in females and 12.7 [3.7] in males). It is also possible that in dysthymic disorder, which has slightly lower response rates to pharmacotherapy,[67] the sex difference in response to imipramine is not as evident.

Because women were overrepresented in this clinical trial, their positive response to sertraline may be overstated. However, the better response of women to SSRIs such as sertraline may also be linked to ovarian hormones. As noted above, there is an association between depressive illnesses in women and periods of declining ovarian hormones. On the other hand, animal research has shown that ovarian hormones, in particular oestradiol, modulate the density of serotonin receptors in the hypothalamus[68] and the density of 5-HT$_2$ receptors in the cortex and nucleus accumbens.[69] Earlier work illustrates that oestradiol enhances antidepressant-induced downregulation of 5-HT$_2$ receptors,[70] further suggesting a biological basis for the response differences seen in this study.

Several reports lend support to the theory that oestrogen-enhanced response to antidepressants, particularly those that are active at 5-HT receptors, may be responsible for the superior response of women to SSRIs such as sertraline. In a multicentre trial of fluoxetine in the treatment of elderly patients, women receiving hormone replacement therapy (HRT) had an enhanced response rate compared with those not undergoing HRT.[71] A second study illustrates that the value of oestrogen to antidepressant response is not limited to postmenopausal women. Postpartum women with MDD experienced a greater degree of symptomatic improvement if oestrogen was administered either with or without concurrent antidepressant treatment.[72]

The results of our multicentre study show a higher placebo response rate in men than in women, a finding that is in accord with the work of others.[45,73] Thus, male subjects appear to be responding to the non-specific features of the study. This may relate to general help-seeking patterns in our society. Men are generally less likely to seek treatment for general medical illness or psychiatric illness,[74,75] but when they finally do seek treatment, they find that the process is itself therapeutic. Given that the suicide rate is higher in males, one might infer that men do not seek treatment often enough and suffer bad consequences of their reticence.

Summary

Dysthymic disorder is a very prevalent affective disorder affecting both women and men in our society. Because of a combination of biological, psychological and socio-cultural factors, dysthymic disorder is most frequently seen in women. Because dysthymic disorder is a chronic condition, the economic and social costs are significant, and may be linked to worker absenteeism and productivity.

Current research suggests that significant differences exist between men and women with early-onset dysthymic disorder, in the comorbid character pathology and response to treatment. Both sertraline and imipramine are more effective than placebo in treating male and female patients with early-onset dysthymic disorder. Women respond better to sertraline and other serotonin agonists than to noradrenergic tricyclics. Men respond somewhat more favourably to noradrenergic tricyclics than to serotonergic agonists. Further studies should be undertaken to elucidate these differences and enhance our knowledge of the pathophysiology of dysthymic disorder among women and their optimal treatment.

References

1. Halbreich U, Premenstrual dysphoric disorders: a diversified cluster of vulnerability traits to depression, *Acta Psychiatr Scand* 1997; **95**:169–76.

2. Weissman MM, Klerman GL, Sex differences and the epidemiology of depression, *Arch Gen Psychiatry* 1977; **34**:98–111.

3. Weissman MM, Bland R, Joyce PR et al, Sex differences in rates of depression: cross-national perspectives, *J Affect Disord* 1993; **29**:77–84.

4. Kessler RC, McGonagle KA, Swartz M et al, Sex and depression in the National Comorbidity Survey. I. Lifetime prevalence, chronicity and recurrence, *J Affect Disord* 1993; **29**:85–96.

5. Links PS, Akiskal HS, Chronic and intractable depressions: terminology, classification, and description of subtypes. In: Zohar J, Belmaker RH, eds, *Treating Resistant Depression* (PMA: New York, 1987) 1–21.

6. Blazer D, Swartz M, Woodbury M et al, Depressive symptoms and depressive diagnosis in a community population. Use of a new procedure for analysis of psychiatric classification, *Arch Gen Psychiatry* 1988; **45**:1078–84.

7. Parry BL, Reproductive factors affecting the course of affective illness in women, *Psychiatr Clin North Am* 1989; **12**:207–20.

8. Weissman MM, Bland RC, Canino GJ et al, Cross national epidemiology of major depression and bipolar disorder. *JAMA* 1996; **276**:293–9.

9. Halbreich U, Lumley LA, The multiple interactional biological processes that might lead to depression and gender differences in its appearance, *J Affect Disord* 1993; **29**:159–73.

10. Halbreich U, Vital-Herne J, Goldstein S et al, Sex differences in biological factors putatively related to depression, *J Affect Disord* 1984; **7**:223–33.

11. Kandel DB, Davis M, Epidemiology of depressive mood in adolescence: an empirical study. *Arch Gen Psychiatry* 1982; **39**:1205–12.

12. Angold A, Worthman CW, Puberty onset of gender differences in rates of depression: a developmental, epidemiological and neuro-endocrine perspective, *J Affect Disord* 1993; **29**:145–58.

13. Halbreich U, Endicott J, Schact S et al, The diversity of premenstrual changes as reflected in the Premenstrual Assessment Form, *Acta Psychiatr Scand* 1982; **65**:45–65.

14. Halbreich U, Alt IH, Paul L, Premenstrual changes. Impaired hormonal homeostasis, *Neurol Clin* 1988; **6**:173–94.

15. Brockington IF, Kumar R, eds, *Motherhood and Mental Illness* (Academic Press: London, 1982).

16. Avis NE, Posner JG, McKinlay JB, Menopause and depression. Paper presented at the Annual Meeting of the American Psychological Association, New Orleans, LA, August 1989. Unpublished.

17. Hochschild AR, *The Second Shift: Working Parents and the Revolution at Home* (Viking: New York, 1989).

18. Nazroo JY, Edwards AC, Brown GW, Gender differences in the onset of depression following a shared life event: a study of couples, *Psychol Med* 1997; **27**:9–19.

19. Sargeant JK, Bruce ML, Florio LP, Weissman MM, Factors associated with 1-year outcome of major depression in the community, *Arch Gen Psychiatry* 1990; **47**:519–26.

20. Costello EJ, Married with children: predictors of mental and physical health in middle-aged women, *Psychiatry* 1991; **54**:292–305.

21. Brown GW, Harris TO, *Social Origins of Depression: A Study of Psychiatric Disorder in*

Women, 1st edn, Vol. 1 (Free Press: New York, 1978).

22. Weissman MM, Leaf PJ, Bruce ML, Florio L, The epidemiology of dysthymia in five communities: rates, risks, comorbidity, and treatment, *Am J Psychiatry* 1988; **145**:815–19.

23. Kessler RC, McGonagle KA, Zhao S et al, Lifetime and 12-month prevalence of DSM-III-R psychiatric disorders in the United States. Results from the National Comorbidity Survey, *Arch Gen Psychiatry* 1994; **51**:8–19.

24. Markowitz JC, Moran ME, Kocsis JH, Frances AJ, Prevalence and comorbidity of dysthymic disorder among psychiatric outpatients, *J Affect Disord* 1992; **24**:63–71.

25. Keller MB, Current concepts in affective disorders, *J Clin Psychiatry* 1989; **50**:157–62.

26. Bakish D, LaPierre YD, Weinstein R et al, Ritanserin, imipramine, and placebo in the treatment of dysthymic disorder, *J Clin Psychopharmacol* 1993; **13**:409–14.

27. Akiskal HS, Dysthymic disorder: psychopathology of proposed chronic depressive subtypes, *Am J Psychiatry* 1983; **140**:11–20.

28. Wells KB, Stewart A, Hays RD et al, The functioning and well-being of depressed patients. Results from the Medical Outcomes Study, *JAMA* 1989; **262**:914–19.

29. Friedman RA, Social impairment in dysthymia, *Psychiatr Ann* 1993; **23**:632–7.

30. Kessler RC, Foster CL, Saunders WB, Stang PE, Social consequences of psychiatric disorders 1: educational attainment, *Am J Psychiatry* 1995; **152**:1026–32.

31. Zisook S, Treatment of dysthymia and atypical depression, *J Clin Psychiatry Monogr* 1992; **10**:15–23.

32. Keller MB, The difficult depressed patient in perspective, *J Clin Psychiatry* 1993; **54**(suppl): 4–8.

33. Weissman MM, Klerman GL, The chronic depressive in the community: unrecognized and poorly treated, *Comp Psychiatry* 1977; **18**:523–32.

34. Harrison WM, Stewart JW, Pharmacotherapy of dysthymic disorder. In: Kocsis JH, Klein DN, eds, *Diagnosis and Treatment of Chronic Depression* (Guilford Press: New York, 1995) 124–45.

35. Gwirtsman HE, Blehar MC, McCullough JP Jr et al, Standardized Assessment of Dysthymia: Report of a National Institute of Mental Health Conference, *Psychopharmacol Bull* 1997; **33**:3–11.

36. American Psychiatric Association, *Diagnostic and Statistical Manual of Mental Disorders DSM-IV*, 4th edn (American Psychiatric Association: Washington, DC, 1994) 327.

37. Thase ME, Fava M, Halbreich U et al, A placebo-controlled, randomized clinical trial comparing sertraline and imipramine for the treatment of dysthymia, *Arch Gen Psychiatry* 1996; **53**:777–84.

38. Yonkers KA, Clark RH, Trivedi MH, The psychopharmacological treatment of nonmajor mood disorders. In: Rush AJ, ed., *Mood Disorders: Systematic Medication Management* (Karger: Basel, 1997) 146–66.

39. Kocsis JH, Frances AJ, Voss C et al, Imipramine treatment for chronic depression, *Arch Gen Psychiatry* 1988; **45**:253–7.

40. Nardi E, Capponi R, Costa DA et al, Moclobemide compared with imipramine in the treatment of chronic depression (dysthymia DSM-III-R): a double-blind placebo controlled trial, *Clin Neuropharmacol* 1992; **15** (suppl 1):430A–4A.

41. Hellerstein DJ, Yanowitch P, Rosenthal J et al, A randomized double-blind study of fluoxetine versus placebo in the treatment of dysthymia, *Am J Psychiatry* 1993; **150**:1169–75.

42. Ravindran AV, Griffiths J, Merali Z, Charbonneau Y, Cognitive-behaviour therapy and sertraline in dysthymia: efficacy and physiology (abstr 15E). Presented at the Annual Meeting of the American Psychiatric Association, Toronto, Ontario, May 1998. Unpublished.

43. Steiner M, Browne G, Roberts J et al, Sertraline and IPT in Dysthymia: One Year Follow-Up. Presented at the Annual Meeting of the NCDEU, 10–14 June 1998.

44. Hamilton JA, Grant M, Jensvold MF, Sex and treatment of depressions: when does it matter? In: Jensvold MF, Halbreich U, Hamilton JA, eds, *Psychopharmacology and Women: Sex, Gender, and Hormones* (American Psychiatric Association: Washington, DC, 1996) 241–60.

45. Steiner M, Wheadon D, Kreider M et al, Antidepressant response to paroxetine by

gender (abstr 462). Presented at the Annual Meeting of the American Psychiatric Association, May 1993, San Francisco, CA. Unpublished.

46. Bakish D, Ravindran A, Hooper C, Lapierre Y, Psychopharmacological treatment response of patients with a DSM-III diagnosis of dysthymic disorder, *Psychopharmacol Bull* 1994; **30**:53–9.

47. Regier DA, Boyd JH, Burke JD Jr et al, One-month prevalence of mental disorders in the United States. Based on five Epidemiologic Catchment Area sites, *Arch Gen Psychiatry* 1988; **45**:977–86.

48. Keller MB, Dysthymia in clinical practice: course, outcome and impact on the community, *Acta Psychiatr Scand Suppl* 1994; **383**:24–34.

49. Kessler RC, McGonagle KA, Zhao S et al, Lifetime and 12-month prevalence of DSM-III-R psychiatric disorders in the United States. Results from the National Comorbidity Survey, *Arch Gen Psychiatry* 1994; **51**:8–19.

50. Spitzer RL, Williams JB, Kroenke K et al, Utility of a new procedure for diagnosing mental disorders in primary care. The PRIME-MD 1000 Study, *JAMA* 1994; **272**:1749–56.

51. Greenberg PE, Stiglin LE, Finkelstein SN, Berndt ER, The economic burden of depression in 1990, *J Clin Psychiatry* 1993; **54**:405–18.

52. Johnson J, Weissman MM, Kerman GI, Service utilization and social morbidity associated with depressive symptoms in the community, *JAMA* 1992; **267**:1478–83.

53. Wells KB, Stewart A, Hays RD et al, The functioning and well-being of depressed patients. Results from the Medical Outcomes Study, *JAMA* 1989; **262**:914–19.

54. Spitzer RL, Kroenke K, Linzer M et al, Health-related quality of life in primary care patients with mental disorders. Results from the PRIME-MD 1000 Study, *JAMA* 1995; **274**:1511–17.

55. Cassano GB, Perugi G, Musetti L, Akiskal HS, The nature of depression presenting concomitantly with panic disorder, *Comp Psychiatry* 1989; **30**:473–82.

56. Lonnqvist J, Sintonen H, Syvalahti E et al, Antidepressant efficacy and quality of life in depression: a double-blind study with moclobemide and fluoxetine, *Acta Psychiatr Scand* 1994; **89**:363–9.

57. Turner R, Quality of life: experience with sertraline, *Int Clin Psychopharmacol* 1994; **9** (suppl 3):27–31.

58. Kocsis JH, Zisook S, Davidson J et al, Double-blind comparison of sertraline, imipramine, and placebo in the treatment of dysthymia: psychosocial outcomes, *Am J Psychiatry* 1997; **154**:390–5.

59. Weissman MM, Bland R, Joyce PR et al, Sex differences in rates of depression: cross-national perspectives, *J Affect Disord* 1993; **29**:77–84.

60. Weissman MM, Leaf PJ, Bruce ML, Florio L, The epidemiology of dysthymia in five communities: rates, risks, comorbidity and treatment, *Am J Psychiatry* 1988; **145**:815–19.

61. Weissman MM, Leaf PJ, Tischler GL et al, Affective disorders in five United States communities, *Psychol Med* 1988; **18**:141–53.

62. Gjerde F, Block J, Block JH, Depressive symptoms and personality during late adolescence: gender differences in the externalization–internalization of symptom expression, *J Abnorm Psychol* 1988; **97**:475–86.

63. Yonkers KA, Halbreich U, Pearlstein T et al, Sex differences in baseline characteristics and treatment response among men and women with dysthymic disorder. In press.

64. Frank E, Carpenter LL, Kupfer DJ, Sex differences in recurrent depression: are there any that are significant? *Am J Psychiatry* 1988; **145**:41–5.

65. Raskin A, Age–sex differences in response to antidepressant drugs, *J Nerv Ment Dis* 1974; **159**:120–30.

66. Davidson J, Pelton S, Forms of atypical depression and their response to antidepressant drugs, *Psychiatr Res* 1986; **17**:87–95.

67. Yonkers KA, Clark RH, Trivedi MH, The psychopharmacological treatment of non-major mood disorders. In: Rush AJ, ed, Mood Disorders. Systematic Medication Management. *Modern Problems of Pharmacopsychiatry* II vol. 25 (S. Karger AG, Basel, 1997) 146–66.

68. Wilson MA, Dwyer KD, Roy EJ, Direct effects of ovarian hormones on antidepressant binding sites, *Brain Res Bull* 1989; **22**:181–5.

69. Summer BE, Fink G, Estrogen increases the density of 5-hydroxytryptamine-2A receptors in cerebral cortex and nucleus accumbens in the female rat, *J Steroid Biochem Mol Biol* 1995; **54**:15–20.

70. Kendall DA, Stancel GM, Enna SJ, The influence of sex hormones on antidepressant-induced alterations in neurotransmitter receptor binding, *J Neurosci* 1982; **2**:354–60.

71. Schneider LS, Small GW, Hamilton SH et al, Estrogen replacement and response to fluoxetine in a multicenter geriatric depression trial, *Am J Geriatr Psychiatry* 1997; **5**:97–106.

72. Gregoire AJ, Kumar R, Everitt B et al, Transdermal oestrogen for treatment of severe postnatal depression, *Lancet* 1996; **347**:930–3.

73. Wilcox CS, Cohn JB, Linden RD et al, Predictors of placebo response: a retrospective analysis, *Psychopharmacol Bull* 1992; **28**: 157–62.

74. Baum C, Kennedy DL, Knapp DE et al, Prescription drug use in 1984 and changes over time, *Med Care* 1988; **26**:105–14.

75. Svarstad BL, Cleary PD, Mechanic D et al, Gender differences in the acquisition of prescribed drugs: an epidemiological study, *Med Care* 1987; **25**:1089–98.

8

Unipolar depression in women

Veronica O'Keane

Major depressive disorder (MDD) is defined as the occurrence of one or more episodes of depression in the absence of manic, mixed or hypomanic episodes. It sometimes represents a recurrent disorder, the frequently chronic nature of which has only been acknowledged recently. The epidemiological evidence demonstrating that rates of depression are higher in women than in men is the subject of Chapter 1. Briefly, studies from many diverse cultures and geographical locations, using comparable methods, show that the rate of depression is almost twice as high in women as in men.[1-4] Some epidemiological points, relevant specifically to unipolar depression, should be highlighted.

Epidemiology

The almost twofold difference in rates of depression between men and women is also seen specifically in the unipolar form of depression.[1] Kessler et al,[2] in a large nationally representative sample from the USA that retro-spectively covered a 40-year period, found that women aged 45–54 years were more likely than men, over a 12-month period, to have recurrent episodes of depression. In a prospective Swiss study conducted over a 7-year period,[3] using different definitions of depression, it was found that women were consistently overrepresented in the more severe forms of depression. Brief recurrent depression occurred equally in both sexes, and recurrence of depression was more likely in women. A study specifically examining the diagnosis of depression in relation to severity of episode found that women reported more symptoms only above a diagnostic threshold.[4] The trend for women to report more symptoms than men does not, therefore, account for the male–female differences in the severe, recurrent form of the disorder.

Thus all the major epidemiological studies demonstrate that there is a real twofold increase in the rates of recurrent depression in women, compared with men. A gender difference in the rates of onset of depression begins in the early teenage years, increases during the childbearing years, and returns to the previous level after 45 years of age.[5] The causes of this discrepancy have been attributed to genetic, environmental, biological and multifactorial models. These will be considered separately.

Aetiology

Genetic

Kendler et al examined the relative importance of genetic and environmental risk factors in a 1-year prevalence of major depression study in 938 adult female–female twin pairs.[6] The subjects were interviewed at two time points, a minimum of 1 year apart, looking at the diagnosis of DSM-III-R MDD. The correlation in liability to have MDD was higher, at the two time points, in monozygotic compared with dizygotic twins. The estimated heritability for the liability to develop MDD over a period of 1 year was 41–46%. They concluded that, while environmental factors played an important role, their effects were transitory and did not result in permanent changes in the liability to become ill.

This study also assessed the lifetime history of MDD and found the estimated heritability for this to be approximately 70%.[7] About half of what appeared to be environmental effects, on first interview, was found to be erroneous when two assessments were included. A more recent, large-scale twin study by this group examined the interaction between onset of MDD and stressful life events.[8] The results suggested that a more sophisticated genetic–environmental interaction may be occurring. The authors concluded that the genetic liability to the development of MDD is mediated by 'a genetic control of sensitivity to the depression-inducing effects of stressful life events.' This is interesting in view of recent biological theories of abnormal stress reactions as a possible cause of depression (see later text).

Personality factors

Personality is most frequently measured using Eysenck's three personality traits of extraversion, neurotocism and psychoticism. The evidence, reviewed below, that high neuroticism scores are a vulnerability factor for the development of MDD is convincing. Women, across different cultures and of all ages, have higher neurotocism scores than men.[9]

A female–female twin study found that neurotocism was strongly correlated with both a lifetime, and a prospective 1-year, prevalence of MDD.[10] This study suggested that: approximately 55% of the genetic liability of MMD was shared with neurotocism and 45% was unique to MDD; neurotocism predisposes to MDD and this is largely the result of genetic factors; and depression predisposes to the development of neurotic traits, the so-called 'scar' effect. This effect has been questioned in an 18-year prospective study, examining neurotocism scores in a group of depressed patients.[11] They found no differential change in neurotocism scores between good and poor outcome groups; nor did the scores change significantly for the group as a whole over this period. Duggan's group, in a study examining the relationship between neuroticism and depressive illness in the first-degree relatives of probands with MDD, found that raised neuroticism scores were associated with both a previous history and a current episode of MDD.[12]

The literature thus indicates that neurotic personality traits predispose individuals to the development of MDD. Recurrent depression may not increase neurotic traits over time. However, those with high neuroticism scores at the start of their illness, and who suffer from the DSM-III melancholic subtype of MDD, tend to have a poor outcome.[13] A caveat of all these studies is that neurotocism is a very broad concept and probably encompasses many vulnerability factors. This point is highlighted in a study that focused on more specific aspects of personality in relation to vulnerability factors for MDD and found that dependency scores remained elevated in recovered depressives.[14] Individuals with high neurotocism scores tend to become distressed because of their increased *reactivity* to stressors, which is more important than the nature of the stressful situation itself.[15] This again could be related to altered stress responses in predisposed individuals.

There may be some relationship between aggressive personality traits and depression. Some workers postulate an association between impulsive aggression and depression, which may be mediated by serotonin (5-HT).[16] This is more likely to be a vulnerability factor for males than for females. The reverse may be true for women: that is, women who display less aggressive behaviour than men are more likely to become depressed (see Chapter 23).[17] This apparent contradiction may be explained by the association between passive-aggressive personality features and certain forms of depression in women.[18] This may also be relevant to helplessness training and socialization, explored later.

Socio-political/developmental factors

Animals consistently not rewarded for trying to escape from adverse circumstances will eventually cease their escape behaviour: a condition labelled 'learned helplessness'.[19] This learned helplessness behaviour may be an animal model for depression, as many of the behaviours mimic depression in humans. This model may be particularly relevant to depression in women, given the political and social conditions experienced by women, compared with men, globally. There is much debate about whether there is an innate typical female psy-

chological structure or whether this results from gender-specific socialization (see Chapters 3 and 31).

Women and men are treated differently in all cultures from childhood onwards, although clearly these differences are more marked in some cultures than others. The influence of early stressors on the development of depression later in life has now been established. The most consistently replicated associations between early life experiences and depression in adulthood are childhood sexual abuse and parental separation or loss. Prolonged separation from both parents has been found to be associated with an increased risk, approximately three- to fourfold, of lifetime depressive episodes in adult women.[20] Prolonged separation from both parents is a stronger risk factor than either parental death or separation/ divorce. Poor maternal care during childhood is also associated with increased rates of depression,[21] and increased severity of depressive episodes,[22] in adult women. Workers in this area suggest a model whereby rates and severity of depression in adult women can be predicted by difficulties in social relationships whose origin can be traced back to early periods that have a continuing effect throughout life.

Women are more likely to be sexually abused as children, and these children have higher rates of depression than children who have not been abused (see Chapter 15).[23] Adult women with a history of sexual abuse are more likely to become depressed than women without such histories.[24] Adult women are more likely to be victimized than men, and a number of studies have described both high rates of depression in women who have been victimized and high rates of victimization in women who are depressed.[25,26]

Women are more likely to experience social adversity during adulthood, and there is convincing epidemiological evidence that the socio-economic status of women may be an important cause of depression in women.[27] More women live in poverty than men, and the relationship between poverty and depression appears to be a particularly important one for women.[28] Kendler et al, in an attempt to develop an integrated aetiological model for the prediction of MDD in women, based on a large epidemiological sample of women, have suggested that the strongest predictor of depression in women is stressful life events.[29] Clearly, any model must take into account that the liability to depression involves several interacting risk factors, but current and past social adversity may be one of the most important risk factors in the development and maintenance of depression in adult women.

Biological factors

Sex steroids and depression

There are many indicators that female sex steroids may predispose to the development of depression, the most obvious one being the epidemiological evidence of a twofold increase in depression in women. The most compelling biological evidence that sex steroids may precipitate mood disturbance is twofold. First, the brain is a major target organ for sex steroids, and they act on discrete regions of the brain in a gender-specific way to modulate behaviours. This is more marked in animals than in humans, where behaviours are modified, rather than altered, by sex steroids. Second, certain forms of mood disturbance are specific to women and associated with altering sex steroid levels: the postpartum blues/depression/psychosis spectrum of mood disorders, premenstrual dysphoria (PMD) and depression associated with the menopause (for more details see Chapters 16, 18 and 22). These periods are marked not only by hormonal shifts but also by major psychosocial stress. This

again serves to emphasize that aetiological models of depression must be multifactorial and interactive. The evidence indicates, however, that there is a specific biological trigger related to these endocrine shifts.

Oestrogen hypothesis

The most convincing evidence indicating that biological triggers are important and specific risk factors for these female-specific mood disorders is related to postpartum psychosis: the strongest predictor of postpartum psychosis is a history of bipolar affective disorder; it has a high rate of recurrence; it has a similar incidence across different cultures, and a singular clinical presentation and course. Postpartum psychosis resolves with either pharmacotherapy or electroconvulsive therapy (ECT). This suggests that biological mechanisms specific to the postpartum period precipitate this illness, and biological mechanisms, perhaps similar to those in bipolar illness, maintain it.

The oestrogen/dopamine hypothesis attempts to explain these observations and suggests that oestrogens exert an inhibitory effect on dopamine neurotransmission, which is removed in the postpartum period and leads to dopamine overdrive and subsequent psychosis in predisposed individuals.[31] This hypothesis is only weakly supported by animal and human studies.[30] Two studies have examined prolactin responses to the dopamine agonist apomorphine in the postpartum period in women with and without postpartum psychoses.[31,32] The paradigm underlying such studies is that prolactin responses to apomorphine reflect central, specifically hypothalamic, dopamine neurotransmitter function. One found that prolactin responses were exaggerated in vulnerable women[31] and the other found similar responses in both groups.[32] A recent study examined dopamine metabolites in the blood at oestrogen-specific phases of the menstrual cycle of healthy women and found no evidence of altered dopamine turnover.[33] It is still unclear whether oestrogens alter dopamine tone and whether this is different in vulnerable women, if such an effect exists.

Progesterone hypothesis

The progesterone hypothesis has its origins in the work of Dalton, which suggested a beneficial effect of progesterone on the symptoms of the premenstrual syndrome (PMS),[34] and stated that progesterone withdrawal was responsible for some sex steroid-related depressions in women. Subsequent controlled clinical trials have not supported the therapeutic efficacy of progesterone in PMS.[35] Postpartum hormone studies have not demonstrated any difference in progesterone levels between women who develop, and women who do not develop, postpartum depression.[36] A caveat of all the studies that simply measure hormone levels is that they do not attempt to account for possible differences occurring at other sites: most importantly, the steroid receptors and post-receptor mechanisms. In relation to this point, one study has suggested that oestrogen receptor mechanisms may be different in women who develop postpartum depression and women who do not.[37]

Sex steroids and unipolar depression

The sex steroid-related mood disorder most closely associated with unipolar depression is postpartum depression. Postpartum depression occurs in 10–15% of new mothers and clinically resembles MDD. A postpartum depression may be an isolated event in a woman's life, may be another episode in a history of recurrent unipolar depression, or may be a harbinger of recurrent MDD. The risk of developing a postpartum depression is increased to approximately 20–30% in women with a prior history of depression. Once a women has suffered a postpartum depression, the risk in subsequent pregnancies of another episode approaches 50%.[5] Apart from a previous history of depression, the most important risk factors for the development of a postpartum depression are psychosocial stressors. Some stressors are specific risk factors for postpartum, as opposed to unipolar depression. These are a previous history of a poor relationship with one's own mother and greater occupational instability.[38]

There are two predictors of postpartum depression that relate to mood disturbance associated with altering sex steroid levels. The first of these is a history of postpartum blues.[39] Postpartum blues is a common and transient mood disturbance seen in new mothers about 3–4 days post-delivery and is attributed to the dramatic endocrine shifts occurring in a woman's physiology. Postpartum blues, especially when severe, is predictive of subsequent postpartum depression.[39] The second of these predictors is a history of PMS, although one study has found that this association is only true when women are examined for depression at the time of resumption of menstruation following childbirth.[40]

Conclusion

Taken together, the above facts suggest that some trigger factor or factors, specific to the postpartum period, can precipitate MDD in vulnerable women. There is some evidence that sex steroids may act as a specific trigger in some women, in that women who experience both PMS and postpartum blues are more likely to have an episode of postpartum depression. Women with a history of unipolar depression are at greater risk of developing postpartum depression than women without such histories. Whether this is secondary to an increased biological vulnerability or to increased social risk factors is not clear. In relation to the latter, there are social stressors specific to the postpartum period that may act in an additive way to the chronic social stressors experienced by women, and thus childbirth may herald the onset of unipolar depression.

Glucocorticoids and depression

One of the most consistently replicated findings in the biology of MDD is that of hypothalamic–pituitary–adrenal (HPA) axis overdrive. Depressed patients have high cerebrospinal fluid levels of corticotrophin-releasing hormone (CRH), loss of diurnal troughs in the pattern of adrenocorticotrophic hormone (ACTH) and cortisol secretion, and hypertrophied adrenal glands.[41] This HPA axis hyperactivity is generally demonstrated in most studies in this field by resistance of blood cortisol levels to suppression by the synthetic glucocorticoid dexamethasone. The rate of dexamethasone non-suppression increases from mild (about 30%) through to severe (about 70%) depression. These endocrine abnormalities tend to normalize with recovery, whereas treatment resistance and future suicide are associated with persistent hypercortisolaemia.[42] Other conditions associated with hypercortisolaemia, such as Cushing's syndrome, have high rates of comorbid depression, and the depression remits when cortisol levels return to normal.[43]

As a result of the now well-established literature demonstrating associations between HPA axis overdrive and depression, recent preliminary clinical trials have examined the efficacy of anti-glucocorticoid drugs in the treatment of depression, with promising results.[44] Some workers in this field now plausibly argue that hypercortisolaemia may be causal in depression, given that depression tends to occur in the context of stressful life events and the HPA axis is activated in almost all situations of stress, both psychological and physiological.

HPA axis stress responses and depression in women

There has been no systematic examination of the glucocorticoid hypothesis in relation to unipolar depression in women. One study has examined HPA axis changes in women during the postpartum period.[45] Of the immense physiological changes occurring during pregnancy, one of the most remarkable is in the function of the HPA axis. Women during the last trimester of pregnancy have cortisol levels in the Cushingoid range, secondary to increased production of placental CRH.[46] Following birth, hypertrophied adrenal glands continue to produce cortisol and cause a transient suppression of endogenous CRH production, as suggested by the finding of transient blunting of ACTH responses to CRH in healthy postpartum women.[45] Although there is a wide spectrum of HPA axis changes associated with MDD, there is much evidence to suggest that abnormalities of CRH drive may be the most important.[47] The above study[45] found that women who develop postpartum depression had HPA axis changes similar to those seen in MDD: namely, sustained (up to 12 weeks) blunting of ACTH responses to CRH. A few studies have examined HPA axis function in PMS, with equivocal results: one has found reduced ACTH levels;[48] another increased cortisol responses to CRH[49] in women with PMS compared with control women.

There is some evidence that stress responses may be different in males and females, and primate work suggests that the submissive stress response in females is associated with altered CRH levels.[50] This submissive stress response may be the corollary of the stress response seen in melancholic depression, in that it is associated with lowered CRH levels and may be an animal model for atypical depression. In atypical depression there is a reversal of the biological symptoms of melancholic depression, and patients suffer from increased sleep, increased appetite and weight gain, and anergia. This form of depression may be associated in humans with lowering of HPA axis function.[51]

HPA axis stress responses may be relevant to the link between parental separation/abuse in childhood and depression in adult women. One study has examined HPA axis responses in adolescent girls with a history of sexual abuse and found that they have blunted ACTH responses to CRH, compared with a control group.[52] This study provides a tentative biological explanation for the occurrence of recurrent unipolar depression in women with histories of abuse or neglect. A model of MDD as an aberrant stress response also explains the occurrence of episodes in the context of stressful life events: a fact very relevant to depression in females. It should be emphasized, however, that the more severe forms of depression are more likely to occur in the absence of life events, and HPA axis disturbances in these cases may be genetically predetermined.[47]

Conclusion
The melancholic type of MDD is associated with hypercortisolaemia and possible central HPA axis overdrive. During the postpartum period, glucocorticoid levels rapidly and dramatically fall from a Cushingoid to a normal range. There is preliminary evidence suggesting that this drop is associated with central overdrive of the HPA axis in women who develop postpartum depression. Abnormal HPA axis responses to stress as a model for MDD may explain the link between stressful life events and depression. Early traumatic experiences may render the HPA axis less plastic and predispose the individual to subsequent aberrant stress responses, thus explaining the association between early childhood trauma and unipolar depression in adult women. Submissive stress responses in female primates are associated

with lowered central HPA axis drive, and this may be an animal model for atypical forms of MDD.

Thyroid axis and depression in women
Thyroid axis function differs between men and women throughout life. Similarly, dysfunction of the thyroid axis differs between the sexes, with women having a lifetime prevalence of thyroid disease of approximately 2.25–4%, which is 4–10 times the estimate for men.[53] The influence of thyroid hormones on the developing brain has been clearly established, and neonates are now routinely screened for hypothyroidism. The effects of hypothyroidism on the adult brain have not been elucidated and have been little investigated, although clearly the brain is a target organ for thyroid hormones. Conditions of gross hypothyroidism are associated with severe depression, and sometimes psychosis and MDD occur with an estimated prevalence of 10–40% in patients being treated for hypothyroidism.[54,55] A neuroendocrine study examining prolactin responses to the d-fenfluramine challenge in hypothyroid women, before and following thyroid hormone replacement therapy, suggests that thyroid hormones may modulate central 5-HT function.[55] Reduced thyroid activity was associated with reduced 5-HT responses, and there was a direct relationship between thyroid-stimulating hormone (TSH) levels and measures of depression.

Thyroid hormone abnormalities in depression are complicated by the fact that some studies suggest that approximately 30% of depressed subjects have blunted TSH responses to thyrotrophin-releasing hormone (TRH), suggesting thyroid axis overdrive.[56] This is probably a transient abnormality and represents a non-specific stress response. A further subgroup of depressed women have exaggerated TSH responses to TRH—a condition known as subclinical hypothyroidism—which lead eventually to clinical hypothyroidism.[53] This may explain why tri-iodothyronine therapy tends to speed recovery from depression in women, but not in men. Thyroid axis abnormalities may underlie some cases of the malignant variant of bipolar affective disorder, known as rapid cycling, since high doses of thyroxine can induce remission in some cases.[54]

Harris et al found that postpartum depression was significantly more common in women who had thyroid hormone antibodies in an antenatal screen, than in women who tested negative for the presence of antibodies antenatally.[57] Another study found that 38% of women with postpartum thyroid disease were depressed and the depression remitted when thyroid function was corrected.[58] Subclinical hypothyroidism also occurs at a greater than expected rate in women with PMS.[59]

Conclusion

Thyroidopathies are 4–10 times more common in women than in men and are frequently associated with affective disturbance. MDD, rapid cycling, PMS and postpartum depression are all associated with thyroid axis abnormalities, and some of these cases respond to thyroid hormone therapy. It is probable that a subgroup of women, from a range of affective disorders, have masked subclinical hypothyroidism. All women with affective disturbance should be screened for thyroid axis function.

Serotonin and depression in women

Several lines of evidence indicate that 5-HT neurotransmitter function is abnormal in depressive illness. These are indirect in human studies and include platelet imipramine binding studies, measures of the 5-HT metabolite 5-hydroxyindoleacetic acid (5-HIAA) in the cerebrospinal fluid, brain 5-HT binding in post-mortem studies and dynamic 5-HT neuro-

endocrine challenge studies.[60] The latter studies provide the most convincing evidence that 5-HT function may be abnormal in depressive illness.[61,62]

Gender differences in 5-HT function are discussed in Chapter 5, but from the point of view of depression, there is evidence to indicate that females may be rendered more vulnerable to depressive illness because of differences in 5-HT responses to stress.[63] Exposure to restraint stress in rats leads to behavioural changes, and these behavioural changes have been widely used as an animal model of depression. With repeated exposure to restraint, these behaviours are reversed, and this adaptive change is associated with alterations in central 5-HT neurotransmitter function.[64] Female rats, in contrast to male rats, fail to adapt to repeated stress, and this is associated with defective 5-HT synthesis in the frontal cortex.[63] This could be related to altered glucocorticoid responses to stress, as these female rats have greater glucocorticoid responses to stress,[65] and glucocorticoids may inhibit 5-HT function in animals[66] and humans.[67] Central 5-HT neurotransmitter function is probably also modulated by sex steroids, especially oestrogens. Animal evidence indicates that oestrogen enhances 5-HT neurotransmission.[68] Prolactin responses to d-fenfluramine throughout the menstrual cycle of healthy women fluctuate directly with blood oestrogen levels.[69] This oestrogen effect probably accounts for the enhanced prolactin responses to d-fenfluramine in women compared with men.[70]

Presentation and course of unipolar depression

Women tend to have more severe depressions as measured by the observer-rated Hamilton Rating Scale for Depression and the self-rated

Beck Depression Inventory.[71] Women also report more functional impairment, particularly in terms of marital and familial adjustment, and have also been found to experience more psychomotor retardation than men.[71] These findings are supported by those of Young et al,[4] who found an excess of women, compared with men, only above a certain diagnostic threshold. The same group of investigators, however, has not found any gender differences in the severity of unipolar depression or in the resulting functional impairment, but increased appetite and weight were more common in women than in men.[72] This may be related to the greater prevalence of atypical depression in women.

The longitudinal course of depression may differ between men and women. Women tend to have an earlier age of onset, usually mid-adolescence, than men, who usually become symptomatic in their mid-twenties.[73] Some evidence suggests that the average length of episodes is longer in women and periods of remission between episodes are shorter.[3] This is not substantiated by a large NIMH prospective study that examined male–female differences in the course of unipolar depression.[74] Over a 15-year period, no differences were found in the time to recovery, time to first recurrence, or the number or severity of recurrences of episodes. Treatment received during follow-up was not controlled for in this study, however, and this may obscure sex differences in the course of depression.

Comorbidity

Up to 50% of patients with MDD have comorbid medical or psychiatric disorders.[75] Women are more likely than men to have high rates of comorbidity. This may be related to high levels of depression in association with psychiatric disorders that are more common in females, such as eating disorders, generalized anxiety and panic disorder.[76] There is also a preponderance of females compared with males who suffer from specific types of medical illnesses that have high rates of comorbid depression: thyroid disorders, rheumatological disorders, irritable bowel syndrome, fybromyalgia and migraine. Reference has been made in the relevant section to possible central 5-HT abnormalities in hypothyroidism and the relationship between this and depression.[55] One study has examined [³H]imipramine binding uptake, as a biochemical indicator of 5-HT uptake, in women with fibromyalgia.[77] [³H]imipramine binding was found to be lower in women with fibromyalgia than in depressed women, suggesting a relative reduction of 5-HT function in the women with fibromyalgia. There is also evidence suggesting 5-HT dysfunction in migraine and irritable bowel syndrome.

There are differences in clinical characteristics between depressions associated with other psychiatric disorders and those associated with medical illnesses. Patients with depressions in association with psychiatric illnesses have an earlier age of onset, are more likely to have suicidal thoughts and to have attempted suicide, are less likely to have memory problems, are less improved with treatment and are more likely to relapse on follow-up than patients with depressions associated with medical illnesses.[75] Overall, however, patients with comorbid disorders have a less successful treatment outcome and a protracted 1-year course compared with those who have uncomplicated depressions.[78]

Treatment of unipolar depression in women
Pharmacotherapies

It is now well established that depression is not a single disorder, with a universal treatment.

Psychotic depression and atypical depression respond preferentially to different pharmacotherapies than MDD. Atypical depression responds better to monoamine oxidase inhibitors (MAOIs) than to tricyclic antidepressants (TCAs).[79] This may be particularly relevant to depression in women, since there is a preponderance of women suffering from atypical symptoms. MAOIs should also be used to treat depression with comorbid panic disorder in women. It has been shown that women with this dual diagnosis respond better to MAOIs than TCAs, whereas the reverse is true for men with these diagnoses.[79] Thyroid therapy can be a useful adjunct for the treatment of depression in women, and this has been discussed in the relevant section earlier in this chapter.

There is evidence to suggest that depression in women may be more responsive to selective serotonin reuptake inhibitors (SSRIs) than to TCAs.[71] This may be due to reduced responsivity of depression in women to TCAs.[80] It may also be related to female-specific 5-HT dysfunction in depression. Interestingly, depression in the premenstrum responds to SSRIs (see Chapter 16) and has been demonstrated in several studies to preferentially respond to SSRIs than to noradrenergic reuptake inhibitors.[81] In relation to this, SSRIs are more effective than TCAs in treating depression in premenopausal years, yet in postmenopausal years this advantage is lost.[72] This suggests that abnormalities of 5-HT neurotransmission, related to sex steroids, may be a shared vulnerability trait for PMD and MDD.

Long-term studies (5 years) indicate that, following response to antidepressant medication, maintenance therapy with a high dose continues to provide a significant prophylactic advantage compared with placebo or low-dose maintenance therapy in both men and women.[82]

Pharmacokinetics

There are few studies investigating gender differences in pharmacodynamics. This is partly the result of exclusion of fertile women from many drug trials. The scant literature suggests that there are differences in absorption, distribution and metabolism of psychotropic drugs and that these factors should be taken into account when treating depression in women (see also Chapter 29). Elderly women consume more psychotropic drugs than other groups, and there is some evidence that elderly women also experience more adverse drug reactions.

Distribution of drug differs between men and women because of the increased ratio of body fat to muscle in women, compared with men.[83] An increased proportion of body fat can increase the volume of distribution. Clearance of a drug is increased as volume of distribution is increased. The ratio of fat to muscle increases with age in women, going from an average of 33% in younger subjects to 48% in the old, versus 18% to 36% in men. This increases the half-life of lipid-soluble drugs in women compared with men: a trend that exaggerates as the population ages.

Women may have reduced secretion of gastric acid compared with men and reduced rates of gastric emptying.[84] Gastrointestinal transit time is influenced by levels of female sex hormones. Oestrogen and progesterone prolong gastric emptying, particularly of liquids. During the menstrual cycle, gastric transit time is maximal at peak progesterone phases.[84]

There are some inconsistent reports of gender differences in liver enzyme systems and one report of altered activity of the P450 isoenzymes throughout the menstrual cycle.[85,86] The isoenzyme CYP 2D6 is responsible for the metabolism of many of the commonly used psychotropic drugs. The limited data available suggest that there are no gender- or age-associated differences in this isoenzyme.[87] CYP 3A4 comprises 60% of the liver's total P450 content and metabolizes most clinically important medications. The activity of this isoenzyme may be greater in young women than in men and may decrease in women with age.[87] This could render the half-lives of triazolam and alprazolam shorter in young women, thereby increasing their addictive liabilities, and increase the side-effect profiles of medications metabolized by CYP 3A4 in elderly women.

Sex steroids alter the activity of the monoamine oxidase enzymes: oestrogen inhibits monoamine oxidase activity, whereas progesterone increases it.[86] Lithium levels have been reported to alter throughout the menstrual cycle but this does not seem to be true for most women.[86] Oral contraceptives have been demonstrated to affect the metabolism of antidepressants and benzodiazepines.[87] There are three negative reports of gender differences in TCA levels, and one that found women had higher levels than men.[88]

These data point to gender differences in the pharmacokinetics of antidepressants, and this is supported by clinical studies demonstrating increased sensitivity to side-effects of TCAs in women compared with men.[71,80] The SSRIs may also be more effective than the TCAs in treating depression in women. Taken together, this suggests that SSRIs should be chosen in preference to the TCAs for the treatment of depression in women.

Psychotherapy

There is scientific research now supporting the long-held belief that psychotherapy is an effective treatment for depression only if neurobiological disturbance is not marked. Specific biological symptoms that have been shown to predict a poor response to psychotherapy are HPA axis overdrive and abnormal sleep profiles.[89,90] Thase et al examined the predictive value of pretreatment sleep EEG profiles in 91 patients who received short-term interpersonal psychotherapy (IPT) and found that subjects with abnormal sleep profiles had significantly poorer clinical outcomes.[89] Seventy-five per cent of the patients who failed to respond to IPT went on to respond to pharmacotherapy. Controlled trials have shown that patients who fail to suppress cortisol following dexamethasone have a poorer response to cognitive-behavioural therapy (CBT) than suppressors.[91]

The time-limited therapies, such as CBT and IPT, have been demonstrated to be effective in treating depression in women (see Chapter 30). One study has compared responses to CBT in depressed men and women.[91] Overall, men and women had generally similar outcomes after a 16-week course of CBT, although men attended fewer appointments than women. Patients with more severe depressive symptomatology had significantly poorer outcomes but, within this subgroup, men were significantly more likely to respond than women. This latter finding may be related to the overall poorer response that depressed patients, with marked biological symptoms, have to CBT. This is also true of depression in the postpartum period: severe depression with psychotic features will not respond to CBT, but moderate depression responds to either pharmacotherapy or CBT.[92] There is a suggestion, from one study, that patients with high pretreatment depression scores may respond better to IPT than to CBT.[93]

Combined interpersonal psychotherapy and pharmacotherapy

As stated above, large-scale studies now indicate that patients suffering from depression characterized by marked biological symptoms tend to respond less well to psychotherapy than those with milder forms of depression.[89] Clinical trials in the more severe forms of unipolar depression suggest that a further treatment advantage can be gained by combining IPT with pharmacotherapy.[82] A 3-year maintenance trial in 128 patients with recurrent depression demonstrated superiority of combined imipramine and IPT over either imipramine or IPT alone.[82]

A 16-week trial comparing responses to combined imipramine and IPT in 50 men and 180 depressed women demonstrated that men were significantly more likely to show a rapid and sustained clinical response than women.[80] The authors hypothesize that females suffering from depression are slower to respond than comparable males because women may require both pharmacotherapy and the slower-acting psychotherapy for complete recovery. This may be an indicator that depression is more interpersonally bound in women than men. The importance of IPT alone, i.e. without pharmacotherapy, in maintaining remission in severe unipolar depression has now been demonstrated.

A study by Spanier et al examined the relationship between the quality of IPT and delta sleep ratios on the length of survival time to recurrence among patients with recurrent unipolar depression over a 3-year period.[94] A high delta sleep ratio was the most specific sleep EEG marker found to be associated with improved outcome in previous studies by this group. They found that, even in those individuals with a low delta sleep ratio, 44% survived the 3-year period without relapse when given monthly IPT of high quality, whereas none of those with this biological marker not given IPT survived.

These studies suggest that although pharmacotherapy is necessary for treatment response in severe depression characterized by marked disturbance of central nervous system arousal, IPT may also be necessary in the acute phase of treatment, especially in women. Combined pharmacotherapy and IPT is superior to pharmacotherapy alone in maintaining remission, and IPT alone may sustain remission, even in those with biological vulnerability for recurrence.

Conclusions

Epidemiological research has established that unipolar depression is about twice as common in women as in men. This is a universal finding and thus cannot be explained by socio-political factors alone, although some development risk factors for depression in adulthood, such as childhood sexual abuse, are universally more common in females than in males. Any model attempting to account for this gender difference in depression must integrate gender differences from the socio-political, through developmental, through personality/behavioural, through life-cycle and experiences, through endocrine to biological differences in brain function. Clearly some biological drives are gender-specific, and it appears to be in the arena of the female-specific role that risk factors for women reside. Women who have not been mothered adequately are vulnerable to developing depression in adulthood. Women are at risk of developing time-limited depressive episodes related to their menstrual cycles and are at their highest lifetime risk of developing depression postnatally. These seemingly endocrine-related depressions can be part of a pattern of unipolar or recurrent depression or can herald the onset of a relapsing disorder. There is convincing evidence that there are specific sex steroid triggers that account for some of the more serious postpartum depressions, which are part of a more general pattern of lifelong affective disorder.

Other biological differences between women and men have not received the same attention as the sex steroids. This is particularly true of gender differences in stress responses and of how these differences may alter the propensity to develop abnormal stress responses: a model for MDD. Although it is now established that there are gender differences in 5-HT function, little attention has been paid to gender differences in glucocorticoid/5-HT interactions. Another endocrine axis that has a profound effect on mood and has marked gender differences in function is the thyroid axis. Dysfunction of this axis in relation to female depression has not been explored systematically.

The most striking sex difference in the presentation and course of depression is the preponderance of comorbidity and the severity of depression in women, compared with men. There has been little systematic research on gender differences in relation to treatment response in women, but there is some evidence indicating that women may respond better to SSRIs than to TCAs. CBT is only an effective therapeutic tool in depressed women when they are not severely depressed. IPT may be a more useful form of psychotherapy in women in the acute phase of treatment, and has been demonstrated to be effective in maintaining remission. Combined IPT and pharmacotherapy is the most effective prophylactic treatment strategy.

References

1. Kessler RC, McGonagle KA, Swartz M et al, Sex and depression in the National Comorbidity Survey I: Lifetime prevalence, chronicity and recurrence, *J Affect Disord* 1993; **29**:85–96.
2. Kessler RC, McGonagle KA, Nelson CB et al, Sex and depression in the National Comorbidity Survey: II. Cohort effects, *J Affect Disord* 1994; **30**:15–26.
3. Ernst C, Angst J, The Zurich Study. XII. Sex differences in depression. Evidence from longitudinal epidemiological data, *Eur Arch Psychiatry Clin Neurosci* 1992; **241**:222–30.
4. Young MA, Fogg LF, Scheftner WA et al, Sex differences in the lifetime prevalence of depression: does varying the diagnostic criteria reduce the male/female ratio? *J Affect Disord* 1990; **18**:187–92.
5. Weissman MM, Olfson M, Depressions in women: implications for healthcare research, *Science* 1995; **269**:799–801.
6. Kendler KS, Neale MC, Kessler RC et al, A longitudinal twin study of 1-year prevalence of major depression in women, *Arch Gen Psychiatry* 1993; **50**:843–52.
7. Kendler KS, Neale MC, Kessler RC et al, The lifetime history of major depression in women: reliability of diagnosis and heritability, *Arch Gen Psychiatry* 1993; **50**:863–70.
8. Kendler KS, Kessler RC, Walters EE et al, Stressful life events, genetic liability, and onset of an episode of major depression in women, *Am J Psychiatry* 1995; **152**:833–42.
9. Lynn R, Martin T, Gender differences in extraversion, neuroticism, and psychoticism in 37 nations, *J Soc Psychol* 1997; **137**:369–73.
10. Kendler KS, Neale MC, Kessler RC et al, A longitudinal twin study of personality and major depression in women, *Arch Gen Psychiatry* 1993; **50**:853–62.
11. Duggan CF, Sham P, Lee AS, Murray RM, Does recurrent depression lead to a change in neuroticism? *Psychol Med* 1991; **21**:985–90.
12. Duggan C, Sham P, Lee A et al, Neurotocism: a vulnerability marker for depression: evidence from a family study, *J Affect Disord* 1995; **35**:139–43.
13. Duggan CF, Lee AS, Murray RM, Do different subtypes of hospitalized depressives have different long-term outcomes? *Arch Gen Psychiatry* 1991; **48**:308–12.
14. Power MJ, Duggan CF, Lee AS, Murray RM,

Dysfunctional attitudes in depressed and recovered depressed patients and their first-degree relatives, *Psychol Med* 1995; **25**:87–93.

15. Bolger N, Schilling EA, Personality and the problems of everyday life: the role of neuroticism in exposure and reactivity to daily stressors, *J Pers* 1991; **59**:355–86.

16. Coccaro EF, Siever LJ, Klar HM et al, Serotonergic studies in patients with affective and personality disorders: Correlates with suicidal and impulsive aggressive behaviour, *Arch Gen Psychiatry* 1989; **46**:587–99.

17. Jakubaschk J, Hubschmid T, Aggression and depression—a reciprocal relationship? *Eur J Psychiatry* 1994; **8**:69–80.

18. McMahon RC, Tyson D, Personality factors in transient versus enduring depression among inpatient alcoholic women: a preliminary analysis, *J Per Disord* 1990; **4**:150–60.

19. Seligman MEP, *Helplessness: on Depression, Development and Death* (WH Freeman: San Francisco, 1975).

20. Oakley Browne MA, Joyce PR, Wells JE et al, Disruptions in childhood parental care as risk factors for major depression in adult women, *Aust NZ J Psychiatry* 1995; **29**:437–48.

21. Oakley-Browne MA, Joyce PR, Wells JE et al, Adverse parenting and other childhood experience as risk factors for depression in women aged 18–44 years, *J Affect Disord* 1995; **34**:13–23.

22. Garnefski N, Van Egmond M, Straatman A, The influence of early and recent life stress on severity of depression, *Acta Psychiatr Scand* 1990; **81**:295–301.

23. Swanston HY, Tebbutt JS, O'Toole BI, Oates RK, Sexually abused children 5 years after presentation: a case-control study, *Pediatrics* 1997; **100**:600–8.

24. Whiffen VE, Clarke SE, Does victimization account for sex differences in depressive symptoms? *Br J Clin Psychol* 1997; **36**:185–93.

25. Carmen EH, Reiker PP, Mills T, Victims of violence and psychiatric illness, *Am J Psychiatry* 1984; **141**:378–83.

26. Jacobson A, Richardson B, Assault experiences of 100 psychiatric inpatients: evidence of the need for routine inquiry, *Am J Psychiatry* 1987; **144**:908–13.

27. Dohrenwend BP, Levav I, Shrout PE et al, Socioeconomic status and psychiatric disorders: the causation–selection issue, *Science* 1992; **255**:946–52.

28. Brown GW, Harris TO, *The Social Origins of Depression: a Study of Psychiatric Disorders in Women* (Tavistock: London, 1987).

29. Kendler KS, Kessler RC, Neale MC et al, The prediction of major depression in women: toward an integrated etiologic model, *Am J Psychiatry* 1993; **150**:1139–48.

30. Wieck A, Hirst AD, Kumar R et al, Growth hormone secretion by human females in response to apomorphine challenge is markedly affected by menstrual cycle phase, *Br J Clin Pharmacol* 1989; **27**:700–1.

31. Wieck A, Kumar R, Hirst AD et al, Increased sensitivity of dopamine receptors and recurrence of affective psychosis after childbirth, *Br Med J* 1991; **303**:613–16.

32. Meakin CJ, Brockington IF, Lynch S, Jones SR, Dopamine supersensitivity and hormonal status in puerperal psychosis, *Br J Psychiatry* 1995; **166**:73–9.

33. Abel KM, O'Keane V, Sherwood RA, Murray RM, Plasma homovanillic acid profile at different phases of the ovulatory cycle in healthy women, *Biol Psychiatry* 1996; **39**:1039–43.

34. Dalton K, Green R, The premenstrual syndrome, *Br Med J* 1953; **1**:1007–13.

35. Dinan TG, O'Keane V, The premenstrual syndrome: a psychoneuroendocrine perspective. In: Grossman A, ed. *Clinical Endocrinology and Metabolism: Psychoneuroendocrinology* (Ballière-Tindall: London, 1991) 143–67.

36. Harris B, Lovett L, Smith J et al, Cardiff puerperal mood and hormone study: III. Postnatal depression at 5 to 6 weeks postpartum, and its hormonal correlates across the peripartum period, *Br J Psychiatry* 1996; **168**:739–44.

37. Bearn JA, Fairhall KM, Robinson IC et al, Changes in a proposed new neuroendocrine marker of oestrogen receptor function in postpartum women, *Psychol Med* 1990; **20**:779–83.

38. Murray D, Cox JL, Chapman G, Jones P, Childbirth: life event or start of a long-term difficulty? Further data from the Stoke-on-Trent controlled study of postnatal depression, *Br J Psychiatry* 1995; **166**:595–600.

39. Fossey L, Papiernik E, Bydlowski M, Postpartum blues: a clinical syndrome and pre-

dictor of postnatal depression? *J Psychosom Obstet Gynaecol* 1997; **18**:17–21.

40. Pop VJ, Essed GG, de Geus CA et al, Prevalence of postpartum depression—or is it post-puerperium depression? *Acta Obstet Gynecol Scand* 1993; **72**:354–8.

41. Dinan TG, Glucocorticoids and the genesis of depressive illness: a psychobiological model, *Br J Psychiatry* 1994; **164**:365–71.

42. APA Task Force on Laboratory Tests in Psychiatry, The dexamethasone suppression test: an overview of its current status in psychiatry, *Am J Psychiatry* 1987; **144**:1253–62.

43. Jeffcoate WJ, Silverstone JT, Edwards CR, Besser GM, Psychiatric manifestations of Cushing's syndrome: response to lowering of plasma cortisol, *Quart J Med* 1979; **48**:465–72.

44. Price LH, Malison RT, McDougle CJ et al, Antiglucocorticoids as treatments for depression, *CNS Drugs* 1996; **5**:311–20.

45. Magiakou MA, Mastorakos G, Rabin D et al, Hypothalamic corticotropin-releasing hormone suppression during the postpartum period: implications for the increase in psychiatric manifestations at this time, *J Clin Endocrinol Metab* 1996; **81**:1912–17.

46. Magiakou MA, Mastorakos G, Webster E, Chrousos GP, The hypothalamic–pituitary–adrenal axis and the female reproductive system, *Ann NY Acad Sci* 1997; **816**:42–56.

47. Holsboer F, Lauer CJ, Schreiber W, Krieg JC, Altered hypothalamic–pituitary–adrenocortical regulation in healthy subjects at high familial risk for affective disorders, *Neuroendocrinology* 1995; **62**:340–7.

48. Redei E, Freeman EW, Preliminary evidence for plasma adrenocorticotropin levels as biological correlates of premenstrual symptoms, *Acta Endocrinol* 1993; **128**:536–42.

49. Rabin DS, Schmidt PJ, Cambell G et al, Hypothalamic–pituitary–adrenal function in patients with the premenstrual syndrome, *J Clin Endocrinol Metab* 1990; **71**:1158–62.

50. Bjorntorp P, Neuroendocrine abnormalities in human obesity, *Metabolism* 1995; **44**:38–41.

51. Cleare AJ, Bearn J, Allain T et al, Contrasting neuroendocrine responses in depression and chronic fatigue syndrome, *J Affect Disord* 1995; **34**:283–9.

52. De Bellis MD, Chrousos GP, Dorn LH et al, Hypothalamic–pituitary–adrenal axis dysregulation in sexually abused girls, *J Clin Endocrinol Metab* 1994; **78**:249–55.

53. Haggerty JJ, Evans DL, Golden RN et al, The presence of anti-thyroid antibodies in patients with affective and non-affective psychiatric disorders, *Biol Psychiatry* 1990; **27**:51–6.

54. Jain VK, A psychiatric study of hypothyroidism, *Psychiatr Clin* 1972; **5**:121–30.

55. Cleare AJ, McGregor A, Chambers SM et al, Thyroxine replacement increases central 5-hydroxytryptamine activity and reduces depressive symptoms in hypothyroidism, *Neuroendocrinology* 1996; **64**:65–9.

56. Calloway SP, Dolan RJ, Fonagy P et al, Endocrine changes and clinical profiles in depression: II. The thyrotropin-releasing hormone test, *Psychol Med* 1984; **14**:759–65.

57. Harris B, Othman S, Davies JA et al, Association between postpartum thyroid dysfunction and thyroid antibodies and depression, *Br Med J* 1992; **305**:152–6.

58. Pop VJ, De Rooy HA, Vader LH et al, Postpartum thyroid dysfunction and depression in an unselected population, *N Engl J Med* 1991; **324**:1815–16.

59. Schmidt PJ, Grover GN, Roy-Byrne PP et al, Thyroid function in women with premenstrual syndrome, *J Clin Endocrinol Metab* 1993; **76**:671–74.

60. O'Keane V, Dynamic serotonin neuroendocrine challenges in depressive disorders: what have we learnt? *J Serotonin Res* 1994; **1**:101–11.

61. O'Keane V, Dinan TG, Prolactin and cortisol responses to d-fenfluramine in major depression: evidence for diminished responsivity of central serotonergic function, *Am J Psychiatry* 1991; **148**:1009–15.

62. Deakin JF, Pennell I, Upadhyaya AJ, Lofthouse R, A neuroendocrine study of 5-HT function in depression: evidence for biological mechanisms of endogenous and psychosocial causation, *Psychopharmacology* 1990; **101**:85–92.

63. Kennett GA, Chaouloff F, Marcou M, Curzon G, Female rats are more vulnerable than males in an animal model of depression: the possible role of serotonin, *Brain Res* 1986; **382**:416–21.

64. Kennett GA, Dickinson SL, Curzon G, Enhancement of some 5-HT-dependent behavioural responses following repeated immobilisa-

tion in rats, *Brain Res* 1985; **330**:253–63.

65. Kant GJ, Lenox RH, Bunnell BN et al, Comparison of stress response in male and female rats: pituitary cyclic AMP and plasma prolactin, growth hormone and corticosterone, *Psychoneuroendocrinology* 1983; **8**:421–8.

66. McEwen BS, Glucocorticoid–biogenic amine interactions in relation to mood and behaviour, *Biochem Pharmacol* 1987; **36**:1755–63.

67. O'Keane V, McLoughlin D, Dinan TG, d-Fenfluramine-induced prolactin and cortisol release in major depression: response to treatment, *J Affect Disord* 1992; **26**:143–50.

68. Biegon A, Bercovitz H, Samuel D, Serotonin receptor concentration during the estrous cycle of the rat, *Brain Res* 1980; **187**:221–5.

69. O'Keane V, O'Hanlon M, Webb M, Dinan TG, d-Fenefluramine/prolactin responses throughout the menstrual cycle: evidence for an oestrogen-induced alteration, *Clin Endocrinol* 1991; **34**:289–92.

70. McBride PA, Tierney H, De Meo M et al, Effects of age and gender on CNS serotonergic responsivity in normal adults, *Biol Psychiatry* 1990; **27**:1143–55.

71. Kornstein SG, Schatzberg AF, Yonkers KA et al, Gender differences in presentation of chronic major depression, *Psychopharmacol Bull* 1995; **31**:711–18.

72. Young MA, Scheftner WA, Fawcett J, Klerman GL, Gender differences in the clinical features of unipolar major depressive disorder, *J Nerv Ment Dis* 1990; **178**:200–3.

73. Jorm AF, Sex and age differences in depression: a quantitative synthesis of published research, *Aust NZ J Psychiatry* 1987; **21**:46–53.

74. Simpson HB, Nee JC, Endicott J, First-episode major depression: few sex differences in course, *Arch Gen Psychiatry* 1997; **54**:633–9.

75. Winokur G, Black DW, Nasrallah A, Depressions secondary to other psychiatric disorders and medical illnesses, *Am J Psychiatry* 1988; **145**:233–7.

76. Van-Valkenburg C, Winokur G, Behar D, Lowry M, Depressed women with panic attacks, *J Clin Psychiatry* 1984; **45**:367–9.

77. Kravitz HM, Katz R, Kot E et al, Biochemical clues to a fibromyalgia–depression link: imipramine binding in patients with fibromyalgia or depression and in healthy controls, *J*

Rheumatol 1992; **19**:1428–32.

78. Keitner GI, Ryan CE, Miller IW et al, 12-Month outcome of patients with major depression and comorbid psychiatric or medical illness (compound depression), *Am J Psychiatry* 1991; **148**:345–50.

79. Davidson J, Pelton S, Forms of atypical depression and their response to antidepressant, *Psychiatry Res* 1986; **17**:87–95.

80. Frank E, Carpenter LL, Kupfer DJ, Sex differences in recurrent depression: are there any that are significant? *Am J Psychiatry* 1988; **145**:41–5.

81. Eriksson E, Hedberg MA, Andersch B, Sundblad C, The serotonin reuptake inhibitor paroxetine is superior to the noradrenaline reuptake inhibitor maprotiline in the treatment of premenstrual syndrome, *Neuropsychopharmacology* 1995; **12**:167–76.

82. Kupfer DJ, Frank E, Perel JM et al, Five-year outcome for maintenance therapies in recurrent depression, *Arch Gen Psychiatry* 1992; **49**:769–73.

83. MacLeod SM, Soldin JJ, Determinants of drug distribution in man, *Clin Biochem* 1986; **19**:67–71.

84. Wald A, Van Thiel DH, Hoechstetter L et al, Gastrointestinal transit: the effect of the menstrual cycle, *Gastroenterology* 1981; **80**:1497–500.

85. Schmucker DL, Woodhouse KW, Wang RK et al, Effects of age and gender on in vitro properties of human liver microsomal monooxygenases, *Clin Pharmacol Ther* 1990; **48**:365–74.

86. Pajer K, New strategies in the treatment of depression in women, *J Clin Psychiatry* 1995; **56**(suppl 2):30–7.

87. Pollock BG, Perel JM, Altieri LP et al, Debrisoquine hydroxylation phenotyping in geriatric psychopharmacology, *Psychopharmacol Bull* 1992; **28**:163–8.

88. Preskorn SH, Mac DS, Plasma levels of amitriptyline: effect of age and sex, *J Clin Psychiatry* 1985; **46**:276–7.

89. Thase ME, Buysse DJ, Frank E et al, Which depressed patients will respond to interpersonal psychotherapy? *Am J Psychiatry* 1997; **154**:502–9.

90. Thase ME, Dube S, Bowler K et al, Hypothalamic–pituitary–adrenocortical activity

and response to cognitive behaviour therapy in unmedicated, hospitalised depressed patients, *Am J Psychiatry* 1996; **153**:886–91.

91. Thase ME, Reynolds CF, Frank E et al, Do depressed men and women respond similarly to cognitive behaviour therapy? *Am J Psychiatry* 1994; **151**:500–5.

92. Appleby L, Warner R, Whitton A, Faragher B, A controlled study of fluoxetine and cognitive-behavioural counselling in the treatment of postnatal depression, *Br Med J* 1997; **314**:932–6.

93. Elkin I, Shea MT, Watkins JT et al, National Institute of Mental Health Treatment of Depression Collaborative Research Programme: general effectiveness of treatment, *Arch Gen Psychiatry* 1989; **46**:971–82.

94. Spanier C, Frank E, McEachran AB et al, The prophylaxis of depressive episodes in recurrent depression following discontinuation of drug therapy: integrating psychological and biological factors, *Psychol Med* 1996; **26**:461–75.

9

Bipolar illness
Ellen Leibenluft

Introduction

A patient with bipolar illness presents, seeking psychiatric care. How should the patient's gender affect his or her assessment and treatment? The purpose of this chapter is to answer that question, from the perspective of the female patient.

Until recently the issue of gender differences in bipolar disorder has been relatively neglected. This neglect may have stemmed from the fact that, while major depressive disorder and dysthymia are both significantly more common in women than in men, bipolar disorder appears to have an approximately 1 : 1 gender ratio. Data from a recent epidemiological study show that the lifetime prevalence of mania is 1.7% in women and 1.8% in men.[1] However, while men and women are equally likely to meet criteria for bipolar disorder, a number of studies indicate that the course of the illness may vary by gender. Specifically, there is evidence that bipolar women may be more likely than bipolar men to develop a rapid cycling course; that, compared with bi-

polar men, bipolar women may be more likely to experience depression and less likely to experience mania; and that bipolar women may be more likely than bipolar men to experience dysphoric, rather than euphoric, mania. These observations highlight a fundamental difference between bipolar disorder and major depressive disorder in terms of the role that gender plays in influencing lifetime risk and course. In the case of bipolar disorder, the lifetime prevalence of the illness does not vary between men and women, but there are gender differences in phenomenology and course. In the case of major depressive disorder, on the other hand, women are more likely than men to develop the illness, but the bulk of the evidence indicates that the course of the illness, and its symptoms, probably do not differ by gender[2,3] (see Chapters 1 and 2).

In bipolar disorder, a gender perspective is useful not only because the phenomenology and course of the illness differ by gender, but also because a bipolar woman's reproductive status can influence the course and treatment of her illness. Women with bipolar disorder are at high risk for developing severe, frequently psychotic, episodes in the postpartum period, a fact that influences their treatment during both the puerperium and pregnancy. The effects of other reproductive events (puberty, menstrual cycle, and menopause) on the course of bipolar illness have received less study, and should be the subject of future research. Women with bipolar illness are likely to have questions about these issues; in addition, given the explosion of research on the genetic underpinnings of bipolar disorder, they frequently inquire about the risk to their children of developing the illness. This, and other reproductive-related issues, will be reviewed below, after a discussion of gender differences in the phenomenology and course of bipolar disorder.

Gender differences in the phenomenology and course of bipolar disorder

Rapid cycling

Introduction
Dunner and Fieve first coined the term 'rapid-cycling bipolar disorder' in a 1974 paper describing patients in a lithium clinic who failed to respond to treatment.[4] The definition that they suggested continues to be used by researchers and clinicians today; it specifies that a patient with bipolar disorder is rapid cycling when he or she has four of more affective episodes in a year (an affective episode being one of hypomania, mania, or depression).[5]

The point prevalence of rapid cycling in research clinics for patients with bipolar disorder is approximately 20%.[4,6,7] However, rapid-cycling patients do not constitute a distinct subpopulation of bipolar disorder, since several longitudinal studies have shown that

only a minority of them continue to have four or more episodes per year in the 1–4 years after ascertainment.[6,8] Thus, bipolar patients go in and out of the 'pool' of rapid-cycling patients, and researchers have studied risk factors for entrance into this pool. While a number of possible risk factors have been examined (age of onset, clinical presentation, family history), only one has been consistently replicated: gender. That is, while exceptions exist, most studies show that bipolar women are approximately three times more likely than bipolar men to develop a rapid-cycling course.[9] This gender difference has been documented in samples of patients who were recruited because they were rapid cycling, as well as in post hoc gender analyses of samples of bipolar patients who were recruited irrespective of cycling frequency. In addition, data from two research clinics[10] (Leibenluft et al, unpublished data) show that the percentage of females in the sample increases with increased episode frequency, so that bipolar patients with more than 24 episodes in a year are almost exclusively female.

Why is rapid cycling more common in bipolar women than in bipolar men?
A number of hypotheses have been suggested to explain the observed gender difference in the prevalence of rapid-cycling bipolar disorder (RCBD). The question is important for at least two reasons. First, since rapid cycling is not a distinct subtype of bipolar disorder, it is probable that the mechanisms underlying mood cycling in women with RCBD are likely to be similar to those underlying mood cycling in other bipolar patients. Second, RCBD is an illness with significant morbidity, and an understanding of the pathogenesis of mood cycling in women with RCBD could pave the way for the development of new, and more effective, treatments.

Among several hypotheses that have been advanced to explain women's increased risk for rapid cycling, the one that has received the most attention posits that hypothyroidism predisposes bipolar patients to develop RCBD.[11] Since, in developed countries, hypothyroidism is more common in women than in men,[12] this hypothesis suggests that the overrepresentation of women in samples of patients with RCBD is secondary to women's increased risk for hypothyroidism. The two types of studies that are relevant to this hypothesis are those comparing the prevalence of hypothyroidism in rapid-cycling and non-rapid-cycling bipolar patients, and those testing the efficacy of exogenous thyroid hormone as a treatment for RCBD. The results of the former line of investigation have been mixed, with approximately half of the studies showing a positive result (see Leibenluft[9] for a compilation of the relevant studies). The interpretation of these data is complicated by the fact that most bipolar patients (and, in particular, most rapid-cycling bipolar patients) have had significant exposure to lithium, which can cause hypothyroidism. Thus, it would be important to control for sex, age and duration of lithium exposure in comparing the thyroid status of rapid-cycling and non-rapid-cycling bipolar patients, but the cumbersome nature of this design means that few studies are able to control for all these variables.

The second line of investigation, that testing the efficacy of exogenous thyroid hormone as a treatment for RCBD, has the advantage of an experimental design that allows for causal conclusions to be drawn. Five groups have reported case series or open trials in which hypermetabolic doses of levothyroxine were used successfully to dampen mood cycling in patients with RCBD.[13–17] In these trials, patients responded favourably irrespective of their pretreatment thyroid status.[13] A placebo-controlled, double-blind trial of high-dose levothyroxine in patients with RCBD is currently ongoing, and its results could have important theoretical and practical implications (Whybrow et al, unpublished data).

A second hypothesis to explain the overrepresentation of women in samples of patients with RCBD implicates the menstrual cycle in the pathogenesis of mood cycling. In at least one clinical population (i.e. women with premenstrual-phase dysphoric disorder), there is a systematic relationship between menstrual cycle and mood.[5] A similar phenomenon among bipolar women might account for the increased prevalence of rapid cycling in female, as opposed to male, bipolar patients. While cases have been described of premenopausal, bipolar women whose mood cycles were synchronized with their menstrual cycle,[18–20] only four studies have examined the question in samples of bipolar women.[21–24] Two of the studies were positive,[21,22] and two negative.[23,24] It is important to note that the two positive studies were retrospective (a methodology that can lead to false-positive findings[25]), while the two negative studies were prospective. In the most recent of these studies,[4] prospective daily mood ratings were obtained in a sample of 25 premenopausal women with RCBD for an average of 13 months, and no consistent relationship was found between menstrual cycle phase and mood. These data indicate that menstrual cycle-related mood changes are unlikely to account for the overrepresentation of women in samples of RCBD. However, they do not rule out other, more subtle ways in which gonadal steroids might be involved in the pathogenesis of mood cycling, such as through their organizational effects on the developing central nervous system. In addition, these data do not rule out the possibility that a subset of bipolar women exists whose mood cycles correspond to their menstrual cycles, and in whom exogenous gonadal steroids might have therapeutic effects.[26–29]

A third hypothesis to explain the increased prevalence of rapid cycling among female bipolar patients relates to gender differences in the use of, or response to, psychotropic medications. Although the data are somewhat controversial, most workers in the field believe that antidepressant medication can not only precipitate mania in bipolar patients, but can also accelerate mood cycles, i.e. cause, or exacerbate, rapid cycling.[30] As outlined below, there is some evidence that bipolar women have more frequent depressive episodes than bipolar men. Therefore, it is conceivable that bipolar women are more likely to take antidepressant medication, thereby increasing their risk for rapid cycling. To test one tenet of this hypothesis, we are currently conducting a study comparing the antidepressant exposure of bipolar men and women.

Alternatively, it is possible that the overrepresentation of women in samples of patients with RCBD results from gender difference in response to psychotropic medications. For example, there is some evidence that women may be more susceptible to the manicogenic (and perhaps, by extension, the cycle-accelerating) side-effects of antidepressants.[30–33] An untested, but also plausible, hypothesis is that women are less responsive than men to the mood-stabilizing effects of lithium. It is important to remember that the first published sample of patients with RCBD, in which two-thirds were female, consisted of non-responders in a lithium clinic.[4] One could speculate that lithium's mood-stabilizing effects may be, in at least some patients, partially counteracted by its thyrotoxic, and therefore mood-destabilizing, effects. Some studies indicate that women may be more sensitive than men to the thyrotoxic effects of lithium.[34,35] It is therefore possible that an increased prevalence of lithium-induced hypothyroidism in women decreases their responsiveness to the medication and puts them at greater risk for rapid cycling, especially in patients who are also prescribed antidepressant medication. A corollary of this hypothesis is that the current gender ratio among patients with RCBD might change with the increased use of other mood-stabilizing medications, such as valproate.

In sum, the observed gender difference in the prevalence of rapid cycling among bipolar patients has led to several intriguing (and not mutually exclusive) hypotheses that raise important questions about the mechanisms underlying mood cycling. Each of the hypotheses requires further amplification and testing. With respect to the hypothyroid hypothesis, for example, it would be important to explain the paradoxical finding that, while the increased prevalence of hypothyroidism in women in community samples results from gender differences in the prevalence of autoimmune thyroiditis, rapid-cycling patients in two research clinics have been found to have relatively low levels of thyroid autoantibodies[11], (Leibenluft et al, unpublished data). With respect to the gonadal steroid hypothesis, the absence of significant menstrually related mood changes in samples of rapid-cycling women makes a straightforward causal relationship unlikely; the challenge at this point is to develop other, testable hypotheses concerning the possible involvement of the hypothalamic–pituitary–gonadal axis in the pathophysiology of mood cycling in bipolar, and other, patients. Finally, the question of gender differences in treatment response, as well as in the prevalence of adverse side-effects, has received very little study in bipolar patients. Given the direct clinical relevance of such findings, this area would clearly bear further exploration.

Depressive symptomatology

In the general population, women are more likely than men to develop clinically significant depressive symptomatology, in the form of major depressive disorder or dysthymic disorder. Interestingly, there is also evidence that bipolar women may be more likely than bipolar men to experience clinically significant depressive symptomatology and a higher prevalence of dysphoric, as opposed to euphoric, mania. While the data here are more limited and mixed than those concerning the gender ratio among rapid-cycling patients, five of seven available studies show an increased risk of depressive symptomatology among women. In one study, for example, Roy-Byrne et al reported that bipolar women had more hospitalizations for depression, and more depressive episodes, than did bipolar men, while bipolar men had more hospitalizations for mania than did bipolar women.[36] Similarly, six of seven available studies show that women are overrepresented among patients with dysphoric, as opposed to euphoric, mania; the interpretation of these studies, however, is complicated by the use of a variety of definitions for dysphoric mania.[37]

We know little about why bipolar women may be at increased risk for depression and dysphoric mania. The question of why unipolar depression is more common in women than in men is itself a complex one; suggested hypotheses range from those centred on cultural or psychological issues to those focusing on hormonal systems such as the gonadal steroid or thyroid axes.[38] Any of these hypotheses may be relevant to the increase in depressive symptomatology that is observed in bipolar women, since the genetic or environmental influences that increase women's risk for depression generally may also be present in bipolar women, skewing the phenotypic expression of

their illness towards the depressive pole.

While depressive symptomatology appears to be more common in bipolar women than in bipolar men, completed suicide is more common in bipolar men, similar to gender differences in the population at large. A survey of all suicides completed in Finland in one year found that 58% ($N = 18$) of the victims with a diagnosis of bipolar disorder were male.[39] The increased suicide risk among bipolar men may be related to their increased risk for comorbid alcohol dependence (again, similar to the trends in the population at large); in the Finnish study, 56% of the male suicide victims, but none of the women, also met criteria for this diagnosis. Interestingly, male bipolar patients tended to commit suicide earlier in the course of their illness than female bipolar patients. In addition, the men were more likely than the women to have had a stressful life event in the week preceding their death (86% of the men versus 37% of the women), although many of those life events appeared to be related to the patient's pathological behaviour.[39]

Treatment implications

What are the treatment implications of these gender differences in the phenomenology and course of bipolar illness? Given the significant morbidity of rapid cycling, a focus on its prevention in bipolar patients, and particularly in bipolar women, is warranted. The hypotheses described above concerning the possible roles of hypothyroidism and/or antidepressant medication of the pathogenesis of RCBD suggest management strategies that might minimize the risk of rapid cycling in bipolar women, or decrease its morbidity.

As noted above, the hypothesis that hypothyroidism predisposes patients to cycle rapidly has led to the use of hypermetabolic doses of levothyroxine in the treatment of the disorder. While the efficacy of this treatment has not yet been demonstrated in a randomized clinical trial, many clinicians feel that it has utility in some treatment-resistant patients with RCBD. The literature indicates that it may be necessary to prescribe high doses of the hormone. For example, in a large clinical trial currently in progress, the patient's free T-4 is titrated to 150% of baseline (unless side-effects intervene), and in the most recent published study the doses used were 0.15–0.40 mg/day of levothyroxine.[13] The apparent need for such high doses raises important questions, both theoretical (are receptors already saturated at a lower dose?) and clinical. The latter centre on possible side-effects of chronic hyperthyroidism, such as osteoporosis and myocardial thickening.[40] A recent follow-up study, however showed that patients with RCBD treated with high-dose levothyroxine for a minimum of 18 months did not develop decreased bone density.[41] High-dose levothyroxine should be used in combination with mood-stabilizing medication, since it otherwise carries a risk of inducing mania.[13]

If antidepressants can precipitate, or exacerbate, rapid cycling, then the use of such medications should be avoided, if possible. If antidepressant use cannot be avoided, then it is advisable to use those antidepressants that have the lowest risk for this adverse effect. In practice, however, both of these seemingly straightforward recommendations are problematic. With respect to the first recommendation, an unfortunate aspect of the current psychopharmacology of bipolar disorder is that the 'first-line' mood stabilizers are all more effective at preventing and treating mania than they are at preventing and treating depression.[42,43] Thus, many rapid-cycling patients on valproic acid or lithium (and, in particular, many women with bipolar illness) experience relatively brief and

manageable hypomanic episodes, but severe, disabling and frequent depressive episodes. Unfortunately, the data for other possible mood stabilizers, including clozapine,[44] levothyroxine[13] and carbamazepine,[45] are similar. Recently, excitement has been generated by the suggestion that lamotrigine, an anticonvulsant now being tested as a possible mood-stabilizing medication in bipolar disorder, may be particularly effective in the treatment of bipolar depression.[46] If this contention is true, and if the medication causes neither hypomania nor rapid cycling, then it would be an important addition to the therapeutic armamentarium. The definitive answer to this question awaits the result of ongoing clinical trials. In addition, other new agents, such as gabapentin,[47] and risperidone,[48,49] may also hold promise as mood stabilizers, but their spectrum of efficacy is currently unclear. Risperidone has been reported to induce mania, particularly at high doses;[50] whether this observation is replicated, and whether the medication has antidepressant effects and/or effects on cycling frequency, remains to be determined.

With respect to the second recommendation (restrict antidepressant use to those agents that are least likely to cause rapid cycling), the literature offers the clinician limited guidance. Since rapid cycling may be a relatively infrequent side-effect, a large, longitudinal study would be required to ascertain the relative risk of the various medications for inducing rapid-cycling. Given that clinical trials of antidepressants are usually short term and often exclude bipolar patients, such data are lacking. Pooling data from a number of studies, Zornberg and Pope recently suggested that tricyclic antidepressants might be significantly more likely than serotonergic reuptake inhibitors to cause switches into mania.[42] Assuming that the mechanism of drug-induced rapid cycling resembles that of drug-induced mania (an assumption that has face validity but has never been tested), the use of tricyclic antidepressants should be avoided, wherever possible, in bipolar patients. Unfortunately, early reports that buproprion might be less likely than other antidepressants to induce hypomania or mania[51,52] have not been confirmed;[53] indeed, all of the available antidepressants have been reported to induce mania. However, one study did indicate that manic episodes induced by monoamine oxidase inhibitors or bupropion might be milder than those that arise spontaneously or are precipitated by tricyclic antidepressants or fluoxetine.[54]

For the clinician treating a rapid-cycling patient, the challenge is not only to prevent antidepressant-induced cycling, but to recognize it when it occurs. The clinician may view the cycle 'up' that usually occurs after the initiation of antidepressant medication as a positive therapeutic response; subsequent depressive episodes may be seen as relapses, without the recognition that they are occurring at greater frequency than before the antidepressant medication was started. Indeed, it is often difficult to detect a change in cycle frequency, because most patients have erratic, irregular cycles. For this reason, all rapid-cycling patients should be asked to maintain a longitudinal, prospective, daily mood log to facilitate both the recognition of antidepressant-induced cycling and the detection of positive treatment responses. Rapid cycling is, by definition, a longitudinal illness, and the clinician who depends solely on a cross-sectional mental status examination to assess treatment response may be misled.

Effects of the female reproductive cycle on the course of bipolar illness

Prevalence, phenomenology, and possible mechanisms

Any of the reproductive milestones in a woman's life—puberty, menarche, pregnancy, the puerperium, lactation, and/or the perimenopause or menopause—could have systematic effects on the symptomatology or course of bipolar illness. With the exception of the postpartum period (which will be discussed below), little is known about whether such effects exist. No information is available concerning the effects of puberty or the menarche on the onset or presentation of bipolar illness, although a recent upsurge of interest in bipolar illness among children and adolescents may mean that relevant studies will be forthcoming soon. As noted above, group data from samples of women with RCBD show no systematic relationship between menstrual cycle phase and mood in postpubertal, premenopausal women. However, these data do not rule out the possibility that such effects may exist in women with non-rapid-cycling bipolar disorder, or in a subgroup (but not the majority) of bipolar women.

Given the clinical importance of such information, it is remarkable how little is known about the course of bipolar illness during pregnancy, during the perimenopause, and after menopause. The one study of pregnant bipolar women indicates that pregnancy is not destabilizing to bipolar women.[55] With respect to the menopause, the two available studies (both retrospective) report either a worsening of mood cycling at that time,[7] or no psychiatric effect of the menopause.[31] It is worth noting that conjugated oestrogen in extremely high doses (e.g. over 4 mg/day) was reported to pre-cipitate rapid cycling in a postmenopausal woman with a history of treatment-resistant depression.[56] However, no systematic studies have examined the effects of hormone replace-ment therapy (or its absence) on the course of bipolar illness; such data would obviously be most welcome.

In contrast to these equivocal (or non-existent) data, it is clear that bipolar women are at high risk of experiencing an acute and, frequently psychotic, affective episode in the postpartum period. A number of studies have shown that approximately 50% of women who require psychiatric hospitalization postpartum are likely to ultimately fit diagnostic criteria for bipolar illness and, conversely, that women with a diagnosis of bipolar illness are at high risk of requiring psychiatric hospitalization postpartum. With regard to the former, a 7–14-year follow-up of women who had had their first psychotic episode within a year of parturition found that approximately half of the women who had recurrences fitted diagnos-tic criteria for bipolar illness.[57] With regard to the latter, Kendall et al found that the risk for psychiatric admission within 30 days of child-birth was 21.4% for women with manic-depressive illness, manic or circular, and 13.3% for women with manic-depressive ill-ness, depressed (the comparable risk for women with schizophrenia was 3.4%).[58] Similarly, Marks et al[59] found that 46% of women with a history of bipolar illness devel-oped a psychotic episode postpartum, while 19% developed a non-psychotic illness and 35% remained well (the comparable numbers for women with a history of major depressive disorder were 0, 29% and 71%, respectively). A number of authors have reported that the postpartum psychoses in bipolar women tend to be characterized by an extreme degree of cognitive disorganization.[60] It is also interesting

to note that the psychosocial risk factors asso-ciated with postpartum affective episodes in women without a prior psychiatric history, such as an unstable relationship with the baby's father, have no predictive value in the case of women with bipolar illness.[59]

The high prevalence of postpartum episodes in bipolar women may yield important clues to the pathophysiology of affective episodes in general; however, given the acuity of these episodes, the phenomenon is not readily acces-sible for study. Virtually all of the physiological systems that have been thought to play a role in the pathophysiology of bipolar disorder (that is, the hypothalamic–pituitary–adrenal axis, the hypothalamic–pituitary–thyroid axis, the hypothalamic–pituitary–gonadal axis, and the sleep–wake cycle) undergo massive pertur-bations in the postpartum period. The litera-ture on the possible physiological under-pinnings of puerperal mood disorders will be reviewed in detail elsewhere in this volume, but the sleep–wake cycle deserves special mention here because of the unique role that it may play in precipitating bipolar, and particularly manic, episodes.

Changes in the sleep–wake cycle are among the classic symptoms of bipolar illness, with patients experiencing severe insomnia when manic, and hypersomnia when depressed. In addition, a number of studies show that alter-ations in the timing and amount of a patient's sleep can influence his or her mood. Specifically, these studies indicate that sleep deprivation, particularly if it occurs in the sec-ond half of the night, can have an antidepres-sant effect or even, in the case of bipolar patients, precipitate mania.[61] The mechanism of this mood-altering effect remains unclear, although there is evidence that the increase in thyroid-stimulating hormone (TSH) secretion that results from sleep deprivation may be involved.[62] Whatever the mechanism of sleep deprivation's euphorigenic effect, sleep loss is probably an important mediator between stress and mood cycling in bipolar patients,[63] and patients frequently report that a manic or hypomanic episode began after their sleep was disrupted by late-night work or study, anxiety, or jet lag. In that context, therefore, it is important to remember that the arrival of an infant is probably the most common cause of severe, prolonged sleep disruption in premenopausal women. In fact, one study did find that disrupted sleep in late pregnancy predicted the development of postpartum blues.[64] Given its possible preventive implications, the role of sleep disruption in the pathogenesis of bipolar postpartum episodes warrants further investigation.

Treatment implications

For several reasons, the management of severe bipolar illness during pregnancy and the postpartum period can be quite problematic. Lithium, valproate and carbamazepine are all relatively contraindicated in pregnancy, although recent data indicate that the risk of severe cardiac malformations with first-trimester lithium exposure may not be as high as originally feared.[65] The situation is further complicated by the fact that both ethical and clinical considerations make it difficult to conduct controlled clinical trials, so the available data are anecdotal and quite limited.

The treatment of pyschiatric disorders during pregnancy and the puerperium is reviewed in detail elsewhere in this book, so only brief mention of the key issues will be made here. Treatment during pregnancy may be indicated either because of the patient's symptoms at that time, and/or in an attempt to prevent a postpartum episode. With regard to the former, we noted above that the magnitude of the problem is unknown, since the clinical course of bipolar illness during pregnancy has not been studied. With regard to the latter, there is evidence that treatment during pregnancy, and/or immediately after delivery, may prevent severe postpartum episodes in women with bipolar disorder.[66] Since the teratogenic risk of lithium is generally considered to be less than that of carbamazepine or valproate, the former is usually used as a mood stabilizer in pregnancy when antipsychotic or antidepressant medications do not suffice.[67] Recently, investigators have been testing the efficacy in bipolar patients of non-pharmacological interventions such as light therapy[68] and social rhythm therapy (a psychotherapy designed to stabilize mood by stabilizing the sleep–wake cycle and other daily rhythms).[69] If these interventions prove to be effective in non-pregnant bipolar patients, their utility in pregnant patients should certainly be explored.

During the postpartum period, the therapeutic challenges include the acuity of the clinical symptoms and the potential interference of pharmacotherapy with nursing (see Chapter 19). It should also be noted that the safety of both mother and child should be carefully monitored during postpartum psychosis, since it is not uncommon for mothers to develop homicidal ideation in the course of these episodes.[60]

Gender and genetics

Data from family, twin and adoption studies demonstrate that genetic factors play a significant role in determining an individual's risk for developing bipolar disorder.[70] Data from such studies indicate that a child who has one parent with bipolar illness (and one without) has an approximately 9% risk for developing the disorder, compared with a 1% risk in the population at large.[71] In applying these data, it is important to remember that the first episode of bipolar illness occurs before age 25 in approximately 50% of cases, and before age 50 in almost all.[71] Therefore, an offspring who has reached 35 years of age without experiencing an episode would have a risk for the illness that is significantly less than 9%.

Because the data indicate a relatively strong genetic component in the aetiology of bipolar illness, the search for gene(s) of risk has been quite active. In the course of these studies, some investigators have reported a parent-of-origin effect, that is, a differential risk to the offspring of developing the illness depending on the sex of the affected parent. Such parent-of-origin effects have been reported in several non-psychiatric illnesses, including deafness, diabetes, and some inherited cancers.[72–74]

At least four genetic mechanisms have been identified that can account for parent-of-origin effects: X linkage, genomic imprinting, mitochondrial inheritance, and trinucleotide repeat expansion. Genomic imprinting occurs when DNA from one parent is methylated (and hence deactivated) during gametogenesis.[75] Thus, for a paternally imprinted gene, only the maternal gene is expressed. This can lead to either increased or decreased transmission of the illness through the maternal line, depending on whether the gene in question is associated with increased or decreased risk. Mitochondrial DNA (mtDNA) is in much greater abundance in oocytes than in sperm, so diseases associated with mtDNA are inherited almost exclusively through the maternal line. There have been several case reports describing mtDNA mutations in patients with unipolar depression or bipolar illness.[76,77] Finally, trinucleotide repeat expansion has been found to occur in Huntington's disease and other neuropsychiatric illnesses.[78] In this genetic mutation, the number of trinucleotide repeats increases in subsequent generations, causing earlier age of onset

('anticipation') and increased disease severity. Anticipation has been reported in some pedigrees affected with bipolar illness.[79] Because the extent of the expansion depends partly on the gender of the affected parent, trinucleotide repeat expansion can also account for parent-of-origin effects.[78]

In bipolar illness, parent-of-origin effects have been studied using both phenotypic and genotypic analyses. Pedigrees must be carefully selected for unilinearity, since the high rates of assortative mating among individuals with affective illness means that probands frequently have affected relatives on both sides. Reporting on a series of 31 unilineal families, McMahon et al,[80] reported a higher than expected frequency of transmitting mothers (63%), a 2.3–2.8-fold increased risk of illness of maternal relatives, and a 1.3–2.5-fold increased risk of illness for the offspring of affected mothers. In addition, in seven large pedigrees, the investigators noted exclusively maternal transmission. Gershon et al[81] replicated the finding of increased maternal transmission in bipolar pedigrees, although this group also reported pedigrees with exclusively paternal transmission. Grigoroiu-Serbanescu et al provided a partial replication, finding that mothers were more likely than fathers to transmit bipolar I illness to male, but not female, offspring.[82] However, Kato et al[83] used both prevalence and age of onset data from offspring and failed to find a parent-of-origin effect for bipolar illness.

Genotypic analyses of possible parent-of-origin effects began with early reports of linkage between bipolar illness and at least three sites on the X chromosome; however, each of these findings failed subsequent replication attempts. To date, the only putative linkage site that has been replicated in bipolar illness is in the pericentromeric region of chromosome 18, a locus that has been reported to demonstrate parent-of-origin effects.[84] Specifically, both Gershon et al[81] and Stine et al[84] have reported that linkage to chromosome 18 is evident only in families with paternal transmission.

Conclusion

In sum, gender does not affect an individual's risk for developing bipolar disorder. However, the gender of bipolar patients does influence the course of his or her illness, and it is possible that a bipolar patient's gender may affect his or her risk for passing the illness on to offspring. In addition, the female bipolar patient is at high risk of developing an affective episode after childbirth.

There is much that we don't know about gender and bipolar illness. Possible gender differences in the response to mood-stabilizing medications, or even to many antidepressants, have not been studied. As noted above, little is known about the effects of reproductive transitions, other than childbirth, on the course of bipolar illness. Adolescent bipolar disorder is

frequently difficult to treat, yet the impact of gender on its presentation or course is unknown. No data exist to guide the clinician who is trying to decide whether, or how, to treat a menopausal bipolar patient with exogenous hormones.

The literature on possible parent-of-origin effects has taught researchers about the importance of analysing genetic data by the sex of the proband and of the transmitting relatives. However, as our genetic studies become more sophisticated, they will be increasingly integrated with an environmental perspective. In that regard, it is interesting to note that some investigators have suggested that gender differences in responses to stress account for the increased prevalence of depression in women.[85] Studies of the relationship between stressful events and bipolar illness are limited, however, and few of them analyse their data by gender.[86] The questions of whether, and how, stress affects the penetrance and course of bipolar illness, and whether those effects differ by gender, should be fertile areas for future research.

References

1. Kessler RC, McGonagle KA, Zhao S et al, Lifetime and 12-month prevalence of DSM-III-R psychiatric disorders in the United States. Results from the national comorbidity survey, *Arch Gen Psychiatry* 1994; **51**:8–19.
2. Simpson HB, Nee JC, Endicott J, First-episode major depression. Few sex differences in course. *Arch Gen Psychiatry* 1997; **54**:633–9.
3. Zlotnick C, Shea MT, Pilkonis PA et al, Gender, type of treatment, dysfunctional attitudes, social support, life events, and depressive symptoms over naturalistic follow-up, *Am J Psychiatry* 1996; **153**:1021–7.
4. Dunner DL, Fieve RR, Clinical factors in lithium carbonate prophylaxis failure, *Arch Gen Psychiatry* 1974; **30**:229–33.
5. American Psychiatric Association, *Diagnostic and Statistical Manual of Mental Disorders, DSM:IV*, 4th edn (American Psychiatric Association: Washington DC, 1994) 390–7.
6. Coryell W, Endicott J, Keller M, Rapid cycling affective disorder. Demographics, diagnosis, family history, and course, *Arch Gen Psychiatry* 1992; **49**:126–31.
7. Kukopulos A, Reginaldi D, Laddomada P et al, Course of the manic-depressive cycle and changes caused by treatment, *Pharma-kopsychiatra* 1980; **13**:156–67.

8. Bauer MS, Calabrese J, Dunner DL et al, Multisite data reanalysis of the validity of rapid cycling as a course modifier for bipolar disorder in DSM-IV, *Am J Psychiatry* 1994; **151:** 506–15.

9. Leibenluft E, Women with bipolar illness: clinical and research issues, *Am J Psychiatry* 1996; **153:**163–73.

10. Bauer MS, Whybrow PC, Rapid cycling bipolar disorder: clinical features, treatment, and etiology. In: Tamminga CA, Schulz SC, eds, *Schizophrenia Research* (Raven Press: New York, 1991) 191–208.

11. Bauer MS, Whybrow PC, Winokur A, Rapid cycling bipolar affective disorder. I. Association with grade I hypothyroidism, *Arch Gen Psychiatry* 1990; **47:**427–32.

12. Tunbridge WMG, Evered DC, Hall R et al, The spectrum of thyroid disease in a community: the Whickham study, *Clin Endocrinol* 1997; 7:481–93.

13. Bauer MS, Whybrow PC, Rapid cycling bipolar affective disorder: II. Treatment of refractory rapid cycling with high-dose levothyroxine: a preliminary study, *Arch Gen Psychiatry* 1990; 47:435–40.

14. Gjessing L, Jenner A, *Contributions to the Somatology of Periodic Catatonia* (Pergamon Press: Oxford, 1976) 116–23.

15. Stancer HC, Persad E, Treatment of intractable rapid-cycling manic-depressive disorder with levothyroxine: clinical observations, *Arch Gen Psychiatry* 1982; 39:311–12.

16. Wakoh TF, Hatotani N, Endocrinological treatment of psychoses. In: Lissak K ed., *Hormones and Brain Function* (Plenum Press: New York, 1973) 491–8.

17. Weeston TF, Constantino J, High-dose T4 for rapid-cycling bipolar disorder, *J Am Acad Child Adolesc Psychiatry* 1996; 35:131–2.

18. Sothern RB, Slover GP, Morris RW, Circannual and menstrual rhythm characteristics in manic episodes and body temperature, *Biol Psychiatry* 1993; 33:194–203.

19. Endo M, Daiguji M, Asano Y et al, Periodic psychosis recurring in association with menstrual cycle, *J Clin Psychiatry* 1978; **39:** 456–61.

20. Brockington IF, Kelly A, Hall P, Deakin W, Premenstrual relapse of puerperal psychosis, *J Affect Disord* 1988; **14:**287–92.

21. Diamond SB, Rubinstein AA, Dunner DL, Fieve RR, Menstrual problems in women with primary affective illness, *Comp Psychiatry* 1976; **17:**541–8.

22. Price WA, DiMarzio L, Premenstrual tension syndrome in rapid-cycling bipolar affective disorder, *J Clin Psychiatry* 1986; **47:**415–17.

23. Wehr TA, Causes and treatments of rapid-cycling affective disorder. In: Amsterdam J, ed., *Pharmacotherapy of Depression: Applications for the Outpatient Practitioner* (Marcel Dekker: New York, 1990) 401–26.

24. Leibenluft E, Ashman SB, Feldman-Naim S, Yonkers KA, Lack of relationship between menstrual cycle phase and mood in women with rapid cycling bipolar disorder, *Biol Psychiatry* 1999; **46:**577–80.

25. Sampson JA, Prescott P, The assessment of the symptoms of premenstrual syndrome and their response to therapy, *Br J Psychiatry* 1981; **138:**399–405.

26. Yui K, The neuroendocrinological investigation of periodic psychosis at adolescence. In: Obiols J, Ballus C, Gonzalez-Monclus E et al, eds, *Biological Psychiatry Today* (Elsevier: Amsterdam, 1979) 746–52.

27. Matsunaga H, Sarai M, Elevated serum LH and androgens in affective disorder related to the menstrual cycle: with reference to polycystic ovary syndrome. *Jpn J Psychiatry Neurol* 1993; **47:**825–42.

28. Hatotani N, Kitayama I, Inoue K, Nomura J, Psychoendocrine studies of recurrent psychoses. In: Hatotani N, Nomura J, eds, *Neurobiology of Periodic Psychoses* (Igaku-Shoin: Tokyo, 1983) 77–92.

29. Price WA, Giannini AJ, Antidepressant effects of estrogen (ltr), *J Clin Psychiatry* 1985; **46:**506.

30. Wehr TA, Goodwin FK, Rapid cycling in manic-depressives induced by tricyclic antidepressants, *Arch Gen Psychiatry* 1979; **36:**555–9.

31. Wehr TA, Sack DA, Rosenthal NE, Cowdry RW, Rapid cycling affective disorder: contributing factors and treatment responses in 51 patients, *Am J Psychiatry* 1988; **145:**179–84.

32. Quitkin FM, Kane J, Rifkin A et al, Prophylactic lithium carbonate with and without imipramine for bipolar I patients. A double

blind study, *Arch Gen Psychiatry* 1981; **38:** 902–7.

33. Lewis JL, Winokur G, The induction of mania. A natural history study with controls, *Arch Gen Psychiatry* 1982; **39:**303–6.

34. Vincent A, Baruch P, Vincent P, Early onset of lithium-associated hypothyroidism, *J Psychiatry Neurosci* 1993; **18:**74–7.

35. Lee S, Chow CC, Wing YK, Shek CC, Thyroid abnormalities during chronic lithium treatment in Hong Kong Chinese: a controlled study, *J Affect Disord* 1992; **26:**173–8.

36. Roy-Byrne P, Post RM, Uhde TW et al, The longitudinal course of recurrent affective illness: life chart data from research patients at the NIMH, *Acta Psych Scand Suppl* 1985; **317:**1–34.

37. McElroy SL, Keck Jr PE, Pope Jr HG et al, Clinical and research implications of the diagnosis of dysphoric or mixed mania or hypomania, *Am J Psychiatry* 1992; **149:**1633–44.

38. Leibenluft E, Sex is complex, *Am J Psychiatry* 1996; **153:**969–72.

39. Isometsa E, Heikkinen M, Henriksson M et al, Recent life events and completed suicide in bipolar affective disorder. A comparison with major depressive suicides, *J Affect Disord* 1995; **33:**99–106.

40. Baran DT, Braverman LE, Thyroid hormones and bone mass, *J Clin Endocrinol Metab* 1991; **72:**1182–3.

41. Gyulai L, Jaggi J, Bauer MS et al, Bone mineral density and 1-thyroxine treatment in rapid cycling bipolar disorder, *Biol Psychiatry* 1997; **41:**503–6.

42. Zornberg GL, Pope Jr HG, Treatment of depression in bipolar disorder: new directions for research, *J Clin Psychopharmacol* 1993; **13:**397–408.

43. McElroy SL, Keck PE, Pope HG Jr, Hudson JI, Valproate in the treatment of bipolar disorder: literature review and clinical guidelines, *J Clin Psychopharmacol* 1992; **12:**42S–52S.

44. Zarate CA Jr, Tohen M, Baldessarini RJ, Clozapine in severe mood disorders, *J Clin Psychiatry* 1995; **56:**411–17.

45. Denicoff KD, Smith-Jackson EE, Disney ER et al, Comparative prophylactic efficacy of lithium, carbamazepine, and the combination in bipolar disorder, *J Clin Psychiatry* 1997;

58:470–8.

46. Calabrese JR, Fatemi SH, Woyshville MJ, Antidepressant effects of lamotrigine in rapid cycling bipolar disorder, *Am J Psychiatry* 1996; **153:**1236.

47. Schaffer CB, Schaffer LC, Gabapentin in the treatment of bipolar disorders, *Am J Psychiatry* 1997; **154:**291–2.

48. Tohen M, Zarate CA Jr, Centorrino F et al, Risperidone in the treatment of mania, *J Clin Psychiatry* 1996; **57:**249–53.

49. Hillert A, Maier W, Wetzel H, Benkert O, Risperidone in the treatment of disorders with a combined psychotic and depressive syndrome—a functional approach, *Pharmacopsychiatry* 1992; **25:**213–17.

50. Dwight MM, Keck Jr PE, Stanton SP et al, Antidepressant activity and mania associated with risperidone treatment of schizoaffective disorder, *Lancet* 1994; **344:**554–5.

51. Haykal RF, Akiskal HS, Bupropion as a promising approach to rapid cycling bipolar II patients, *J Clin Psychiatry* 1990; **51:**450–5.

52. Wright G, Galloway L, Kim J et al, Bupropion in the long-term treatment of cyclic mood disorders: mood stabilizing effects, *J Clin Psychiatry* 1985; **46:**22–5.

53. Sachs GS, Lafer B, Stoll AL et al, A double-blind trial of bupropion versus desipramine for bipolar depression, *J Clin Psychiatry* 1994; **55:**391–3.

54. Stoll AL, Mayer PV, Kolbrener M et al, Antidepressant-associated mania: a controlled comparison with spontaneous mania, *Am J Psychiatry* 1994; **151:**1642–5.

55. Lier L, Kastrup M, Rafaelsen OJ, Psychiatric illness in relation to pregnancy and childbirth II: diagnostic profiles and perinatal aspects, *Nordisk Psykiatrisk Tidsskrift* 1989; **43:**535–42.

56. Oppenheim G, A case of rapid mood cycling with estrogen: implications for therapy, *J Clin Psychiatry* 1984; **45:**34–5.

57. Videbech P, Gouliaev G, First admission with puerperal psychosis: 7–14 years of follow-up, *Acta Psychiatr Scand* 1995; **91:**167–73.

58. Kendell RE, Chalmers JC, Platz C, Epidemiology of puerperal psychoses, *Br J Psychiatry* 1987; **150:**662–73.

59. Marks MN, Wieck A, Checkley SA, Kumar R, Contribution of psychological and social factors to psychotic and non-psychotic relapse after child-

birth in women with previous histories of affective disorders, *J Affect Disord* 1992; **24**:253–63.

60. Wisner KL, Peindl K, Hanusa BH, Symptomatology of affective and psychotic illness related to childbearing, *J Affect Disord* 1994; **30**:77–87.

61. Wehr TA, Effects of sleep and wakefulness in depression and mania. In: Montplaisir J, Godbout R, eds, *Sleep and Biological Rhythms* (Oxford University Press: London, 1990) 42–86.

62. Sack DA, Rosenthal NE, Duncan WC et al, Early versus late partial sleep deprivation therapy of depression, *Acta Psychiatr Scand* 1988; **77**:219–24.

63. Wehr TA, Sack DA, Rosenthal NE, Sleep reduction as a final common pathway in the genesis of mania, *Am J Psychiatry* 1987; **144**:201–4.

64. Wilkie G, Shapiro CM, Sleep deprivation and the postnatal blues, *J Psychosomat Res* 1992; **36**:309–16.

65. Cohen LS, Friedman JM, Jefferson JW et al, A reevaluation of risk of in utero exposure to lithium, *J Am Med Assoc* 1994; **271**:146–50.

66. Cohen LS, Sichel DA, Robertson LM et al, Postpartum prophylaxis for women with bipolar disorder, *Am J Psychiatry* 1995; **152**:1641–5.

67. Altshuler LL, Cohen L, Szuba MP et al, Pharmacologic management of psychiatric illness during pregnancy: dilemmas and guidelines, *Am J Psychiatry* 1996; **153**:592–606.

68. Leibenluft E, Turner EH, Feldman-Naim S et al, Light therapy in patients with rapid cycling bipolar disorder: preliminary results, *Psychopharmacol Bull* 1995; **31**:705–10.

69. Frank E, Kupfer DJ, Ehlers CL et al, Interpersonal and social rhythm therapy for bipolar disorder: integrating interpersonal and behavioural approaches, *Behav Ther* 1994; **17**:143–9.

70. NIMH Genetics Initiative Bipolar Group, Genomic survey of bipolar illness in the NIMH genetics initiative pedigrees: a preliminary report, *Am J Med Genet* 1997; **74**:227–37.

71. Nurnberger JI, Berrettini WH, *Psychiatric Genetics* (Chapman & Hall Medical: London, 1998).

72. Kadowaki T, Kadowaki H, Mori Y et al, A subtype of diabetes mellitus associated with a mutation of mitochondrial DNA, *N Engl J Med* 1994; **330**:962–8.

73. Feinberg AP, Genomic imprinting and gene activation in cancer, *Nat Genet* 1993; **4**:110–13.

74. Prezant TR, Agapian JV, Bohlman MC et al, Mitochondrial ribosomal RNA mutation associated with both antibiotic-induced and non-syndromic deafness, *Nature Genet* 1993; **4**:289–94.

75. Hall JG, Genomic imprinting: review and relevance to human diseases, *Am J Hum Genet* 1990; **46**:857–73.

76. Ciafoaloni E, Shanske S, Apostolski S et al, Multiple deletions of mitochondrial DNA, *Neurol Suppl* 1991; **41**:207.

77. Suomalainen A, Majander A, Haltia M et al, Multiple deletions of mitochondrial DNA in several tissues of a patient with severe retarded depression and familial progressive external ophthalmoplegia, *J Clin Invest* 1992; **90**:61–6.

78. La Spada AR, Paulson HL, Fischbeck KH, Trinucleotide repeat expansion in neurological disease, *Ann Neurol* 1994; **36**:814–22.

79. McInnis MG, McMahon FJ, Chase GA et al, Anticipation in bipolar affective disorder, *Am J Hum Genet* 1993; **53**:385–90.

80. McMahon FJ, Stine OC, Meyers DA et al, Patterns of maternal transmission in bipolar affective disorder, *Am J Hum Genet* 1994; **56**:1277–86.

81. Gershon ES, Badner JA, Detera-Wadleigh SD et al, Maternal inheritance and chromosome 18 allele sharing in unilineal bipolar illness pedigrees, *Am J Med Genet* 1996; **67**:202–7.

82. Grigoroiu-Serbanescu M, Nothen M, Propping P et al, Clinical evidence for genomic imprinting in bipolar I disorder, *Acta Psychiatr Scan* 1995; **92**:365–70.

83. Kato T, Winokur G, Coryell W et al, Parent-of-origin effect in transmission of bipolar disorder, *Am J Med Genet* 1996; **67**:546–50.

84. Stine OC, Xu J, Koskela R et al, Evidence for linkage of bipolar disorder to chromosome 18 with a parent-of-origin effect, *Am J Hum Genet* 1995; **57**:1384–94.

85. Nolen-Hoeksema S, Responses to depression and their effects on the duration of depressive episodes, *J Abnorm Psychol* 1991; **100**:569–82.

86. Johnson SL, Roberts JE, Life events and bipolar disorder: implications from biological theories, *Psychol Bull* 1995; **117**:434–49.

10
Seasonal affective disorder
Alexander Neumeister and Siegfried Kasper

Seasonal rhythms of sleep, energy, anxiety and mood levels are found in depressed and non-depressed individuals; the rhythms are of a lower amplitude in the latter group. These findings are compatible with the assumption that seasonality is a dimension which spans the general population. Although seasonal depression was recorded by physicians in the era of Hippocrates (460?–365? BC), the effect of the physical environment on human behaviour has been neglected for centuries. In recent years, though, researchers, physicians and patients have shown an increasing interest in how seasonal variations can influence the course of some affective disorders. In addition, researchers and patients have been fascinated by the possibility of treating some depressed patients with light. Over the past 15 years, speculation and anecdotes have been bolstered by scientific inquiry. This chapter summarizes the current knowledge and what remains unclear about seasonal affective disorders.

Diagnostic assessment

The first set of diagnostic criteria for winter seasonal affective disorder (SAD) used the seasons as their point of reference.[1] Patients had to have depressive symptoms regularly during fall and winter and have the symptoms remit during spring and summer. Other psychiatric diagnoses and clear-cut psychosocial variables that could account for the seasonal variability in mood and behaviour had to be excluded. The DSM-III-R[2] introduced diagnostic criteria for mood disorders with seasonal patterns specifiers. These included recurrent depressive episodes which began and ended within a 60-day window of one another. In addition, the ratio of seasonal to non-seasonal depressions had to be at least 3 : 1. However, it was argued by some that these diagnostic criteria did not represent an advance on the original description. In the more recent DSM-IV, the diagnostic criteria for seasonal pattern specifier (Table 10.1) were again revised,[3] but further evaluation of the original[1] description in contrast with the DSM-IV criteria is required.[4]

Table 10.1 Criteria for SAD (seasonal pattern specifier).³

With seasonal pattern (can be applied to the pattern of major depressive episodes in bipolar I disorder, bipolar II disorder, or major depressive disorder, recurrent)

A. There has been a regular temporal relationship between the onset of major depressive episodes in bipolar I or bipolar II disorder or major depressive disorder, recurrent, and a particular time of the year (e.g. regular appearance of the major depressive episode in the fall or winter)

   Note: Do not include cases in which there is an obvious effect of seasonal-related psychosocial stressors (e.g. regularly being unemployed every winter)

B. Full remissions (or a change from depression to mania or hypomania) also occur at a characteristic time of the year (e.g. depression disappears in the spring)

C. In the last 2 years, two major depressive episodes have occurred that demonstrate the temporal seasonal relationships defined in criteria A and B, and no non-seasonal major depressive episodes have occurred during the same period

D. Seasonal major depressive episodes (as described above) substantially outnumber the non-seasonal major depressive episodes that may have occurred over the individual's lifetime

---

Emil Kraepelin was perhaps the first to suggest that behavioural changes seen in seasonal cases of manic depressive illness might represent an exaggeration of seasonal fluctuations that can also be observed in healthy people.[5] This concept has since been investigated, and it is now evident that behavioural and mood changes seen in patients with SAD during the winter, such as low energy level, overeating, weight gain, and hypersomnia, are also found in a certain percentage of normal subjects, albeit to a lesser degree.[6] Thus the propensity for seasonal fluctuations is a dimension which spans the population; SAD patients fall at one end of the spectrum, normal individuals without any seasonal changes fall at the other (Figure 10.1), and there are individuals that fall in between the two extremes with troublesome, albeit subsyndromal, SAD symptoms (S-SAD) (Table 10.2).

Goel et al found that two structured interviews—the Hypomania Interview Guide for Seasonal Affective Disorder (HIGH-SAD) and its successor, the Hypomania Interview Guide, Retrospective Assessment Version (HIGH-R)—are useful and valid for the assessment of non-depressed spring/summer mood states in patients with DSM-III-R or DSM-IV diagnoses of recurrent bipolar disorder or recurrent major depressive disorder, both with seasonal pattern.[7]

Clinical features

Characteristic symptoms of winter depression in patients with SAD are: changes in affect such as sadness, increased irritability and anxiety which are usually accompanied by concentration difficulties, decreased activity, daytime

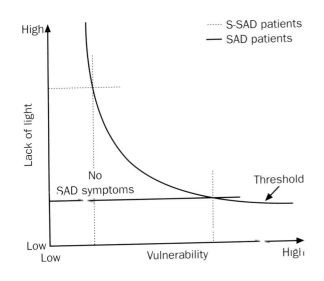

Figure 10.1 Relationships between the likelihood of developing SAD symptoms and the amount of lack of light. The dotted lines represent the possible relationships in S-SAD individuals and the solid lines represent the relationships in SAD patients. Vertical lines indicate the development and involution of SAD symptoms with the amount of lack of light.

Table 10.2 Criteria for subsyndromal SAD (S-SAD).[6]

1) Subjects have a history of some difficulty during the winter months that had occurred on a regular basis (at least two consecutive winters) and had lasted for a sustained period of time (at least 4 weeks). Examples of these difficulties are decreased energy, decreased efficiency at work (e.g. concentration, completing tasks), decreased creativity or interest in socializing, change in eating habits (e.g. eating more carbohydrates), weight (gaining weight) or sleep patterns (more sleep)

2) Subjects regard themselves as 'normal', i.e. not suffering from an illness or disorder

3) Subjects have not sought medical or psychological help specifically for their difficulties, and nor has anyone else suggested that they do so

4) People who do not know the subjects well do not recognize that they have a problem, or if they do, easily attribute it to circumstances such as 'flu or overwork'.

5) The symptoms experienced by the subjects have not disrupted their functioning to a major degree, e.g. calling in sick several times per winter, or severe marital discord

6) Subjects have no history of major affective disorder in wintertime

7) Subjects have no serious medical illness

drowsiness, social withdrawal and decreased libido. Unlike most depressed patients, many patients with SAD complain of so-called 'atypical' depressive symptoms of increased fatigue, increased appetite and increased sleep.[1,8] Typically, patients not only report carbohydrate craving, but actually eat more carbohydrate-rich foods at these times, which is usually followed by weight gain.[9] Many patients are more disturbed by their atypical symptoms, especially during the early phases of their winter depressions, than by the mood changes themselves. The effects of the depressive episodes on patients' daily functioning and quality of life are sometimes underestimated. It must be pointed out that although the depression is usually classified as being mild to moderate, the majority of patients report interpersonal difficulties and difficulties at work. Suicidality in persons with SAD seems to be a rare, although not a negligible, phenomenon, especially during the initial weeks of treatment, when a dissociation of mood and drive may occur.[10]

Depressive episodes typically begin in fall and resolve by springtime,[1] although some patients do not fully recover before the early summer. The onset and offset of the depressive episodes seem to be influenced by the total amount of hours of available daylight. It is of interest that many patients report relief from their symptoms when they travel to latitudes nearer to the equator during fall and winter or when they are up in the mountains during their 'critical' period of the year. Patients with SAD may experience a reversal of their winter symptoms during the spring and summer months: mainly mild hypomania with elated mood, increased social activity and energy, increased libido, diminished sleep and appetite and decreased weight.[11] SAD has also been seen in children and adolescents, who typically present with fatigue, increased irritability, difficulty getting out of bed in the morning and a seasonal pattern of difficulties at school.[12]

Patients with SAD can also present with the opposite pattern of mood changes, that is, with summer depressions and winter hypomania.[13] This has been termed summer SAD, as opposed to the aforementioned winter SAD. Wehr et al have hypothesized that temperature may influence some patients' clinical states.[14]

Epidemiology

Investigators in several continents have found that the majority of the general population notices (to various degrees) seasonal changes of mood and behaviour (Table 10.3). These variations fall mainly within the bounds of normalcy; however, a substantial portion of the general population meet the diagnostic criteria for SAD or S-SAD.[15] The data suggest that SAD and S-SAD represent a considerable public health problem.

Results of North American and Australian studies

In a monocentre study, Kasper et al surveyed the population of Montgomery County (Washington, DC; 39° latitude north of the equator) and found that 4.3% of the population met criteria for SAD and that 13.5% of the population met criteria for S-SAD; only 7.6% reported no changes in mood and behaviour across the seasons.[16] In the Washington DC area, recurrent winter depression typically begins in November and ends in March, whereas Alaskan (64° northern latitude) volunteers complained of symptom onset by late August; the Alaskan subjects experienced peak symptomatology in October or early November.[17] Notably, one of the main findings

Table 10.3 Prevalence rates (point prevalence) of SAD and its subsyndromal form (S-SAD) in different countries of the world (%).

	Latitude	SAD	S-SAD	SAD + S-SAD
USA				
Kasper et al 1989[16]	39°	4.3	13.5	17.8
Rosen et al 1990[18]	43°	9.7	11.0	20.7
	40°	4.7	12.4	17.1
	39°	6.3	10.4	16.7
	27°	1.4	2.6	4.0
Booker and Hellekson 1992[17]	64°	9.2	19.1	28.3
Australia				
Lack et al 1992[19]	37°a	=USA	>USA	>USA
Switzerland				
Wicki et al 1991[21]	47°	–	–	10.4
Wirz-Justice et al 1992[22]	47°	–	–	10.1
Finland				
Hagfors et al 1995[23]	66°	7.1	11.8	18.9
Sweden				
Hagfors et al 1995[23]	?	3.9	13.9	17.8
Netherlands				
Mersch et al 1995[24]	53°	3	8.2	11.2
Norway				
Lingjaerde and Reichborn-Kjennerud 1993[25]	60°	11b	–	–
Iceland				
Magnussen and Stefansson 1993[20]	63°–67°	3.8	7.5	11.3

aSouth of equator.
bIn 70 unselected hospital employees.

of this study was that seasonality scores, which describe the magnitude of seasonal changes in mood and behaviour, are significantly higher in women than in men between 21 and 40 years of age.

The first multicentre study, published by Rosen et al, compared demographic and symptomatological data at four different latitudes in North America (43°, 40°, 39°, 27° respectively, north of the equator).[18] The combined point prevalence of winter SAD and S-SAD ranged from 4% to 20.7%. The most important result was the positive correlation between latitude and prevalence of SAD, with significantly higher rates of winter SAD and S-SAD in more northern latitudes. Similar to the findings of Kasper et al,[16] women were more frequently affected than men. To our knowledge, only one investigation has attempted to study prevalence rates of SAD and S-SAD in the southern hemisphere (Australia).[19] The results showed similar point prevalence rates of SAD in both hemispheres, but there was a higher rate of the subsyndromal form in the southern hemisphere.

Results of European studies

Recently reported prevalence rates of SAD and S-SAD in Europe are somewhat different from those reported in American studies.

Magnussen and Stefansson found a lower than expected prevalence rate of SAD and S-SAD of 11.3% in Iceland (63°–67° northern latitude).[20] The long dark winter in Iceland results in substantial light deprivation during this period; light deprivation is considered to be one of the major aetiological factors for SAD. This relatively low rate of SAD and S-SAD has been interpreted as a population selection towards increased tolerance of winter darkness, since Iceland is a locale of emigration and not immigration. The low prevalence rate of winter SAD in this area might also be explained by the relatively mild and stable climate all year round; that is, temperature changes and not just light deprivation may play a role in the pathogenesis of SAD.

Epidemiological studies in Switzerland,[21,22] Finland,[23] Sweden,[23] The Netherlands[24] and Norway[24,25] (47°–69° northern latitude) have shown prevalence rates for winter SAD and S-SAD between 10.1% and 18.9%, a range

which is lower than in comparable regions in the USA. Wirz-Justice et al suggested that seasonal changes of mood and behaviour may not only result from the number of hours of available sunshine in a given region but may also depend on the number of hours that an individual spends outdoors.[22] Cultural differences may also contribute to the lower prevalence rates. Wicki et al[21] reported that 23% of depressed patients 27–28 years of age reported an increased susceptibility in fall/winter and that 10.4% of the population suffered from seasonal changes of mood. These rates may be similar to those reported for SAD and S-SAD. The authors correctly pointed out that the diagnosis of SAD should be based on prospective assessment and that additional information should also be obtained from a collateral source (e.g. a partner or family members).

In conclusion, there is substantial evidence that the prevalence of SAD and S-SAD is closely related to geographical location and that there is a higher prevalence of SAD and S-SAD in the northern latitudes. No relationship between prevalence rates and longitude could be found. Taken together, these findings suggest that light deprivation may play a major role in the pathogenesis of SAD and S-SAD.

Gender-specific issues in the epidemiology of SAD

Studies from across the world have shown that women are particularly vulnerable to SAD. The sex ratio between women and men as shown in the literature varies between 2 : 1 and 4 : 1.[4,16,18,21–29] There have been different explanations for this finding. The high proportion of women found in research clinics may result from selection bias and may overstate the true relative prevalence of the disorder among women. Interestingly, in a Japanese study of middle-aged patients with SAD, a female/male ratio closer to 1 : 1 has been observed, and is being regarded as one of the characteristics of SAD in Japan.[30] Alternatively, the preponderance of women in some studies may be accounted for by gender differences in the underlying biology of SAD such as monoamine metabolism, hormonal fluctuations or biological clock mechanisms.[31,32]

Treatment

Light therapy

Based on the observation that many animals exhibit seasonal changes in behaviour and physiology (e.g. reproduction, migration, and hibernation), researchers have explored the possibility that rhythms in humans might also be controlled by environmental light. The suppression of human melatonin secretion with exposure to bright artificial light or sunlight suggested that environmental light might affect human circadian and seasonal rhythms.[33] Researchers have also demonstrated that light can induce antidepressant[1] and circadian phase shifting effects.[34]

Although the beneficial effects of exposing patients to artificial bright light have been known for some time, the modern era of light therapy began in the 1980s, when a 63-year-old man with recurrent depressive episodes during the fall/winter period and with euthymic or hypomanic episodes during the spring/summer period presented to the National Institute of Mental Health in Bethesda, MD. The patient himself had reached the conclusion that the changes in length and intensity of environmental light might contribute to the pathogenesis of his depressive episodes. He was treated with light therapy, and after 4 days of treatment his depression lifted.[35]

Since the early anecdotal observations and the first systematic study,[1] experience with light therapy for SAD and S-SAD has increased rapidly.[36] Numerous groups around the world have documented robust antidepressant responses to bright artificial light in patients with SAD.[37] Whereas most observations obtained in uncontrolled settings would support the treatment of SAD patients throughout the whole fall and winter, there is some evidence that bright light therapy administered before the beginning of winter when subjects are still free of symptoms can also be used as a preventative measure.[38,39] It is noteworthy that several studies have reported the most favourable outcomes with bright light therapy in patients with predominantly atypical symptoms. The antidepressant response to light therapy usually appears within the first week of treatment, and when the lights are withdrawn, relapse into depression frequently occurs within a few days (Fig. 10.2).

In addition, some investigators have questioned whether bright light therapy also has a

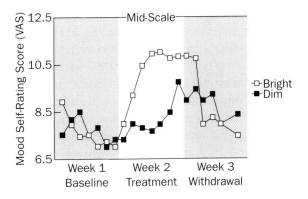

Figure 10.2 Characteristic course under light therapy with either bright light (light intensity: 2500 lux) or dim light (light intensity: <300 lux) in patients with SAD. VAS, visual analogue scale.

psychological effect on patients with S-SAD or on normal subjects. Results of studies conducted with both groups have shown that enhancement of ambient light is beneficial only for patients with S-SAD.[6] Individuals with no history of winter depression or recurrent depressive symptoms do not seem to profit from light treatment. Caution is also advised when plans are considered to enhance lighting in public facilities, because it has not been demonstrated that such a manipulation is beneficial for everybody.

Clinical issues of light therapy for SAD and S-SAD

Light intensity and duration of treatment
Currently, standard light therapy involves exposing patients with SAD and S-SAD to 10 000-lux light intensity for 45 min in the morning and 45 min in the evening. There is considerable variation in the way that light therapy is administered, and the optimal duration of daily treatment depends on the individual patient, on the time of year, and on the geographical location.

Mode of administration
Controversy surrounds the optimal time of day for treatment administration. Several researchers have demonstrated the superiority of morning light therapy over evening light therapy.[33,40–43] However, others have found the treatment also to be beneficial when administered at times of day other than the morning.[44] In everyday practice, the convenience and special needs of the individual patient must be considered in designing an optimal treatment regimen. Frequently, patients do best if the light therapy dosage is spread over the day.

Side-effects
There is general agreement that light therapy is mostly free of side-effects; the more common complaints include headaches, eyestrain, increased irritability, and sleep disturbance, especially when the treatment is administered late at night. When side-effects do occur, they are usually mild and transient and can be handled by decreasing the duration of treatments or asking the patient to increase the distance between the light box and the eyes (thus decreasing the light intensity).[45] However, most reports of side-effects were based on treatment with 2500 lux. As previously mentioned, in recent years it has become common practice to use brighter 10 000-lux exposure when treating patients with SAD. A recent report showed that 10 000-lux light therapy often produced mild but transient side-effects (as noted above) early in the treatment but that the side-effects did not interfere with treatment outcome.[46]

What to do if light therapy does not work
Although bright light therapy has been shown to be remarkably successful for the treatment of SAD and S-SAD,[37] not all patients show a favourable outcome or complete remission of depressive symptoms following light therapy. Based on analyses of large data sets, it is estimated that about 20% of SAD patients treated with light have a partial response and that 20% have little or no response. To date, there are no published studies on strategies for dealing with light therapy non-responders or partial responders. However, the first strategy for improving response is to increase the duration of daily treatment. If light therapy alone is unsuccessful in alleviating the patient's depressive symptoms, psychopharmacological treatment either in conjunction with or instead of light therapy should be tried. L-Tryptophan may also be an effective augmentation strategy for patients with SAD showing a limited or a poor response to bright light therapy.[47] Further placebo-controlled trials are warranted to demonstrate the efficacy of this treatment com-

bination. Thus far, the possibility cannot be ruled out that L-tryptophan alone may be as effective as the combination treatment.[48] In clinical practice, light therapy and antidepressants are often combined with good effect.

Pharmacotherapy for SAD

Recent studies reporting on the use of antidepressants in SAD are summarized in Table 10.4.

Open studies

Early studies used serotonergic compounds such as L-tryptophan, fluoxetine or d-fenfluramine,

and all of them have been shown to be effective.[48–50] A small study also showed modest efficacy with the partial benzodiazepine agonist alprazolam.[51] Winter depression responded to treatment with the monoamine oxidase inhibitor tranylcypromine,[52] whereas Lingjaerde and Haggag used the reversible monoamine oxidase A inhibitor moclobemide (400 mg daily), and also reported an improvement in mood.[53] More recently, mirtazapine (30 mg daily) (a novel antidepressant drug with a dual mechanism of action involving noradrenergic and serotonergic transmitter systems) has been shown to be effective and well tolerated by patients.[54] A longitudinal single case study

---

Table 10.4 Antidepressant medication in patients with seasonal affective disorder (SAD).

Author	Number of patients	Antidepressants
Open studies		
McGrath et al 1990[48]	$n = 9$	L-Tryptophan
Jacobson et al 1989[49]	$n = 3$	Fluoxetine, trazodone
O'Rourke et al 1989[50]	$n = 7$	d-Fenfluramine
Teicher and Glod 1990[51]	$n = 6$	Alprazolam
Dilsaver and Jaeckle 1990[52]	$n = 14$	Tranylcypromine
Lingjaerde and Haggag 1992[53]	$n = 5$	Moclobemide
Heßelmann et al 1999[54]	$n = 8$	Mirtazapine
Wirz-Justice et al 1992[55]	$n = 1$	Citalopram
Controlled studies		
Ruhrmann et al 1993[56]	$n = 40$	Fluoxetine versus bright light
Martinez et al 1994[57]	$n = 20$	Hypericum ± bright light
Partonen and Lönnqvist 1996[58]	$n = 32$	Fluoxetine versus moclobemide
Placebo-controlled studies		
Lingjaerde et al 1993[59]	$n = 34$	Moclobemide versus placebo
Lam et al 1995[60]	$n = 78$	Fluoxetine versus placebo
Blashko 1995[61]	$n = 187$	Sertraline versus placebo
Oren et al 1994[62]	$n = 25$	Levodopa + carbidopa versus placebo
Schlager 1994[63]	$n = 23$	Propranolol versus placebo
Thorell et al 1999[64]	$n = 8$	Light + citalopram versus placebo

showed that light and citalopram both selectively reduced intake of sweet carbohydrates parallel with the improvement in depression, implicating serotonergic mechanisms in the interaction of mood and food in winter.[55] However, the results of these studies have to be considered as preliminary, since all were open trials and only small sample sizes of patients with SAD were included.

Controlled studies
Several controlled studies involved comparison of two treatments but did not include a placebo. One study compared fluoxetine with bright light therapy,[56] another compared St John's wort with bright light therapy,[57] and a third compared fluoxetine with moclobemide.[58] In the study by Ruhrmann et al, 40 patients were exposed to either bright light and placebo capsules or to dim light conditions and fluoxetine (20 mg daily).[56] The results revealed that after 4 weeks of treatment, fluoxetine was as effective as bright light therapy. In comparison with fluoxetine, the bright light group experienced faster onset of antidepressant action and reported less side-effects.

In the controlled study by Martinez et al, St Johns' wort (900 mg daily) was used in combination with bright light or with dim light therapy. The treatment conditions were equally efficacious, although differences between the treatment groups may have been masked by the small sample size.[57]

A multicentre, 6-week randomized controlled trial of 32 SAD patients compared moclobemide (300–450 mg daily) with fluoxetine (20–40 mg daily) and showed no difference in outcome between the two treatment groups. While 79% of patients with SAD had a favourable outcome with either treatment, the authors also demonstrated that moclobemide was somewhat better in terms of improving the patient's quality of life.[58]

Placebo-controlled trials
Thus far, six placebo-controlled trials of antidepressants in the treatment of SAD have been published.[59-64]

Lingjaerde et al tracked patients' health status over a period of 14 weeks following administration of moclobemide.[59] Moclobemide, but not placebo, resulted in a significant decrease of atypical symptoms after 1 week of treatment. However, no significant difference between moclobemide and placebo was found on the Montgomery–Asberg Depression Rating Scale or the Clinical Global Impression rating. When patients were dichotomized according to the median age (45 years), there was a somewhat better effect of moclobemide as compared with placebo in the older age group.

The multicentre, placebo-controlled study of fluoxetine in the treatment of SAD included 78 patients treated with either fluoxetine (20 mg daily) or placebo for 5 weeks.[60] At the end of the treatment, both groups displayed significant improvement; however, the proportion of clinical responders (defined as 50% reduction in depression scores) was higher in the fluoxetine group than in the placebo group (59% and 34% respectively). Post hoc analyses showed that the most pronounced fluoxetine responses were in the more severely depressed patients and that the overall response was greater for patients studied later in the season. The authors concluded that fluoxetine might be an effective, well-tolerated treatment for SAD.

To date, there has been only one large-scale study which has addressed the efficacy of antidepressants in the treatment of SAD. In an 8-week multicentre controlled trial, 187 patients were prospectively randomized to receive either sertraline 50–200 mg daily ($n = 70$) or placebo ($n = 72$).[61] A significantly greater proportion of those receiving placebo as compared with those receiving sertraline withdrew due to inadequate response (15% and 3% respectively). There was a non-significant difference between groups regarding the number of patients discontinuing due to adverse events. Overall, sertraline was found to be clinically and statistically superior to placebo treatment. The mean final daily dose of sertraline was 111 mg. These results are the first to clearly demonstrate the superiority of an antidepressant over placebo in the treatment of SAD.

Oren et al explored the role of dopaminergic deficiency in the pathogenesis of SAD and tested the efficacy of levodopa (up to 7 mg/kg daily) plus carbidopa (100 mg daily) as a treatment for SAD.[62] Following a 2-week wash out period, patients were treated for 2 weeks with the dopaminergic compounds. There was no difference in the rates of responses between the active compound groups and the placebo group. Based on their findings, the authors concluded that a model of systemic dopaminergic deficiency does not readily explain the pathophysiology of SAD.

Testing the role of melatonin in the pathophysiology of SAD, Schlager administered propanolol (60 mg or less per day) to 23 SAD patients.[63] Propranolol is known to block melatonin secretion which was believed to play a role in the development of depressive symptoms in SAD. Propranolol was administered daily between 5:30 and 6:00 a.m., with the intention of truncating nocturnal melatonin secretion, which the author postulated should be linked to antidepressant action. After open treatment with a daily mean dose of 33 mg propranolol, patients were randomly assigned either to placebo or to continuation treatment with propranolol. Patients who received the placebo relapsed significantly more often than those who were being treated with propranolol. The author concluded that these findings are consistent with the hypothesis that the duration of nocturnal melatonin secretion is a critical seasonal time cue in humans. However,

the results of this study may only be valid for a small subgroup of SAD patients who respond to propranolol treatment.

A recent placebo-controlled, double-blind, one-year pilot study investigated the possible clinical advantages of combining light therapy with the selective serotonin reuptake inhibitor citalopram in patients with SAD.[64] Eight women were randomized to receive either 40 mg citalopram or placebo daily in addition to initial light treatment. The results of this small but carefully designed study suggest that light therapy with concomitant continuous treatment with citalopram is a useful strategy to achieve long-term remissions in patients with SAD.

Altogether, the use of antidepressants with a strong sedating component, such as the tri- and tetracyclic antidepressants, is not recommended for the treatment of SAD. Evidence from studies published thus far suggests that antidepressants with a serotonergic mechanism of action might be the first treatment alternative to light therapy in the treatment of SAD.

Biological basis of SAD and light therapy

Neither the aetiology of SAD nor the mechanisms mediating the antidepressant effects of light therapy are fully understood, and both areas are the focus of ongoing research. Although no-one knows exactly how light therapy works, there are some active areas of research that have yielded promising results. These include: (1) brain monoaminergic systems, (2) hypothalamic–pituitary–adrenal (HPA) axis functioning, (3) abnormal circadian rhythms, and (4) aberrant profiles of nocturnal melatonin secretion.

The role of brain monoamine systems in SAD and light therapy

In recent years, there has been increasing interest in the role that brain monoaminergic systems play in the pathophysiology of SAD and also in the mechanism of action of light therapy. Multiple lines of evidence taken together suggest that brain serotonin (5-HT) may be involved in both. These include: (1) seasonal rhythms of (a) human hypothalamic 5-HT concentrations, (b) platelet 5-HT uptake and ^{3}[H]imipramine binding, and (c) levels of 5-HT and its metabolites in plasma and cerebrospinal fluid; (2) abnormal activation-euphoria responses induced by the predominantly 5-HT_{2c} receptor agonist meta-chlorophenylpiperazine (m-CPP) in symptomatic depressed SAD patients, but not after successful light therapy or during summer or in healthy controls; (3) abnormal hormonal responses after administration of m-CPP or the 5-HT_{1D} receptor agonist sumatriptan in depressed SAD patients; and (4) the efficacy of serotonergic agents such as fenfluramine or the selective 5-HT reuptake inhibitors such as fluoxetine or sertraline in the treatment of SAD (for review see Kasper et al[65]).

The investigation of catecholaminergic systems in SAD showed (1) resting plasma noradrenaline levels to be inversely correlated with the level of depression,[66] (2) light therapy decreased the urinary output of noradrenaline,[67] (3) decreased basal plasma prolactin levels;[68] (4) an increased eyeblink rate;[69] and (5) that the combination of carbidopa plus levodopa was not superior to placebo in the treatment of SAD.[62] Thus, studies of catecholamine systems in SAD have been less consistent in implicating abnormalities of these transmitter systems than has been the case with the indolamine systems.

Several groups around the world have been involved in studies investigating serotonergic and catecholaminergic mechanisms in SAD and light therapy using tryptophan depletion (TD) and catecholamine depletion (CD) paradigms.[70] TD was induced by a 24-h low-tryptophan diet and by ingestion of a tryptophan-free amino acid beverage. During sham depletion in the TD studies, the diet and the amino acid beverage were supplemented with tryptophan. Administration of the tyrosine hydroxylase inhibitor alpha-methyl-para-tyrosine (AMPT) was used to deplete catecholamines. Diphenhydramine was used as an active placebo during sham depletion. The effects of these interventions were evaluated with measures of depression, plasma tryptophan levels and plasma catecholamine metabolites. Results indicate that TD does not exacerbate the depressive syndrome in untreated symptomatic depressed patients with SAD,[71] but disrupts the antidepressant effects of light therapy,[72] and causes a depressive relapse in patients during summer.[73] Taken together, the evidence suggests that serotonergic dysfunction may be a trait marker in SAD and that light therapy may compensate for this dysfunction. However, these studies do not rule out the possibility that other systems might be playing a role as well. To investigate the relative contributions of 5-HT and catecholamines in the mechanisms underlying light therapy, the effects of TD combined with CD were compared versus placebo in a randomized, controlled, crossover study of patients with SAD who responded well to light therapy. Both active depletions (TD and CD) but not sham depletion caused a transient recurrence of depressive symptoms,[74] thus confirming previous work showing that serotonin plays an important role in the mechanism of action of light therapy, and providing new evidence that brain catecholaminergic systems may also be involved. In all of these aforementioned studies, no gender-specific behavioural or biochemical effects were observed. The authors concluded that the behavioural responses to monoamine depletion are not gender-specific.

Other hypotheses of SAD

Other theories about the pathophysiology underlying SAD involve abnormalities in HPA axis functioning. Patients with SAD frequently report impaired ability to respond to psychological stress. Unlike typically depressed patients, patients with SAD do not show elevated cortisol levels or failure to suppress cortisol secretion in response to dexamethasone administration,[75,76] which suggests that the HPA axis in patients with SAD is not over-aroused as it is in melancholic depressives. Nevertheless, there is evidence of impaired pituitary corticotrophin (ACTH) response to a variety of stimuli, including corticotrophin-releasing hormone (CRH), m-CPP infusion,[77,78] and ipsapirone administration.[79] These findings suggest that the HPA axis may be underactive in SAD. This could be secondary to decreased brain serotonergic transmission, since 5-HT is one of the neurotransmitters responsible for CRH release.

Some researchers have suggested that the symptoms of SAD might be a result of abnormally delayed circadian rhythms and that light therapy may work by shifting these rhythms to a normal phase position.[33] However, other investigators support the hypothesis that abnormal profiles of nocturnal melatonin secretion might influence the development of symptoms in SAD.[80] Despite these promising leads, there is no consensus on how light therapy works in the treatment of SAD or on the pathophysiological basis of this disorder.[81]

Gender-specific aspects in the pathophysiology of SAD

SAD is a cyclical disorder which predominantly affects women. Thus, it may serve as a model for a better understanding of the contribution of reproductive hormones in the pathophysiology of mood disorders in general. A large proportion (about 70%) of women suffering from SAD also report mood changes closely associated with their menstrual cycle. The authors and others have shown that light therapy has beneficial effects on premenstrual symptomatology. A large proportion of patients have also reported seasonal changes in the severity of their premenstrual complaints, mostly in parallel with the overall seasonal changes of mood, and light therapy seems to be an effective treatment for patients with a seasonal premenstrual syndrome.[82] Interestingly, light therapy has also benefited patients with non-seasonal premenstrual syndrome.[83]

Conclusions

There is substantial agreement among researchers around the world that SAD is a common condition, and that for the majority of subjects, who are mostly female, the clinical symptoms of this illness can be effectively treated with environmental light. Beyond these fundamental points of agreement, many other aspects of this area remain controversial. Most notable among these is the mechanism of action of light therapy. In addition, the biological and psychological mechanisms that may be involved in the pathogenesis of SAD are not yet fully understood. Clearly, family studies are needed to explore the possible role of genetic and environmental factors that might contribute to this illness. Future epidemiological studies should also address the question of the socio-economic impact of SAD on society. Forthcoming epidemiological studies will need to address the question of whether patients with a history of seasonal depressions are at higher risk for further depressive episodes. Biological markers which could delineate patients at risk have also not yet been identified. However, the behavioural response to TD by patients in full remission and off therapy during the summer may be a promising strategy to identify those patients who may experience further winter depressions.[84] Moreover, controlled therapeutic trials are warranted to

explore whether maintainance light therapy throughout the year might prevent the recurrence of winter depression. In addition, there are, as yet, no systematic studies which address effective interventions for patients refractory to light therapy. Researchers and clinicians all around the world are attracted by SAD, possibly because it offers an outstanding model to better understand the relative contributions of biological mechanisms and environmental factors in the pathophysiology of affective disorders.

References

1. Rosenthal NE, Sack DA, Gillin JC et al, Seasonal affective disorder: a description of the syndrome and preliminary findings with light therapy, *Arch Gen Psychiatry* 1984; **41**:72–80.
2. American Psychiatric Association, *Diagnostic and Statistical Manual of Mental Disorders*, 3rd edn, Revised (American Psychiatric Association: Washington, DC, 1987) 131–2.
3. American Psychiatric Association, *Diagnostic and Statistical Manual of Mental Disorders*, 4th edn (American Psychiatric Association: Washington, DC, 1994) 389–90.
4. Wesson VA, Levitt AJ. Light therapy for seasonal affective disorders. In: Lam RN, ed., *Seasonal Affective Disorder and Beyond. Light Treatment for SAD and non SAD Conditions* (American Psychiatric Press, Inc.: Washington, DC, 1998) 45–89.
5. Kraepelin E, *Manic-Depressive Insanity and Paranoia* (Livingstone: Edinburgh, 1921) 139.
6. Kasper S, Rogers SLB, Yancey A et al, Phototherapy in individuals with and without subsyndromal seasonal affective disorder, *Arch Gen Psychiatry* 1989; **46**:837–44.
7. Goel N, Terman M, Terman JS, Williams JBW, Summer mood in winter depressives: validation of a structured interview, *Depress Anxiety* 1999; **9**:83–91.
8. Rosenthal NE, Sack DA, Carpenter CJ et al, Antidepressant effects of light in seasonal affec-

tive disorder, *Am J Psychiatry* 1985; **142**:163–70.
9. Kräuchi K, Wirz-Justice A, The four seasons: food intake frequency in seasonal affective disorder in the course of a year, *Psychiatry Res* 1988; **25**:323–38.
10. Praschak-Rieder N, Neumeister A, Hesselmann B et al, Suicidal tendencies as a complication of light therapy for seasonal affective disorder: a report of three cases, *J Clin Psychiatry* 1997; **58**:389–92.
11. Jacobsen FM, Rosenthal NE, Seasonal affective disorder. In: Georgotas A, Cancro R, eds, *Depression and Mania: A Comprehensive Textbook* (Elsevier Science: New York, 1988) 104–16.
12. Rosenthal NE, Carpenter CJ, James SP et al, Seasonal affective disorder in children and adolescents, *Am J Psychiatry* 1986; **143**:356–8.
13. Srivastava S, Sharma M, Seasonal affective disorder: report from India, *J Affect Disord* 1998; **49**:145–50.
14. Wehr TA, Sack DA, Rosenthal NE, Seasonal affective disorder with summer depression and winter hypomania, *Am J Psychiatry* 1987; **144**:1602–3.
15. Kasper S, Neumeister A, Epidemiology of seasonal affective disorder (SAD) and its subsyndromal form (S-SAD). In: Beigel A, Lopez Ibor JJ, Costa de Silva JA, eds, *Past, Present and*

Future of Psychiatry. IX. World Congress of Psychiatry (World Scientific: Singapore, New Jersey, 1994) 300–5.

16. Kasper S, Wehr TA, Bartko JJ et al, Epidemiological findings of seasonal changes in mood and behavior, *Arch Gen Psychiatry* 1989; **46**:823–33.

17. Booker JM, Hellekson CJ, Prevalence of seasonal affective disorder in Alaska, *Am J Psychiatry* 1992; **149**:1176–82.

18. Rosen LN, Targum SD, Terman M et al, Prevalence of seasonal affective disorder at four latitudes, *Psychiatry Res* 1990; **31**:131–44.

19. Lack L, Aurora Australis, SAD, rhythm disorders and light therapy in Australia, *Bull Soc Light Treatment Biol Rhythms* 1992; **4**:46–9.

20. Magnusson A, Stefansson JG, Prevalence of seasonal affective disorder in Iceland, *Arch Gen Psychiatry* 1993; **50**:941–6.

21. Wicki W, Angst J, Merikangas KR, The Zurich study, XIV. Epidemiology of seasonal depression, *Eur Arch Psychiatry Clin Neurosci* 1991; **241**:301–6.

22. Wirz-Justice A, Kräuchi K, Graw P et al, Seasonality in Switzerland: an epidemiological survey. Abstract, Society for Light Treatment and Biological Rhythms, Annual Meeting 1992; **4**:33.

23. Hagfors C, Thorell LH, Arned M, Seasonality in Finland and Sweden, an epidemiologic study, preliminary results. Abstract, Society for Light Treatment and Biological Rhythms, Annual Meeting 1995; **7**:33.

24. Mersch PP, Middendorp H, Bouhuys AL et al, The prevalence of seasonal affective disorders in the Netherlands, *Acta Neuropsychiatrica* 1995; **7**:47–9.

25. Lingjaerde O, Reichborn-Kjennerud T, Characteristics of winter depression in the Oslo area, *Acta Psychiatr Scand* 1993; **88**:111–20.

26. Weissman MM, Leaf PJ, Holzer CE III et al, The epidemiology of depression: an update on sex differences in rates, *J Affect Disord* 1984; **7**:179–88.

27. Low KG, Feissner JM, Seasonal affective disorder in college students: prevalence and latitude, *J Am Coll Health* 1998; **47**:135–7.

28. Dam H, Jakobsen K, Mellerup E, Prevalence of winter depression in Denmark, *Acta Psychiatr Scand* 1998; **97**:1–4.

29. Saarijarvi S, Lauerma H, Helenius H, Saarilehto S, Seasonal affective disorders among rural Finns and Lapps, *Acta Psychiatr Scand* 1999; **99**:95–101.

30. Okawa M, Shirakawa S, Uchiyama M et al, Seasonal variation of mood and behaviour in a healthy middle-aged population in Japan, *Acta Psychiatr Scand* 1996; **94**:211–16.

31. Partonen T, Estrogen could control photoperiodic adjustment in seasonal affective disorder, *Med Hypotheses* 1995; **45**:35–6.

32. Parry BL, Mood disorders linked to the reproductive cycle in women. In: Bloom FE, Kupfer DJ, eds, *Psychopharmacology. The Fourth Generation of Progress* (Raven Press: New York, 1995) 1029–42.

33. Lewy AJ, Sack RL, Miller LS, Hoban TM, Antidepressant and circadian phase-shifting effects of light, *Science* 1987; **235**:352–4.

34. Van Cauter E, Sturis J, Byrne MM et al, Demonstration of rapid light-induced advances and delays of the human circadian clock using hormonal phase markers, *Am J Physiol* 1994; **266**:E953–63.

35. Rosenthal NE, Lewy AJ, Wehr TA et al, Seasonal cycling in a bipolar patient, *Psychiatry Res* 1983; **8**:25–31.

36. Kasper S, Neumeister A, Non-pharmacological treatments for depression—focus on sleep deprivation and light therapy. In: Briley M, Montgomery S, eds, *Antidepressant Therapy at the Dawn of the Third Millennium* (Martin Dunitz: London, 1998) 255–78.

37. Terman M, Terman JS, Quitkin FM et al, Light therapy for seasonal affective disorder. A review of efficacy, *Neuropsychopharmacology* 1989; **2**:1–22.

38. Meesters Y, Lambers PAS, Jansen JHC et al, Can winter depression be prevented by light treatment? *J Affect Disord* 1991; **23**:75–9.

39. Partonen T, Lönnqvist J, Prevention of winter seasonal affective disorder by bright-light treatment, *Psychol Med* 1996; **26**:1075–80.

40. Eastman C, Young M, Fogg L et al, Bright light treatment of winter depression. A placebo-controlled trial, *Arch Gen Psychiatry* 1998; **55**:883–9.

41. Avery DH, Khan A, Dager SR et al, Bright light treatment of winter depression: morning versus evening light, *Acta Psychiatr Scand* 1990; **82**:335–8.

42. Sack RL, Lewy AJ, White DM et al, Morning vs evening light treatment for winter depression: evidence that the therapeutic effects of light are mediated by circadian phase shifts, *Arch Gen Psychiatry* 1990; **47**:343–51.

43. Terman M, Terman JS, Ross DC, A controlled trial of timed bright light and negative air ionization for treatment of winter depression, *Arch Gen Psychiatry* 1998; **55**:875–82.

44. Wirz-Justice A, Graw P, Kräuchi K et al, Light therapy in seasonal affective disorder is independent of time of day or circadian phase, *Arch Gen Psychiatry* 1993; **50**:929–37.

45. Oren DA, Shannon NJ, Carpenter CJ, Rosenthal NE, Usage patterns of phototherapy in seasonal affective disorder, *Compr Psychiatry* 1991; **32**:147–52.

46. Kogan AO, Guilford PM, Side effects of short-term 10,000-lux light therapy, *Am J Psychiatry* 1998; **155**:293–4.

47. Lam RW, Levitan RD, Tam EM et al, L-tryptophan augmentation of light therapy in patients with seasonal affective disorder, *Can J Psychiatry* 1997; **42**:303–6.

48. McGrath RE, Buckwald B, Resnick EV, The effect of L-tryptophan on seasonal affective disorder, *J Clin Psychiatry* 1990; **51**:162–3.

49. Jacobsen FM, Murphy DL, Rosenthal NE, The role of serotonin in seasonal affective disorder and the antidepressant response to phototherapy. In: Rosenthal NE, Blehar MC, eds, *Seasonal Affective Disorder and Phototherapy* (Guilford Press: New York, 1989) 333–41.

50. O'Rourke D, Wurtman JJ, Wurtman RJ et al, Treatment of seasonal depression with d-fenfluramine, *J Clin Psychiatry* 1989; **50**:343–7.

51. Teicher MH, Glod CA, Seasonal affective disorder: rapid resolution by low-dose alprazolam, *Psychopharmacol Bull* 1990; **26**:197–202.

52. Dilsaver SC, Jaeckle RS, Winter depression responds to an open trial of tranylcypromine, *J Clin Psychiatry* 1990; **51**:326–9.

53. Lingjaerde O, Haggag A, Moclobemide in winter depression: some preliminary results from an open trial, *Nord J Psychiatry* 1992; **46**:201–3.

54. Heßelmann B, Habeler A, Praschak-Rieder N et al, Mirtazapine in seasonal affective disorder (SAD)—a preliminary report, *Hum Psychopharmacol Clin Exp* 1999; **14**:59–62.

55. Wirz-Justice A, van der Velde P, Bucher A, Nil R, Comparison of light treatment with citalopram in winter depression: a longitudinal single case study, *Int Clin Psychopharmacol* 1992; **7**:109–16.

56. Ruhrmann S, Kasper S, Hawellek B et al, Fluoxetine as a treatment alternative to light therapy in seasonal affective disorder (SAD), *Pharmacopsychiatry* 1993; **26**:193.

57. Martinez B, Kasper S, Ruhrmann S, Möller HJ, Hypericum in the treatment of seasonal affective disorders, *J Geriatr Psychiatry Neurol* 1994; **7**(suppl 1):S29–33.

58. Partonen T, Lönnqvist J, Moclobemide and fluoxetine in treatment of seasonal affective disorder, *J Affect Disord* 1996; **41**:93–9.

59. Lingjaerde O, Reichborn-Kjennerud T, Haggag A et al, Treatment of winter depression in Norway. II. A comparison of the selective monoamine oxidase A inhibitor moclobemide and placebo, *Acta Psychiatr Scand* 1993; **88**:372–80.

60. Lam RW, Gorman CP, Michalon M et al, Multi-centre, placebo-controlled study of fluoxetine in seasonal affective disorder, *Am J Psychiatry* 1995; **152**:1765–70.

61. Blashko CA, A double-blind, placebo-controlled study of sertraline in the treatment of outpatients with seasonal affective disorders, *Eur Neuropsychopharmacol* 1995; **5**:258.

62. Oren DA, Moul DE, Schwartz PJ et al, A controlled trial of levodopa plus carbidopa in the treatment of winter seasonal affective disorder: a test of the dopamine hypothesis, *J Clin Psychopharmacol* 1994; **14**:196–200.

63. Schlager DS, Early-morning administration of short-acting beta-blockers for treatment of winter depression, *Am J Psychiatry* 1994; **151**:1383–5.

64. Thorell LH, Kjellman B, Arned M et al, Light treatment of seasonal affective disorder in combination with citalopram or placebo with 1-year follow-up, *Int Clin Psychopharmacol* 1999; **14**(suppl 2):S7–11.

65. Kasper S, Neumeister A, Rieder N, Ruhrmann S, Serotonergic mechanisms in the pathophysiology and treatment of seasonal affective disorder. In: Holick MF, ed., *Biologic Effects of Light 1995* (Walter de Gruyter: Berlin, 1996) 325–31.

66. Rudorfer MV, Skwerer RE, Rosenthal NE,

Biogenic amines in seasonal affective disorder: effects of light therapy, *Psychiatry Res* 1993; **46**:19–28.

67. Anderson JL, Vasile RG, Mooney JJ et al, Changes in norepinephrine output following light therapy for fall/winter seasonal depression, *Biol Psychiatry* 1992; **32**:700–4.

68. Oren DA, Levendosky AA, Kasper S et al, Circadian profiles of cortisol, prolactin, and thyrotropin in seasonal affective disorder, *Biol Psychiatry* 1996; **39**:157–70.

69. Depue RA, Arbisi P, Krauss S et al, Seasonal independence of low prolactin concentration and high spontaneous eye blink rates in unipolar and bipolar II seasonal affective disorder, *Arch Gen Psychiatry* 1990; **47**:356–64.

70. Neumeister A, Praschak-Rieder N, Heßelmann B et al, Der Tryptophandepletionstest–Grundlagen und klinische Relevanz, *Der Nervenarzt* 1997; **68**:556–62.

71. Neumeister A, Praschak-Rieder N, Heßelmann B et al, Rapid tryptophan depletion in drug-free depressed patients with seasonal affective disorder, *Am J Psychiatry* 1997; **154**:1153–5.

72. Neumeister A, Praschak-Rieder N, Heßelmann B et al, Effects of tryptophan depletion on drug-free patients with seasonal affective disorder during a stable response to bright light therapy, *Arch Gen Psychiatry* 1997; **54**:133–8.

73. Neumeister A, Praschak-Rieder N, Heßelmann B et al, Effects of tryptophan depletion in fully remitted patients with seasonal affective disorder during summer, *Psychol Med* 1998; **28**: 257–64.

74. Neumeister A, Turner EH, Matthews JR et al, Effects of tryptophan depletion vs catecholamine depletion in patients with seasonal affective disorder in remission with light therapy, *Arch Gen Psychiatry* 1998; **55**:524–30.

75. Joseph-Vanderpool JR, Rosenthal NE, Chrousos GP et al, Abnormal pituitary–adrenal responses to corticotropin-releasing hormone in patients with seasonal affective disorder: clinical and pathophysiological implications, *J Clin Endocrinol Metab* 1991; **72**:1382–7.

76. Oren DA, Levendosky AA, Kasper S et al, Circadian profiles of cortisol, prolactin, and thyrotropin in seasonal affective disorder, *Biol Psychiatry* 1996; **39**:157–70.

77. Schwartz PJ, Murphy DL, Wehr TA et al, Effects of m-CPP infusions in patients with seasonal affective disorder and healthy control subjects: diurnal responses and nocturnal regulatory mechanisms, *Arch Gen Psychiatry* 1997; **54**: 375–85.

78. Jacobsen FM, Mueller EA, Rosenthal NE et al, Behavioral responses to intravenous metachlorophenylpiperazine in patients with seasonal affective disorder and control subjects before and after phototherapy, *Psychiatry Res* 1994; **52**:181–97.

79. Schwartz PJ, Turner EH, Garcia-Bonneguero D et al, Serotonin hypothesis of winter depression, *Psychiatry Res* 1999; **86**:9–28.

80. Rosenthal NE, Sack DA, Jacobsen FM et al, Melatonin in seasonal affective disorder and phototherapy, *J Neural Transm (Suppl)* 1986; **21**:257–67.

81. Rosenthal NE, The mechanism of action of light in the treatment of seasonal affective disorder. In: Holick MF, ed., *Biologic Effects of Light 1995* (Walter de Gruyter: Berlin, 1996) 317–24

82. Parry BL, Rosenthal NE, Tamarkin L, Wehr TA, Treatment of a patient with seasonal premenstrual syndrome, *Am J Psychiatry* 1987; **144**:762–6.

83. Lam RW, Carter D, Misri S et al, A controlled study of light therapy in women with late luteal phase dysphoric disorder, *Psychiatry Res* 1999; **86**:185–92.

84. Neumeister A, Habeler A, Praschak-Rieder N et al, Tryptophan depletion: a predictor of future depressive episodes in seasonal affective disorder? *Int Clin Psychopharmacol* 1999; **14**:313–15.

11

Depression in the elderly

Carl-Gerhard Gottfries

Introduction

The number of elderly people in the population is increasing rapidly throughout the developed and developing world. This is due to increasing life-expectancy, as a result of improved health and social conditions. Currently, 6% of the global population is more than 65 years of age. It is anticipated that by the year 2000, 5% of the population will be over 80 years old.[1]

Depression is a common condition in the elderly, occurring either on its own or in association with other diseases. Depressive illness has a substantial negative impact on the quality of life of patients and their relatives. In addition, there is a strong link between depression and suicide.

Depression in elderly patients has a complex aetiology and may have a different symptomatology from that in younger patients. Thus, all depressed elderly patients require accurate diagnosis and effective treatment.

In this chapter, our current understanding of depression in later life is reviewed, with the focus on women.

Epidemiology

Depression may occur on its own or in association with other diseases. The elderly are particularly at risk of depressive illness, as they are more likely to suffer from impaired health compared with younger individuals. Thus, it is of paramount importance that the possible presence of depression be considered by all health-care professionals caring for elderly patients.

General population

Depression is a widespread disease, with an overall prevalence of 5–8% in the world as a whole. The cumulative incidence of depression in people aged up to 70 years is 26.9% for men and 45.2% for women.[2]

A well-documented finding in psychiatric epidemiology is that women have higher rates of major depression than men. This has been found in community epidemiological studies and is also consistent with data from the US National Comorbidity Survey,[3] a structured

Table 11.1 The prevalence of depression in the elderly: depression according to the DSM criteria.

Study	Place	Age	Diagnosis	Men (%)	Women (%)	Total (%)
Skoog et al[4]	Göteborg	85	MDD	5.6	8.5	7.7
			Dysthymia	5.6	4.0	4.5
Fichter et al[5]	Munich	85+	MDD	0	1.8	
			Dysthymia	4.9	5.1	
	ECA, USA	85+	MDD	0.9	1.4	
			Dysthymia	0.9	2.9	
Lobo et al[6]	Zaragoza	65+	All	3.4	5.7	4.8
Henderson et al[7]	Canberra	70+	MDD	0.4	1.5	
			Dysthymia	0.2	0.8	
Kivelä et al[8]	Ähtäri	70+	All	21.0	32.7	26.8
Bland et al[9]	Edmonton	65+	MDD	0.9	1.4	1.2
			Dysthymia	1.8	4.3	3.3

MDD, major depressive disorder.

Table 11.2 The prevalence of depression in the elderly: depression according to the AGECAT diagnosis.

Study	Place	Age	Men (%)	Women (%)	Total (%)
Magnússon[10]	Iceland	87	5.3	9.3	7.8
Copeland et al[11]	New York	65+	13.0	18.3	16.2
	London	65+	13.1	22.8	19.4
Copeland et al[12]	Liverpool	65+	7.6	13.6	11.3
Saunders et al[13]	Liverpool	65+	7.6	11.6	10.0
		90+	4.7	7.6	

psychiatric interview of a representative sample of the US general population. Women are approximately 1.7 times as likely as men to report a lifetime history of mood disorders, including a major depressive episode. Age-at-onset analyses show that this sex difference begins in early adolescence and persists up to the mid-fifties.

There is a marked variation in the prevalence of depression among different studies and certain groups of elderly patients (Tables 11.1–11.3).[18] This variation may be explained,

Table 11.3 The prevalence of depression in the elderly: depression according to other diagnostic criteria.

Study	Place	Age	Criteria	Men (%)	Women (%)	Total (%)
Livingston et al[14]	London	65+	CARE			15.9
		80+		16.4	16.5	16.5
Lindesay et al[15]	London	65–74		8.8	15.4	
		75+		7.5	18.7	
Woo et al[16]	Hong Kong	70+	GDS	29.2	41.1	35.0
		85+		41.7	42.1	41.9
Beekman et al[17]		70–74	CES-D	10.6	18.0	14.3
		75–79		14.6	22.9	18.6
		80–85		13.8	24.7	19.4

at least in part, by the fact that depressive disorders in later life are not necessarily the same as those seen in younger people, and they may have different aetiologies. The estimation of the prevalence of depression based on the Diagnostic and Statistical Manual for Mental Disorders (DSM-III-R[19] and DSM-IV[20]) criteria varies between 0% and 33%, depending on what kinds of diagnoses are included. The prevalence of major depressive disorder according to the DSM criteria varies between 0% and 5.6% for men and between 1.4% and 8.5% for women. Dysthymia varies between 0.2% and 5.6% for men and between 0.8% and 5.1% for women. In a study by Kevelä et al,[21] which included patients above 70 and where all types of depression were sampled in one group, the prevalence was 21% for men and 32.7% for women. When the computerized psychiatric diagnostic system Automated Geriatric Examination for Computer Assisted Taxonomy (AGECAT)[22] for depression is used, the prevalence varies between 4.7% and 13.7% for men and between 7.2% and 22.8% for women in

age groups above 65 years. When other methods are used for diagnosis of depression, the prevalence figures vary between 7.5% and 41.7% for men and between 15.4% and 42.1% for women in various age groups above 65 years (Table 11.3). There is good evidence that females develop a more complex and more severe depression with a more severe course than males.[23] There may be many reasons for this phenomenon, either biological (androgens may be a partial protection against depression) or social. In addition, the gender ratio changes with increasing age. Beekman et al[17] confirmed a preponderance of females (18.3% females versus 11.2% males) in a group of people (n = 3056) 55–85 years of age. However, there is also evidence which suggests that the sex difference is less marked or even non-existent in elderly depressives.[24] A neglected factor affecting the sex distribution of prevalence rates is the definition of affective disorders. It is generally acknowledged that men report fewer complaints and symptoms on checklists and at interviews.[25]

The mental status of elderly people was assessed by Haller et al[26] in a European study. Assessment instruments were the Mini-Mental State Examination (MMSE) and the 15-item Geriatric Depression Scale (GDS). Both sexes had an MMSE mean score of 26.7, and 8.5% of the men and 10.9% of the women had an MMSE score below 23. The overall mean GDS score was 3.9, with a mean score of 3.2 for the men and 4.6 for the women. GDS scores above the cut-off score of 5 were found in 11.6% of the men and 27.5% of the women. In this investigation of 880 subjects, there were significant correlations between the MMSE and GDS scores and education, Katz[9] Activities of Daily Living (ADL)[27] scores, subject health and plasma micronutrient levels.

Thus prevalence data show that 10–15% of the elderly suffer from depressive disorders, if all types of depression are included, and older women tend to have a somewhat higher prevalence of depression than older men. The female preponderance is most accentuated in the middle of life and decreases with age.[28,29]

Elderly outpatients

In elderly outpatients who seek medical care, the prevalence of depression varies between 13% and 40%. Evans and Katona[30] used the GDS[31] to identify depression in a series of elderly people who consulted their primary care physicians. They found that 30% of the men and 40% of the women showed signs of depression. A modification of the GDS was used as a screening instrument in a recent Swedish study of a random sample of elderly outpatients in primary care; the prevalence of significant depression was found to be 13%.[32] In this study, 58% of the consecutive outpatients were women. There was, however, no difference between the sexes in the frequency of depression. In a related study, data obtained on 4302 women, between the ages of 43 and 89 years, who participated in a breast cancer screening programme showed that correlations for age, anxiety, anger and depression are generally weak.[33]

Hospitalized elderly patients

Depression is a common finding in hospitalized patients, with a prevalence of 10–45% being reported in medical inpatients over the age of 65 years.[34] Cancer, predominantly a disease of the elderly, is associated with significant depression in up to 50% of cases.[35] Lansky et al,[36] in a multicentre study of 500 female patients with cancer, found that a subgroup of women with cancer and major depressive disorder had significantly more pain and greater physical disability and also was more likely to have had prior episodes of depression.

Another common reason for hospitalization of elderly people is cardiovascular disease. This is also associated with a profound degree of depression that cannot be explained by psychological factors or chance alone.[37] In Denmark, Weeke et al[38] demonstrated, in a sample of 6000 depressed patients who were followed for an average of 5 years, that there was a 50% increase in cardiovascular death compared with the general population. This was true for both male and female depressed patients.

People in nursing homes and geriatric institutions

In 1985, about 12% of all people in Sweden ≥80 years of age lived in institutions. In this same year and country, the mean age at death was 79 years for women and 73 years for men, and the ratio of men to women 80–85 years of age was 0.6. One study[39] found a similar distribution in nursing homes, where the male/female ratio was 0.48. A detailed study investigating depressive symptoms in elderly nursing home residents showed that 20% of patients met DSM-III criteria for major depressive disorder and that 30% were dysphoric;[40] overall, there were indications of a significant degree of depression in 44% of the patients. Two other studies based on the populations of geriatric institutions[41,42] have estimated the prevalence of depression at approximately 30%.[30,31] In the detailed study by Andersson[21] of nursing home patients, 63% were considered to be depressed and 42% to be suffering from anxiety; no differences between the sexes in the frequency of depression were found.

Depression and neurodegenerative disorders

In dementia, depression is a variable but common finding, and the prevalence rate in samples of hospitalized demented patients has been reported to be as high as 51.7%.[43]

Irritability, agitation and aggression, together with depressed mood, were found in 81% of patients afflicted by Alzheimer's disease.[44] Among patients with Alzheimer-type dementia, about 25% have symptoms that fulfil the criteria for major depressive disorder, and if other types of depression are also included, the prevalence increases to 50%.[45] Several investigators have reported a significantly higher prevalence in individuals with dementia due to vascular disease than in those with Alzheimer's disease,[46–48] and depression has been reported in 38% of patients with senile dementia of Lewy body type.[49] There is also a high prevalence of depression in patients who have suffered a cerebrovascular accident.[50] Based on a critical review of the literature, it has been estimated that up to 60% of stroke patients suffer from clinically significant depression during the first 2 years after the

event.[51] In these reports, sex differences are either not studied or were not found.

The reported prevalence of depression associated with Parkinson's disease varies from 5% to 70%, with a rate of approximately 20% if only patients with major depressive disorders are included.[52,53] Importantly, the occurrence of depressive symptoms may precede motor symptoms, and they are often combined with anxiety. In a study of 50 male and 50 female patients with Parkinson's disease, 23 patients were diagnosed with major depressive disorder according to the DSM-III-R criteria; 10 of these 23 were women.[54]

Suicide in the elderly

There is a strong link between depression and suicide, with 70% of suicides following depressive illness.

Two of the most common risk factors for suicide are age and male gender. Although the suicide rates differ from country to country, they generally rise with increasing age (Fig. 11.1),[55] the highest rates being reported in males aged 65 years or more. In a survey of statistics reported to the World Health Organization from 1988 to 1991, Poland was found to be the only country recording the highest prevalence of male suicides in younger age groups, namely those in the 45–54-year bracket.[56]

Increasing age is also an important risk factor for suicide among women. In most countries, the highest prevalence of female suicides is found in the 75+ age group. However, in some Scandinavian countries, Ireland, The Netherlands, Poland, Sri Lanka, New Zealand, Canada, the USA and South America, peak female suicide rates occur in age groups below 75 years. The reasons for this remain unclear.

Age-adjusted rates for various industrialized nations, published in 1995, showed that Hungary had the highest prevalence of suicide

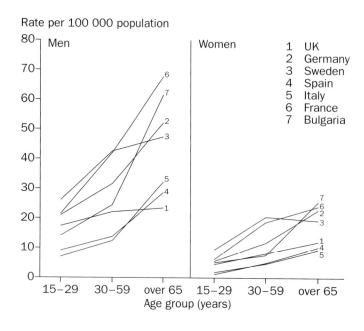

Rate per 100 000 population

Figure 11.1 In most industrialized countries, suicide rates increase with advancing age.[55]

and that Northern Ireland had the lowest (Fig. 11.2).[57] In all countries, men were more likely to commit suicide than women. The ratio of male to female suicides in the USA increased from 3.1 : 1 in 1979 to 4.2 : 1 in 1990.[58] There are also racial differences, with over 70% of all suicides in the USA being white men.

Despite improved medical care, suicide rates have remained relatively constant in many countries for the past 20 years or more. For example, in Japan, which has a suicide rate as high as 50–90 per 100 000 men, the rate has been stable since 1965.[59] There are, however, seasonal and circadian variations in the suicide rate. A study of suicides committed by elderly people in Kawasaki between 1979 and 1990 found that most suicides occurred between April and July, and the lowest rate was recorded in December.[59] In addition, there was a tendency to fewer suicides from 18.00 to 23.00 hours compared with the rest of each 24-h period.[59]

Aetiology

The aetiology of depression is more heterogeneous in the elderly than in younger people. Risk factors that have been identified include the normal ageing process, deficiencies in essential nutrients, dementia disorders, other degenerative disorders, cardiac disease, endocrine disease, and neoplasia.

Depression is also a potential side-effect of some medications in general, and elderly people use a great many pharmaceuticals. Psychosociogenic and genetic influences are of significance as well.

It has been hypothesized that the cerebral metabolism of monoamines, particularly serotonin (5-HT) and noradrenaline (NA), is of importance in emotional disturbances, especially mood disorders. Neurotransmitter metabolism and the activity of the various enzyme systems involved in metabolism undergo change during the normal ageing

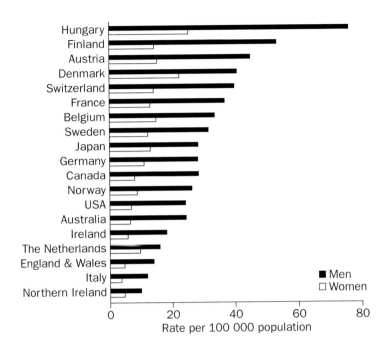

Figure 11.2 Age-adjusted suicide rates per 100 000 population aged 15–74 years in selected industrialized nations, for 1987 or the most recent year available.[57]

process. The acetylcholinergic system is particularly sensitive to ageing, with reduced activity of cholineacetyl transferase and changes in muscarinic and nicotinic receptors in discrete brain areas. The concentrations of dopamine (DA), NA and 5-HT are reduced in discrete brain areas in individuals over 65 years of age. There are also reports of age-related reductions in homovanillic acid, but these are less convincing.[60] The concentrations of 5-hydroxyindoleacetic acid (5-HIAA) do not appear to decrease with age. As 5-HT is considered to be a marker of the number of neuron terminals and 5-HIAA a marker of metabolic activity, these findings suggest that there is a reduction in the number of nerve terminals in normal ageing, but that increasing metabolic activity in the remaining terminals maintains the end metabolite concentration. Interestingly,

monoamine oxidase (MAO)-B activity increases significantly with age. One possible explanation of the increased MAO-B activity is that this form of the enzyme is primarily localized in extraneuronal tissue (whereas the A-form is found intracellularly in the neurons), and age-related gliosis increases the relative amount of extraneuronal tissue. Studies of the brains of patients with Alzheimer's disease and vascular dementia have shown that severe disturbances of the monoaminergic systems are associated with these disorders.[61,62]

In the hypothalamus, there is a significant positive correlation between age and the concentration of corticotrophin-releasing factor (CRF).[63] A study by Raadsheer[64] found that CRF neurons in the paraventricular nucleus of the hypothalamus were overactive and expressed vasopressin in elderly people. This finding may explain the high activity in the hypothalamic–pituitary–adrenal (HPA) axis seen in elderly people. In addition, in post-mortem studies of human brains, age-related reductions in the concentration of 5-HIAA in the hypothalamus have been recorded.[65] Together, these findings indicate that the serotonergic system has a reduced impact on the hypothalamus in elderly people. Heuser et al[66] compared cortisol secretion in young and old volunteers. After dexamethasone treatment, cortisol secretion was higher in the old age group, but none of the subjects escaped suppression of cortisol. After additional corticotrophin-releasing hormone administration to the dexamethasone-treated volunteers, the release of cortisol increased significantly more in the old subjects than in their younger counterparts. Gender profoundly affected the test outcomes: females, regardless of age, had an increased hormonal secretion in comparison with males.

Increased basal thyroid-stimulating hormone (TSH) concentrations are more common in older people, especially women.[67] This may be related to an increased incidence of thyroiditis in the elderly, resulting in reduced thyroid gland function. However, in elderly people without thyroid or other systemic disease, thyroid function remains reasonably normal. These changes suggest that hypothalamic thyrotrophin-releasing hormone (TRH) production may be compensatorily increased in some elderly subjects with reduced thyroid function. TRH has been shown to be colocalized with the classic neurotransmitter serotonin and with substance P in the raphe nucleus and medulla, and TRH receptors are widely distributed in the CNS. Thus, TRH has effects in addition to its effects on the pituitary. It has been shown that TRH is increased in the cerebrospinal fluid (CSF) of depressed patients,[68] and 25–30% of depressed patients may show a blunted TSH response to TRH.[69] Treatment studies have found that the antidepressant effect is mixed. It is possible that there is an effect in the form of acceleration or potentiation of the antidepressant response to other drugs.[70]

Changes in hypothalamic-pituitary–gonadal (HPG) axis function with ageing have also been reported. The female menopause represents the most dramatic alteration. The decline in ovarian gonadal steroid output results in loss of negative feedback from these steroids to the pituitary and the CNS. Thus, there is an increased output of gonadotrophin-releasing hormone (GnRH) and gonadotrophins. In men, there is a gradual decrease in HPG axis function, leading to decreased free testosterone concentrations. In major depression, the HPG axis has been the focus of a few studies. Significantly lower basal concentrations of luteinizing hormone (LH) in postmenopausal depressed women compared with age-matched controls have been reported.[71] Studies of the pituitary response to administered GnRH in major depression have not shown age or sex differences in gonadotropin secretion or growth hormone response.[72]

It is obvious that the steroid hormones are of great importance for depressive disorders. These hormones are indeed able to influence mental functions in a rather dramatic way. For instance, premenstrual depression, contraceptive pill depression and menopausal depression are examples where the depressive mood swings are related to changing sexual hormones. There is a relationship between high levels of testosterone and depression in women; however, in men depressed mood is related to low levels of testosterone. The interaction of sexual hormones and serotonin in the brain requires further examination.

Recent data indicate an association between myocardial infarction (MI) and depression.[73]

There is a high prevalence of depression in post-MI patients, and some patients with this combination of somatic and psychiatric illness initially present with depression. In addition, patients with a combination of MI and depression have a higher mortality rate than MI patients without depression.[37]

Vitamin B_{12} (cobalamin) is an essential nutrient with important coenzymatic functions in the metabolism of most tissues, including those of the nervous system. A wide range of neuropsychiatric symptoms has been associated with vitamin B_{12} deficiency, including depression and dementia.[74] Low vitamin B_{12} levels are found in elderly people without concomitant anaemia, and 32% of the elderly seem to have insufficient uptake of vitamin B_{12}. This may be due to atrophic gastritis, reduced levels of intrinsic factor, and disturbed B_{12} transport.[75] In a study by Regland,[76] the CSF/serum B_{12} ratios were investigated in patients with a mixed form of dementia. In the group with a low CSF/serum B_{12} ratio, there was a male predominance (81%). From this observation, the author concluded that men are more predisposed than women to disturbance of the transportation of vitamin B_{12} from the serum into the CNS, which could be due to men being more exposed to toxic agents.

Folate deficiency is also linked to depressive disorders. In 1962, Herbert[77] reported data supporting an association between folate deficiency and depressive symptoms in human beings. In patients with megaloblastic anaemia due to folate deficiency, depressive symptoms are the most common psychiatric symptoms, and cognitive impairment is also seen.[78] In addition, investigations have shown that 15–38% of depressed patients show low serum or red blood cell folate concentrations.[79,80] In a study by Heilmann,[81] it was shown that, during the two first decades of life, men and women have equally high folate concentrations in the serum. In the third decade, there is an increase in the serum folic acid levels in both sexes. In men the levels are highest between 31 and 40 years of age, and in women between 41 and 50 years. After the age of 60, there is a fall in folic acid levels in both sexes in the normal population. In most of the older normal population, the folic acid levels are below the lower reference limit of 5 ng/ml, and the difference from the younger normal population is significant. The only significant difference between the sexes with regard to folic acid levels in the normal population has been found in the age span of 51 60 years, where women have higher folic acid levels than men.

When looking at the outcome of lithium treatment and treatment with electroconvulsive therapy (ECT), antidepressants and selective serotonin reuptake inhibitors (SSRIs), a better response to the treatment is found if the folate levels are normal or if the treatment is combined with folate substitution.[80,82–84]

Vitamin B_{12} and folate are both important for 1-carbon cycle activity (Fig. 11.3). Deficiency of these vitamins causes reduced activity of methionine synthetase, thus leading to an accumulation of homocysteine and reduced formation of S-adenosylmethionine (SAM). Decreased levels of SAM have been reported in the CSF of depressed and demented patients.[85] Moreover, in a controlled study, the addition of methylfolate to traditional antidepressant treatment was significantly more favourable than the addition of placebo.[86] Thus, in the elderly, a deficiency of vitamin B_{12} and/or folate may be an important risk factor for depression and cognitive impairment. The outcome of antidepressant treatment may also be suboptimal if these vitamins are deficient.

Psychosociogenic influences are also implicated in the aetiology of depression. Large numbers of adverse life events have been reported in patients with late-in-life depression.

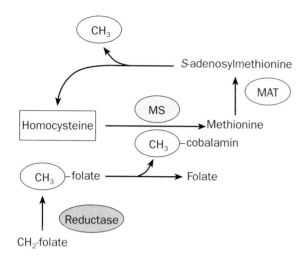

Figure 11.3 The 1-carbon cycle. MS, methionine synthetase; MAT, methionine adenosyltransferase.

Social factors may have a major influence, particularly chronic financial and health problems.[87] Married adults are at lower risk of depression than unmarried ones, although at least 30% of spouses of the demented patients themselves develop depressive disorders.

Despite the consistency of correlation between adverse life events and depression in the elderly, the magnitude of the relationship is usually modest. However, a combination of these psychosocial and biological factors best explains the onset of depressive syndromes in elderly people.

Symptomatology

Few studies have examined gender differences within older depressed subjects. Kivelä and Pahkala[88] noted that somatic and hypochondriacal symptoms among elderly depressed people were more marked in women than in men. The former also showed more sleep disturbances, worrying, crying and helplessness, whereas depressed men expressed more loss of interest and low mood.

In contrast to younger depressed patients, elderly patients often avoid reporting or showing that their mood level is reduced, as they experience guilt associated with these symptoms. If they enjoy life less than before, they may think that this is an inevitable consequence of ageing. Thus, reduced mood may be less evident in elderly people, whereas anxiety and somatic symptoms—which are more willingly admitted—are more prominent. In addition, suicidal symptoms and symptoms of reduced sexual activity may be difficult to recognize. Good contact with the patient and an atmosphere of trust are needed to detect these symptoms.

Thoughts and ideas are always influenced by depression, becoming increasingly pessimistic as the mood lowers. Interpretations may eventually reach the level of paranoia. In elderly people with severe depression, concern about relatives and recovery often has the form of true paranoid psychotic symptoms. Hypochondriacal symptoms are considered common by many authors, but recent studies have yielded somewhat contradictory results.[89] Hallucinations may occur in severely depressed elderly people. The content of both paranoid ideas and hallucinations is always affected by the depressed mood. Psychotic symptoms and hallucinations sometimes suggest a paranoid psychosis, but the depressive nature of the psychotic symptoms reveals the underlying depression.

The prevalence of anxiety among the elderly is estimated at around 15%,[90] which is similar to that of depression. There is also a higher rate of anxiety in elderly patients with major depressive disorders than in younger depressive patients.[91] This high coexistence of anxiety and depression suggests that depression in the elderly is part of a depression–anxiety syndrome, in which either reduced mood or anxiety is the predominant symptom. It has been stated that there is generally a higher prevalence of anxiety in women,[92] although this was not confirmed by Lindesay et al.[15]

Depression in the elderly is often hidden behind somatic symptoms, because of either somatization of the disorder or accentuation of symptoms of a concomitant physical illness.[93] The most common somatic symptom is asthenia. Pain in different parts of the body is also common. Constipation is often seen in elderly people, and reduced appetite with weight loss may be prominent. Worsening of the symptoms in the morning is not a regular feature in elderly depressive people with somatic complaints, but this may be helpful in the differential diagnosis between a somatic disorder and depression.

The presence of cognitive impairment as part of the depressive syndrome in the elderly is often of special importance, as elderly people may already have cognitive impairment caused by ageing or degenerative disorders.[94] The cognitive impairment caused by depression is usually referred to as 'pseudo-dementia' or 'depression with dementia', and it is important to differentiate this condition from true dementia.

Diagnosis

Depression in the elderly is usually a chronic disorder, which is more readily diagnosed as dysthymic disorder, although this term was originally attributed to a disorder with onset at younger ages. In a review of the symptom pattern of depression in the elderly, it has been claimed that minor depression (a poorly defined DSM-IV diagnosis intended for research and including fewer criteria than major depressive disorder) is common in the elderly and predominates in patients over 80 years of age.[95] In the elderly, it is often difficult to fit the symptoms of depression to the diagnostic criteria of the DSM-IV or the International Classification of Diseases, 10th revision (ICD-10). That there is a need for diagnoses specific to elderly people is evident from the use of terms such as 'old age melancholia with or without psychotic symptoms', 'old age depression with hypochondria', 'organic depression' and 'depression–anxiety syndrome'. The comorbidity with anxiety states is high among the elderly, further supporting the notion that the types of depression seen in elderly people differ from those seen in younger people.

Several studies have shown that depression is underdiagnosed in the elderly. The reason may be that patients, care-givers and health-care providers regard the symptoms as manifestations of normal ageing and are unable to identify the disorder as an illness. Elderly people have difficulties in describing depressive symptoms, and the manifestations of the disorder often afford an atypical clinical picture. Of course, concomitant somatic disease and/or organic brain damage may make diagnosis more difficult. Elderly people preferentially seek a somatic explanation of their complaints.

A significant problem in the diagnosis of depression in old age is that many elderly patients are not seen by specialists. Most of the patients do not seek medical help at all. Some patients are seen by district nurses and district doctors. The latter are often pressed for time and do not always consider the possible existence of a depressive illness in an older patient who presents with somatic symptoms.

Rating scales which screen for depression may be valuable aids for general practitioners. The 15-item Geriatric Depression Scale (GDS-15) has been used in several studies and is easy to apply.[96] The scale has been modified by the addition of five items (GDS-20) and was used in a Swedish study in which 1184 patients were evaluated with respect to depression. The added symptoms included sleep disturbance, anxiety, panic, pain and hypochondria. The use of the GDS-20 revealed previously undiagnosed depressive disorders in the elderly cohort. As the scale was easy to apply, the district doctors subsequently adopted it for continuous use. No difference in the prevalence of depressive disorders between the sexes was found.

For a more sophisticated quantification of symptoms of depression, the Montgomery–Åsberg Depression Rating Scale (MADRS)[97] or the Hamilton Depression Scale (HDS)[98] may be used.

In diagnosing depression in the elderly, laboratory analyses should be undertaken that focus on thyroid dysfunction and deficiency of essential nutrients.[99]

Importantly, the dexamethasone suppression test (DST), which measures activity in the hypothalamic–pituitary–adrenal axis, may be abnormal in both depression and dementia disorders. Thus, the test cannot be used to reliably distinguish between these two conditions.

For a complete diagnostic work-up, computed tomography, electroencephalograms and psychological tests may also be performed.

Treatment

Treatment of depression in the elderly is largely the same as that offered to younger people. However, different life situations, concomitant diseases and drug reactions bring about special problems in the treatment of depression in later life.

Although biological factors may be linked to the development of depressive disorders in the elderly, this does not rule out psychotherapeutic treatment strategies. The recommended type is cognitive psychotherapy. Elderly people often have a stiff, negative and illogical train of thought, which may be positively influenced by cognitive psychotherapy.

Families are generally a very important source of support for depressed patients. The family members have to help the patients to adhere to their treatment regimens. They should also be able to understand how the patients think and feel. The burden of depressive illness extends to other family members, and treatment should therefore aim at providing support for care-giving relatives as well.

Some elderly patients may not have relatives, or have relatives who are unable to provide the amount of support required, and society, therefore, has a prominent role in treatment. Elderly people who have suffered bereavement or who live alone often need help to find something to fill their time, and social workers and district nurses are key contacts for them.

Pharmacological intervention is important in treating depression in the elderly. Different classes of drugs may be prescribed (Table 11.4). The risk of adverse advents is usually greater in the elderly than in younger patients, and any side-effects that do occur may be less well tolerated. Drug interactions are also more likely in the elderly, as the older patient may be taking several medications.

Treatment with tricyclic antidepressants (TCAs) has been proven successful in relieving depressive disorders in younger individuals. However, tricyclic antidepressants have several other effects, for example inhibition of the cholinergic neurotransmitter system, antihistaminergic effects and cardiotoxicity. As the cholinergic system in the ageing brain has a reduced capacity, elderly people are vulnerable to drugs with anticholinergic effects. In addition to unwanted anticholinergic effects, the

Table 11.4 Drugs that may be used in the treatment of depression.

Drug class	Mode of action	Examples
Tricyclic antidepressants	Activates noradrenaline	Desipramine Lofepramine Maprotiline Nortriptyline Protriptyline
	Activates 5-HT and noradrenaline	Amitriptyline Clomipramine Dothiepin Doxepin Imipramine Trimipramine
Selective serotonin reuptake inhibitors	Activates 5-HT (serotonin)	Citalopram Fluoxetine Fluvoxamine Paroxetine Sertraline
Others	Activates 5-HT	Nefazodone Trazodone
	Activates noradrenaline	Mianserin
	Activates 5-HT and noradrenaline	Moclobemide Venlafaxine Lithium

5-HT, 5-hydroxytryptamine.

most common side-effects of TCAs are impaired cognitive functions, delirium, weight gain, hypotension and confusion.[100–102] Moreover, several of these side-effects enhance susceptibility to falls, with potentially disastrous consequences, especially in women with osteoporosis.

SSRIs have comparable effectiveness to TCAs, and response rates can be as high as 65%. They have improved tolerability profiles, with fewer and milder side-effects compared with TCAs. Among these side-effects are nausea, difficulty in falling asleep, sedation and reduced sexual activity. The side-effects seem less common in older people and do not preclude successful treatment of this category. Thus, SSRIs represent a major advance and are now the first choice for treatment of geriatric depressed patients.

In a study based on 98 patients with Alzheimer-type dementia or vascular dementia, citalopram produced significant improvements with respect to confusion, irritability, anxiety, depressed mood and restlessness, according to the Gottfries–Bråne–Steen (GBS) scale, a geriatric rating scale.[103] The mood level was improved, as assessed by the MADRS. In a further study of 133 depressed elderly patients, including those with somatic disorders and dementia, citalopram provided significantly greater improvement than placebo,[104] as measured using the HDS, MADRS and Clinical Global Impression scales.[105] The GBS scale results indicated that the citalopram-treated group of patients with dementia had significantly greater improvement in emotional functioning than the placebo-treated group.

Thus, there is evidence that SSRIs are highly beneficial in the treatment of depressed mood and other emotional disturbances, such as anxiety, fear/panic, aggressiveness and agitation, in the elderly and in patients with dementia. Post-stroke pathological crying and post-stroke depression have also been successfully treated with citalopram in controlled trials.[106,107]

Open studies have shown that elderly people do not seem to develop tolerance to the SSRIs.[108] This is of interest, as the treatment of depression in elderly people may well be lifelong.

As discussed earlier, activity in the 1-carbon cycle may be of importance in the outcome of antidepressant treatment. Vitamin B_{12} and folate, in the form of either folic acid or methylfolate, should be prescribed if laboratory data show low levels of these vitamins or high levels of serum homocysteine. The indication for this additional treatment should be broad,

as patients with normal serum folate levels and with no megaloblastic anaemia have improved on folate therapy.

Monamine oxidase inhibitors (MAOIs) have been used to treat depression, and moclobemide, an MAOI, has been tested in Alzheimer patients.[109] Improvement was seen concerning mood levels.

Trazodone therapy is associated with hypotension, ventricular arrhythmias, priapism and confusion, all of which limit its use in later life. In addition, the wide dose range makes optimal therapy difficult to determine and achieve.[102]

Studies of the treatment of depressed elderly people with other new antidepressants, such as venlafaxine, nefazodone and mirtazapine, are extremely limited, but the fact that these drugs lack anticholinergic properties suggests that they may be suitable for the elderly.

In the treatment of affective disorders, lithium has been proven to have prophylactic effects. However, lithium is usually used only in recurrent uni- and bipolar affective psychoses, which are relatively rare in the elderly, and the use of lithium in elderly patients is restricted mainly to those who are refractory to other types of treatment. There is little literature on the treatment of severe depression in the elderly. The new drugs that influence both 5-HT and noradrenaline metabolism have not, as yet, been investigated with this population. Clinical experience suggests that addition of a noradrenergic-active drug, for example mianserin, may increase the response rate in those who do not respond to SSRIs alone. In patients with severe depression, administration of TCAs may also be considered.

Relapse after cessation of treatment is common in the elderly, although it may be minimized by the early introduction of appropriate and effective antidepressant treatment.[110] The high degree of degenerative changes in the ageing brain may induce a more chronic course of depression in elderly people. Treatment with current medications will reduce the depressive symptoms, but cannot cure an underlying organic disorder. Long-term treatment should therefore be considered in chronic depression in the elderly, or when an underlying organic disorder can be assumed. This makes it essential to find a treatment strategy with a low side-effect profile.

Short depressive episodes in the elderly should be treated in the same way as depressive episodes in younger people, with withdrawal of the drug after 6–12 months. If the patient has had previous depressive episodes, 1–2 years of therapy should be considered, and if episodes have been frequent or severe, lifelong prophylaxis is recommended.[111] The literature on pharmacological treatment of depression in young as well as old people is extensive. However, with regard to the outcome, no substantial differences between the sexes have been reported.

Electroconvulsive therapy (ECT) is effective in 70–80% of depressed patients. Age and dementia are not contraindications for ECT; up to 80% of elderly patients with symptoms of depression with a psychotic dimension respond favourably to ECT, although the treatment sometimes causes mild confusion.[112] If so, the interval between treatments should be extended and the number of treatments increased. As ECT is usually administered only in hospital, it is not the first choice for the treatment of severe depression in elderly people.

Anxiety and depression are often seen together in the elderly, especially in women. Environmental stress, such as problems with housing and financial difficulties, bereavement, retirement and physical illness, are also associated with anxiety and depression. The use of anxiolytics is not always feasible or appropriate in the treatment of elderly people. In the acute situation, such drugs should be used with care and only temporarily, for instance, in the case of insomnia. Anxiety will often respond to the same medications used in the treatment of depression. Although frequently prescribed, benzodiazepines can cause serious side-effects in geriatric patients. Long-term use may increase depression, delirium, ataxia and falls, particularly in elderly people with degenerative brain disorders.

Buspirone, a 5-HT$_1$ receptor agonist, has anti-anxiety effects in elderly people, and the combination of this drug with SSRIs may further increase the antidepressant effects.

It has been suggested that there is overuse of anxiolytic drugs in older populations. Indeed, a US study showed that 11% of men and 25% of women aged 60–74 years used anxiolytic drugs[113] and the 65+ age group, which constitutes 10% of the population in the USA, accounted for 21% of all prescriptions for diazepam.[114]

References

1. Warner JP, Depression in older people: what does the future hold? *Int J Geriatr Psychiatry* 1996; **11**:831–5.
2. Gräsbeck A, The epidemiology of anxiety and depressive syndromes. A prospective, longitudinal study of a geographically defined, total population: the Lundby study. Doctoral thesis, University of Lund, 1996.
3. Kessler RC, McGonagle KA, Swartz M et al, Sex and depression in the National Comorbidity Survey 1: lifetime prevalence, chronicity and recurrence, *J Affect Disord*

1993; **29**:85–96.

4. Skoog I, Nilsson L, Palmertz B et al, A population-based study of dementia in 85-year-olds, *N Engl J Med* 1993; **328**:153–8.

5. Fichter MM, Bruce ML, Schroppel H et al, Cognitive impairment and depression in the oldest old in a German and in US communities, *Eur Arch Psychiatry Clin Neurosci* 1995; **245**:319–25.

6. Lobo A, Saz P, Marcos G et al, The prevalence of dementia and depression in the elderly community in a southern European population. The Zaragoza study, *Arch Gen Psychiatry* 1995; **52**:497–506.

7. Henderson AS, Jorm AF, MacKinnon A et al, The prevalence of depressive disorders and the distribution of depressive symptoms in later life: a survey using Draft ICD-10 and DSM-III-R, *Psychol Med* 1993; **23**:719–29.

8. Kivelä S, Pahkala K, Laippala P, Prevalence of depression in an elderly population in Finland, *Acta Psychiatr Scand* 1988; **78**:401–3.

9. Bland RC, Orn H, Newman SC, Lifetime prevalence of psychiatric disorders in Edmonton, *Acta Psychiatr Scand* 1988; **338** (suppl):24–32.

10. Magnússon H, Mental health of octogenarians in Iceland. An epidemiological study, *Acta Psychiatr Scand* 1989; **79** (suppl):1–112.

11. Copeland JR, Gurland BJ, Dewey ME et al, Is there more dementia, depression and neurosis in New York? A comparative study of the elderly in New York and London using the computer diagnosis AGECAT, *Br J Psychiatry* 1987; **151**:466–73.

12. Copeland JR, Dewey ME, Wood N et al, Range of mental illness among the elderly in the community. Prevalence in Liverpool using the GMS-AGECAT package, *Br J Psychiatry* 1987; **150**:815–23.

13. Saunders PA, Copeland JR, Dewey ME et al, The prevalence of dementia, depression and neurosis in later life: the Liverpool MRC-ALPHA Study, *Int J Epidemiol* 1993; **22**:838–47.

14. Livingston G, Hawkins A, Graham N et al, The Gospel Oak study: prevalence rates of dementia, depression and activity limitation among elderly residents in inner London, *Psychol Med* 1990; **20**:137–46.

15. Lindesay J, Briggs K, Murphy E, The Guy's Age Concern survey. Prevalence rates of cognitive impairment, depression and anxiety in an urban elderly community, *Br J Psychiatry* 1989; **155**:317–29.

16. Woo J, Ho SC, Lau J et al, The prevalence of depressive symptoms and predisposing factors in an elderly Chinese population, *Acta Psychiatr Scand* 1994; **89**:8–13.

17. Beekman AT, Deeg DJ, van Tilburg T et al, Major and minor depression in late life: a study of prevalence and risk factors, *J Affect Disord* 1995; **36**:65–75.

18. Palsson S, Skoog I, The epidemiology of affective disorders in the elderly: a review, *Int Clin Psychopharmacol* 1997; **12** (suppl 7):S3–13.

19. American Psychatric Association, *Diagnostic and Statistical Manual of Mental Disorders*, 3rd rev edn (APA: Washington, DC, 1987).

20. American Psychiatric Association, *Diagnostic and Statistical Manual of Mental Disorders*, 4th edn (APA: Washington DS, 1994).

21. Kivelä SL, Pahkala K, Eronen A, Depressive symptoms and signs that differentiate major atypical depression from dysthymic disorder in elderly Finns, *Int J Geriatr Psychiatry* 1989; **155**:330–6.

22. Copeland JR, Dewey ME, Griffiths-Jones HM, A computerized psychiatric diagnostic system and case nomenclature for elderly subjects GMS and AGECAT, *Psychol Med* 1986; **16**:89–99.

23. Blehar MC, Oren DA, Gender differences in depression, *Medscape Womens Health* 1997; **2**:3.

24. Pahkala K, Kesti E, Köngäs-Saviaro P et al, Prevalence of depression in an aged population in Finland, *Soc Psychiatry Psychiatr Epidemiol* 1995; **30**:99–106.

25. Angst J, Dobler-Mikola A, Do the diagnostic criteria determine the sex ratio in depression? *J Affect Disord* 1984; **7**:189–98.

26. Haller J, Weggemans RM, Ferry M, Guigoz Y, Mental health: Mini-Mental State Examination and Geriatric Depression score of elderly Europeans in the SENECA study of 1993, *Eur J Clin Nutr* 1996; **50** (suppl 2):S112–16.

27. Katz S, Ford AB, Moskowitz RW et al, Studies of illness in the aged. The index of ADL: a

standardized measure of biological and psychosocial function, *JAMA* 1963; **185**: 914–19.

28. Jorm AF, Sex and age differences in depression: a quantitative synthesis of published research, *Aust NZ J Psychiatry* 1987; **21**:45–53.

29. Fuhrer R, Antonucci TC, Gagnon M et al, Depressive symptomatology and cognitive functioning: an epidemiological survey in an elderly community sample in France, *Psychol Med* 1992; **22**:159–72.

30. Evans S, Katona C, Epidemiology of depressive symptoms in elderly primary care attenders, *Dementia* 1993; **4**:327–33.

31. Yesavage JA, Brink TL, Rose TL et al, Development and validation of a geriatric depression screening scale: a preliminary report, *J Psychiatr Res* 1982–83; **17**:37–49.

32. Gottfries CG, Noltorp S, Nørgaard N, Experience with a Swedish version of the Geriatric Depression Scale in primary care centers, *Int J Geriatr Psychiatry* 1997; **12**:1029–34.

33. Bleiker EM, van der Ploeg HM, Mook J, Kleijn WC, Anxiety, anger and depression in elderly women, *Psychol Rep* 1993; **72**:567–74.

34. Rapp SR, Parisi SA, Walsh DA, Psychological dysfunction and physical health among elderly medical inpatients, *J Consult Clin Psychol* 1988; **56**:851–5.

35. Spiegel D, Cancer and depression, *Br J Psychiatry (Suppl)* 1996; **30**:109–16.

36. Lansky SB, List MA, Herrmann CA et al, Absence of major depressive disorder in female cancer patients, *J Clin Oncol* 1985; **3**:1553–60.

37. Anda R, Williamson D, Jones D et al, Depressed affect, hopelessness, and the risk of ischemic heart disease in a cohort of US adults, *Epidemiology* 1993; **4**:285–94.

38. Weeke A, Juel K, Vaeth M, Cardiovascular death and manic-depressive psychosis, *J Affect Disord* 1987; **13**:287–92.

39. Andersson M, Elderly patients in nursing homes and in home care. Doctoral thesis, Göteborg University 1989.

40. Katz IR, Lesher E, Kleban M et al, Clinical features of depression in the nursing home, *Int Psychogeriatr* 1989; **1**: 5–15.

41. Harrison R, Savla N, Kafetz K, Dementia, depression and physical disability in a London borough: a survey of elderly people in and out of residential care and implications for future developments, *Age Ageing* 1990; **19**:97–103.

42. Phillips CJ, Henderson AS, The prevalence of depression among Australian nursing home residents: results using draft ICD-10 and DSM-III-R criteria, *Psychol Med* 1991; **21**:739–48.

43. Ballard CG, Bannister C, Oyebode F, Depression in dementia sufferers, *Int J Geriatr Psychiatry* 1996; **11**:5007–15.

44. Jast BC, Grossberg GT, The evolution of psychiatric symptoms in Alzheimer's disease: a natural history study, *J Am Geriatr Soc* in press.

45. Blazer D, Williams CD, Epidemiology of dysphoria and depression in an elderly population, *Am J Psychiatry* 1980; **137**:439–44.

46. Cummings JL, Dementia and depression, an evolving enigma, *J Neuropsychiatry Clin Neurosci* 1989; **1**:236–42.

47. Cummings JL, Miller B, Hill MA et al, Neuropsychiatric aspects of multi-infarct dementia and dementia of the Alzheimer type, *Arch Neurol* 1987; **44**:389–93.

48. Rovner BW, Broadhead J, Spencer M, Neshkes R, Depression and Alzheimer's disease, *Am J Psychiatry* 1989; **146**:350–3.

49. McKeith IG, Perry RH, Fairbairn AF et al, Operational criteria for senile dementia of Lewy body type, *Psychol Med* 1992; **22**:911–22.

50. Agrell B, Dehlin O, Depression in stroke patients with left and right hemisphere lesions. A study in geriatric rehabilitation inpatients, *Aging* 1994; **6**:49–56.

51. Primeau F, Post-stroke depression: a critical review of the literature, *Can J Psychiatry* 1988; **33**:757–65.

52. Ågren H, Symptom patterns in unipolar and bipolar depression correlating with monoamine metabolites in the cerebrospinal fluid: II. suicide, *Psychiatr Res* 1980; **3**:225–36.

53. Åsberg M, Nordstrøm P, Träskman-Bendz L, Cerebrospinal fluid studies in suicide: an overview, *Ann NY Acad Sci* 1986; **487**:243–55.

54. Hoogendijk WJG, Sommer IEC, Tissingh G et al, Depression in Parkinson's disease: the impact of symptom overlap on the prevalence, *Psychosomatics* 2000; in press.

55. Lovestone S, Howard R, *Depression in Elderly People* (Martin Dunitz: London 1996) 7.

56. Pearson JL, Conwell Y, Suicide in late life. Challenges and opportunities for research, *Int Psychogeriatr* 1995; 7:131–6.

57. Moscicki EK, Epidemiology of suicide, *Int Psychogeriatr* 1995; 7:137–48.

58. National Center for Health Statistics, *Advance report of final mortality statistics 1990. Monthly Vital Statistics Report*, Vol. 41, No. 7 Suppl (Hyattsville, Maryland: Public Health Service, 1993).

59. Watanabe N, Hasegawa K, Yoshinaga Y, Suicide in later life in Japan: urban and rural differences, *Int Psychogeriatr* 1995; 7:253–61.

60. Gottfries CG, Neurochemical aspects of aging and diseases with cognitive impairment, *J Neurosci Res* 1990; 27:541–7.

61. Raskind MA, Peskind ER, Neurobiologic basis of noncognitive behavioral problems in Alzheimer's disease, *Alzheimer Dis Assoc Disord* 1994; 8 (suppl 3):54–60.

62. Gottfries CG, Adolfsson R, Aquilonius SM et al, Biochemical changes in dementia disorders of Alzheimer type (AD/SDAT), *Neurobiol Aging* 1983; 4:261–71.

63. Wallin A, Gottfries CG, Biochemical substrates in normal aging and Alzheimer's disease, *Pharmacopsychiatry* 1990; 23 (suppl):37–43.

64. Raadsheer FC, Increased activity of hypothalamic corticotrophin-releasing hormone: neurons in aging, Alzheimer's disease and depression, Doctoral thesis, University of Amsterdam, 1994.

65. Arranz B, Blennow K, Ekman R et al, Brain monoaminergic and neuropeptidergic variations in human aging, *J Neural Transm* 1996; 103:101–15.

66. Heuser IJ, Gotthardt U, Schweiger U et al, Age-associated changes of pituitary–adrenocortical hormone regulation in humans: importance of gender, *Neurobiol Aging* 1994; 15:227–31.

67. Spaulding SW, Age and the thyroid, *Endocrinol Metab Clin North Am* 1987; 16:1013–25.

68. Kirkegaard C, Faber J, Hummer L, Rogowski P, Increased levels of TRH in cerebrospinal fluid from patients with endogenous depression, *Psychoneuroendocrinology* 1979; 4:227–35.

69. Loosen PT, Prange AJ Jr, Serum thyrotropin response to thyrotropin-releasing hormone in psychiatric patients: a review, *Am J Psychiatry* 1982; 139:405–16.

70. Prange AJ Jr, The therapeutic use of hormone of the thyroid axis in depression. In: Post RM, Ballenger JC, eds, *Neurobiology of Mood Disorders* (Williamsen & Wilkins: Baltimore, 1984) 311–22.

71. Altman N, Sachar EJ, Gruen PH et al, Reduced plasma LH concentration in postmenopausal depressed women, *Psychosomat Med* 1975; 37:274–6.

72. Sadow TF, Rubin RT, Effects of hypothalamic peptides on the aging brain, *Psychoneuroendocrinology* 1992; 17:293–314.

73. Anda RF, Williamson DF, Jones D et al, Depressed affect, hopelessness and the risk of ischemic heart disease in a cohort of US adults, *Epidemiology*, 1993; 4:285–94.

74. Lindenbaum J, Healton EB, Savage DG et al, Neuropsychiatric disorders caused by cobalamin deficiency in the absence of anaemia or macrocytosis, *N Engl J Med* 1988; 318:1720–8.

75. Regland B, Abrahamsson L, Blennow K et al, Vitamin B_{12} in CSF: reduced CSF/serum B_{12} ratio in demented men, *Acta Neurol Scand* 1992; 85:276–81.

76. Regland R, Vitamin B_{12} deficiency in dementia disorders, Doctoral thesis, University of Göteborg, 1991.

77. Herbert V, Experimental nutritional folate deficiency in man, *Trans Assoc Am Physicians* 1962; 75:307–20.

78. Shorvon SD, Carney MW, Chanarin I, Reynolds EH, The neuropsychiatry of megaloblastic anaemia, *Br Med J* 1980; 281:1036–8.

79. Carney MW, Chary TK, Laundy M et al, Red cell folate concentrations in psychiatric patients, *J Affect Disord* 1990; 19:207–13.

80. Reynolds EH, Preece JM, Bailey J, Coppen A,

Folate deficiency in depressive illness, *Br J Psychiatry* 1970; **117**:287–92.

81. Heilmann E, Folsäuremangel: Ergebnisse eigener Untersuchungen an gesunden Probanden in verschiedenen Altersstufen und bei unterschiedlichen Erkrankungen. In: von Pietrzik K, ed., *Folsäuremangel: Fachgespräch am 5. Juli 1986 in Rottach-Egern* (W. Zuckschwerdt Verlag: München, 1987) 41–55.

82. Coppen A, Abou-Saleh MT, Plasma folate and affective morbidity during long-term lithium therapy, *Br J Psychiatry* 1982; **141**:87–9.

83. Fava M, Borus JS, Alpert JE et al, Folate, vitamin B$_{12}$ and homocysteine in major depressive disorder, *Am J Psychiatry* 1997; **154**:426–8.

84. Alpert M, Silva R, Pouget B, Folate as a predictor of response to sertraline and nortryptiline in geriatric depression. Presented at the 36th Annual Meeting of the NCDEU, Boca Raton FL, USA, 28–31 May 1996.

85. Bottiglieri T, Godfrey P, Flynn T et al, Cerebrospinal fluid S-adenosylmethionine in depression and dementia. Effects of treatment with parenteral and oral S-adenosylmethionine, *J Neurol Neurosurg Psychiatry* 1990; **53**:1096–8.

86. Godfrey PS, Toone BK, Carney MW et al, Enhancement of recovery from psychiatric illness by methylfolate, *Lancet* 1990; **336**: 392–5.

87. Georges LK, Social factors and depression in late life. In: Schneider LS, Reynolds III CF, Lewbowitz BD, Friedhoff AJ, eds, *Diagnosis and Treatment of Depression in Late Life. Results of the NIH Consensus Development Conference* (American Psychiatric Press: Washington DC, 1994) 131–53.

88. Kivelä SL, Pahkala K, Symptoms of depression in old people in Finland, *Z Gerontol* 1988; **21**:257–63.

89. Barsky AJ, Frank CB, Cleary PD et al, The relation between hypochondriasis and age, *Am J Psychiatry* 1991; **148**:923–8.

90. Katona CLE, *Depression in Old Age* (Wiley: Chichester, 1994) 29–41.

91. Baldwin RC, Tomenson B, Depression in later life. A comparison of symptoms and risk factors in early and late onset cases, *Br J Psychiatry* 1995; **167**:649–52.

92. Regier DA, Narrow WE, Rae DS, The epidemiology of anxiety disorders: the epidemiologic catchment area (ECA) experience, *J Psychiatr Res* 1990; **24**:3–14.

93. Tebbs VM, Martin AJ, Affective disorders in the elderly: 1000-patient GP trial on a new drug, *Geriatr Med* 1987; **17**:17–21.

94. Magni E, Frisoni GB, Rozzini R et al, Depression and somatic symptoms in the elderly: the role of cognitive function, *Int J Geriatr Psychiatry* 1996; **11**:517–22.

95. Tannock C, Katona C, Minor depression in the aged. Concepts, prevalence and optimal management, *Drugs Aging* 1995; **6**:278–92.

96. Mitchell AJ, Dening TR, Depression-related cognitive impairment: possibilities for its pharmacological treatment, *J Affect Disord* 1996; **36**:79–87.

97. Montgomery SA, Åsberg M, A new depression scale designed to be sensitive to change, *Br J Psychiatry* 1995; **167**:649–52.

98. Hamilton M, A rating scale for depression, *J Neurol Neurosurg Psychiatry* 1960; **23**:50–62.

99. Lindenbaum J, Healton EB, Savage DG et al, Neuropsychiatric disorder caused by cobalamin deficiency in the absense of anaemia or macrocytosis, *N Engl Med* 1988; 1720–8.

100. Branconnier RJ, DeVitt DR, Cole JO, Spera KF, Amitriptyline selectively disrupts verbal recall from secondary memory of the normal aged, *Neurobiol Aging* 1982; **3**:55–9.

101. Feinberg M, The problems of anticholinergic effects in older patients, *Drugs Aging* 1993; **3**:335–48.

102. Rothschild AJ, The diagnosis and treatment of late-life depression, *J Clin Psychiatry* 1996; **57** (suppl 5):5–10.

103. Nyth AL, Gottfries CG, The clinical efficacy of citalopram in treatment of emotional disturbances in dementia disorders. A Nordic multicentre study, *Br J Psychiatry* 1990; **157**: 894–901.

104. Nyth AL, Gottfries CG, Lyby K et al, A controlled multicenter clinical study of citalopram and placebo in elderly depressed patients with and without concomitant dementia, *Acta Psychiatr Scand* 1992; **86**:138–45.

105. Guy W, *ECDEU Assessment Manual for Psychopharmacology. Clinical Global Impressions (028-CGI)* (USGPO: Washington, DC, 1976) 216–22.

106. Andersen G, Vestergaard K, Riis JO, Citalopram for post-stroke pathological crying, *Lancet* 1993; **342**:837–9.

107. Andersen G, Vestergaard K, Lauritzen L, Effective treatment of post-stroke depression with the selective serotonin reuptake inhibitor citalopram, *Stroke* 1994; **25**:1099–104.

108. Ragneskog H, Eriksson S, Karlsson I, Gottfries CG, Long-term treatment of elderly individuals with emotional disturbances—an open study with citalopram, *Int Psychogeriatr* 1996; **8**:659–68.

109. Roth M, Mountjoy CQ, Amrein R, Moclobemide in elderly patients with cognitive decline and depression. An international double-blind, placebo-controlled trial, *Br J Psychiatry* 1996; **168**:149–57.

110. Bonner D, Howard R, Treatment resistant depression in the elderly, *Int J Geriatr Psychiatry* 1995; **10**:259–64.

111. Newhouse PA, Use of selective serotonin reuptake inhibitors in geriatric depression, *J Clin Psychiatry* 1996; **57** (suppl 5):12–22.

112. Mulsant BH, Rosen J, Thornton JE, Zubenko GS, A prospective naturalistic study of electroconvulsive therapy in late-life depression, *J Geriatr Psychiatry Neurol* 1991; **4**:3–13.

113. Martin LM, Fleming KC, Evans JM, Recognition and management of anxiety and depression in elderly patients, *Mayo Clin Proc* 1995; **70**:999–1006.

114. Abrams R, Anxiety and personality disorders. In: Sadavoy J, Lazarus LV, Jarvik LS, eds, *Comprehensive Review of Geriatric Psychiatry* (American Psychiatric Press: Washington DC, 1991) 369–86.

12

Female sex steroids, the brain and behaviour

Torbjörn Bäckström, Patrik Appelblad, Marie Bixo, David Haage,
Staffan Johansson, Sven Landgren, Lena Seippel, Inger Sundström,
Mingde Wang and Göran Wahlström

Introduction

Female sex steroids profoundly influence the brain. Apart from the symptoms characterizing female-specific mood disorders such as irritability, dysphoria, affect lability, and changes in appetite,[1-7] other aspects of brain function, such as sexual activity,[5] cognitive capabilities, sensorimotor function, and seizure susceptibility,[8] are also related to serum levels of oestrogens, progesterone and various progesterone metabolites. Whereas the phenomenology and treatment of conditions such as premenstrual syndrome (PMS) and menopausal-related complaints are presented thoroughly in other chapters of this book (see Chapters 13, 16 and 22), in the present chapter these and other conditions will be discussed as illustrative examples of how the brain is being regulated by female sex steroids.

Theoretical aspects

The concentrations of female sex steroids in brain reflect the concentrations in serum. The level of progesterone in the cerebral cortex is hence 300 times higher during the luteal phase than during the follicular phase in pseudo-pregnant rat;[9] moreover, the concentrations of oestrogen, progesterone and progesterone metabolites in the central nervous system (CNS) are higher in women of fertile age than in postmenopausal women.[10,11] Sex steroids can, however, also be produced in the brain, as illustrated by the finding that stress increases allopregnanolone concentration in the brain before the serum levels of this hormone are changed.[12]

Specific intracellular receptors for oestradiol and progesterone have been identified in certain brain regions. The steroids[13-15] and their receptors[16-19] are not evenly distributed in the brain, but concentrated in certain regions, such as the hypothalamus, where the regulation of gonadotrophin release takes place. Other brain regions in which steroids are accumulated, and steroid receptors are abundant, are the amygdala, which is related to mood and emotionality, and the hippocampus, which is related to memory and cognitive functions.

The classical mechanism of action of a steroid is to act (in conjunction with the steroid receptor) as a genomic transcription factor, hence influencing protein synthesis. Such effects are relatively slow; thus, it usually takes 5–15 min, but sometimes days, before an effect of the hormonal stimulation may be observed.[16,20] The influence on sexual behaviour in experimental animals is one example of a genomic effect of female sex steroids.

In addition to the relatively slow effects of sex steroids on protein synthesis, these substances may also exert rapid effects, via a direct interaction with membrane-bound receptors or ion channels.[20] Such an effect usually occurs within fractions of a second; for example, oestradiol has been shown to inhibit the firing rate of certain hypothalamic nerve cells within milliseconds after application,[21] and the effect of allopregnanolone on epileptic discharges in rat brain has been shown to occur within seconds.[22]

Many of the functional effects of these hormones could probably, at least in part, be explained in terms of an interaction between the hormone and certain neurotransmitter systems. The well-established sedative and antiepileptic effects of various progesterone derivatives may hence be due to a non-genomic influence on GABAergic transmission; the epileptogenic effects of oestrogens, on the other hand, may be related to an effect on glutamate. Whereas the influence of female sex steroids on symptoms such as irritability and depressed mood may be related to the effect of sex steroids on serotonergic transmission, the effect of oestrogen on motor control may be dopamine-mediated. That female sex steroids influence various aspects of the monoaminergic activity in experimental animals has been

revealed by a large number of studies,[23–33] and is further discussed in Chapter 5.

Variation in mood symptoms during the menstrual cycle

PMS (or premenstrual dysphoric disorder, PMDD) is characterized by mental symptoms such as depressed mood, irritability, lack of energy, tension, and changes in appetite, and by somatic symptoms such as bloatedness and breast tenderness.[2–4,6] An analysis of the exact relationship between symptom development and hormonal variations during the menstrual cycle reveals that the cluster of symptoms characterizing PMS is usually most severe during the last 5 days prior to menstruation.[34] When the menstrual period starts, the symptoms rapidly decrease, and 3–4 days after the onset of menstruation they have usually disappeared (Figure 12.1). Although the symptoms thus develop in parallel with the development of the corpus luteum, the symptom peak is reached within 5–6 days after the peak in serum progesterone levels. On the other hand, the increase in symptoms occurs before the onset of the rapid premenstrual decline in hormonal levels, indicating that the symptoms cannot be provoked solely by progesterone withdrawal. At the end of the luteal phase, when oestradiol and progesterone reach follicular phase levels, the symptoms disappear.[34] During the preovulatory oestradiol peak there is a period of wellbeing, which appears to be closely related to the oestradiol peak (see Figure 12.1).

In anovulatory cycles, the corpus luteum is not formed, and progesterone and other substances synthesized by the corpus luteum are not being produced. Symptoms caused by factors produced by the corpus luteum should thus not be present in anovulatory cycles. Anovulation occurs spontaneously in about

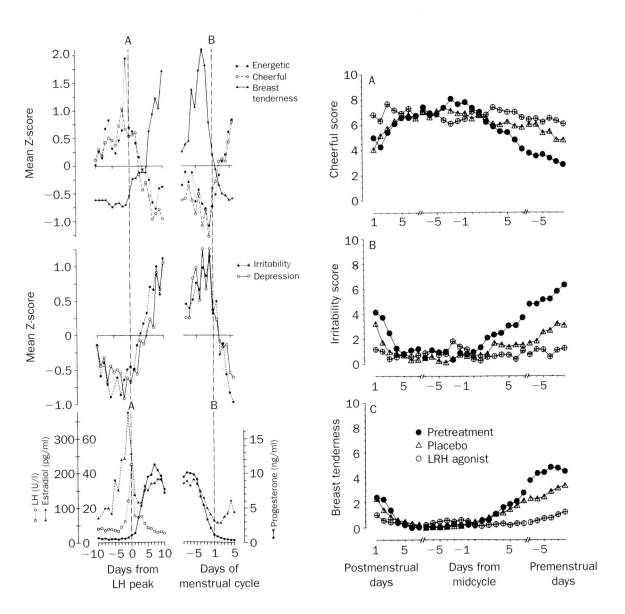

Figure 12.1 Mean Z-scores for mood and physical symptoms and hormonal data during the menstrual cycle in patients with PMS (*n* = 12). (A) The data are synchronized around the day of luteinizing hormone (LH) surge. (B) The data are synchronized around the first day of menstrual bleeding (Day 0). (Reprinted from Bäckstrom et al,[34] with kind permission from Lippincott Williams & Wilkins, Baltimore, MD, USA. © 1983.)

Figure 12.2 Mean scores for the items cheerfulness, irritability and breast tenderness for a group of PMS patients during a pretreatment cycle, a cycle on placebo, and a cycle on a GnRH agonist. The data are centred around the day of ovulation or mid-cycle and the day of onset of menstrual bleeding. (Reprinted from Hammarbäck and Bäckstrom[38] with kind permission from Munksgaard International Publishers Ltd, Copenhagen, Denmark. © 1988.)

10% of menstrual cycles,[35] and can be induced by treatment with gonadotrophin-releasing hormone (GnRH) analogues administered nasally or subcutaneously. A prospective study comprising daily symptom ratings and hormone measurements in women with both ovulatory and spontaneously anovulatory cycles revealed that cycle-related symptoms are present in ovulatory cycles only.[36] Similarly, artificial induction of anovulation by means of a GnRH analogue diminishes the cyclical mood changes more effectively than placebo.[37-40] Other ways of manipulating the ovarian cycle have also been reported to reduce the symptoms of PMS. Oestradiol implants in high doses causing anovulation,[41] and ovulation-inhibiting doses of danazol, are thus reported to be effective.[42] Oophorectomy has also been reported to effectively abolish the symptoms of PMS,[43,44] but not hysterectomy, where the ovaries are left intact. After hysterectomy, the cyclical symptom variations continue, with symptoms recurring during the late luteal phase, although the severity may decrease.[45] The presence of symptoms during the late luteal phase can thus not be due to the anticipation of an approaching menstrual period, but must be due to some factor produced by the corpus luteum (see also Chapter 16). The severity of the symptoms may, however, be influenced by psychological factors; notably, the placebo effect in PMS is considerable.[38,46,47]

Although it is not yet known which factors from the corpus luteum are responsible for the symptoms characterizing PMS, the hypothesis that progestagens may be involved derives support from studies in which sex steroids have been given to postmenopausal women and to women in which the premenstrual complaints have been abolished by means of an ovulation inhibitor.[40] Interestingly, it seems that women with PMS may be more sensitive to ovarian steroids than controls. As discussed below (and in Chapter 5), the effects of progestagens on

the brain, like the effects of benzodiazepines, may partly be mediated by GABA-A receptors; hence, the observation that women with PMS display a different sensitivity not only with regard to compounds such as pregnenolone, but also with regard to benzodiazepines,[48,49] is of interest in this context. This difference in CNS sensitivity to sex steroids could be the reason why only certain women show mood changes related to hormone variations.[40]

Relation between luteal phase steroid production and symptom severity

In a study investigating daily serum hormone levels and symptomatology for two consecutive menstrual cycles, PMS women reported more symptoms in a cycle with higher luteal phase concentrations of progesterone, and, in particular, oestrogen, than in a cycle with lower hormonal concentrations.[50] These results clearly contradict the theory that PMS is due to low levels of progesterone.[1] The correlation between symptom severity and high luteal phase oestradiol is in line with the finding (in a placebo-controlled trial) that the addition of exogenous oestradiol during the luteal phase may increase the severity of symptoms in women with PMS, contrary to what was expected.[51] Moreover, a symptom-provoking effect, not only of progesterone, but also of oestrogen, has been observed in PMS women pretreated with a GnRH analogue.[40]

As discussed below, not only oestrogens and progesterone, but also several sex steroid precursors and metabolites, exert an influence on the brain. In humans, serum levels of the first and second 5-reduced metabolites of progesterone, 5α-pregnane-3,20-dione (5-DHP) and

3α-hydroxy-5α-pregnane-20-one (3OH-THP), increase during the luteal phase of the cycle. The variation of these metabolites, which are produced by the corpus luteum, during the menstrual cycle is highly correlated with progesterone level.[52–55] The enzymes necessary for 5-reduction of progesterone have also been identified in the brain;[56] and the brain concentrations of 5-DHP are much higher than in plasma during progesterone-induced anaesthesia.[57] In addition to 5-DHP and 3OH-THP, two other progesterone derivatives, pregnenolone and pregnenolone sulphate, display significant fluctuations within menstrual cycles that are also correlated with progesterone level.[55] Other steroids produced by the corpus luteum might also be active in the brain; new methods to measure steroids may give us new insights into the various CNS active progesterone metabolites that are being produced by the ovary.[58] As discussed below, many progesterone derivatives interact with brain GABAergic transmission in an anxiolytic-like manner; however, some of them, like pregnenolone sulphate, may instead be anxiogenic.

In the above-mentioned study on the relationship between serum hormone levels and symptomatology in women with PMS, daily plasma pregnenolone, pregnenolone sulphate, 5-DHP and 5-THP were also studied. More severe symptoms occurred in cycles with relatively high luteal phase plasma pregnenolone and pregnenolone sulphate concentrations; in contrast, higher luteal phase 5-DHP and 5-THP levels were associated with low symptom rating.[55] The symptom scores were correlated with hormone levels, but the symptom peak showed a delay of 3–4 days from the peaks of progesterone, pregnenolone, 5-DHP and 5-THP in plasma, whereas the plasma pregnenolone sulphate peak appeared on the same day or 1 day before the symptom peak.

In plasma, oestradiol is largely bound to transport proteins, sex hormone-binding globulin (SHBG) and albumin; only a small fraction (1–3%) is unbound.[59] Progesterone is bound to transcortin and albumin, up to 10% being unbound.[8] It is generally considered that it is the unbound fraction that exerts the hormonal effects in peripheral organs. The 5-reduced progesterone metabolites are not known to bind to specific plasma binding proteins, but only to albumin, with low affinity.[60]

In the above-mentioned study,[55] there were no differences in concentrations between patients and controls with respect to the various progesterone derivatives, which is in agreement with findings by Schmidt et al.[61] Notably, however, Rapkin et al have reported lower levels (in the luteal phase) of allopregnanolone in PMS subjects compared with controls.[62] With respect to serum levels of oestradiol and progesterone, most studies suggest that PMS patients do not differ from controls[40,55] (see also Chapter 16). It may probably be concluded that PMS patients do not differ from controls with respect to absolute plasma levels of sex steroids, but rather in the way in which their brains react to these hormones.[40]

Mood effects of oral contraceptives

Negative mood symptoms are well-known side-effects of oral contraceptives (OCs),[63,64] and about 30% of women report mental side-effects as the main reason for discontinuing OC use.[63] Women experiencing mental side-effects on OCs also report severe PMS when not taking OCs,[63–66] whereas women with mild premenstrual complaints have, in contrast, been reported to benefit from treatment with OCs;[67] a superiority of OCs over placebo has, however, not been established in controlled trials.[47]

Studies on women taking combined OCs suggest unexpectedly that a contraceptive with a low progestagen concentration may be more symptom-provoking than one with a high concentration.[64,67,68] Qualitative differences between different progestagenic compounds have been reported: desorgestrel seems to be less symptom-provoking than levonor-gestrel.[64,67]

Mood effects of oestrogen and progestagens

Mood changes in relation to menopausal transition are often discussed in the lay press and among patients. Longitudinal studies, however, have failed to demonstrate an increase in frequency of major depression or severe mood changes in relation to transition.[69–71] Some studies, however, suggest that milder mood changes, expressed as decreased wellbeing, are more common after the menopause than before;[70,72,73] data in this field are not unanimous[65,74–78] (see also Chapters 13 and 22).

A possible antidepressant effect of oestrogen has been evaluated in menopausal women suffering from depression. Several controlled, randomized studies, however, showed no antidepressant effect of oestrogen, in the doses used for hormone replacement therapy (HRT),[79–81] whereas one controlled study suggests that oestrogen may improve mood in mildly depressed, menopausal women.[82] In one double-blind study, a high dose of oestrogen was shown to be effective for postpartum depression.[83] Moreover, according to an earlier study, a high dose of oestrogen may be useful for the treatment of severely depressed patients;[84] this study still awaits replication (for reviews see Archer[85] and Panay and Studd[86]).

In younger oophorectomized patients, the antidepressant effects of oestrogen seem more pronounced than in women following a natural menopause. Four controlled studies thus show a significant oestrogen-induced reduction in depressive symptoms in oophorectomized, depressed women;[82,87–89] in one of these studies, the effect of oestrogen was found to be dose-dependent.[89] It should be remembered that the ovary continues to produce steroids several years after the menopause; oophorectomized women thus have less oestrogen than those who are naturally postmenopausal, presumably explaining why the mood-lifting effects of oestrogen replacement are more evident in oophorectomized patients than in those who are naturally menopausal.

Some women on sequential HRT will develop negative mood changes (depression and irritability) related to the progestagen component of the treatment (Figure 12.3).[90,91] In these women, the symptoms appear shortly after the progestagen has been added to the treatment, and increase gradually throughout treatment. The symptoms usually disappear within 2 or 3 days following the discontinuation of the progestagen.[90] Although the mechanism underlying these symptoms remains unknown, there can be no doubt that the negative mood change is related to the progestagen component of the HRT. The symptoms resemble those reported by women with PMS during the luteal phase of ovulatory cycles, as well as those provoked by gestagen administration to women with PMS pretreated with a GnRH agonist.[40] The negative effects of progestagen in menopausal women seem to be dose-related, higher doses causing more symptoms than lower ones.[91] This is the major cause for discontinuation of HRT in this population.[92]

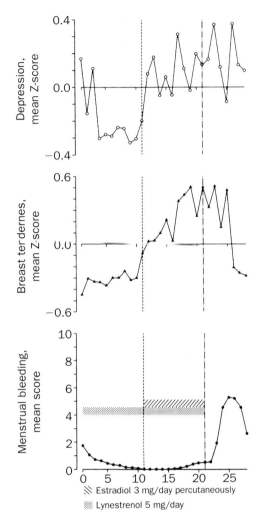

Figure 12.3 Mean depression and breast tenderness Z-scores, and menstrual bleeding scores, during one cycle in 11 postmenopausal women on sequential oestrogen/progestagen replacement therapy. (Reprinted from Hammarbäck at al[90] with kind permission from Munksgaard International Publishers Ltd, Copenhagen, Denmark. © 1985.)

Effect of oestrogens on sensorimotor functions

Behavioural studies in animals and humans have shown that the oestrogen-dominated follicular phase is related to increased activity and wakefulness.[93] A higher rapidity of fine motor skills in both hands and legs has been noted during the follicular phase, when compared with the luteal phase;[94] also, high levels of oestrogen were reported to enhance the control of movements.[95] Both animal experiments and clinical studies suggest that increased oestradiol concentrations are related to increased two-points discrimination ability, touch sensitivity, visual function, hearing, and olfactory function;[96] in addition, an improvement in postural balance has been reported in postmenopausal women on oestrogen replacement therapy when compared with women without treatment.[97] That oestrogen influences the control of movements is further supported by the finding that high doses of oestrogen may induce chorea-like involuntary movements as a side-effect;[98] tentatively, such an effect may be related to the influence of oestrogen on brain dopaminergic neurotransmission (see Chapter 5). Whereas the animal experiments regarding the influence of oestrogen on sensorimotor function cited above have usually been controlled and have revealed clear-cut results, human studies in this field have been mostly observational and non-controlled (with the exception of those regarding balance).

Effects of oestrogen on cognitive function and on the development of Alzheimer's disease

Several studies have investigated the effect of HRT on memory in non-demented subjects (for reviews, see Hogervoorst et al[99] and Haskell et al[100]). Whereas several studies suggest that oestrogen treatment improves cognitive function,[101–106] no such effect has been detected in others.[107–111]

A deterioration of memory function has been reported in patients receiving GnRH agonists for treatment of endometriosis, but the memory has been restored to normal baseline in subjects who received oestrogen add-back.[112]

Effects of oestrogens on memory function and on the possibility of coping with daily activities have also been investigated in patients with Alzheimer's dementia. A few studies, mostly uncontrolled and comprising only a few patients, suggest that oestrogen may cause a moderate improvement in memory in patients with mild to moderate dementia, but not in those with severe dementia.[113–118]

Recent epidemiological case-control studies have addressed the issue of whether oestrogen replacement therapy may reduce the risk of developing Alzheimer's disease; they are, however, often marred by methodological problems related to the diagnosis of Alzheimer's disease, to the doses and duration of the oestrogen treatment, and to the possibility of differences between oestrogen users and non-users (not related to treatment) influencing the results. Some of these studies reveal a clear-cut protective effect, whereas in others, the effects are less evident.[111,119–127] In a cohort study of 8877 women, the risk of developing Alzheimer's disease was not significantly lower among the oestrogen users, but women with a higher dose had a significantly lower risk compared with those given a lower dose.[125] A prospective longitudinal study, in which 1124 postmenopausal elderly women were followed for 1–5 years, the incidence of Alzheimer's disease was significantly lower in the oestrogen-treated group when compared with the group not taking oestrogen.[126] These results are encouraging, but more studies are needed in order to confirm that oestrogen replacement reduces the risk for Alzheimer's disease.

Several effects of oestrogen on the brain, observed mostly in animal studies, may be of importance for the tentative effects of this hormone on memory, and for the protective effect with respect to the development of Alzheimer's disease. For example, a morphological reduction in neuronal connections has been observed in the hippocampus 6 days after oophorectomy, reaching a maximum at 40 days after the operation. Following oestrogen replacement, the number of synapses is fully restored. This effect of oestrogen, which is in all likelihood a genomic effect, is apparent 24 h after initiation of treatment.[128] Given the well-established role of acetylcholine in memory function, and in the pathophysiology of Alzheimer's disease, the finding that oestrogen influences cholinergic activity may also be of importance in this context.[23,128,129] Of additional possible relevance for the tentative protective effects of oestrogen on the brain are the observations that the hormone increases the production and action of β-amyloid peptides,[130,131] that brain circulation is enhanced within 10 min after an oestradiol injection,[132] and that activation of certain brain areas (measured using magnetic resonance imaging (MRI)) during working memory tasks is increased in non-demented menopausal women after 3 weeks of oestrogen treatment.[133] Moreover, animal experiments have revealed a facilatory effect of oestrogen on learning and memory[134] and on the electrophysiological event that is believed to form the basis for learning (long-term potentiation).[135]

Effects of female sex steroids on excitability and epilepsy

Oestradiol has been shown to decrease the seizure threshold in a dose-dependent fashion.[136] An acute increase in frequency of epileptic discharges from an epileptic focus was noted in 11 of 14 women following an intravenous injection of a high dose (40 mg) of conjugated oestrogens. In four patients, a grand mal seizure occurred within 15 min after the injection.[137] Also, it has been shown that an epileptic focus can be induced by application of oestradiol directly onto the cerebral cortex.[138] Notably, certain women with partial epilepsy show a fluctuation in epileptic seizures in relation to the fluctuations of oestrogen and progesterone during the menstrual cycle, with a low seizure frequency at times of high progesterone levels, and a high seizure frequency at times of high oestrogen levels.[8,139]

Of possible relevance for these observations is the finding that oestradiol seems to have a facilatory effect on the excitatory transmitter substance glutamate in the brain (via an interaction with glutamate receptors of non-NMDA subtypes).[140–144] This influence has been shown in both the hippocampus and the cerebellum, and may be of importance not only for the epileptogenic effects of the hormone, but also for effects on memory, movement control, and balance.

Certain progesterone metabolites, especially 3α-hydroxy-5α-pregnan-20-one, allopregnanolone, and its 5β-derivative (3α-hydroxy-5β-pregnan-20-one) pregnenolone, display potent CNS-depressing effects when given at pharmacological doses; in fact, they are more potent in this respect than barbiturates.[145,146] In both humans and animals, these substances have been shown to exert anti-epileptic, anaesthetic and anxiolytic effects, and derivatives of them are now being evaluated as potential drugs for epilepsy and sleeping disorders, and as anaesthetics.[22,147–151] As discussed above, pregnenolone and certain similar progesterone metabolites are produced by the corpus luteum of the ovary, and they are also formed as metabolites of the progestagens that are being used in HRT. Oral administration of micronized progesterone leads to high serum concentrations of several of these metabolites,[152,153] resulting in a sedative effect.[154] Also, the observation that progesterone enhances the effect of benzodiazepines could be explained by the formation of these metabolites.[155]

In all likelihood, the anxiolytic, sedative and anti-epileptic effects of certain progesterone derivatives are due to an interaction with the inhibitory transmitter γ-aminobutyric acid (GABA). Various progesterone derivatives, like benzodiazepines and barbiturates, hence bind to the GABA-A/chloride ion channel complex, thereby enhancing the effect of GABA on chloride transport.[151,156] Indeed, data from patch clamp studies suggest that allopregnanolone prolongs GABA-mediated postsynaptic currents.[157] Whereas chronic progestagen treatment has been shown to reduce the sensitivity to benzodiazepines of hippocampal GABA-A receptors,[158,159] progestagen withdrawal in experimental animals elicits withdrawal symptoms that appear to be related to a certain subunit of the GABA receptor complex.[160]

Although many progesterone derivatives may display anxiolytic effects, some of them, such as pregnenolone sulphate, have been suggested to be anxiogenic.[161] In low doses, pregnenolone sulphate exerts an inhibitory influence on synaptic transmission in CA1 hippocampus slices, acting via the GABA-A receptor, but in higher doses it exerts a stimulatory influence, which is not inhibited by picrotoxin.[141] Notably, pregnenolone sulphate has been shown to augment an NMDA receptor-mediated increase in intracellular Ca^{2+}.[162]

Conclusions

Both oestrogen and various progesterone derivatives have been shown to interact with the receptors for the amino acid neurotransmitters glutamate and GABA. Such rapid, non-

genomic effects may influence seizure susceptibility, anxiety and wakefulness, and they may
also contribute to the anaesthetic effects of certain progesterone derivatives. Tentatively,
mood symptoms related to PMS, or to the
addition of a progestagen to HRT, could be
related to the formation of anxiogenic progestagen metabolites.

Acknowledgements

This work was supported by the Swedish
Medical Research Council, projects 11198 and
11202, Samverkansnämden Norra Regionen,
Systembolagets forskningsfond.

References

1. Dalton K, *The Premenstrual Syndrome and
Progesterone Therapy* (William Heineman
Medical Books Ltd: London, 1984).
2. Andersch B, Wendestam C, Hahn L, Ohman
R, Premenstrual complaints. I. Prevalence of
premenstrual symptoms in a Swedish urban
population, *J Psychosom Obstet Gynaecol*
1986; 5:39–49.
3. Halbreich U, Endicott J, Classification of premenstrual syndromes. In: Friedman RC, ed.,
Behaviour and the Menstrual Cycle (Marcel
Dekker: New York, 1982) 243–65.
4. Moos RH, Typology of menstrual cycle symptoms, *Am J Obstet Gynecol* 1969; **103**:
390–402.
5. Sanders D, Warner P, Bäckstrom T, Bancroft
J, Mood, sexuality, hormones and the menstrual cycle I. Changes in mood and physical
state: description of subjects and method,
Psychosom Med 1983; 45:487–501.
6. American Psychiatric Association, *Diagnostic
and Statistical Manual of Mental Disorders*,
4th edn (DSM-IV) (American Psychiatric
Association: Washington, 1994) 714–18.
7. Mortola JF, Issues in the diagnosis and
research of premenstrual syndrome, *Clin
Obstet Gynecol* 1992; **35**:587–98.
8. Bäckstrom T, Epileptic seizures in women
related to plasma estrogen and progesterone
during the menstrual cycle, *Acta Neurol Scand*
1976; 54:321–47.
9. Bixo M, Bäckstrom T, Winblad B, Andersson
A, Comparison between pre- and postovula-
tory distributions of oestradiol and progesterone in the brain of the PMSG-treated rat,
Acta Physiol Scand 1986; **128**:241–6.
10. Bixo M, Bäckstrom T, Winblad B, Andersson
A, Estradiol and testosterone in specific
regions of the human female brain in different
endocrine states, *J Steroid Biochem Mol Biol*
1995; 55:297–303.
11. Bixo M, Andersson A, Winblad B et al,
Progesterone, 5alpha-pregnane-3,20-dione
and 3alpha-hydroxy-5alpha-pregnane-20-one
in specific regions of the human female brain
in different endocrine states, *Brain Res* 1997;
764:173–8.
12. Purdy RH, Morrow AL, Moore Jr PH, Paul
SM, Stress-induced elevations of gamma-
aminobutyric acid type A receptor-active
steroids in the rat brain, *Proc Natl Acad Sci
USA* 1991; **88**:4553–7.
13. Appelgren LE, Sites of steroid hormone formation, *Acta Physiol Scand (Suppl)* 1967;
301:1–108.
14. Pfaff D, Keiner M, Atlas of estradiol-concen-
trating cells in the central nervous system of
the female rat, *J Comp Neurol* 1973;
151:121–58.
15. Pfaff DW, Gerlach JL, McEwen BS et al,
Autoradiographic localization of hormone-
concentrating cells in the brain of the female
rhesus monkey, *J Comp Neurol* 1976;
170:279–93.
16. McEwen BS, Steroid hormone actions on the
brain: when is the genome involved? *Horm
Behav* 1994; 28:396–405.
17. MacLusky NJ, Lieberburg I, Krey LC,
McEwen BS, Progestin receptors in the brain
and pituitary of the bonnet monkey (*Macaca
Radiata*): differences between the monkey and
the rat in the distribution of progestin receptors, *Endocrinology* 1980; **106**:185–91.
18. Simerley RB, Chang C, Muramatsu M,
Swanson LW, Distribution of androgen and
estrogen receptor mRNA-containing cells in
the rat brain: an in situ hybridization study, *J*

Comp Neurol 1990; **294**:76–95.

19. Osterlund M, Kuiper GG, Gustafsson JA, Hurd YL, Differential distribution and regulation of estrogen receptor-alpha and -beta mRNA within the female rat brain, *Brain Res Mol Brain Res* 1998; **54**:175–80.

20. Joels M, Steroid hormones and excitability in the mammalian brain, *Front Neuroendocrinol* 1997; **18**:2–48.

21. Kelly MJ, Moss RL, Dudley CA, Fawcett CP, The specificity of the response of preoptic-septal area neurons to estrogen: 17alpha-estradiol versus 17beta-estradiol and the response of extrahypothalamic neurons, *Exper Brain Res* 1977; **30**:43–52.

22. Landgren S, Aasly J, Bäckstrom T et al, The effect of progesterone and its metabolites on the interictal epileptiform discharge in the cat's cerebral cortex, *Acta Physiol Scand* 1987; **131**:33–42.

23. Luine V, Khylchevskaya RI, McEwen BS, Effect of gonadal steroids on activities of monoamine oxidase and choline acetylase in rat brain, *Brain Res* 1975; **86**:293–306.

24. Breuer H, Koster G, Interaction between oestrogens and neurotransmitters: biochemical mechanism, *Adv Biosci* 1975; **15**:287–300.

25. Belmaker RH, Murphy DL, Wyatt RJ, Loriaux DL, Human platelet monoamine oxidase changes during the menstrual cycle, *Arch Gen Psychiatry* 1974; **31**:553–6.

26. Lofstrom A, Bäckstrom T, Relationship between plasma estradiol and brain catecholamine content in the diestrous female rat, *Psychoneuroendocrinology* 1978; **3**:103–7.

27. Lofstrom A, Bäckstrom T, Plasma steroid–tissue catecholamine relationships in limbic and related areas of the brain. In: Fuxe K, Gustafsson J-A, Wetterberg L, eds, *Steroid Hormone Regulation of the Brain* (Wenner-Gren Symposium Series, Pergamon Press: Oxford, 1981) 147–60.

28. Ladisch W, Influence of progesterone on serotonin metabolism: a possible causal factor for mood changes, *Psychoneuroendocrinology* 1977; **2**:257–66.

29. Hruska RE, Silbergeld EK, Increased dopamine receptor sensitivity after estrogen treatment using the rat rotation model, *Science* 1980; **208**:1466–8.

30. Fernandez-Ruiz JJ, de Miguel R, Hernandez ML, Ramos JA, Time-course of the effects of ovarian steroids on the activity of limbic and striatal dopaminergic neurons in female rat brain, *Pharmacol Biochem Behav* 1990; **36**:603–6.

31. Morissette M, Di Paolo T, Effect of chronic estradiol and progesterone treatments of ovariectomized rats on brain dopamine uptake sites, *J Neurochem* 1993; **60**:1876–83.

32. Rubinow DR, Schmidt PJ, Roca CA, Estrogen–serotonin interactions: implications for affective regulation, *Biol Psychiatry* 1998; **44**:839–50.

33. Saigusa T, Takada K, Baker SC et al, Dopamine efflux in the rat nucleus accumbens evoked by dopamine receptor stimulation in the entorhinal cortex is modulated by oestradiol and progesterone, *Synapse* 1997; **25**:37–43.

34. Bäckstrom T, Sanders D, Leask R et al, Mood, sexuality, hormones and the menstrual cycle. II. Hormone levels and their relationship to the premenstrual syndrome, *Psychosom Med* 1983; **45**:503–7.

35. Metcalf MG, Incidence of ovulation from the menarche to the menopause. *NZ Med J* 1983; **96**:645–8.

36. Hammarbäck S, Ekholm UB, Bäckstrom T, Spontaneous anovulation causing disappearance of cyclical symptoms in women with the premenstrual syndrome, *Acta Endocrinol* 1991; **125**:132–7.

37. Bancroft J, Boyle H, Warner P, Fraser HM, The use of an LHRH agonist, buserelin, in the long term management of premenstrual syndromes, *Clin Endocrinol* 1987; **27**:171–82.

38. Hammarbäck S, Bäckstrom T, Induced anovulation as treatment of premenstrual tension syndrome: a double-blind crossover study with GnRH-agonist versus placebo, *Acta Obstet Gynaecol Scand* 1988; **67**:159–66.

39. Muse KN, Cetel NS, Futterman LA, Yen SC, The premenstrual syndrome: effects of 'medical ovariectomy', *N Engl J Med* 1984; **311**:1345–9.

40. Schmidt PJ, Nieman LK, Danaceau MA et al, Differential behavioral effects of gonadal steroids in women with and in those without premenstrual syndrome, *N Engl J Med* 1998; **338**:209–16.

41. Magos AL, Brincat M, Studd JW, Treatment of the premenstrual syndrome by subcutaneous estradiol implants and cyclical oral norethisterone: placebo controlled study, *Br Med J* 1986; 292:1629–33.

42. Halbreich U, Rojansky N, Palter S, Elimination of ovulation and menstrual cyclicity (with danazol) improves dysphoric premenstrual syndromes, *Fertil Steril* 1991; 56:1066–9.

43. Casper RF, Hearn MT, The effect of hysterectomy and bilateral oophorectomy in women with severe premenstrual syndrome, *Am J Obstet Gynecol* 1990; 162:105–9.

44. Casson P, Hahn PM, Van Vugt DA, Reid RL, Lasting response to ovariectomy in severe intractable premenstrual syndrome, *Am J Obstet Gynecol* 1990; 162:99–105.

45. Bäckström T, Boyle H, Baird DT, Persistence of symptoms of premenstrual tension in hysterectomized women, *Br J Obstet Gynaecol* 1981; 88:530–6.

46. Freeman EW, Rickels K, Characteristics of placebo responses in medical treatment of premenstrual syndrome, *Am J Psychiatry* 1999; 156:1403–8.

47. Graham CA, Sherwin BB, A prospective treatment study of premenstrual symptoms using a triphasic oral contraceptive, *J Psychosom Res* 1992; 36:257–66.

48. Sundstrom I, Ashbrook D, Bäckström T, Reduced benzodiazepine sensitivity in patients with premenstrual syndrome, a pilot study, *Psychoneuroendocrinology* 1997; 22:25–38.

49. Sundstrom I, Andersson A, Nyberg S et al, Patients with premenstrual syndrome have a different sensitivity to a neuroactive steroid during the menstrual cycle compared to control subjects, *Neuroendocrinology* 1998; 67:126–38.

50. Hammarbäck S, Damber J-E, Bäckström T, Relationship between symptom severity and hormone changes in women with premenstrual syndrome, *J Clin Endocrinol Metab* 1989; 68:125–30.

51. Dhar V, Murphy BE, Double-blind randomized crossover trial of luteal phase estrogens (Premarin) in the premenstrual syndrome (PMS), *Psychoneuroendocrinology* 1990; 15: 489–93.

52. Bäckström T, Andersson A, Baird DT, Selstam G, The human corpus luteum secretes 5alpha-pregnane-3,20-dione, *Acta Endocrinol* 1986; 111:116–21.

53. Ichikawa S, Sawada T, Nakamura Y, Morioka H, Ovarian secretion of pregnane compounds during the estrous cycle and pregnancy in rats, *Endocrinology* 1974; 94:1615–20.

54. Purdy RH, Moore PH Jr, Rao PN et al, Radioimmunoassay of 3alpha-hydroxy-5alpha-pregnan-20-one in rat and human plasma, *Steroids* 1990; 55:290–6.

55. Wang M, Seippel L, Purdy RH, Bäckström T, Relationship between symptom severity and steroid variation in women with premenstrual syndrome: study on plasma pregnenolone, pregnenolone sulfate, 5alpha-pregnane-3,20-dione and 3alpha-hydroxy-5alpha-pregnane-20-one, *J Clin Endocrinol Metab* 1996; 81:1076–82.

56. Karavolas HJ, Progesterone processing by neuroendocrine structures. In: Celotti F, Naftolin F, Martini L, eds, *Metabolism of Hormonal Steroids in the Neuroendocrine Structures* (Raven Press: New York, 1984) 149–70.

57. Bixo M, Bäckström T, Regional distribution of progesterone and 5alpha-pregnane-3,20-dione in rat brain during progesterone induced 'anaesthesia', *Psychoneuroendocrinology* 1990; 15:159–62.

58. Appelblad P, Pontén E, Jaegfeldt H et al, Derivatization of steroids with dansylhydrazine using trifluoromethanesulfonic acid as catalyst, *Anal Chem* 1997; 69:4905–11.

59. Sodergard R, Bäckström T, Shanbhag V, Carstensen H, Calculation of free and bound fractions of testosterone and estradiol-17beta to human plasma proteins at body temperature, *J Steroid Biochem* 1982; 16:801–10.

60. Westphal U, *Steroid Protein Interactions* (Springer-Verlag: New York, 1971) 164–225.

61. Schmidt PJ, Purdy RH, Moore PH Jr et al, Circulating levels of anxiolytic steroids in the luteal phase in women with premenstrual syndrome and in control subjects, *J Clin Endocrinol Metab* 1994; 79:1256–60.

62. Rapkin AJ, Morgan M, Goldman L et al, Progesterone metabolite allopregnanolone in women with premenstrual syndrome, *Obstet Gynecol* 1997; 90:709–14.

63. Milsom I, Sundell G, Andersch B, A longitudinal study of contraception and pregnancy outcome in a representative sample of young Swedish women, *Contraception* 1991; **43**: 111–19.

64. Cullberg J, Mood changes and menstrual symptoms with different gestagen/estrogen combinations. A double blind comparison with placebo, *Acta Psychiat Scand (Suppl)* 1972; **236**:1–86.

65. Graham CA, Sherwin BB, The relationship between retrospective premenstrual symptom reporting and present oral contraceptive use, *J Psychosom Res* 1987; **31**:45–53.

66. Hammarbäck S, Bäckstrom T, A demographic study in subgroups of women seeking help for premenstrual syndrome, *Acta Obstet Gynaecol Scand* 1989; **68**:247–53.

67. Bäckström T, Hansson-Malmstrom Y, Lindhe BA et al, Oral contraceptives in premenstrual syndrome: a randomized comparison of triphasic and monophasic preparations, *Contraception* 1992; **46**:253–68.

68. Bancroft J, Sanders D, Warner P, Loudon N, The effects of oral contraceptives on mood and sexuality: comparison of triphasic and combined preparations, *J Psychosom Obstet Gynaecol* 1987; **7**:1–8.

69. Hällstrom T, Samuelsson S, Mental health in the climacteric. The longitudinal study of women in Gothenburg, *Acta Obstet Gynaecol Scand* 1985, 130 (suppl):13–18.

70. Kaufert PA, Gilbert P, Tate R, The Manitoba Project; a re-examination of the link between menopause and depression, *Maturitas* 1992; **14**:143–55.

71. Avis NE, Brambilla D, McKinlay SM, Vass K, A longitudinal analysis of the association between menopause and depression. Results from the Massachusetts Women's Health Study, *Ann Epidemiol* 1994; **4**:214–20.

72. Hunter M, The South-east England longitudinal study of the climacteric and post-menopause, *Maturitas* 1992; **14**:117–26.

73. Holte A, Influences of natural menopause on health complaints; a prospective study of healthy Norwegian women, *Maturitas* 1992; **14**:127–41.

74. Ballinger CB, Psychiatric aspects of the menopause, *Br J Psychiatry* 1990; **156**: 773–87.

75. Dennerstein L, Smith AM, Morse C et al, Menopausal symptoms in Australian women, *Med J Aust* 1993; **159**:232–6.

76. McKinlay JB, McKinlay SM, Brambilla D, The relative contributions of endocrine changes and social circumstances to depression in mid-aged women, *J Health Soc Behav* 1987; **28**:345–63.

77. McKinlay SM, Brambilla DJ, Posner JG, The normal menopause transition, *Maturitas* 1992; **14**:103–15.

78. Collins A, Landgren BM, Reproductive health, use of estrogen and experience of symptoms in perimenopausal women: a population-based study, *Maturitas* 1994; **20**:101–11.

79. Coope J, Is oestrogen therapy effective in the treatment of menopausal depression? *JR Coll Gen Pract* 1981; **31**:134–40.

80. Campbell S, Double blind psychometric studies on the effects of natural oestrogens on postmenopausal women. In: Campbell S, ed., *Management of the Menopause and the Postmenopausal Years* (MTP Press: Lancaster, 1976) 149–58.

81. Thomson J, Oswald I, Effect of oestrogen on the sleep, mood and anxiety of menopausal women, *Br Med J* 1977; **2**:1317–19.

82. Ditkoff EC, Crary WG, Cristo M, Lobo RA, Estrogen improves psychological function in asymptomatic postmenopausal women, *Obstet Gynecol* 1991; **78**:991–5.

83. Gregoire AJ, Kumar R, Everitt B et al, Transdermal oestrogen for treatment of severe postnatal depression, *Lancet* 1996; **347**: 930–3.

84. Klaiber EL, Broverman DM, Vogel W, Kobayashi Y, Estrogen therapy for severe persistent depressions in women, *Arch Gen Psychiatry* 1979; **36**:550–4.

85. Archer JS, Relationship between estrogen, serotonin, and depression, *Menopause* 1999; **6**:71–8.

86. Panay N, Studd JW, The psychotherapeutic effects of estrogens, *Gynecol Endocrinol* 1998; **12**:353–65.

87. Dennerstein L, Burrows GD, Hyman GJ, Sharpe K, Hormone therapy and affect, *Maturitas* 1979; **1**:247–59.

88. Montgomery JC, Appleby L, Brincat M et al,

Effect of oestrogen and testosterone implants on psychological disorders in the climacteric, *Lancet* 1987; 1:297–9.

89. Sherwin BB, Gelfand MM, Sex steroids and affect in the surgical menopause: a double-blind, cross-over study, *Psychoneuroendocrinology* 1985; 10:325–35.

90. Hammarbäck S, Bäckström T, Holst J et al, Cyclical mood changes as in the premenstrual tension syndrome during sequential estrogen–progestagen postmenopausal replacement therapy, *Acta Obstet Gynaecol Scand* 1985; 64:393–7.

91. Magos AL, Brewster E, Singh R et al, The effects of norethisterone in postmenopausal women on oestrogen replacement therapy: a model for the premenstrual syndrome, *Br J Obstet Gynaecol* 1986; 93:1290–6.

92. Bäckström T, Bixo M, Seippel L et al, Progestins and behavior. In: Genazzani AR, Petraglia F, Purdy RH, eds, *The Brain: Source and Target for Sex Steroid Hormones* (Parthenon: New York, 1996) 277–91.

93. Asso D, Braier JR, Changes with the menstrual cycle in psychophysiological and self-report measures of activation, *Biol Psychol* 1982; 15:95–107.

94. Broverman DM, Klaiber EL, Kobayashi Y et al, Roles of activation and inhibition in sex differences in cognitive abilities, *Psychol Rev* 1968; 75:23–50.

95. Zimmerman E, Parlee MB, Behavioral changes associated with the menstrual cycle: an experimental investigation, *J Appl Soc Psychol* 1973; 3:335–44.

96. Hampson E, Kimura D, Reciprocal effects of hormonal fluctuations on human motor and perceptual–spatial skills, *Behav Neurosci* 1988; 102:456–9.

97. Hammar ML, Lindgren R, Berg GE et al, Effects of hormonal replacement therapy on the postural balance among postmenopausal women, *Obstet Gynecol* 1996; 88:955–60.

98. Maggi A, Perez J, Role of female gonadal hormones in the CNS. Clinical and experimental aspects, *Life Sci* 1985; 37:893–906.

99. Hogervorst E, Boshuisen M, Riedel W et al, The effect of hormone replacement therapy on cognitive function in elderly women, *Psychoneuroendocrinology* 1999; 24:43–68.

100. Haskell SG, Richardson ED, Horwitz RI, The effect of estrogen replacement therapy on cognitive function in women: a critical review of the literature, *J Clin Epidemiol* 1997; 50: 1249–64.

101. Fedor-Freybergh P, The influence of oestrogens on the wellbeing and mental performance in climacteric and postmenopausal women, *Acta Obstet Gynaecol Scand* 1977; 64 (suppl):1–91.

102. Sherwin BB, Estrogen and/or androgen replacement therapy and cognitive functioning in surgically menopausal women, *Psychoneuroendocrinology* 1988; 13:345–57.

103. Phillips SM, Sherwin BB, Effects of estrogen on memory function in surgically menopausal women, *Psychoneuroendocrinology* 1992; 17:485–95.

104. Resnick SM, Metter EJ, Zonderman AB, Estrogen replacement therapy and longitudinal decline in visual memory. A possible protective effect? *Neurology* 1997; 49:1491–7.

105. Jacobs DM, Tang MX, Stern Y et al, Cognitive function in nondemented older women who took estrogen after menopause, *Neurology* 1998; 50:368–73.

106. Wolf OT, Kudielka BM, Hellhammer DH et al, Two weeks of transdermal estradiol treatment in postmenopausal elderly women and its effect on memory and mood: verbal memory changes are associated with the treatment induced estradiol levels, *Psychoneuroendocrinology* 1999; 24:727–41.

107. Polo-Kantola P, Portin R, Polo O et al, The effect of short-term estrogen replacement therapy on cognition: a randomized, double-blind, cross-over trial in postmenopausal women, *Obstet Gynecol* 1998; 91:459–66.

108. Greendale GA, Reboussin BA, Hogan P et al, Symptom relief and side effects of postmenopausal hormones: results from the Postmenopausal Estrogen/Progestin Interventions Trial, *Obstet Gynecol* 1998; 92: 982–8.

109. Rauramo L, Lagerspetz K, Engblom P, Punnonen R, The effect of castration and peroral estrogen therapy on some psychological functions, *Front Horm Res* 1975; 3:94–104.

110. Vanhulle R, Demol R, A double-blind study into the influence of estriol on a number of

psychological tests in post-menopausal women. In: van Keep PA, Greenblatt RB, Albeaux-Fernet M, eds, *Consensus on Menopause Research* (MTP: Lancaster, 1976) 94–9.

111. Barret-Connor E, Kritz-Silverstein D, Estrogen replacement therapy and cognitive function in older women, *JAMA* 1993; **269**:2637–41.

112. Sherwin BB, Tulandi T, 'Add-back' estrogen reverses cognitive deficits induced by a gonadotropin-releasing hormone agonist in women with leiomyomata uteri, *J Clin Endocrinol Metab* 1996; **81**:2545–9.

113. Ohkura T, Isse K, Akazawa K et al, Long-term estrogen replacement therapy in female patients with dementia of the Alzheimer type: 7 case reports, *Dementia* 1995; **6**:99–107.

114. Honjo H, Ogino Y, Naitoh K et al, In vivo effects by estrone sulfate on the central nervous system—senile dementia (Alzheimer's type), *J Steroid Biochem* 1989; **34**:521–5.

115. Fillit H, Weinreb H, Cholst I et al, Observations in a preliminary open trial of estradiol therapy for senile dementia–Alzheimer's type, *Psychoneuroendocrinology* 1986; **11**:337–45.

116. Ohkura T, Isse K, Akazawa K et al, Low-dose estrogen replacement therapy for Alzheimer disease in women, *Menopause* 1994; **1**:125–30.

117. Costa MM, Reus VI, Wolkowitz OM et al, Estrogen replacement therapy and cognitive decline in memory-impaired post-menopausal women, *Biol Psychiatry* 1999; **46**:182–8.

118. Asthana S, Craft S, Baker LD et al, Cognitive and neuroendocrine response to transdermal estrogen in postmenopausal women with Alzheimer's disease: results of a placebo-controlled, double-blind, pilot study, *Psychoneuroendocrinology* 1999; **24**:657–77.

119. Heyman A, Wilkinson WE, Stafford JA et al, Alzheimer's disease: a study of epidemiological aspects, *Ann Neurol* 1984; **15**:335–41.

120. Amaducci LA, Fratiglioni L, Rocca WA et al, Risk factors for clinically diagnosed Alzheimer's disease: a case-control study of an Italian population, *Neurology* 1986; **36**:922–31.

121. Broe GA, Henderson AS, Creasey H et al, A case-control study of Alzheimer's disease in Australia, *Neurology* 1990; **40**:1698–707.

122. Graves AB, White E, Koepsell TD et al, A case-control study of Alzheimer's disease, *Ann Neurol* 1990; **28**:766–74.

123. Henderson VW, Paganini-Hill A, Emanuel CK et al, Estrogen replacement therapy in older women. Comparisons between Alzheimer's disease cases and nondemented control subjects, *Arch Neurol* 1994; **51**:896–900.

124. Paganini-Hill A, Henderson VW, Estrogen deficiency and risk of Alzheimer's disease in women, *Am J Epidemiol* 1994; **140**:256–61.

125. Brenner DE, Kukull WA, Stergachis A et al, Postmenopausal estrogen replacement therapy and the risk of Alzheimer's disease: a population-based case-control study, *Am J Epidemiol* 1994; **140**:262–7.

126. Tang MX, Jacobs D, Stern Y et al, Effect of oestrogen during menopause on risk and age at onset of Alzheimer disease, *Lancet* 1996; **348**:429–32.

127. Waring SC, Rocca WA, Petersen RC et al, Postmenopausal estrogen replacement therapy and risk of AD: a population-based study, *Neurology* 1999; **52**:965–70.

128. McEwen BS, Alves SE, Bulloch K, Weiland NG, Ovarian steroids and the brain: implications for cognition and aging, *Neurology* 1997; **48** (suppl 7):S8–15.

129. Gibbs RB, Hashash A, Johnson DA, Effects of estrogen on potassium-stimulated acetylcholine release in the hippocampus and overlying cortex of adult rats, *Brain Res* 1997; **749**:143–6.

130. Xu H, Gouras GK, Greenfield JP et al, Estrogen reduces neuronal generation of Alzheimer beta-amyloid peptides, *Nat Med* 1998; **4**:447–51.

131. Pike CJ, Estrogen modulates neuronal Bcl-xL expression and beta-amyloid-induced apoptosis: relevance to Alzheimer's disease, *J Neurochem* 1999; **72**:1552–63.

132. Goldman H, Skelley EB, Sandman CA et al, Hormones and regional brain blood flow, *Pharmacol Biochem Behav* 1976; **5** (suppl 1): 165–9.

133. Shaywitz SE, Shaywitz BA, Pugh KR et al, Effect of estrogen on brain activation patterns in postmenopausal women during working memory tasks, *JAMA* 1999; **281**:1197–202.

134. Packard MG, Teather LA, Intra-hippocampal estradiol infusion enhances memory in ovariectomized rats, *Neuroreport* 1997; 8:3009–13.

135. Cordoba Montoya DA, Carrer HF, Estrogen facilitates induction of long term potentiation in the hippocampus of awake rats, *Brain Res* 1997; 778:430–8.

136. Wooley DE, Timiras PS, The gonad–brain relationship: effects of female sex hormones on electro-shock convulsions in the rat, *Endocrinology* 1962; 70:196–209.

137. Logothetis J, Harner R, Morrell F, Torres F, The role of estrogens in catamenial exacerbation of epilepsy, *Neurology* 1959; 9:352–60.

138. Marcus EM, Watson CW, Simon SA, An experimental model of some varieties of petit mal epilepsy. Electrical–behavioral correlations of acute bilateral epileptogenic foci in cerebral cortex, *Epilepsia* 1968; 9:233–48.

139. Laidlaw J, Catamenial epilepsy, *Lancet* 1956; 271:1235–7.

140. Landgren S, Selstam G, Interaction between 17 beta oestradiol and 3alpha-hydroxy-5alpha-pregnane-20-one in the control of neuronal excitability in slices from CA1 hippocampus in vitro of guinea-pigs and rats, *Acta Physiol Scand* 1995; 154:165–76.

141. Wang MD, Landgren S, Bäckstrom T, The effects of allopregnanolone, pregnenolone sulphate and pregnenolone on the CA1 population spike of the rat hippocampus after 17beta-oestradiol priming, *Acta Physiol Scand* 1997; 159:343–4.

142. Smith SS, Estrogen administration increases neuronal responses to excitatory amino acids as a long-term effect, *Brain Res* 1989; 503:354–7.

143. Weiland NG, Estradiol selectively regulates agonist binding sites on the N-methyl-D-aspartate receptor complex in the CA1 region of the hippocampus, *Endocrinology* 1992; 131:662–8.

144. Wong M, Moss RL, Patch-clamp analysis of direct steroidal modulation of glutamate receptor-channels, *J Neuroendocrinol* 1994; 6:347–55.

145. Norberg L, Wahlstrom G, Bäckstrom T, The anaesthetic potency of 3alpha-hydroxy-5alpha-pregnan-20-one and 3alpha-hydroxy-5beta-pregnan-20-one determined with an intravenous EEG-threshold method in male rats, Pharmacol Toxicol 1987; 61:42–7.

146. Korkmaz S, Wahlstrom G, The EEG burst suppression threshold test for the determination of CNS sensitivity to intravenous anaesthetics in rats, *Brain Res Protoc* 1997; 1:378–84.

147. Belelli D, Bolger MB, Gee KW, Anticonvulsant profile of the progesterone metabolite 5alpha-pregnan-3alpha-ol-20-one, *Eur J Pharmacol* 1989; 166:325–9.

148. Bitran D, Hilvers RJ, Kellogg CK, Anxiolytic effects of 3alpha-hydroxy-5alpha[beta]-pregnan-20-one: endogenous metabolites of progesterone that are active at the GABA-A receptor, *Brain Res* 1991; 561:157–61.

149. Wieland S, Lan NC, Mirasedeghi S, Gee KW, Anxiolytic activity of the progesterone metabolite 5alpha-pregnan-3alpha-ol-20-one, *Brain Res* 1991; 565:263–8.

150. Carl P, Hogskilde S, Nielsen JW et al, Pregnenolone emulsion: a preliminary pharmacokinetic and pharmacodynamic study of a new intravenous anaesthetic agent, *Anaesthesia* 1990; 45:189–97.

151. Finn DA, Gee KW, The significance of steroid action on the GABA-A receptor complex. In: Berg G and Hammar M, eds, *The Modern Management of the Menopause* (The Parthenon Publishing Group: New York, 1994) 301–13.

152. de Lignieres B, Dennerstein L Bäckstrom T, Influence of route of administration on progesterone metabolism, *Maturitas* 1995; 21:251–7.

153. Arafat ES, Hargrove JT, Maxson WS et al, Sedative and hypnotic effects of oral administration of micronized progesterone may be mediated through its metabolites, *Am J Obstet Gynecol* 1988; 159:1203–9.

154. Freeman EW, Purdy RH, Coutifaris C et al, Anxiolytic metabolites of progesterone: correlation with mood and performance measures following oral progesterone administration to healthy female volunteers, *Neuroendocrinology* 1993; 58:478–84.

155. McAuley JW, Reynolds IJ, Kroboth FJ et al, Orally administered progesterone enhances sensitivity to triazolam in postmenopausal women,

J Clin Psychopharmacol 1995; **15**: 3–11.

156. Majewska MD, Harrison NL, Schwartz RD et al, Steroid hormone metabolites are barbiturate-like modulators of the GABA receptor, *Science* 1986; **232**:1004–7.

157. Haage D, Johansson S, Neurosteroid modulation of synaptic and GABA-evoked currents in neurons from the rat medial preoptic nucleus, *J Neurophysiol* 1999; **82**:143–51.

158. Costa AM, Spence KT, Smith SS, ffrench-Mullen JM, Withdrawal from the endogenous steroid progesterone results in GABAA currents insensitive to benzodiazepine modulation in rat CA1 hippocampus, *J Neurophysiol* 1995; **74**:464–9.

159. Friedman L, Gibbs TT, Farb DH, Gamma-aminobutyric acid A receptor regulation: chronic treatment with pregnenolone uncouples allosteric interactions between steroid and benzodiazepine recognition sites, *Mol Pharmacol* 1993; **44**:191–7.

160. Smith SS, Gong QH, Hsu FC et al, GABA(A) receptor alpha4 subunit suppression prevents withdrawal properties of an endogenous steroid, *Nature* 1998; **392**:926–30.

161. Paul SM, Purdy RH, Neuroactive steroids, *FASEB J* 1992; **6**:2311–22.

162. Irwin RP, Maragakis NJ, Rogawski MA et al, Pregnenolone sulfate augments NMDA receptor-mediated increases in intracellular Ca^{2+} in cultured rat hippocampal neurons, *Neurosci Lett* 1992; **141**:30–4.

13

Oestrogens, progestins and mood

Kimberly A Yonkers, Karen D Bradshaw and Uriel Halbreich

Oestrogens, progestins and mood

There is a common belief in medicine that exogenous progestins or oral contraceptives (OCs) can cause disturbances in mood or precipitate mood disorders such as major depressive disorder (MDD);[1,2] conversely, some researchers and clinicians advocate the use of oestrogens[3,4] or progesterone[5] to treat mood disturbances. Exogenous gonadal steroids are commonly prescribed to women for contraceptive purposes or to palliate postmenopausal symptoms such as hot flushes and vaginal dryness. They are also prophylactic against long-term complications occurring during the postmenopausal years, including osteoporosis, cerebrovascular or cardiovascular disease and dementia. It is currently estimated that 10 million postmenopausal women in the USA take hormone replacement therapy (HRT),[6] and 15 million women aged 15–44 receive OCs.[7] Given the frequency with which these agents are prescribed, there is a need to critically evaluate any risks associated with them, including the risk of mood disorder or symptoms associated with mood disturbances. The aim of this chapter is to review existing data on the psychological effects of exogenous oestrogens and progestins.

In order to evaluate existing data, a literature search was conducted using Medline data sets between 1966 and 1997. Keywords used in this search included hormones, oestrogen, progestin, progestogen, oral contraceptives, mood, depression, menopause and premenstrual syndrome. In addition, bibliographies of all articles were examined and articles relevant to this topic were reviewed. Because of the difficulty in extrapolating unbiased results from studies that were conducted openly, the focus of this chapter is on placebo-controlled investigations; case-control studies and open studies are noted when appropriate.

The mood-modifying effects of oestrogen

The major circulating oestrogen in women of reproductive age is 17β-oestradiol. The other significant oestrogen is oestrone, which is produced from both direct ovarian secretion and peripheral aromatization of ovarian and adrenal-derived androstenedione in the adipose tissue. During the normal menstrual cycle, oestradiol levels vary between 40 and 400 pg/ml. Oestrogen circulates while bound to sex hormone-binding globulin (SHBG), which is produced by the liver; the quantity produced is under partial control of oestrogen. After the menopause, oestradiol and oestrone production by the ovaries dramatically declines. Oestradiol levels decrease to less than 40 pg/ml, while testosterone production declines by only 25% at the time of the natural menopause. Although adrenal steroid production is gradually reduced with age, there is still substantial androstenedione production for peripheral conversion. Therefore, oestrone is the major circulating oestrogen in the menopause. Due to an increased androgen to oestrogen ratio, SHBG declines.

Oestrogens are available in both oral and parenteral forms. The oestrogens commonly used for OCs are ethinyl oestradiol and mestranol. The addition of an ethinyl group at the 17 position of oestradiol made this a pharmacologically potent oral oestrogen. Mestranol is the 3-methyl ether of ethinyl oestradiol and is converted to ethinyl oestradiol in the body. Today, all low-dose OCs contain ethinyl oestradiol in doses of 20, 30 or 35 μg. These doses range from three to four times the potency of replacement therapy oestrogens. OCs containing 75–100 μg of ethinyl oestradiol or mestranol are no longer on the market.

The most commonly used oestrogen for HRT is conjugated equine oestrogen, a combination of oestrone (50%), equilin (23%), 17α-dihydroequilin (13%) and various other oestrogens extracted from the urine of pregnant mares.[8] This formulation has been available in the USA for more than 50 years; thus, most of the data regarding the safety and effi-

cacy of oestrogen therapy have been gathered from women taking conjugated oestrogens. Several other oestrogen preparations have been developed, and data are accumulating regarding their comparable effectiveness. There is, at present, no compelling reason for the clinician to recommend one preparation over others based on risks or side-effects.

Other oral oestrogens include piperazine oestrone sulphate and micronized 17β-oestradiol. Oestrogens are used orally as the first-line therapy in most women. Although transdermal oestradiol patches have also been found to be effective, there are several potential drawbacks to this approach. On a physiological level, it is uncertain whether similar reductions in cardiovascular risks occur with the transdermal oestrogens, as they avoid the 'first pass' through the liver and hence have less effect on low-density lipoprotein (LDL) and high-density lipoprotein (HDL).[9] Also, patches are more expensive than oral preparations and result in some skin irritation in about 30% of users. Indications for transdermal delivery include non-toleration of oral therapy and the development of hypertriglyceridaemia on an oral preparation. Standard dosages of commonly used oestrogens and progestins are listed in Table 13.1.

Conjugated oestrogens are also available in cream form, and rates of vaginal absorption are similar to those of oral absorption.[10] Oestrogen gels, implants and injections are available but used infrequently due to the erratic absorption and wide expanses in blood levels with use. So-called 'natural oestrogens' are available in health food markets, in the forms of soy oestrogens or yam extracts. The exact chemical nature of these products is not well known, and nor is the appropriate dosing regimen for the short- and long-term treatment of postmenopausal symptoms.

Oestrogen has a number of effects on neuro-

Table 13.1 Standard dosages of commonly used oestrogens and progestins.

	Dosage range
Oestrogens	
Oral	
Conjugated oestrogens	0.625–1.25 mg/day
Ethinyl oestradiol	0.025–0.035 mg/day
Piperazine oestrone sulphate	1.0 mg/day
Micronized 17β-oestradiol	0.5–2.0 mg/day
Mestranol	0.05 mg/day
Parenteral	
Transdermal oestradiol	0.05–1.0-mg patch once or twice weekly
Vaginal conjugated oestrogens	0.2–0.625 mg, 2–7 times weekly
Vaginal 17β-oestradiol	1.0 mg, 1–3 times weekly
Progestins	
Oral	
Medroxyprogesterone	2.5–5.0 mg/day or 10 mg 10–14 days per month
Norethindrone	1–5 mg/day
Norethindrone acetate	1–5 mg/day
Norgestrel	0.15 mg/day
Micronized progesterone	100–300 mg/day

transmitter systems[11–13] which are described in greater detail in other chapters. The relationship between oestrogen and the serotonergic (5–HT) system is of particular interest. In rat brain, oestrogen treatment decreases 5–HT$_1$ receptor density[14] and increases 5-HT$_2$ receptor density in frontal cortex,[14–17] as well as nucleus accumbens, cingulate cortex and olfactory cortex.[15,16,18] In raphe cells, oestrogen increases serotonin content via stimulation of tryptophan hydroxylase mRNA.[19] Further, oestrogen inhibits monoamine oxidase activity[20] and decreases the turnover of 5-HT[21] in rodents. In humans, oestrogen increases platelet 5-HT$_2$ binding and is associated with increased binding in the platelet serotonin transporter.[22] Finally, both endogenous and exogenous oestrogens increase the prolactin response to serotonin agonists.[23,24]

More recent evidence has shown that oestrogen has activational effects. As noted by Smith,[25] oestrogen increases locomotor activity and enhances the activity of excitatory amino acids in the central nervous system of rodents. It is suggested that the latter property is responsible for cognition-enhancing effects, but may also relate to mood effects.[26–28] These various properties in humans and animals are similar to those found with antidepressant agents, and thus strengthen the position that oestrogens may have mood-elevating properties.

Treatment of mood disturbances associated with the menopause

It is estimated that approximately 35% of women will seek medical treatment for symptoms associated with the menopause.[1] The complaints most commonly noted by women include hot flushes, muscle and joint pain, headaches, weight gain, decreased libido, fatigue, low mood and irritability.[29] Oestrogen preparations are used to treat menopausal symptoms, including mood symptoms, which often accompany physical symptoms. While oestrogen is effective in the treatment of hot flushes, evidence for its therapeutic efficacy in ameliorating mood symptoms is less concrete. In part, this may be due to the heterogeneity in clinical trials, which include: (1) investigations in women who are at various menopausal stages, including the perimenopause, non-surgical postmenopause and surgical menopause; (2) examination in groups which varied in severity of their mood disturbance; (3) inclusion of women suffering from concurrent psychiatric illness; (4) utilization of different types of oestrogens with or without a progestin; and (5) the use of different outcome measures, including single-symptom measures as well as scales measuring a variety of depressive symptoms. In the following review of oestrogen's efficacy in menopausal-related mood disturbances, these factors are considered.

An excellent, quantitative review of the effect of oestrogen on depressed mood was published

in 1997.[30] The present review is qualitative rather than quantitative and we discuss additional variables and considerations. However, the results of the quantitative review are presented when appropriate. This report also differs from the previous quantitative review in that we include additional studies published since the earlier review.

Twenty-one placebo-controlled studies have evaluated the therapeutic efficacy of oestrogen for depressive symptoms or depressive disorders associated with the menopause (Tables 13.2–13.5). Of these studies, five[31–35] included only women who were surgically rendered postmenopausal, nine studies included women who experienced natural menopause,[4,36–43] five studies included both peri- and postmenopausal women,[44–48] one trial included only perimenopausal women,[49] one study did not define the exact menopausal status of women included in the protocol,[50] and one study included both surgically and naturally menopausal women.[41]

Surgically induced menopause

Three[33,35,51] of the five studies conducted on surgically postmenopausal women found that oestrogen was superior to placebo for mood symptoms. The oestrogen preparations used in these positive studies included conjugated oestrogens,[33] ethinyl oestradiol[51] and oestradiol valerate.[35] The two negative trials employed either oestrogen sulphate[31] or conjugated oestrogen.[34] The sample sizes in the positive studies were larger ($n = 49, 36, 43$) than those in the negative studies ($n = 28, 13$), and thus a type-two error cannot be ruled out in the two studies which found oestrogen and placebo to be equivalent. The negative study by Coppen et al[31] was also heterogeneous in terms of illness severity at baseline, a characteristic which may

Table 13.2 Studies evaluating the effects of oestrogen in peri- and postmenopausal women: Perimenopausal studies.

Author	Duration (months)	Design	Hormonal preparation	Post-treatment placebo	Post-treatment active	Comments
Aylward et al[44] $N = 55$	1	Parallel	Piperazine oestrone sulphate	HRS-D change $= +20\%$	HRS-D change $= -20\%$	Peri- and postmenopausal women included. Oestrone significantly better than placebo; tryptophan levels higher with oestrone Rx
Coope et al[45] $N = 30$	1	Crossover	Conjugated oestrogens; no progestogen	24% with complete relief	29% with complete rel ef	Differences between conditions not found. Hot flushes appeared with withdrawal of oestrogen unblinding investigators. Two Ss on oestrogen withdrew because of depression
Coope et al[46] $N = 55$	4		Piperazine oestrone sulphate no progestogen	BDI change $= -11$	BDI change $= -9$	No significant Rx effect. Mildly depressed Ss allowed; two Ss developed severe depression on oestrogen
Montgomery et al[47] $N = 70$	4	Parallel	Two active Rx: oestradiol; oestradiol and testosterone; 5 mg norethisterone for final week of month	Oestradiol/ testosterone change score $= 11$	Placebo change score $= 18$	Rx differences significant at 2 months but not at 4 months
Strickler et al[48] $N = 70$	6	Crossover	Conjugated oestrogens	Author Scale $=$ no difference between active and placebo	Author Scale $=$ no difference between active and placebo	Three were manic and nine were depressed at some point before study; nine taking psychotropics
Thomson and Oswald[49] $N = 34$	2	Crossover	Piperazine oestrone sulphate	HRS-D change $= -10.4$	HRS-D change $= -13.7$	No significant difference in Rx conditions; oestrogen did not decrease the number of awakenings in perimenopausal women

HSR-D, Hamilton Rating Scale for Depression; BDI, Beck Depression Inventory; Rx, treatment; Ss, subjects.

Table 13.3 Studies evaluating the effects of oestrogen in peri- and postmenopausal women: postmenopausal studies.

Author	Duration	Design	Hormonal preparation	Post-treatment placebo	Post-treatment active	Comments
Brincat et al[36] N = 55	4 months	Parallel and single-blind	100 mg testosterone and oestradiol implant 50 mg; 5 mg norethisterone last week of month	Change in depression item −0.1 at 2 months and −0.3 at 4 months	Change in depression item −1.3 at 2 months and −1.1 at 4 months	Return of symptoms after 4 months oestrogen and testosterone significantly better than placebo for all symptoms except 'aches and pains'
Campbell[37] N = 64	2 months	Crossover	Conjugated oestrogens; no progestin	BDI change = −4	BDI change = −5	No significant Rx effect No baseline assessment of psychopathology
Campbell and Whitehead[53] N = 56	6 months					
Derman et al[38] N = 82	16 weeks	Parallel	β-oestradiol; sequential norethindrone acetate	BDI change = (=)0.1	BDI change = −2.0	The most profound change occurred in vasomotor symptoms but mild mood symptoms improved with active treatment
Fedor-Freybergh[39] N = 50	3 months	Parallel	Oral oestradiol; progestin added days 13–22	HRS-D change = +3	HRS-D change = −9	Oestrogen significantly better than placebo Ss with baseline psychopathology excluded
Furuhjelm et al[40] N = 48 (three groups)	2 months	Crossover	Oral oestradiol and oestriol; norethisterone during final week	Change scores: severe = 1.2; moderate = 1.1; minimal = 0.7	Change scores: severe = 5.5; moderate = 1.3; minimal = 1.9	Ss grouped by severity at baseline. Group 1 most and group 3 least symptomatic Rx effect for depression strongest in most symptomatic group
Klaiber et al[4]	1 month	Parallel	Oestropipate and placebo or oestropipate and norethindrone, placebo	HRS-D change = −8.8	HRS-D change = −7.7	Mood and anxiety slightly worsened in oestrogen and progesterone cycle (non-significant)
Saletu et al[42] N = 64	3 months	Parallel	Transdermal oestradiol; no progestin	HRS-D change = −10.3	HRS-D change = −9.6	All Ss met criteria for MDD High non-specific response rate in placebo group
Wiklund et al[43] N = 242	3 months	Parallel	Transdermal oestradiol; no progestin	Psychological wellbeing change = −6.5	Psychological wellbeing change = −13.5	Significant improvement in several measures of psychological health, including depression Ss with psychiatric illness excluded

BDI, Beck Depression Inventory; HRS-D, Hamilton Rating Scale for Depression; Rx, treatment; Ss, subjects.

Table 13.4 Studies evaluating the effects of oestrogen in peri- and postmenopausal women: postsurgical menopause studies.

Author	Duration	Design	Hormonal preparation	Post-treatment control	Post-treatment active	Comments
Coppen et al[31] N = 28	6 months with follow-up	Parallel	Piperazine oestrone sulphate; no progestin	BDI change = −4.5 in matched group at 6 months	BDI change = −5.6 in matched group at 6 months	Groups differed greatly at baseline Response in matched groups not significantly different
	1 year with follow-up					
Dennerstein and Burrows[51] N = 49	3 months	Crossover	Three active Rxs; ethinyl oestradiol; levonorgestrel; ethinyl oestradiol and levonorgestrel	HRS-D change = +4.3	HRS-D change = −3.4 levonorgestrel; −1.9 ethiny oestradiol; −2.8 combined	Excluded Ss with psychiatric illness Best response in Ss on oestrogen
Ditkoff et al[33] N = 13	3 months	Parallel	Conjugated oestrogens; no progestogen	BDI change = +2	BDI change = −2	Included only 'asymptomatic' Ss at baseline Significant difference between groups
George et al[34] N = 13	1 month	Crossover	Conjugated oestrogens; no progestogen	BDI change = −13	BDI change = −11	All Ss were started on active and then switched to oestrogen or placebo No significant difference in treatment conditions
Sherwin and Gelfand[35] N = 43	3 months	Crossover	Oestrogen or androgen or combination	MAACL change = +3	MAACL change = −3	Significant Rx difference Groups evaluated by the MAACL at baseline
Paterson[41] N = 20	3 months	Crossover	Mestranol and norethisterone	Author Scale group 1 = −0.6 group 2 = 0	Author Scale group 1 = 0 group 2 = −0.3	Mood scores showed sxs improved in the first 3 months regardless of treatment conditions

BDI, Beck Depression Inventory; HRS-D, Hamilton Rating Scale for Depression; MAACL, Multiple Affect Adjective Check List; Rx, treatment; Ss, subjects.

Table 13.5 Studies evaluating the effects of oestrogen in peri- and postmenopausal women: Other postmenopausal study.

Author	Duration	Design	Hormonal preparation	Post-treatment placebo	Post-treatment active	Comments
Gerdes et al[50] N = 38	5 months	Parallel	Conjugated oestrogens; medroxyprogesterone days 16–21	Not enough information	Not enough information	Improvement in mood symptoms significantly greater in the oestrogen versus placebo group

have further obfuscated a difference between active and placebo treatments.

A number of the specific aspects of these studies are informative. In a study reporting a benefit for oestradiol valerate,[52] researchers compared placebo to oestradiol valerate, testosterone enanthate or a combination of the two. Baseline levels for all oophorectomized women were equivalent to those of a hysterectomized but non-oophorectomized control group. The placebo condition was associated with a deterioration in mood ,whereas all hormonal treatments led to improved mood. The testosterone-only treatment had the most robust effect on decreasing mood symptoms, but it also increased hostility scores.

A second positive study was conducted in Hispanic-American women.[33] Care was taken to exclude women who were suffering from substantial mood or physical symptoms prior to treatment. None the less, the group taking conjugated oestrogens still exhibited greater improvement in mood than the placebo group.

Finally, the third study to show benefit for oestrogen had four cells: ethinyl oestradiol alone, ethinyl oestradiol in combination with levonorgestrel, levonorgestrel alone, and placebo.[51] Depression rating scales at baseline showed that one woman was moderately to severely depressed, while eight women were moderately depressed; the remainder were not depressed. The group assigned to oestrogen fared most favourably, while the placebo group did least well. The severity of mood disturbance at baseline did not influence drug effect. There was no particular association with any treatment condition (e.g. oestrogen only, progestin only, or the combination) or with the onset of moderate to severe depressive symptoms during the course of the study.

Naturally occurring postmenopause

Seven studies in this group included women who were naturally postmenopausal,[36–40,42,43] and one trial included a mixed group of surgically and naturally postmenopausal women.[41] Five studies[36,38–40,43] found a benefit of oestrogen over placebo. Medication used in these studies included parenteral and oral oestradiol. In one trial, 17β-oestradiol administered parenterally with testosterone was significantly better than placebo on all menopausal symptoms evaluated (somatic as well as psychological), with the exception of aches and pains.[36] Oral oestradiol with sequential norethisterone was also helpful for mood symptoms, although the greatest difference between active and placebo conditions occurred for hot flushes.[38]

These findings are reinforced by results of a large study ($n = 223$) evaluating transdermal oestradiol in a group of mildly symptomatic women.[43] A dose of 50 μg 17β-oestradiol was significantly more beneficial than placebo for psychological wellbeing, anxiety and depression, as well as vasomotor symptoms.

Oral micronized oestrogen was used in a study[40] which divided baseline symptoms of 'depression' and 'mental distress' into three levels of severity: mild, moderate and severe. All three groups experienced improvement in 'mental distress'. However, only the severely depressed group showed greater improvement with oestrogen compared with placebo, and women in this group continued to experience symptoms that were considered moderate in severity even after treatment.

A small crossover study of 20 naturally and surgically menopausal women compared placebo to the synthetic oestrogen mestranol, followed by addition of norethisterone.[41] Active treatment was superior to placebo for night sweats and flushing but not for mood symptoms. The author found no changes in depression or anxiety during the course of the trial.

A relative lack of benefit for oestrogen over placebo was found in another study which specifically evaluated postmenopausal women with MDD.[42] This trial enrolled 69 women who were given either 50 μg of transdermal 17β-oestradiol or placebo. Sixty-three per cent of the active-treatment group and 65% of the placebo group were considered to be responders; a high non-specific response rate was also found in an earlier study of 64 minimally symptomatic women receiving either conjugated oestrogen or placebo.[37,53] Statistically significant improvements over baseline in the Beck Depression Inventory (BDI) and General Health Questionnaire (GHQ) scores were found for both groups, although the magnitude of these effects did not differ between the oestrogen and placebo cells. It should be mentioned that the null finding in these studies was not due to low efficacy of oestrogen but to a high non-specific response.

Perimenopause

A total of six studies evaluated the response of low mood during the perimenopause. Five studies with perimenopausal women also included postmenopausal subjects,[44–48] while one study included perimenopausal women only.[49] Two trials showed benefit for the oestrogen condition.[44,47] In one investigation, oestrone sulphate improved mood, and this correlated with an increase in free tryptophan levels.[44] In a second study, 17β-oestradiol alone or β-oestradiol in conjunction with testosterone was compared to placebo.[47] At baseline, 86% of subjects had symptom scores consistent with psychiatric illness. Improvement occurred in both the peri- and postmenopausal women

in all treatment cells, but was significantly greater in the active-treatment groups at two months. The benefit with hormonal treatment was lost in both peri- and postmenopausal women by four months. This may have occurred either because hormone levels were diminished at this point or because placebo-treated patients continued to improve.

In studies which failed to find a benefit of oestrogen over placebo, the oestrogen preparation used included conjugated equine oestrogen (two studies)[45,48] and oestrone sulphate.[46,49] Results from several of these trials are difficult to interpret, since some, but not all, women had concurrent psychiatric illnesses[46,48] and were allowed to continue psychotropic medication during the trials. It is probable that in these two studies, the underlying psychopathology made a greater contribution to mood symptoms than did the effect of menopause. The same issue of a high non-specific response rate occurred in several studies which found significant improvement over baseline in both the oestrogen and placebo conditions.[45,49]

Other studies

Gerdes et al[50] published a trial of 38 women who were given daily conjugated oestrogen and 14 days of medroxyprogesterone versus clonidine. These groups were compared to a no-treatment group. The HRT group, compared to the other groups, showed improvement on a variety of personality measures and on a self-report mood measure.

Oestrogen treatment of longer duration may be more palliative in terms of mood. In a longitudinal study, one group found that women who remained on oestrogen for 1 year had improved mood and sexual functioning, compared to women who discontinued treatment.[54] In a cross-sectional epidemiological study, nearly 1200 women over the age of 50 were evaluated. Depressive symptoms occurred more often in women between 50 and 60 but they were lower in the over-60 group.[55] The authors suggested that women who were symptomatic sought treatment and hence had higher initial rates in the 50–60-year-old hormone replacement group. Over time and with treatment, these women felt more improved, explaining why women in the >60-year age group felt better when they were undergoing HRT.

Summary of studies using oestrogen in peri- and postmenopausal women

A quantitative review found that oestrogen treatment of menopausal women had a moderate to large benefit on mood, compared to control or placebo conditions.[30] That review found a greater effect among perimenopausal than among postmenopausal women. In addition, the effect was larger for naturally versus surgically induced menopause. Finally, women who were treated for longer than 8 months exhibited the greatest improvement. Although our review was qualitative, our conclusions differ in that the benefits of oestrogen treatment appeared to be more consistent in surgically menopausal women. However, most women included in these studies were mildly symptomatic. Thus, the efficacy of oestrogen in hysterectomized and oophorectomized women with severe depressive symptoms (such as those seen in MDD) could not be determined from these trials.

Of the studies investigating the utility of oestrogen in natural menopause, the most methodologically sound studies showed significantly greater benefit of oestrogen over placebo. Among the negative studies in natural menopause and perimenopausal women, the non-specific (placebo) response rate was unusually high, thus obscuring the benefit of the active agent.

Our review included several negative studies not in the quantitative review cited and was limited to placebo-controlled studies. A quantitative review can be advantageous in estimating overall effect sizes summed from a number of studies. However, results must be tempered by the fact that studies have substantial differences in design and outcome criteria and vary in the inclusion criteria of women (for example, some included women with current psychiatric illness and heterogeneous symptom severity).

While studies did not generally compare one oestrogen preparation to another, the trials which were most reliably able to detect a drug–placebo difference employed parenteral or transdermal oestradiol as a treatment. Only one of six studies using parenteral or transdermal oestradiol was negative, whereas negative findings occurred in 9 of 12 studies using an oestrogen compound that predominantly yielded oestrone. 17β-oestradiol is the more biologically active oestrogen, whereas oestrone has one-tenth of the biological activity. This review suggests that it is possible that 17β-oestradiol is more effective at ameliorating mood symptoms associated with the menopause.

Progestins in the treatment of menopausal mood disorders

Progesterone is made by the corpus luteum in ovulatory women of reproductive age. Progesterone is released in a pulsatile manner, and levels range from 1 to 50 mg/ml from the day of ovulation until the next menstruation. Peak progesterone levels occur in the mid-luteal phase. Follicular-phase progesterone levels, as well as levels in anovulatory and menopausal women, are extremely low.

Progesterone is poorly absorbed by the intestine. Two approaches have been utilized to make it orally active. One is to micronize the preparation. This product has been available in Europe for years and is just starting to be widely used in the USA. Progesterone has also been modified at C-17 and C-6 to make potent oral progestins (medroxyprogesterone acetate, megestrol acetate). Another manipulation that is used to make progestins for OCs is the modification of testosterone. Removing the C-18 carbon and adding an ethinyl group at C-17 is the base modification for norethindrone, norethindrone acetate and norgestrel.[56] Progestins are available in several different formulations (Table 13.1). The most common progestin used for postmenopausal women is oral medroxyprogesterone acetate. However, no single progestin is clearly superior to another. If a woman has significant side-effects with one progestin dose, a lower dose or a different progestin formulation is recommended.

Progesterone has also been shown to influence neurotransmitter systems. In part, progesterone may temper the effects of oestrogen.[19,25] An important property of selected progesterone metabolites is sedation.[25,57,58] The α-reduced progesterone compound allopregnanolone binds to a specific site on the GABA–benzodiazepine receptor and increases the duration of channel opening. This activity is similar to that of barbiturates, which bind at a different site on the receptor complex.[25] In rat models of anxiety, this compound decreases anxiety.[59] In humans, administration of progesterone can increase allopregnanolone levels and increase fatigue.[60]

Progesterone without oestrogen decreases the density of 5-HT$_1$ receptors and increases 5-HT$_2$ receptor density in frontal cortex,[14] but this effect is less pronounced than it is with oestrogen. Progesterone also increases serotonin turnover in brain.[61] As with oestrogen, progesterone increases serotonin content in the raphe, although to a lesser extent than does oestrogen.[19] In sum, progesterone and its metabolites have some modulating effects on oestrogen, but progesterone alone has important properties; it is not known whether synthetic progestins share any of these properties.

Some workers suggest that oestrogen improves mood in menopausal mood disorders but stipulate that this effect is reversed by the addition of a progestational agent.[1,3] Seven studies have evaluated the effects of progestin on menopausal mood symptoms.[62–68] Four studies used combination oestrogen followed by progestin or placebo,[63,64,67,68] while three studies included placebo-controlled treatment with either progestin or placebo but no oestrogen[62,65,66] (Table 13.6). An earlier open study, reported in three papers, showed a mild deterioration in mood among women openly treated with percutaneous oestradiol followed by a progestin.[1,69,70] The results of several double-blind placebo-controlled studies which followed this report are mixed. One group of investigators treated 58 postmenopausal women with subcutaneous oestradiol daily followed by norethisterone at a dose of 2.5 mg daily or 5.0 mg daily, or placebo for 7 days. Daily ratings for concentration and negative affect were slightly but significantly worse on norethisterone.[64]

Support for a deleterious effect of progestin is also found in a report by Sherwin,[67] although the results are not easy to explain. These investigators randomized 48 women to four groups: high-dose (1.25 mg daily) conjugated oestrogens plus placebo, high-dose conjugated oestrogens and 5 mg daily of medroxyprogesterone (days 15–25), low-dose (0.625 mg daily) conjugated oestrogens plus placebo, and low-dose

Table 13.6 Studies evaluating the mood effects of progestins in peri- and postmenopausal women.

Author	Duration (months)	Design	Hormonal preparation	Post-treatment placebo	Post-treatment active	Comments
Bullock et al N = 69	6	Parallel	Depot medroxy-progesterone	10% with side effect of depressed mood	10% with side effect of depressed mood	No difference between groups in onset of depression
Kirkham et al[63] N = 48 (surgical postmenopausal)	1	Crossover	Transdermal oestrogen days 1–25 and medroxy-progesterone days 12–15	BDI = 7.2 in former PMS group; BDI = 5.4 in non-PMS group	BDI = 6.3 in former PMS group; BDI = 5.5 in non-PMS group	Half of Ss had a history of prospectively documented PMS No difference in Rx condition (placebo versus progestogen) for either the former or non-PMS group
Magos et al[64] N = 70 (surgical postmenopausal)	1	Parallel	Group 1: transdermal oestradiol with 5 mg norethisterone versus placebo (50 Ss) Group 2: 2.5 mg norethisterone versus placebo (20 Ss)	MDQ Negative affect did not increase on placebo in groups 1 or 2	MDQ Negative affect increased; down 0.25 on 5 mg and 0.05 on 2.5 mg	Somatic symptoms and negative affect worsened in group 1 Differences were very small
Prior et al[66] N = 11 (postmenopausal)	2	Crossover	Medroxyprogesterone	Author Daily Diary Mood worsened 1 point	Author Daily Diary Mood improved 1 point	No significant worsening of somatic symptoms No mood worsening on progestin Very small sample size
Sherwin et al[67] N = 48	12	Parallel	0.625 mg conjugated oestrogen and medroxyprogesterone or placebo; 1.25 mg conjugated oestrogen and medroxyprogesterone	Daily Rating Calendar Addition of placebo—positive mood score in third month of 12 months; increased by 5.5 in 0.625 CEE group; 6.1 in 1.25 CEE group	Daily Rating Calendar Addition of progestin—positive mood score in third week by 4.8 in 0.625 CEE group; increased by 4.8 in 1.25 CEE group	Despite intermittent administration of progestin, scores differed between groups with added progestin and placebo
Morrison et al[65] N = 48	3	Parallel	Depot medroxy-progesterone	Side-effect of depression = 25%	Side effect of depression = 6%	Results are from side-effect data; wellbeing and somatic symptoms improved more with medroxyprogesterone

BDI, Beck Depression Inventory; PMS, premenstrual syndrome; MDQ, Menstrual Distress Questionnaire; Rx, treatment; Ss, subjects.

conjugated oestrogens and 5 mg daily medroxyprogesterone (days 15–25). Mood scores were worse in the medroxyprogesterone groups throughout the month, even though medroxyprogesterone was only given for 10 days. All groups had cyclical variation in mood, and the women who had the most cyclical mood variation were in the high-dose oestrogen and placebo groups.

Several investigators failed to find an association between progestin and mood worsening, despite using similar methodology.[4,63] In surgically menopausal women, mood deterioration was compared among those who did or did not have a history of premenstrual syndrome (PMS).[63] Neither women with a history of PMS nor asymptomatic women felt worse on oestrogen and progestin compared with oestrogen and placebo. Similarly, there was no significant mood deterioration when progestin was added to treatment with oestrone piperazine.[4]

Progestins have been used as monotherapy for menopausal complaints in three studies that provide information on mood symptoms. A placebo-controlled crossover trial investigated the mood-altering effects of medroxyprogesterone.[66] Eleven women were included in this 2-month study. Mood neither improved nor deteriorated in women taking progestin in this study.

In a heterogeneous group (surgical and non-surgical) of postmenopausal women, depot medroxyprogesterone ($n = 57$) or placebo ($n = 12$) was given for 6 months to control menopausal symptoms.[62] Hot flushes were diminished by the active treatment, and the rate of transient depression was the same in the active-treatment and placebo groups. This same agent was used in a second study of 48 women in whom the rate of depressive symptoms was no higher in the active-treatment than in the placebo cells.[65]

In sum, several but not all trials showed support for mood worsening after addition of progestin to oestrogen. However, the magnitude of mood worsening was not large. Second, some postmenopausal women appear to manifest monthly mood variation, even if they are only taking the oestrogen component of HRT. Third, the most problematic mood deterioration occurred with high-dose oestrogen plus progestin versus low-dose oestrogen plus progestin.

When the addition of progestin to ongoing oestrogen treatment was subjected to quantitative review, the results supported our qualitatively described findings.[30] Oestrogen in combination with progestin still had a more mitigating effect on mood, but it was less pronounced than was found with oestrogen alone.

Oestrogen in the treatment of non-menopausal mood disorders

Oestrogen has been tested as a treatment for non-menopausal mood disorders in nine studies, including two monotherapy trials for MDD,[71,72] three adjunct therapy trials for MDD,[73–75] one trial of postpartum MDD[76] and three trials of PMS[77–79] (Table 13.7).

Oestrogen as monotherapy for severe MDD was tested in an inpatient study of 40 women.[71] This trial employed extremely high doses of conjugated oestrogen; the starting dose was 5 mg daily, and the maximum dose was 25 mg daily. While the 23 women in the oestrogen group improved significantly more than women in the placebo group, post-treatment depression scores in the oestrogen group were still moderate to severe, suggesting that this intervention was not satisfactory by itself. This study has not been replicated.

Table 13.7 Studies evaluating the effects of oestrogen on non-reproductive-related mood disorders.

Author	Disorder	Duration	Design	Hormonal preparation	Post-treatment placebo/no HRT	Post-treatment active	Comments
Dhar and Murphy[79] N = 11	PMS	3 months	Crossover	Conjugated oestrogen	Authors Scale (range 62–239) Endpoint Score = 86	Authors Scale (range 62–239) Endpoint Score = 114	No significant differences among conditions; higher scores indicate increased symptoms
Gregoire et al[76] N = 51	Postpartum MDD	12 weeks	Adjunct trial	Oestradiol	EPDS decrease of 10.5	EPDS decrease of 16	Oestradiol was significantly better than placebo; 50% of Ss were also on antidepressants
Klaiber et al[71] N = 40	MDD	12 weeks	Parallel	Conjugated oestrogens 5–25 mg daily	Change in HRS-D = 0	Change in HRS-D = –9	Oestrogen dose was extremely high Actively treated Ss remained very symptomatic
Magos et al[64] N = 68	PMS	12 weeks	Parallel	Oestradiol	MDQ Change after 2 months = 0.12	Questionnaire change after 2 months = 0.25	(HRS-D = 22 post-Rx) Oestradiol was significantly better than placebo for total MDQ
Michael et al[72] N = 50	No diagnosis	38 months	Parallel	Conjugated oestrogen	HAS = 80 at 38 months	HAS = 74 at 38 months	Depressive sxs per se were not queried; Ss felt better on oestrogen, as reflected by lower score
Prange et al[73] N = 30	MDD	42 weeks	Adjunct trial	Conjugated oestrogen	HRS-D = 7	HRS-D = 7	Ss receiving oestrogen augmentation fared least well
Shapira et al[74] N = 11	MDD		Adjunct trial	200 mg imipramine; conjugated oestrogen 1.25–3.75 mg	No overall improvement with oestrogen or placebo	No overall improvement with oestrogen or placebo	Ss were Rx resistant
Schneider et al[75] N = 367	MDD	6 weeks	Adjunct trial	Various oestrogen preparations	Fluoxetine/no HRT change = –36%; placebo/no HRT change = –30%	Fluoxetine/HRT change = –40%; placebo/HRT change = –17%	Difference between HRT and no HRT was only a trend Placebo and HRT had least improvement
Watson et al[78] N = 40	PMS	3 months	Crossover	Oestradiol	PDQ Active Rx—placebo depressed mood increase 0.60	PCQ Placebo—active Rx depressed mood decrease 0.6	Oestradiol was significantly better than placebo

PMS, premenstrual syndrome; MDD, major depressive disorder; EPDS, Edinburgh Postnatal Depression Scale; HSR-D, Hamilton Rating Scale for Depression; HAS, Hospital Adjustment Scale; MDQ, Menstrual Distress Questionnaire; PDQ, Premenstrual Distress Questionnaire; HRT, hormone replacement therapy; Rx, treatment; Ss, subjects.

Oestrogen has also been evaluated as an adjunct therapy for MDD. An early study tested the benefit of adding oestrogen to a tricyclic antidepressant (TCA).[73] Although improvement in a TCA plus high-dose oestrogen group was initially greater than that in a low-dose oestrogen plus TCA or a TCA-alone group, this benefit was lost by 2 weeks, and the high-dose oestrogen plus TCA patients ultimately fared less well than the low-dose oestrogen plus TCA or the TCA-alone group. Similar results were reported in a small study of 11 women who were treated with imipramine and then randomized to conjugated oestrogen (in doses up to 3.75 mg/day) or placebo as an adjunct treatment.[74] There was no benefit with oestrogen augmentation compared with placebo augmentation. Finally, in a placebo-controlled trial of fluoxetine for MDD, older women on fluoxetine who were undergoing oestrogen replacement therapy (ORT) showed slightly greater improvement than the fluoxetine-treated group who were not receiving ORT.[75] However, women on ORT without fluoxetine did less well than women on no ORT. This makes the results of the study difficult to interpret.

An earlier investigation evaluated the effects of oestrogen versus placebo on personality and functioning in older women (60–91).[72] The Hospital Adjustment Scale (HAS) measured changes in interpersonal relationships, self-care, social responsibilities and activities. Women assigned to oestrogen improved and sustained better functioning. However, it is not clear whether the benefit of oestrogen was secondary to mood improvement or effects on cognitive functioning.[12,80]

There may be a role for oestrogen in the treatment of postpartum MDD. Sixty-four women with postpartum MDD were treated with either transdermal 17β-oestradiol or with placebo.[76] The 17β-oestradiol-treated women

had a significantly greater response, both statistically and clinically, compared to the placebo group. However, one-half of the women in this trial were also undergoing concurrent treatment with antidepressant agents. It is not known whether 17β-oestradiol was effective as an adjunct treatment or as monotherapy in this disorder.

Oestrogen has been used to treat the mood symptoms seen with PMS or premenstrual dysphoric disorder (PMDD). Two studies[77,78] compared transdermal 17β-oestradiol followed by 7 days of norethisterone to placebo. A third study used conjugated oestrogens[79] for this condition. 17β-Oestradiol was more effective than placebo for premenstrual dysphoria in both studies, but there was no difference between oestrogen and placebo in the study which used conjugated oestrogens. This latter study incorporated only 11 women, and thus the lack of significant difference may be due to a lack of power.

In sum, oestrogen does not appear to be effective for non-reproductive-related mood symptoms or disorders. The only study finding benefit for oestrogen treatment required doses that were 5–10 times as high as doses used in ORT, and women still remained very symptomatic. Similarly, oestrogen was not more beneficial than placebo as an adjunct treatment. The results of trials for postpartum depression and PMDD are more promising, however. Of note is the fact that positive trials employed 17β-oestradiol rather than formulations yielding predominantly oestrone.

Progesterone and progestins in the treatment of non-menopausal mood disorders

Although progesterone has not been used to treat MDD in double-blind studies, it has been used to treat women with PMS and PMDD (Table 13.8). To date, over 400 women have been included in 10 placebo-controlled trials investigating the efficacy of progesterone for the treatment of premenstrual symptoms.[81–90] One trial did not report post-treatment mood scores.[87] Of the remaining studies, only one investigation of 23 women found that progesterone was superior to placebo for mood symptoms[81] (Table 13.8).

The consistency of this body of work is impressive. It unequivocally shows that progesterone is no more beneficial than placebo for the treatment of premenstrual mood symptoms. On the other hand, given a postulated association between mood symptoms and progestins, it is reasonable to ask if women assigned to progesterone were more likely to develop either depressive symptoms or a depressive illness. This was not the case in these studies. In fact, women who received both placebo and progesterone experienced mild relief from their premenstrual mood symptoms.

The utility of several progestins in the treatment of premenstrual mood symptoms has also been tested, and although the results are not as consistent as those of the trials using progesterone, they are generally negative. The progestin most commonly used was dydrogesterone, which was evaluated in four studies.[91–94] In one study,[94] data were not presented in a way that allowed for evaluation of mood symptoms. The other three studies failed to show any benefit of dydrogesterone over placebo for premenstrual mood symptoms.

Two studies were conducted to test the bene-fit of medroxyprogesterone versus placebo[95,96] for PMS. In the first, medroxyprogesterone was compared to norethisterone and placebo in 48 women. Women were given either norethisterone versus placebo or medroxyprogesterone versus placebo and crossed over to another condition. There was significantly greater improvement in psychological symptoms with medroxyprogesterone treatment compared to placebo, while norethisterone treatment was not superior to placebo.[96] Because medroxyprogesterone disrupted menstrual cyclicity while norethisterone did not, the authors hypothesized that changes in the menstrual cycle may underlie the therapeutic effect of medroxyprogesterone. On the other hand, the placebo response was highest in the cycle comparing norethisterone to placebo, and it is likely that this obscured any benefit for norethisterone.

A three-way crossover study compared medroxyprogesterone, spironolactone and placebo for premenstrual symptoms.[95] This study enrolled 43 women and found that medroxyprogesterone was significantly better than placebo for depression, while spironolactone was significantly better than placebo for bloatedness. The two active treatments were not different from each other for clusters of physical or mood symptoms.

The studies with medroxyprogesterone suggest that this compound may be somewhat better than progesterone or dydrogesterone for mood symptoms associated with the premenstrual period. Importantly, none of these studies showed mood deterioration to be associated with the progestin.

Oral contraceptives and mood

OCs are commonly thought to cause mood disorders. However, most of the evidence support-

Table 13.8 Placebo-controlled studies evaluating the effects of progesterone on non-menopausal mood disorders.

Reference	N	Condition	Drug	Duration	Outcome measures	Results	Comments
Andersch and Hahn[82]	17	PMS	Progesterone 100 mg twice daily or placebo	1 month	CPRS Scale	Progesterone = placebo	Crossover; luteal phase Rx
Baker et al[83]	17	PMS	Progesterone 100 mg twice daily or placebo	2 months	STAI, POMS, SCL-90, HRS-D, SAD-C, BPRS, BDI	Progesterone = placebo on STAI, HRS-D, BID, POMS, SCL-90	Crossover after two cycles with washout; luteal phase Rx
Dennerstein et al[81]	23	PMS	Progesterone or placebo 300 mg	2 months	MDQ, BDI, STAI, MACL, DRS	Progesterone > placebo	Crossover; luteal phase Rx
Freeman et al[84]	121	PMS	Progesterone 400 mg or 800 mg or placebo	2 months	DRS, Global Improvement, SCL-90	Progesterone = placebo; mood symptoms improved in both groups	Crossover; luteal phase Rx; 49 dropped
Freeman et al[84]	24	Normal controls	Progesterone 300, 600, 1200 mg versus placebo	1 day	POMS	Progesterone was no more likely to cause depression than placebo	Plasma levels were as high as 58 ng/ml
Freeman et al[85]	170	PMS	Progesterone 900–2700 mg; alprazolam 0.75–2.5 mg or placebo	3 months	DSR	Progesterone = placebo; alprazolam > progesterone or placebo	Luteal phase Rx; parallel design; 49 dropped
Maddocks et al[86]	20	PMS	Progesterone 400 mg versus placebo	3 months	BDI, Buss-Durkee, STAI, MDQ, PMTS	Progesterone = placebo	Luteal phase Rx
Richter et al[88]	22		Progesterone 800 mg versus placebo	2 months	DRS	Progesterone = placebo	Luteal phase Rx
Sampson et al[89]	35/25		Progesterone 400 mg versus placebo then 800 mg versus placebo	2 months	MDQ	Progesterone = placebo	Luteal phase Rx; crossover
van der Meer et al[90]	13		Progesterone 400 mg versus placebo	2 months	Author Daily Ratings	Progesterone = placebo	Luteal phase Rx

PMS, premenstrual syndrome; HRS-D, Hamilton Rating Scale for Depression; BDI, Beck Depression Inventory; CPRS, Comprehensive Psychopathological Rating Scale; STAI, State–Trait Anxiety Inventory; POMS, Profile of Mood States; SCL, Symptom Checklist 90; SAD-C, Schedule for Affective Disorders and Schizophrenia – Change Scale; BPRS, Brief Psychiatric Rating Scale; MDQ, Menstrual Distress Questionnaire; MACL, Multiple Adjective Checklist; PMTS, Premenstrual Tension Scale; DRS, Daily Rating Scale; DSR, Daily Sympton Ratings; Rx, treatment.

ing this contention is based upon cross-sectional, uncontrolled studies rather than either longitudinal studies or placebo-controlled studies. This literature received a thorough review in the early 1980s.[97] Since that time, there have been two notable additions to the literature,[98,99] to yield four placebo-controlled studies that have specifically evaluated the effects of OC agents on mood (Table 13.9). One of the studies evaluated mood in women with PMS.[100]

The first placebo-controlled study utilized four different hormonal preparations, including a high-dose oestrogen–sequential progestin pill, a high-dose oestrogen–progestin combination pill, a low-dose oestrogen combination pill, and a progestin-only pill.[101,102] Subjects (about 80 per cell) were treated for four cycles, and some women were crossed over to an alternative pill. The percentage of patients complaining of depressed mood during the first three cycles was approximately equal in all groups. Rates for nervousness were higher than for depression among all treatment conditions, including placebo. Women given the high-dose oestrogen combination pill were slightly more likely to develop either depressed or anxious mood. In general, complaints of depressed mood gradually diminished over the 6 months of the study. This study did not support an overall deleterious effect for OCs on mood.

A similar strategy was employed in a second study that used three different combination OC preparations.[103] Four groups, each of approximately 80 women, were treated with either placebo or 1.0 mg, 0.5 mg or 0.06 mg norgestrel daily with a fixed dose of ethinyl oestradiol. This was a carefully designed study which used several outcome measures, including an assessment of whether mood improved or deteriorated. Between 40% and 60% of women reported some type of mood change among all groups, and the degree of change was predominantly negative for all conditions.

When 'depressed mood' was evaluated specifically, placebo-treated women experienced the least degree of change (5%) compared to hormone-treated women (8% in the high-dose group, 5% in the intermediate-dose group and 6% in the low-dose group). The group that experienced the most negative mood change was the low dose oestrogen/progestin group, and this difference was statistically significant. In this cell, 18% of women had negative mood changes, compared with 8% in the high-dose progestin group, 6% in the intermediate-progestin group and 1% in the placebo group. 'Dysphoric' changes were greater than those for 'depressed mood' for all groups, but were still significantly higher in the hormone groups than in the placebo group. Thus, this investigation shows that mood worsening is common in women placed on either placebo or hormonal therapy; however, the likelihood is slightly greater in women treated with OCs. In contrast to findings from the Goldzieher et al study,[101] mood worsening was found to be most pronounced when the OC was administered with lower dosages of progestin and oestrogen. However, the lowest dose used by Goldzieher et al[101] (0.1 mg ethinyl oestradiol) was not as low as the dose employed by Cullberg[103] (0.05 mg ethinyl oestradiol). However, current pill dosage is limited to 0.02–0.035 mg ethinyl oestradiol, with only rare use of 0.05-mg doses.

A third placebo-controlled OC study was conducted in two cohorts from two countries (Edinburgh and Manila).[98] This trial, supported by the World Health Organization, included 25 women in each condition from each centre: placebo, combined ethinyl oestradiol (0.03 mg) and levonorgestrel (0.15 mg) or progestin-only therapy (levonorgestrel 0.03 mg). Women were treated for 4 months, and at study endpoint the main treatment effect as reflected by the BDI was a reduction in mood symptoms for the women placed in the progestin-only group. The

Table 13.9 Placebo-controlled studies evaluating the effects of oral contraceptives on mood and other selected symptoms.

Author	Disorder	Duration (months)	Design	Hormonal preparation	Post-treatment placebo	Post-treatment active	Comments
Goldzieher et al[101] N = 398	Not ill	1	Crossover	Sequential ethinyl oestradiol 0.1 mg/dimethisterone 25 mg	0.42	0.47	Symptoms varied slightly cycle by cycle. No significant differences in rates of depressive sxs. Higher score means more symptoms
				Mestranol 0.1 mg/ethynodial diacetate 1 mg	0.42	0.62	Somewhat higher rate of nervousness in high-oestrogen preparations
				Mestranol 0.5 mg/ norethindrone 1 mg	0.42	0.49	The crossover part of the study showed that Ss who had symptoms on placebo continued to have symptoms when they were crossed over to placebo
				0.5 mg chormadinone daily and continuously	0.42	0.33	
Silbergeld[105] N = 8	Not ill	2	Crossover	Enovid (norethindrone 5 mg/mestranol 0.75 mg)	Mood adjective checklist; MDQ = 1.15	Mood adjective checklist; MDQ = 1.43	Significant decrease in irritability and aggression, and increase in regretfulness on OC; only 8 Ss
Cullberg et al[103] N = 240	Not ill			Norgestrel 1.0 mg/ EO 0.05 mg	Mean score = +0.2	Mean score = +0	The differences between conditions was very small. Ss on 'oestrogen-dominant' compound fared the least well overall
				Norgestrel 0.5 mg/ EO 0.05 mg	Mean score = +0.2	Mean score = +0	
				Norgestrel 0.6 mg/EO 0.05 mg	Mean score = +0.2	Mean Score = -0.4	Higher score means more depression
Graham and Sherwin[100] N = 82	Not ill	3	Parallel	EO 0.035 mg plus norethindrone	N/A	N/A	Group with depressive symptoms at baseline did significantly better on OCs than on placebo
Graham et al[98] N = 150	Not ill	4	Parallel	EO 0.03 mg plus levongestrel 0.15 mg	Manila Site change = +0.1; Edinburgh Site change = 0.1	Manila Site change = -0.1; Edinburgh Site change = -0.15	Study conducted in Manila and Edinburgh. Mood evaluated with daily ratings
				Levongestrel 0.03 mg	Manila Site change = +0.1; Edinburgh Site change = +0.1	Manila Site change = -0.1; Edinburgh Site change = -0.15	An increase in ratings indicates worse mood. Greatest reduction in mood scores
				Placebo			

PMS, premenstrual syndrome; OC, oral contraceptive; EO, ethinyl oestradiol; MDQ, Menstrual Distress Questionnaire; Ss, subjects; N/A, not applicable.

Edinburgh group showed worse premenstrual mood disturbance on the combination pill, compared to progestin only or placebo. The last placebo-controlled study to investigate the effects of an OC on mood was carried out in women with PMS.[100] An OC with sequential increase of progestin was used. There was no difference between the effects of placebo and the OC on mood during the premenstrual phase of the cycle; however, women on the OC had more mood symptoms during the early follicular phase.

These results show limited support for OC-induced mood deterioration. The study by Cullberg[103] illustrated that mood worsening was more likely to occur in women on the lowest dose of progestin with oestrogen. Similarly, Graham and Sherwin[100] found that mood symptoms were more severe when women took oestrogen and the lowest progestin dose. It is difficult to explain why mood deterioration was more likely to occur with lower doses. One possible explanation is that the relatively higher dose of progestin was conferring some benefit against the mood-worsening effects of oestrogen. On the other hand, it could be that the higher-dose pills and progestin-only pills are more effective in the treatment of mild premenstrual symptoms.

The lack of dose-related mood effects is necessarily inconsistent with the findings of Goldzieher et al,[101] since, in that study, the group faring least well took hormonal combinations that consisted of higher doses of both oestrogen and progestin. It may be that when oestrogen is given in higher doses, the progestin may not be able to counteract the deleterious effects on mood. Both Goldzieher et al[101] and Sherwin[67] found that higher doses of oestrogen were associated with mood changes, regardless of progestin dose.

Treatment recommendations

It appears that women who are surgically menopausal benefit from oestrogen therapy in terms of protection against and treatment of mood disturbances. In this group, the type of oestrogen preparation employed appears to matter less. However, if women fail to respond to conjugated oestrogens or to other preparations that predominantly deliver oestrone, and if there are no contraindications to parenteral or transdermal oestrogen, they should be changed to a preparation that delivers 17β-oestradiol. Women who are naturally menopausal are also likely to derive mood-lifting effects after oestrogen administration, particularly if the oestrogen is 17β-oestradiol. There is no support for the use of oestrogen as monotherapy for severe menopausal mood symptoms. Furthermore, there is no support for the use of oestrogen as monotherapy or adjunct therapy for non-reproductive-related mood disorders. 17β-Oestradiol appears to be useful as a treatment for postpartum depression or premenstrual dysphoria, but its efficacy needs to be compared to that of standard antidepressant therapy. Finally, clinicians should not be wary of using OCs in women because of mood-altering effects. It is likely that if a mood disorder occurs, it would have occurred in any case. Women in this latter group should be treated with standard antidepressant therapy while they are undergoing hormonal therapy.

Summary

There is some support for the contention that oestrogen is helpful for mood disturbances in reproductive-related conditions, but there is little support for the view that progestins lead to mood worsening. The strongest benefit for oestrogen is found for postpartum depression and premenstrual dysphoria. These positive findings, however, are tempered by the fact that the postpartum depression study has not been replicated, and the studies finding oestrogen helpful for premenstrual dysphoria have all been conducted by the same research group. There is also strong evidence that oestrogen is helpful for menopausal mood symptoms, although the most consistent findings are in women who are surgically menopausal and in women who have mild symptoms. The oestrogen preparations most highly associated with positive mood changes are percutaneous and transdermal β-oestradiol. If the difference in response is due to the type of oestrogen used, this would explain the mixed findings for menopausal mood symptoms compared to premenstrual dysphoria.

The effects of progestin on mood are not, by and large, negative. There is some support for progestin-induced dysphoria in the menopause literature, although the findings are inconsistent. There is no support for this hypothesis in the literature on premenstrual dysphoria, and, if anything, progestin-only contraceptive pills appear to induce fewer mood changes than combination pills. In terms of the effects of OCs on mood, the widely held belief that OCs induce negative mood changes is not uniformly supported. Rather, placebo-controlled trials favour the findings of a large British epidemiological study of over 16 000 women.[104] Mood disorders in those using OCs, a diaphragm or an intrauterine device were compared. The rate of mood disorders was approximately 3% in each group and did not differ significantly among groups.

References

1. Backstrom T, Symptoms related to the menopause and sex steroid treatments, *Ciba Found Symp* 1995; **191**:171–86.
2. Studd J, Chakravarti S, Oram D, The climacteric, *Clin Obstet Gynecol* 1977; **4**:3–29.
3. Studd JWW, Smith RNJ, Estrogens and depression in women. Menopause, *J North Am Menopause Soc* 1994; **1**:33–7.
4. Klaiber EL, Broverman DM, Vogel W et al, Individual differences in changes in mood and platelet monoamine oxidase (MAO) activity during hormonal replacement therapy in menopausal women, *Psychoneuroendocrinology* 1996; **21**:575–92.
5. Dalton K, Prospective study into puerperal depression, *Br J Psychiatry* 1971; **118**:689–92.
6. Lobo RA, ed., Preface. In: Lobo R, ed., *Treatment of the Postmenopausal Woman: Basic and Clinical Aspects*, Vol. xvii (Raven Press: New York, 1994).
7. Ortho Pharmaceutical Corporation, ed., *Annual Birth Control Study* (Philadelphia, 1996).
8. Lyman GW, Johnson RN, Assay for conjugated estrogens in tablets using fused-silica capillary gas chromatography, *J Chromatogr* 1982; **234**:234–9.
9. Stanczyk FZ, Shoupe D, Nunez V et al, A randomized comparison of nonoral estradiol delivery in postmenopausal women, *Am J Obstet Gynecol* 1988; **159**:1540–6.
10. Dickerson J, Bressler R, Christian CD, Hermann HW, Efficacy of estradiol vaginal cream in postmenopausal women, *Clin Pharmacol Ther* 1979; **26**:502–7.
11. Halbreich U, Lumley LA, The multiple interactional biological processes that might lead to depression and gender differences in its appearance, *J Affect Disord* 1993; **29**:159–73.
12. Halbreich U, Role of estrogen in postmenopausal depression, *Neurology* 1997; **48** (suppl 7):S16–19.
13. Steiner M, Lepage P, Dunn EJ, Serotonin and gender-specific psychiatric disorders, *Int J Psychiatry Clin Practice* 1997; **1**:3–13.

14. Biegon A, Reches A, Snyder L, McEwen BS, Serotonergic and noradrenergic receptors in the rat brain: modulation by chronic exposure to ovarian hormones, *Life Sci* 1983; **32:** 2015–21.
15. Sumner BE, Fink G, Estrogen increases the density of 5-hydroxytryptamine-2A receptors in cerebral cortex and nucleus accumbens in the female rat, *J Steroid Biochem Mol Biol* 1995; **54:**15–20.
16. Jarrett RB, Comparing and combining short-term psychotherapy and pharmacotherapy for depression. In: Bekham EE, Leber WR, eds. *Handbook of Depression,* 2nd edn (The Guilford Press: New York, 1995) 435–64.
17. Fischette CT, Biegon A, McEwen BS, Sex differences in serotonin 1 receptor binding in rat brain, *Science* 1983; **222:**333–5.
18. Fink G, Sumner BE, Rosie R et al, Estrogen control of central neurotransmission: effect on mood, mental state, and memory, *Cell Mol Neurobiol* 1996; **16:**325–44.
19. Pecins-Thompson M, Brown NA, Kohama SG, Bethea CL, Ovarian steroid regulation of tryptophan hydroxylase mRNA expression in rhesus macaques, *J Neurosci* 1996; **16:**7021–9.
20. Jones EE, Naftolin F, Estrogen effects on the tuberoinfundibular dopaminergic system in the female rat brain, *Brain Res* 1990; **510:**84–91.
21. Shimizu H, Bray GA, Effects of castration, estrogen replacement and estrus cycle on monoamine metabolism in the nucleus accumbens, measured by microdialysis, *Brain Res* 1993; **621:**200–6.
22. Rojansky N, Halbreich U, Zander K et al, Imipramine receptor binding and serotonin uptake in platelets of women with premenstrual changes, *Gynecol Obstet Invest* 1991; **31:**146–52.
23. Halbreich U, Rojansky N, Palter S et al, Estrogen augments serotonergic activity in postmenopausal women, *Biol Psychiatry* 1995; **37:**434–41.
24. O'Keane V, O'Hanlon M, Webb M, Dinan T, d-Fenfluramine/prolactin response throughout the menstrual cycle: evidence for an estrogen-induced alteration, *Clin Endocrinol* 1991; **34:**289–92.
25. Smith SS, Female sex steroid hormones from

26. Sherwin BB, Estrogenic effects on memory in women, *Ann NY Acad Sci* 1994; **743:** 213–30.
27. Phillips SM, Sherwin BB, Effects of estrogen on memory function in surgically menopausal women, *Psychoneuroendocrinology* 1992; **17:**485–95.
28. Kampen DL, Sherwin BB, Estrogen use and verbal memory in healthy postmenopausal women, *Obstet Gynecol* 1994; **83:**979–83.
29. Stuenkel CA, Menopause and estrogen replacement therapy, *Psychiatr Clin North Am* 1989; **12:**133–52.
30. Zweifel JE, O'Brien WH, A meta-analysis of the effect of hormone replacement therapy upon depressed mood, *Psychoneuroendocrinology* 1997; **22:**189–212.
31. Coppen A, Bishop M, Beard RJ, Effects of piperazine oestrone sulphate on plasma tryptophan, oestrogens, gonadotrophins and psychological functioning in women following hysterectomy, *Curr Med Res Opin* 1977; **4:**29–36.
32. Dennerstein L, Mood and menopause. In: Sitruk-Ware R, Utian WH, eds, *The Menopause and Hormonal Replacement Therapy. Facts and Controversies* (Marcel Dekker Inc.: New York, 1991) 101–18.
33. Ditkoff EC, Crary WG, Cristo M, Lobo RA, Estrogen improves psychological function in asymptomatic postmenopausal women, *Obstet Gynecol* 1991; **78:**991–5.
34. George GC, Utian WH, Beaumont PJ, Beardwood CJ, Effect of exogenous oestrogens on minor psychiatric symptoms in postmenopausal women, *S Afr Med J* 1973; **47:**2387–8.
35. Sherwin BB, Gelfand MM, Sex steroids and affect in the surgical menopause: a double-blind, cross-over study, *Psychoneuroendocrinology* 1985; **10:**325–35.
36. Brincat M, Magos A, Studd JW et al, Subcutaneous hormone implants for the control of climacteric symptoms, *Lancet* 1984; **1:**16–18.
37. Campbell S, Double blind psychometric studies on the effects of natural estrogens on post-

menopausal women. In: Campbell S, ed., *The Management of Menopause and Postmenopausal Years* (MTP: Lancaster, 1976) 149–58.

38. Derman RJ, Dawood MY, Stone S, Quality of life during sequential hormone replacement therapy—a placebo-controlled study, *Int J Fertil* 1995; **40**:73–8.

39. Fedor-Freybergh P, The influence of oestrogen on the wellbeing and mental and mental performance in climacteric and postmenopausal women, *Acta Obstet Gynecol Scand* 1977; **64** (suppl):1–91.

40. Furuhjelm M, Karlgren E, Carlstrom K, The effect of estrogen therapy on somatic and psychical symptoms in postmenopausal women, *Acta Obstet Gynecol Scand* 1984; **63**:655–61.

41. Paterson ME, A randomized, double-blind, cross-over study into the effect of sequential mestranol and norethisterone on climacteric symptoms and biochemical parameters, *Maturitas* 1982; **4**:83–94.

42. Saletu B, Brandstatter N, Metka M et al, Double-blind, placebo-controlled, hormonal, syndromal and EEG mapping studies with transdermal oestradiol therapy in menopausal depression, *Psychopharmacology* 1995; **122**:321–9.

43. Wiklund I, Karlberg J, Mattsson LA, Quality of life of postmenopausal women on a regimen of transdermal estradiol therapy: a double-blind placebo-controlled study, *Am J Obstet Gynecol* 1993; **168**:824–30.

44. Aylward M, Holly F, Parker RJ, An evaluation of clinical response to piperazine oestrone sulphate ('Harmogen') in menopause patients, *Curr Med Res Opin* 1974; **2**:417–23.

45. Coope J, Thomson JM, Poller L, Effects of 'natural oestrogen' replacement therapy on menopausal symptoms and blood clotting, *Br Med J* 1975; **4**:139–43.

46. Coope J, Is oestrogen therapy effective in the treatment of menopausal depression? *J R Coll Gen Practitioners* 1981; **31**:134–40.

47. Montgomery JC, Appleby L, Brincat M et al, Effect of oestrogen and testosterone implants on psychological disorders in the climacteric, *Lancet* 1987; **1**:297–9.

48. Strickler RC, Borth R, Cecutti A et al, The role of oestrogen replacement in the climacteric syndrome, *Psychol Med* 1977; **7**:631–9.

49. Thomson J, Oswald I, Effect of oestrogen on the sleep, mood, and anxiety of menopausal women, *Br Med J* 1977; **2**:1317–19.

50. Gerdes LC, Sonnendecker EW, Polakow ES, Psychological changes effected by estrogen–progestogen and clonidine treatment in climacteric women, *Am J Obstet Gynecol* 1982; **142**:98–104.

51. Dennerstein L, Burrows GD, Affect and the menstrual cycle, *J Affect Disord* 1979; **1**: 77–92.

52. Sherwin BB, Gelfand MM, Brender W, Androgen enhances sexual motivation in females: a prospective, crossover study of sex steroid administration in the surgical menopause, *Psychosom Med* 1985; **47**:339–51.

53. Campbell S, Whitehead M, Oestrogen therapy and the menopausal syndrome, *Clin Obstet Gynaecol* 1977; **4**:31–47.

54. Maoz B, Durst N, The effects of oestrogen therapy on the sex life of post-menopausal women, *Maturitas* 1980; **2**:327–36.

55. Palinkas LA, Barrett-Connor E, Estrogen use and depressive symptoms in postmenopausal women, *Obstet Gynecol* 1992; **80**:30–6.

56. Whitehead MI, Hillard TC, Crook D, The role and use of progestogens, *Obstet Gynecol* 1990; **75**(suppl):59S-76S.

57. Majewska MD, Harrison NL, Schwartz RD et al, Steroid hormone metabolites are barbiturate-like modulators of the GABA receptor, *Science* 1986; **232**:1001–7.

58. Mahesh VB, Brann DW, Hendry LB, Diverse modes of action of progesterone and its metabolites, *J Steroid Biochem Mol Biol* 1996; **56**:209–19.

59. Bitran D, Purdy RH, Kellogg CK, Anxiolytic effect of progesterone is associated with increases in cortical allopregnanolone and GABAa receptor function, *Pharmacol Biochem Behav* 1993; **45**:423–8.

60. Freeman EW, Purdy RH, Coutifaris C et al, Anxiolytic metabolites of progesterone: correlation with mood and performance measures following oral progesterone administration to healthy female volunteers, *Neuroendocrinology* 1993; **58**:478–84.

61. Gereau IV RW, Kedzie KA, Renner KJ, Effect of progesterone on serotonin turnover in rats primed with estrogen implants into the ventromedial hypothalamus, *Brain Res Bull* 1993; **32**:293–300.

62. Bullock JL, Massey FM, Gambrell RD, Use of medroxyprogesterone acetate to prevent menopausal symptoms, *Obstet Gynecol* 1975; **46**:165–8.

63. Kirkham C, Hahn PM, Van Vugt DA et al, A randomized, double-blind, placebo-controlled, cross-over trial to assess the side effects of medroxyprogesterone acetate in hormone replacement therapy, *Obstet Gynecol* 1991; **78**:93–7.

64. Magos AL, Brewster E, Singh R et al, The effects of norethisterone in postmenopausal women on oestrogen replacement therapy: a model for the premenstrual syndrome, *Br J Obstet Gynaecol* 1986; **93**:1290–6.

65. Morrison JC, Martin DC, Blair RA et al, The use of medroxyprogesterone acetate for relief of climacteric symptoms, *Am J Obstet Gynecol* 1980; **138**:99–104.

66. Prior JC, Alojado N, McKay DW, Vigna YM, No adverse effects of medroxyprogesterone treatment without estrogen in postmenopausal women: double-blind, placebo-controlled, crossover trial, *Obstet Gynecol* 1994; **83**:24–8.

67. Sherwin BB, The impact of different doses of estrogen and progestin on mood and sexual behavior in postmenopausal women, *J Clin Endocrinol Metab* 1991; **72**:336–43.

68. Siddle NC, Fraser D, Whitehead MI et al, Endometrial physical and psychological effects of postmenopausal oestrogen therapy with added dydrogesterone, *Br J Obstet Gynaecol* 1990; **97**:1101–7.

69. Hammarback S, Backstrom T, Holst J et al, Cyclical mood changes as in the premenstrual tension syndrome during sequential estrogen–progestogen postmenopausal replacement therapy, *Acta Obstet Gynecol Scand* 1985; **64**:393–7.

70. Holst J, Backstrom T, Hammarback S, von Schoultz B, Progestogen addition during oestrogen replacement therapy—effects on vasomotor symptoms and mood, *Maturitas* 1989; **11**:13–20.

71. Klaiber EL, Broverman DM, Vogel W, Kobayashi Y, Estrogen therapy for severe persistent depressions in women, *Arch Gen Psychiatry* 1979; **36**:550–4.

72. Michael CM, Kantor HI, Shore H, Further psychometric evaluation of older women—the effect of estrogen administration, *J Gerontol* 1970; **25**:337–41.

73. Prange AJ, Lipton MA, Nemeroff CB, Wilson IC, The role of hormones in depression, *Life Sci* 1977; **20**:1305–18.

74. Shapira B, Oppenheim G, Zohar J et al, Lack of efficacy of estrogen supplementation to imipramine in resistant female depressives, *Biol Psychiatry* 1985; **20**:576–9.

75. Schneider LS, Small GW, Hamilton SH et al, Estrogen replacement and response to fluoxetine in a multicenter geriatric depression trial, *Am J Geriatr Psychiatry* 1997; **5**:97–106.

76. Gregoire AJ, Kumar R, Everitt B et al, Transdermal oestrogen for treatment of severe postnatal depression, *Lancet* 1996; **347**:930–3.

77. Magos AL, Brincat M, Studd JW, Treatment of the premenstrual syndrome by subcutaneous oestradiol implants and cyclical oral norethisterone: placebo controlled study, *Br Med J* 1986; **292**:1629–33.

78. Watson NR, Studd JW, Savvas M et al, Treatment of severe premenstrual syndrome with oestradiol patches and cyclical oral norethisterone, *Lancet* 1989; **ii**:730–2.

79. Dhar V, Murphy BEP, Double-blind randomized crossover trial of luteal phase estrogens (Premarin) in the premenstrual syndrome (PMS), *Psychoneuroendocrinology* 1990; **15**:489–93.

80. Barrett-Connor E, Kritz-Silverstein D, Estrogen replacement therapy and cognitive function in older women, *JAMA* 1993; **269**:2637–41.

81. Dennerstein L, Spencer-Gardner C, Gotts G et al, Progesterone and the premenstrual syndrome: a double blind crossover trial, *Br Med J* 1985; **290**:1617–21.

82. Andersch B, Hahn L, Progesterone treatment of premenstrual tension—a double-blind study, *J Psychosom Res* 1985; **29**:489–93.

83. Baker ER, Best RG, Manfredi RL et al, Reproductive endocrinology. Efficacy of progesterone vaginal suppositories in alleviation of nervous symptoms in patients with premenstrual syndrome, *J Assist Reprod Genet* 1995; **12**:205–9.

84. Freeman E, Sondheimer SJ, Rickels K, Polansky M, Ineffectiveness of progesterone suppository treatment for premenstrual syndrome, *JAMA* 1990; **264**:349–53.

85. Freeman EW, Rickels K, Sondheimer SJ, Polansky M, A double-blind trial of oral progesterone, alprazolam, and placebo in treatment of severe premenstrual syndrome, *JAMA* 1995; **274**:51–7.

86. Maddocks S, Hahn P, Moller F, Reid RL, A double-blind placebo-controlled trial of progesterone vaginal suppositories in the treatment of premenstrual syndrome, *Am J Obstet Gynecol* 1986; **154**:573–81.

87. Magill PJ, Investigation of the efficacy of progesterone pessaries in the relief of symptoms of premenstrual syndrome, *Br J Gen Practice* 1995; **45**:589–93.

88. Richter MA, Haltvick R, Shapiro SS, Progesterone treatment of premenstrual syndrome, *Curr Therapeut Res* 1984; **36**:840–50.

89. Sampson GA, Premenstrual syndrome: a double-blind controlled trial of progesterone and placebo, *Br J Psychiatry* 1979; **135**:209–15.

90. Van der Meer YG, Benedek-Jaszmann LJ, Van-Loenen AC, Effect of high-dose progesterone on the premenstrual syndrome, *J Psychosom Obstet Gynaecol* 1983; **2**:220–2.

91. Dennerstein L, Morse C, Gotts G et al, Treatment of premenstrual syndrome. A double-blind trial of dydrogesterone, *J Affect Disord* 1986; **11**:199–205.

92. Kerr GD, Day JB, Munday MR et al, Dydrogesterone in the treatment of the premenstrual syndrome, *Practitioner* 1980; **224**:852–5.

93. Sampson G, Heathcote P, Wordsworth J et al, Premenstrual syndrome: a double-blind crossover study of treatment with dydrogesterone and placebo, *Br J Psychiatry* 1988; **153**:232–5.

94. Williams JGC, Martin AJ, Hulkenberg-Tromp TEML, PMS in four European countries: Part 2. A double-blind placebo controlled study of dydrogesterone, *Br J Sexual Med* 1983; **10**: 8–18.

95. Hellberg D, Claesson B, Nilsson S, Premenstrual tension: a placebo-controlled efficacy study with spironolactone and medroxy-progesterone acetate, *Int J Gynaecol Obstet* 1991; **34**:243–8.

96. West CP, Inhibition of ovulation with oral progestins—effectiveness in premenstrual syndrome, *Eur J Obstet Gynecol Reprod Biol* 1990; **34**:119–28.

97. Slap GB, Oral contraceptives and depression: impact, prevalence and cause, *J Adolescent Health Care* 1981; **2**:53–64.

98. Graham CA, Ramos R, Bancroft J et al, The effects of steroidal contraceptives on the well-being and sexuality of women: a double-blind, placebo-controlled, two-centre study of combined and progestogen-only methods, *Contraception* 1995; **52**:363–9.

99. Kumar R, Robson KM, A prospective study of emotional disorders in childbearing women, *Br J Psychiatry* 1984; **144**:35–47.

100. Graham CA, Sherwin BB, The relationship between mood and sexuality in women using an oral contraceptive as a treatment for premenstrual symptoms, *Psychoneuroendocrinology* 1993; **18**:273–81.

101. Goldzieher JW, Moses LE, Averkin E et al, Nervousness and depression attributed to oral contraceptives: a double-blind, placebo-controlled study, *Am J Obstet Gynecol* 1971; **111**:1013–20.

102. Goldzieher JW, Moses LE, Averkin E et al, A placebo-controlled double-blind crossover investigation of the side effects attributed to oral contraceptives, *Fertil Steril* 1971; **22**:609–23.

103. Cullberg J, Mood changes and menstrual symptoms with different gestagen/estrogen combinations. A double blind comparison with a placebo, *Acta Psychiatr Scand* 1972; **236** (suppl):1–86.

104. Vessey MP, McPherson K, Lawless M, Yeates D, Oral contraception and serious psychiatric illness: absence of an association, *Br J Psychiatry* 1985; **146**:45–9.

105. Silbergeld, S, Brast N, Noble EP, The menstrual cycle: a double-blind study of symptoms, mood and behavior, and biochemical variables using enovid and placebo, *Psychosom Med* 1971; **33**:411–28.

14

Behavioural effects of androgens in women

Elias Eriksson, Charlotta Sundblad, Mikael Landén and Meir Steiner

Introduction

The influence of androgens on the female organism is currently gaining increasing attention; thus, a large number of recent studies suggest an important role of testosterone in somatic conditions such as recurrent miscarriages,[1,2] hirsutism,[3] acne,[4] the polycystic ovary syndrome (PCO),[5,6] and the combination of abdominal obesity and insulin resistance (also known as the metabolic syndrome).[7] In comparison, studies on the effect of androgens in behaviour and mood in women are sparse; however, data have recently been presented suggesting that androgen deficiency in oophorectomized or naturally menopausal women may be associated with a reduction in libido, cognitive function, and vigilance; on the other hand, androgen excess in women has been suggested to be associated with depression, irritability and compulsive behaviour (including binge eating). In this chapter, the current literature regarding the putative impact of androgens on brain and behaviour in females will be reviewed and discussed.

Androgen production in females

The production of androgens in women takes place both in the ovary and in the adrenal gland.[8] Whereas androstendione is the major ovarian androgen, dehydroepiandrosterone (DHEA) is the most important of the androgens formed in the adrenal gland; however, androstendione is also, to a considerable extent, of adrenal origin. The production of testosterone in the ovary and the adrenal gland is relatively low; thus, 75% of the circulating testosterone in women is formed by conversion from androstendione or DHEA (via androstendione) in organs such as the liver and the skin.

Normal serum testosterone concentrations in women are 10–30 times lower than in men. Approximately 75–80% of the circulating testosterone is bound to sex hormone-binding globulin (SHBG); another 20–25% is loosely bound to albumin. The free, unbound, biologically active testosterone thus represents only about 1% of the total amount of testosterone.[8]

The ovarian production of androstendione is influenced by luteinizing hormone and hence fluctuates during the menstrual cycle, with higher levels in the luteal than in the follicular phase. In contrast, the adrenal production of DHEA appears to be independent of the pituitary and does not vary markedly during the cycle. The testosterone levels in serum are much more stable than are the levels of oestradiol or progesterone; however, usually, a peak in serum testosterone is observed around ovulation.[9–12]

How androgens influence the brain

The androgen receptor is a cytoplasmatic receptor that acts by regulating gene transcription within the cell nucleus.[13] The biological effects of testosterone are to a great extent preceded by conversion to the very effective androgen receptor agonist dihydrotestosterone (DHT) within the effector cell (enzyme: alpha-reductase); however, testosterone also displays affinity for the androgen receptor per se. Notably, DHT may be formed not only from testosterone but also from other androgens, such as androstendione.

Androgen receptors are widely distributed in the brain of both males and females, with high concentrations in the hypothalamus and the amygdala.[14] In most brain areas, the expression of androgen receptors is similar in the two sexes; however, in certain areas, such as the medial preoptic area and the principal portion of the bed nucleus of the stria terminalis, the expression is considerably lower in females than in males.[15]

The effect of androgens on the androgen receptor can be effectively counteracted by androgen receptor antagonists (such as cypro-

terone acetate or flutamide);[16] such compounds are today frequently used not only for the treatment of prostate carcinoma in men, but also for reducing hirsutism in women.[17]

Importantly, testosterone is also converted to oestradiol by aromatization; thus, many effects of androgens may in fact be mediated by the oestrogen receptors rather than by the androgen receptor. In both females and males, oestrogen receptors of two subtypes are expressed throughout the brain, with high concentrations in the hypothalamus.[14,18]

Animal experiments suggest that both the androgen and the oestrogen receptors may be involved in mediating the effects of testosterone on androgen-dependent masculine behaviours, such as male sexual activity and aggression.[19–22] In females, as in males, androgens have been shown to stimulate aggression and sexual behaviour (see below); as in males, both androgen and oestrogen receptors are believed to be important in mediating these effects.[23–28]

Apart from influencing protein synthesis by interacting with androgen and oestrogen receptors, like other steroid hormones,[29,30] various androgen derivatives probably also influence membrane-bound receptors, hence exerting a rapid effect on neuronal firing.[31,32]

Role of androgens in sexual differentiation

Many studies suggest that the intrinsic developmental programme for the brain as well as for the rest of the body is female rather than male. To force it into a male direction, high levels of androgens (or oestrogens) at critical phases during early development are required.[33–38] In line with this assumption, sex differences in brain morphology (see Chapter 4)—such as differences in the sexually dimorphic nucleus

(SDN) in the hypothalamus,[35] the medial nucleus of the amygdala, and the bed nucleus of the stria terminalis[39]—seem to be dependent on the presence of androgens during gestation or in the neonatal period. Likewise, exposure of female rats to androgens prenatally or shortly after parturition leads to a more masculine behaviour of the adult animal with respect to sexual behaviour and aggression; conversely, neonatal administration of an androgen antagonist to a male rat leads to a femininization at adult age. Such permanent effects of androgens on brain morphology and behaviour are called 'organizational effects'.[33–38,40] Early androgen exposure may exert a permanent influence on behaviour not only in experimental animals but also in humans, as illustrated by studies showing that increased prenatal androgen exposure may masculinize social play in girls[41–43] and influence psychosexual function in the adult woman.[44]

The importance of organizational effects of androgens on sex differences in brain neurochemistry and behaviour is thus well established, as is the fact that neonatal exposure of females to supraphysiological doses of sex steroids may lead to permanent changes. However, it is still unknown to what extent subtle interindividual differences in androgen exposure during fetal life (within the normal female range) may influence brain and behaviour at adulthood. Interestingly, animal experiments do suggest that minor, physiological differences in androgen exposure may have functional consequences; for example, female pups with male siblings (hence exposed to somewhat higher levels of testosterone neonatally) display more aggressive behaviour as adults than do females with female siblings.[45,46]

Apart from the organizational effects, sexual steroids also may exert short-lasting effects on brain neurotransmission that are dependent on the presence of the hormone; these effects are termed 'activational effects'.[38] The effects on sexual and aggressive behaviour induced by modulation of serum testosterone concentrations in adult animals are due to such activational effects, which may or may not require that the animal has previously been exposed to the organizational effects of the hormone. In the subsequent sections of this chapter, we will discuss the possibility that activational and/or organizational effects of androgens on the female human brain may influence cognitive function, sexual behaviour, irritability and aggression, compulsive behaviour, and mood.

Androgens and cognitive function

An increasing body of evidence supports the notion that men and women differ with respect to various aspects of cognitive function. Thus, whereas women—as a group—usually perform better on tests reflecting verbal skill, perceptual speed and manual dexterity, men often obtain higher scores on tests reflecting visuospatial and mathematical ability.[47,48] Moreover, the brain lateralization with respect to spatial and verbal processing is reported to be more pronounced in men than in women.

Women with congenital adrenal hyperplasia have been shown to display a male-like cognitive profile, suggesting that prenatal steroid exposure may influence cognitive function later in life.[49] In line with these data, Roof and Havens[50] reported enhanced performance with respect to a spatial navigation task—as well as a masculinized hippocampal morphology—in female rats that were administered testosterone neonatally. The influence of androgens on cognitive function seems, however, not to be restricted to the prenatal phase; supporting the idea that androgens may influence cognitive function also as an activational effect, van Goozen et al[47,51] reported that testosterone administration to female-to-male transsexuals leads to a reduction in the outcome of verbal fluency tests, but to an improvement with respect to visuospatial abilities.

To what extent fluctuations and interindividual variations in serum testosterone levels within the normal female range influence cognitive function is less thoroughly investigated; however, Gouchie and Kimura[52] have reported a correlation between salivary testosterone levels and spatial/mathematical ability in women. Also supporting the assumption that androgens at concentrations normally occurring in females may affect cognition, replacement of androgen (as well as oestrogens) in oophorectomized women has been shown to improve cognitive function.[53,54] The effect of testosterone antagonism on the performance in various cognitive tests in women has, to our knowledge, not been investigated.

Androgens and female sexual behaviour

Whereas the importance of the female sex steroids oestradiol and progesterone for sexual behaviour in female rodents is well established, the possible influence of androgens on female sexual behaviour has been less thoroughly investigated. However, several reports do support the assumption that androgens may facilitate sexual drive not only in male but also in female rats.[23–28]

Although the literature is not unanimous, many clinical studies suggest that androgens may also influence libido in women.[55–58] Several studies thus indicate that libido in premenopausal women correlates with fluctuations in serum levels of testosterone, and that women with high levels of serum testosterone generally display higher libido and sexual arousability than those with low levels.[59–62] Furthermore, in ovariectomized or naturally menopausal women, a combined replacement with oestradiol plus testosterone has been shown to improve sexual function more effectively than replacement with female sex steroids only;[63–65] tentatively, androgens may also be effective for the treatment of subnormal libido in premenopausal women.[66] In female-to-male transsexuals, administration of relatively high doses of testosterone has been shown to induce a clearcut increase in sexual arousability.[48]

If androgens stimulate sexual interest in females, the possibility that the administration of a testosterone antagonist may lead to a reduction in libido should be taken into consideration. Treatment of hirsutism with cyproterone acetate—which is both an antiandrogen and a progestogen—has indeed been reported to reduce libido;[67] in contrast, a reduction in female libido has, to our knowledge, not been reported as a major side-effect of the selective androgen antagonist flutamide. However, reduced libido is seldom spontaneously reported; thus, unless the possible presence of sexual dysfunction has been actively inquired for, data should be interpreted with caution.

Androgens and irritability/aggression

Animal studies indicate that androgens increase aggressive behaviour in both males and females.[37,68–71] The role of androgens in human aggression has been less thoroughly investigated; however, studies on sex differences with respect to human aggressive behaviour,[47] on the relationship between testosterone levels and aggression,[72–78] and on the psychotropic effects of anabolic steroid abuse,[79] all support a facilitory effect of androgens on aggression and irritability in men.[80,81]

In transsexual women, administration of high doses of testosterone (equal to male levels) leads to an increase in irritability;[47] moreover, an increase in irritability and aggression has been observed in women exposed to high androgen levels neonatally, owing to congenital adrenal hyperplasia.[82] Thus supranormal levels of androgens seem to be related to enhanced irritability in women, but the possible significance of fluctuations (and interindividual differences) within the normal female range on this aspect of human behaviour has been less thoroughly investigated. Sherwin and Gelfand[63] have, however, reported enhanced hostility in oophorectomized women when exposed to relatively low testosterone replacement doses. Moreover, a correlation between testosterone levels and aggression in women has been reported by several authors;[12,83–85] however, studies in this field are still sparse and the results are far from unanimous. Noteworthy in this context is the fact that the perimenopause is often characterized by both an increase in irritability and androgen secretion (see Chapter 22).

Many women experience heightened irritability during the luteal phase of the menstrual cycle; indeed, many researchers regard irritability (rather than depressed mood) as the cardinal symptom of premenstrual dysphoric disorder (see Chapter 16). Supporting the assumption that high levels of androgens may promote irritability in women, two studies have revealed slightly (but significantly) elevated levels of serum testosterone in women with severe premenstrual irritability when compared to controls.[86,87] Also supporting an influence of testosterone on premenstrual irritability, administration of the testosterone (and aldosterone) antagonist spironolactone

has been reported to reduce premenstrual dysphoria in women with high luteal levels of testosterone;[88,89] moreover, preliminary results suggest that the androgen antagonists cyproterone acetate[90] and flutamide (Landén et al, unpublished) may also reduce premenstrual dysphoria. Other groups have, however, not observed abnormal levels of serum testosterone in women with premenstrual complaints;[12,91–93] tentatively, this discrepancy in results may be due to differences in symptom profile of the populations studied. Supporting the possibility that serum levels of testosterone may be elevated in women with premenstrual irritability, but not in women with other premenstrual complaints, Steiner et al[94] have reported a strong correlation between irritability and testosterone levels within a group of patients all fulfilling the diagnostic criteria of premenstrual dysphoric disorder.

Androgens and mood

In oophorectomized women, androgen plus oestrogen replacement has been reported to improve wellbeing and depressed mood more effectively than replacement with oestrogen only.[57] Although subnormal levels of androgens may lead to a reduction in wellbeing, preliminary data suggest that relatively high levels of androgens may also be associated with depressed mood. Supporting this assumption, Baischer et al have reported elevated levels of free testosterone in premenopausal depressed women when compared to age-matched controls.[95] Also, in a group of hirsute women, Shulman et al[96] observed a marked correlation between depressed mood and serum levels of androgens; in contrast, mood did not correlate with the degree of hirsutism. Women with a combination of abdominal obesity, insulin resistance and high serum levels of lipids (the so-called metabolic syndrome) often display high levels of serum testosterone[7] and are more prone to depression, irritability and anxiety than controls.[97,98] Moreover, since depressed mood is a prominent finding in premenstrual dysphoria, bulimia nervosa, and the perimenopause, the observation that all these conditions may be associated with elevated levels of testosterone (see above and below) supports the assumption that elevated androgens may be associated with depressed mood.

Although several reports suggest that enhanced androgenicity may be associated with depressed mood, the possible causal relationship between elevated serum levels of testosterone and depression remains to be elucidated. Obviously, elevated levels of androgens do not uniformly lead to depressed mood; thus, many women with polycystic ovaries display very high levels of testosterone, but do not suffer from depression; also, as discussed above, administration of testosterone to ovariectomized or menopausal women generally does not lead to an increase in depressive symptoms, but rather to enhanced wellbeing.

Androgens in obsessive-compulsive behaviour and bulimia nervosa

To our knowledge, no studies have been published on androgen levels in patients with obsessive-compulsive disorder (OCD). However, in one open trial, a marked symptom reduction was observed following the administration of an antiandrogen (cyproterone acetate) to women with OCD,[99] supporting the possibility that obsessive-compulsive behaviour may be related to an enhanced androgenic influence on the brain. Moreover, the antiandrogen flutamide has shown some symptom-

reducing effects in another disorder characterized by compulsive behaviour, Gilles de la Tourette's syndrome.[100]

Bulimia nervosa is characterized by compulsive behaviour in the form of binge eating and purging. In a preliminary study, levels of free testosterone were found to be higher in women with normal-weight bulimia nervosa than in age-matched controls;[101] in addition, several studies have suggested a relationship between binge eating and polycystic ovaries.[101–104] A reduction in bulimic symptoms in two women treated with the testosterone antagonist flutamide was recently reported;[105] an interim analysis of an ongoing controlled trial suggests that flutamide may indeed be superior to placebo for the treatment of this disorder.[106]

Possible interactions between androgens and serotonin

As discussed above, a large number of reports have shown that exposure of female rodents to androgens in the neonatal period, or later in life, may lead to masculinization with respect to aggressive and sexual behaviour; reciprocally, castration of neonatal or adult male rodents has opposite effects. The behavioural effects of compounds inhibiting the synthesis of the brain neurotransmitter serotonin in rodents, or destroying serotonergic neurons, are to some extent similar to those induced by administration of androgens; thus, in both male and female rats, serotonin depletion causes an increase in both aggressive and sexual behaviour.[71,107–110]

Androgens and serotonin also appear to exert opposite effects on behaviour in humans. Thus, whereas androgens promote sexual drive in both men and women, a reduction in libido and anorgasmia is the most common side-effect of the serotonin reuptake inhibitors.[111,112] Androgens may tentatively promote compulsive behaviour, binge eating, depressed mood, and premenstrual irritability in women; all these symptoms are also known to respond to treatment with serotonin reuptake inhibitors.[113,114]

Given the fact that serotonin appears to influence testosterone-regulated behaviour, the hypothesis that some of the behavioural effects of androgens are partly mediated by a reduction in serotonin activity seems plausible. Indeed, several studies have revealed a difference between male and female rats with respect to brain serotonergic neurotransmission; moreover, both neonatal and adult androgenization of female rats have been shown to influence serotonergic activity.[115–118]

Relating androgen levels to behaviour: methodological considerations

As discussed above, the available information regarding the possible psychotropic effect of androgens in women is to a great extent based on studies in which serum levels of testosterone have been shown to correlate with various aspects of behaviour. However, when interpreting studies that are based on the measurement of serum testosterone levels—and in particular when the data are negative—one should consider that the androgenic influence on the brain may be regulated by a variety of factors apart from the actual production of testosterone and testosterone precursors in the ovary and the adrenal gland.

The extent to which testosterone is bound (to SHBG and albumin) may be of critical importance in this context; thus, many researchers have argued that the measurement of the free fraction of testosterone is more informative than the assessment of total testosterone.[8] Notably, in most reports relating androgen levels to behaviour in women, total testosterone rather than the free fraction has been measured.

Although steroid hormones are generally assumed to penetrate the blood–brain barrier easily, and although a correlation between testosterone concentrations in serum and in the cerebrospinal fluid (CSF) has been reported,[119] the possibility cannot be excluded that serum testosterone levels do not always accurately reflect testosterone levels in the brain. Indeed, some researchers have therefore elected to measure testosterone levels in the CSF rather than in serum.[78]

The genes for the alpha-reductase (type I) and the aromatase responsible for conversion of testosterone into active metabolites (DHT and oestradiol, respectively)[120] may display polymorphisms of functional significance; thus, tentatively, the effectiveness of the conversion of testosterone to DHT and oestradiol—and hence the physiological effect of the hormone—may vary considerably between individuals with similar serum testosterone levels.

Also, the androgen and oestrogen receptors may display considerable interindividual variations in density, structure, and responsiveness. The androgenic influence on the brain may be partly dependent on the number and state of these receptors.

Finally, the behavioural effects of testosterone may be counteracted or augmented by the action of oestradiol and progesterone.[25] Thus, simultaneous measurement of testosterone and the female sex steroids—as well as of certain physiologically active androgen derivatives—may yield more information regarding the androgenic influence on the brain than do measurements of testosterone only.

In order to further clarify the influence of testosterone on the brain in females, studies investigating the behavioural effects of androgen antagonism are clearly warranted. Androgen antagonists must, however, be administered to women with caution since they may influence the development of a fetus, and they may also exert a negative influence on hepatic function.[17]

Summary

To date, little is known regarding the possible influence of androgens on behaviour and mood in women. Recent data, however, suggest that androgen replacement in women with subnormal levels of the hormone may improve sexual function, cognition and wellbeing; on the other hand, preliminary reports suggest that high levels of androgens may be associated with symptoms such as irritability, depressed mood, compulsive behaviour and binge eating.

References

1. Okon MA, Laird SM, Tuckerman EM, Li TC, Serum androgen levels in women who have recurrent miscarriages and their correlation with markers of endometrial function, *Fertil Steril* 1998; **69**:682–90.
2. Tulppala M, Stenman UH, Cacciatore B, Ylikorkala O, Polycystic ovaries and levels of gonadotrophins and androgens in recurrent miscarriage: prospective study in 50 women, *Br J Obstet Gynaecol* 1993; **100**:348–52.
3. Redmond GP, Clinical evaluation of the woman with an androgenic disorder. In: Redmond GR, ed., *Androgenic Disorders* (Raven Press: New York, 1995) 1–20.
4. Rothman KF, Acne vulgaris. In: Redmond GR, ed., *Androgenic Disorders* (Raven Press: New York, 1995) 231–50.
5. Pugeat M, Nicolas MH, Craves JC et al, Androgens in polycystic ovarian syndrome, *Ann NY Acad Sci* 1993; **687**:124–35.
6. Futterweit W, Pathophysiology of the polycystic ovarian syndrome. In: Redmond GR, ed., *Androgenic Disorders* (Raven Press: New York, 1995) 77–166.
7. Björntorp P, The android woman—a risky condition, *J Intern Med* 1996; **239**:105–10.
8. Demers LM, Biochemistry and laboratory measurement of androgens in women. In:

Redmond GR, ed., *Androgenic Disorders* (Raven Press: New York, 1995) 21–34.
9. Epstein MT, McNeilly AS, Murray MA, Hockaday TD, Plasma testosterone and prolactin in the menstrual cycle, *Clin Endocrinol* 1975; **4**:531–5.
10. Vermeulen A, Verdonck L, Plasma androgen levels during the menstrual cycle, *Am J Obstet Gynecol* 1976; **125**:491–4.
11. Guerrero R, Aso T, Brenner P-F et al, Studies on the pattern of circulating steroids in the normal menstrual cycle. I. Simultaneous assays of progesterone, pregnenolone, dehydroepiandrosterone, testosterone, dihydrotestosterone, androstenedione, oestradiol and oestrone, *Acta Endocrinol* 1976; **81**:133–49.
12. Dougherty DM, Bjork JM, Moeller FG, Swann AC, The influence of menstrual-cycle phase on the relationship between testosterone and aggression, *Physiol Behav* 1997; **62**:431–5.
13. Sawaya ME, Androgen action at the cellular level. In: Redmond GR, ed., *Androgenic Disorders* (Raven Press: New York, 1995) 35–48.
14. Simerley RB, Chang C, Muramatsu M, Swanson LW, Distribution of androgen and estrogen receptor mRNA-containing cells in

the rat brain: an in situ hybridization study, *J Comp Neurol* 1990; **294:**76–95.

15. McAbee MD, DonCarlos LL, Ontogeny of region-specific sex differences in androgen receptor messenger ribonucleic acid expression in the rat forebrain, *Endocrinology* 1998; **139:**1738–45.

16. Sufrin G, Coffey DS, Flutamide. Mechanism of action of a new nonsteroidal antiandrogen, *Invest Urol* 1976; **13:**429–34.

17. Conn JJ, Jacobs HS, The clinical management of hirsutism, *Eur J Endocrinol* 1997, **136:**339–48.

18. Osterlund M, Kuiper GG, Gustafsson JA, Hurd YL, Differential distribution and regulation of estrogen receptor-alpha and -beta mRNA within the female rat brain, *Brain Res Mol Brain Res* 1998; **54:**175–80.

19. Brain PF, Simon V, Hasan S et al, The potential of antiestrogens as centrally-acting anti-hostility agents: recent animal data, *Int J Neurosci* 1988; **41:**169–77.

20. Zumpe D, Bonsall RW, Michael RP, Effects of the nonsteroidal aromatase inhibitor, fadrozole, on the sexual behavior of male cynomolgus monkeys (Macaca fascicularis), *Horm Behav* 1993; **27:**200–15.

21. Clancy AN, Zumpe D, Michael RP, Intracerebral infusion of an aromatase inhibitor, sexual behavior and brain estrogen receptor-like immunoreactivity in intact male rats, *Neuroendocrinology* 1995; **61:**98–111.

22. Vagell ME, McGinnis MY, The role of aromatization in the restoration of male rat reproductive behavior, *J Neuroendocrinol* 1997; **9:**415–21.

23. van de Poll NE, van Zanten S, de Jonge FH, Effects of testosterone, estrogen, and dihydrotestosterone upon aggressive and sexual behavior of female rats, *Horm Behav* 1986; **20:**418–31.

24. van de Poll NE, Taminiau MS, Endert E, Louwerse AL, Gonadal steroid influence upon sexual and aggressive behavior of female rats, *Int J Neurosci* 1988; **41:**271–86.

25. Fernandez-Guasti A, Vega-Matuszczyk J, Larsson K, Synergistic action of estradiol, progesterone and testosterone on rat proceptive behavior, *Physiol Behav* 1991; **50:**1007–11.

26. Vega-Matuszczyk J, Larsson K, Role of androgen, estrogen and sexual experience on the female rat's partner preference, *Physiol Behav* 1991; **50:**139–42.

27. Sodersten P, Eneroth P, Hansson T et al, Activation of sexual behaviour in castrated rats: the role of oestradiol, *J Endocrinol* 1986; **111:**455–62.

28. de Jonge FH, Kalverdijk EH, van de Poll NE, Androgens are specifically implicated in female rat sexual motivation. The influence of methyltrienelone (R1881) on sexual orientation, *Pharmacol Biochem Behav* 1986; **24:**285–9.

29. McEwen BS, Steroid hormone actions on the brain: when is the genome involved? *Horm Behav* 1994; **28:**396–405.

30. Joels M, Steroid hormones and excitability in the mammalian brain, *Front Neuroendocrinol* 1997; **18:**2–48.

31. Wilson MA, Biscardi R, Influence of gender and brain region on neurosteroid modulation of GABA responses in rats, *Life Sci* 1997; **60:**1679–91.

32. Imamura M, Prasad C, Modulation of GABA-gated chloride ion influx in the brain by dehydroepiandrosterone and its metabolites, *Biochem Biophys Res Commun* 1998; **243:**771–5.

33. Saal FS, Gandelman R, Svare B, Aggression in male and female mice: evidence for changed neural sensitivity in response to neonatal but not adult androgen exposure, *Physiol Behav* 1976; **17:**53–7.

34. Gandelman R, Gonadal hormones and the induction of intraspecific fighting in mice, *Neurosci Biobehav Rev* 1980; **4:**133–40.

35. Gorski RA, Sexual differentiation of the brain: possible mechanisms and implications, *Can J Physiol Pharmacol* 1985; **63:**577–94.

36. Hoepfner BA, Ward IL, Prenatal and neonatal androgen exposure interact to affect sexual differentiation in female rats, *Behav Neuroscience* 1988; **102:**61–5.

37. Compaan JC, van Wattum G, de Ruiter AJ et al, Genetic differences in female house mice in aggressive response to sex steroid hormone treatment, *Physiol Behav* 1993; **54:**899–902.

38. Pilgrim C, Hutchison JB, Developmental regulation of sex differences in the brain: can the

role of gonadal steroids be redefined? *Neuroscience* 1994; **60**:843–55.

39. Hines M, Allen LS, Gorski RA, Sex differences in subregions of the medial nucleus of the amygdala and the bed nucleus of the stria terminalis of the rat, *Brain Res* 1992; **579**:321–6.

40. Phoenix CH, Goy RW, Gerall AA, Young WC, Organizing action of prenatally administered testosterone proprionate on the tissues mediating mating behaviour in the female guinea pig, *Endocrinology* 1959: **65**:369–82.

41. Meaney MJ, The sexual differentiation of social play, *Psychiatr Dev* 1989; **7**:247–61.

42. Sato T, Koizumi S, Effects of fetal androgen on childhood behavior, *Acta Paediatr Jpn* 1991; **33**:639–44.

43. Hines M, Kaufman FR, Androgen and the development of human sex-typical behavior: rough-and-tumble play and sex of preferred playmates in children with congenital adrenal hyperplasia (CAH), *Child Dev* 1994; **65**:1042–53.

44. Zucker KJ, Bradley SJ, Oliver G et al, Psychosexual development of women with congenital adrenal hyperplasia, *Horm Behav* 1996; **30**:300–18.

45. Kinsley CH, Konen CM, Miele JL et al, Intrauterine position modulates maternal behaviors in female mice, *Physiol Behav* 1986; **36**:793–9.

46. Palanza P, Parmigiani S, vom Saal FS, Urine marking and maternal aggression of wild female mice in relation to anogenital distance at birth, *Physiol Behav* 1995; **58**:827–35.

47. van Goozen SH, Cohen-Kettenis PT, Gooren LJ et al, Gender differences in behaviour: activating effects of cross-sex hormones, *Psychoneuroendocrinology* 1995; **20**:343–63.

48. Collaer ML, Hines M, Human behavioural sex differences: a role for gonadal hormones during early development, *Psychol Bull* 1995; **118**:55–107.

49. Helleday J, Bartfai A, Ritzen EM, Forsman M, General intelligence and cognitive profile in women with congenital adrenal hyperplasia (CAH), *Psychoneuroendocrinology* 1994; **19**:343–56.

50. Roof RL, Havens MD, Testosterone improves maze performance and induces development

of a male hippocampus in females, *Brain Res* 1992; **572**:310–3.

51. van Goozen SH, Cohen-Kettenis PT, Gooren LJ et al, Activating effects of androgens on cognitive performance: causal evidence in a group of female-to-male transsexuals, *Neuropsychologia* 1994; **32**:1153–7.

52. Gouchie C, Kimura D, The relationship between testosterone levels and cognitive ability patterns, *Psychoneuroendocrinology* 1991; **16**:323–34.

53. Sherwin BB, Estrogen and/or androgen replacement therapy and cognitive functioning in surgically menopausal women, *Psychoneuroendocrinology* 1988; **13**:345–57.

54. Morrison MF, Androgens in the elderly: will androgen replacement therapy improve mood, cognition, and quality of life in aging men and women, *Psychopharmacol Bull* 1997; **33**:293–6.

55. Bancroft J, Sanders D, Davidson D, Warner P, Mood, sexuality, hormones, and the menstrual cycle. III. Sexuality and the role of androgens, *Psychosom Med* 1993; **45**:509–16.

56. Hutchinson KA, Androgens and sexuality, *Am J Med* 1995; **98**:111S-5S.

57. Sands R, Studd J, Exogenous androgens in postmenopausal women, *Am J Med* 1995; **98**:76S-9S.

58. Warnock JK, Bundren JC, Morris DW, Female hypoactive sexual desire disorder due to androgen deficiency: clinical and psychometric issues, *Psychopharmacol Bull* 1997; **33**:761–6.

59. Persky H, Dreisbach L, Miller WR et al, The relation of plasma androgen levels to sexual behaviors and attitudes of women, *Psychosom Med* 1982; **44**:305–19.

60. Morris NM, Udry JR, Khan-Dawood F, Dawood MY, Marital sex frequency and midcycle female testosterone, *Arch Sex Behav* 1987; **16**:27–37.

61. Alexander GM, Sherwin BB, Sex steroids, sexual behavior, and selection attention for erotic stimuli in women using oral contraceptives, *Psychoneuroendocrinology* 1993; **18**:91–102.

62. van Goozen SH, Wiegant VM, Endert E et al, Psychoendocrinological assessment of the menstrual cycle: the relationship between hormones, sexuality, and mood, *Arch Sex Behav* 1997; **26**:359–82.

63. Sherwin BB, Gelfand MM, Sex steroids and affect in the surgical menopause: a double-blind, cross-over study, *Psychoneuroendocrinology* 1985; **10**:325–35.

64. Sherwin BB, Gelfand MM, The role of androgen in the maintenance of sexual functioning in oophorectomized women, *Psychosom Med* 1987; **49**:397–409.

65. Davis SR, McCloud P, Strauss BJ, Burger H, Testosterone enhances estradiol's effects on postmenopausal bone density and sexuality, *Maturitas* 1995; **21**:227–36.

66. Bancroft J, Skakkebaek NE, Androgens and human sexual behaviour, *Ciba Found Symp* 1978; **62**:209–26.

67. Appelt H, Strauss B, Effects of antiandrogen treatment on the sexuality of women with hyperandrogenism, *Psychother Psychosom* 1984; **42**:177–81.

68. Whalen RE, Edwards DA, Hormonal determinants of the development of masculine and feminine behavior in male and female rats, *Anat Rec* 1967; **157**:173–80.

69. Simon NG, Whalen RE, Sexual differentiation of androgen-sensitive and estrogen-sensitive regulatory systems for aggressive behavior, *Horm Behav* 1987; **21**:493–500.

70. Albert, DJ, Jonik RH, Walsh ML, Hormone-dependent aggression in male and female rats: experimental, hormonal, and neural foundations, *Neurosci Biobehav Rev* 1992; **16**:177–92.

71. Brain PF, Haug M, Hormonal and neuro-chemical correlates of various forms of animal 'aggression', *Psychoneuroendocrinology* 1992; **17**:537–51.

72. Herrmann WM, Beach RC, Psychotropic effects of androgens: a review of clinical observations and new human experimental findings, *Pharmakopsychiatr Neuropsychopharmakol* 1976; **9**: 205–19.

73. Rose RM, Neuroendocrine correlates of sexual and aggressive behaviour in humans. In: Lipton MA, DiMascio A, Killam KF, eds, *Psychopharmacology: A Generation of Progress* (Raven Press: New York, 1978) 541–52.

74. Dent RR, Endocrine correlates of aggression, *Prog Neuropsychopharmacol Biol Psychiatry* 1983; **7**:525–8.

75. Christiansen K, Knussman R, Androgen levels and components of aggressive behaviour in men, *Horm Behav* 1987; **21**:170–80.

76. Dabbs JM, Frady RL, Carr TS, Besch NF, Saliva testosterone and criminal violence in young adult prison inmates, *Psychosom Med* 1987; **49**:174–82.

77. Olweus D, Mattsson Å, Schalling D, Löw H, Circulating testosterone levels and aggression in adolescent males: a causal analysis, *Psychosom Med* 1988; **50**:261–72.

78. Virkkunen M, Kallio E, Rawlings R et al, Personality profiles and state aggressiveness in Finnish alcoholic, violent offenders, fire setters, and healthy volunteers, *Arch Gen Psychiatry* 1994; **51**:28–33.

79. Lukas SE, CNS effects and abuse liability of anabolic-androgenic steroids, *Annu Rev Pharmacol Toxicol* 1996, **36**:333–57.

80. Archer J, The influence of testosterone on human aggression, *Br J Psychol* 1991; **82**: 1–28.

81. Rubinow DR, Schmidt PJ, Androgens, brain, and behavior, *Am J Psychiatry* 1996; **153**: 974–84.

82. Berenbaum SA, Resnick SM, Early androgen effects on aggression in children and adults with congenital adrenal hyperplasia, *Psychoneuroendocrinology* 1997; **22**:505–15.

83. Ehlers CL, Richter KC, Hovey JE, A possible relationship between plasma testosterone and aggressive behaviour in a female outpatient population. In: Grigis M, Kiloh IG, eds, *Limbic Epilepsy and Dyscontrol Syndrome* (Elsevier: Amsterdam, 1980) 183–94.

84. Harris JA, Rushton JP, Hampson E, Jackson DN, Salivary testosterone and self-report aggressive and pro-social personality characteristics in men and women, *Aggressive Behav* 1996; **22**:321–31.

85. Dabbs JM Jr, Hargrove MF, Age, testosterone, and behavior among female prison inmates, *Psychosom Med* 1997; **59**:477–80.

86. Eriksson E, Sundblad C, Lisjo P et al, Serum levels of androgens are higher in women with premenstrual irritability and dysphoria than in controls, *Psychoneuroendocrinology* 1992; **17**:195–204.

87. Eriksson E, Alling C, Andersch B et al, Cerebrospinal fluid levels of monoamine

metabolites, *Neuropsychopharmacology* 1994; **11**:201–13.

88. Rowe T, Sasse V, Androgens and premenstrual symptoms—the response to therapy. In: Deneerstein L, Frazer, I, eds, *Hormones and Behaviour* (Elsevier Science Publishers: New York, 1986) 160–5.

89. Burnet RB, Radden HS, Easterbrook EG, McKinnon RA, Premenstrual syndrome and spironolactone, *Aust NZ J Obstet Gynaecol* 1991; **31**:366–8.

90. Itil TM, Cora R, Akpinar S et al, 'Psychotropic' action of sex hormones: computerized EEG in establishing the immediate CNS effects of steroid hormones, *Curr Ther Res Clin Exp* 1974; **16**:1147–70.

91. Bäckström T, Aakvaag A, Plasma prolactin and testosterone during the luteal phase in women with premenstrual tension syndrome, *Psychoneuroendocrinology* 1981; **6**:245–51.

92. Rubinow DR, Hoban MC, Grover GN et al, Changes in plasma hormones across the menstrual cycle in patients with menstrually related mood disorder and in control subjects, *Am J Obstet Gynecol* 1988; **158**:5–11.

93. Bloch M, Schmidt PJ, Su TP et al, Pituitary–adrenal hormones and testosterone across the menstrual cycle in women with premenstrual syndrome and controls, *Biol Psychiatry* 1998; **43**:897–903.

94. Steiner M, Coote M, Wilkins A, Dunn E, Biological correlates of irritability in women with premenstrual dysphoria, *Eur Neuropsychopharmacol* 1997; 7 (suppl 2):S172.

95. Baischer W, Koinig G, Hartmann B et al, Hypothalamic–pituitary–gonadal axis in depressed premenopausal women: elevated blood testosterone concentrations compared to normal controls, *Psychoneuroendocrinology* 1995; **20**:553–9.

96. Shulman LH, DeRogatis L, Spielvogel R et al, Serum androgens and depression in women with facial hirsutism, *J Am Acad Dermatol* 1992; **27**:178–81.

97. Björntorp P, Body fat distribution, insulin resistance, and metabolic diseases, *Nutrition* 1997; **13**:795–803.

98. Wing RR, Matthews KA, Kuller LH et al, Waist to hip ratio in middle-aged women. Associations with behavioral and psychosocial factors and with changes in cardiovascular risk factors, *Arterioscler Thromb* 1991; **11**: 1250–7.

99. Casas M, Alvarez E, Duro P et al, Antiandrogenic treatment of obsessive-compulsive neurosis, *Acta Psychiatr Scand* 1986; **73**:221–2.

100. Peterson BS, Zhang H, Anderson GM, Leckman JF, A double-blind, placebo-controlled, crossover trial of an antiandrogen in the treatment of Tourette's syndrome, *J Clin Psychopharmacol* 1998; **18**:324–31.

101. Sundblad C, Bergman L, Eriksson E, High levels of free testosterone in women with bulimia nervosa, *Acta Psychiatr Scand* 1994; **90**:397–8.

102. Raphael FJ, Rodin DA, Peattie A et al, Ovarian morphology and insulin sensitivity in women with bulimia nervosa, *Clin Endocrinol* 1995; **43**:451–5.

103. Jahanfar S, Eden JA, Nguyent TV, Bulimia nervosa and polycystic ovary syndrome, *Gynecol Endocrinol* 1995; **9**:113–17.

104. McCluskey S, Evans C, Lacey JH et al, Polycystic ovary syndrome and bulimia, *Fertil Steril* 1991; **55**:287–91.

105. Bergman L, Eriksson E, Marked symptom reduction in two women with bulimia nervosa treated with the testosterone receptor antagonist flutamide, *Acta Psychiatr Scand* 1996; **94**:137–9.

106. Landén M, Sundblad C, Bergman L et al, The role of androgens and serotonin for the pathophysiology and treatment of bulimia nervosa, *Nordic J Psychiatry* 1999; **53**:96.

107. Meyerson BJ, Carrer H, Eliasson M, 5-Hydroxytryptamine and sexual behavior in the female rat, *Adv Biochem Psychopharmacol* 1974; **11**:229–42.

108. Larsson K, Fuxe K, Everitt BJ et al, Sexual behavior in male rats after intracerebral injection of 5,7-dihydroxytryptamine, *Brain Res* 1978; **141**:293–303.

109 Pucilowski O, Kostowski W, Aggressive behaviour and the central serotonergic systems, *Behav Brain Res* 1983; **9**:33–48.

110. Vergnes M, Depaulis A, Boehrer A, Kempf E, Selective increase of offensive behavior in the rat following intrahypothalamic 5,7-DHT-induced serotonin depletion, *Behav Brain Res* 1988; **29**:85–91.

111. Monteiro WO, Noshirvani HF, Marks IM, Lelliott PT, Anorgasmia from clomipramine in obsessive-compulsive disorder. A controlled trial, *Br J Psychiatry* 1987; **151**:107–12.

112. Segraves RT, Antidepressant-induced sexual dysfunction, *J Clin Psychiatry* 1998; **59** (suppl 4):48–54.

113. Eriksson E, Humble M, Serotonin in psychiatric pathophysiology. A review of data from experimental and clinical research, *Prog Basic Clin Pharmacol* 1990; **3**:66–119.

114. Eriksson E, Hedberg MA, Andersch B, Sundblad C, The serotonin reuptake inhibitor paroxetin is superior to the noradrenaline reuptake inhibitor maprotiline in the treatment of premenstrual syndrome, *Neuropsychopharmacology* 1995, **12**:167–76.

115. Martinez-Conde E, Leret ML, Diaz S, The influence of testosterone in the brain of the male rat on levels of serotonin (5-HT) and hydroxyindole-acetic acid (5-HIAA), *Comp Biochem Physiol C* 1985; **80**:411–14.

116. Bitar MS, Ota M, Linnoila M, Shapiro BH, Modification of gonadectomy-induced increases in brain monoamine metabolism by steroid hormones in male and female rats, *Psychoneuroendocrinology* 1991; **16**:547–57.

117. Gonzáles MI, Leret ML, Extrahypothalamic serotonergic modification after masculinization induced by neonatal gonadal hormones, *Pharmacol Biochem Behav* 1992; **41**:329–32.

118. Sundblad C, Eriksson E, Reduced extracellular levels of serotonin in the amygdala of androgenized female rats, *Eur Neuropsychopharmacol* 1997; **7**:253–9.

119. Bäckström T, Carstensen H, Sodergard R, Concentration of estradiol, testosterone and progesterone in cerebrospinal fluid compared to plasma unbound and total concentrations, *J Steroid Biochem* 1976; **7**:469–72.

120. Celotti F, Negri-Cesi P, Poletti A, Steroid metabolism in the mammalian brain: 5alpha-reduction and aromatization, *Brain Res Bull* 1997; **44**:365–75.

15

Menarche and mood disorders in adolescence

Meir Steiner, Leslie Born and Peter Marton

Introduction

Gender differences in the prevalence of mood disorders have been well documented. Epidemiological studies consistently show that, beginning at menarche, mood disorders are at least twice as common in women as in men (see also Chapters 1 and 2). Why these gender differences exist and why they start at puberty is perhaps one of the most intriguing and least understood phenomena in clinical psychiatry.[1] Gender is relevant in this context because of the known relationship between female reproductive milestones and psychiatric illness. The associations of mood disorders with the menstrual cycle (e.g. premenstrual dysphoria), with pregnancy and the postpartum period and with the perimenopause continue to be the focus of ongoing research in North America and around the world. Menarche seems to be the forgotten milestone.

Prior to adolescence, the rates of depression are similar in girls and boys (or are slightly higher in boys); yet, with the onset of puberty, the gender proportion of depression dramati-cally shifts to a 2:1 female/male ratio[1–4] (Figure 15.1). This chapter will address the relationship between menarche and mood disorders in adolescence. The role of puberty and other precipitating factors, as well as gender differences in the presentation of depressive disorders, will be examined. Clinical information regarding the management of depression in adolescent and young adult women will be provided, including instruments to assist with diagnosis, treatment options, and long-term follow-up. Practical treatment-related differences between males and females will be highlighted.

Epidemiology

Lifetime prevalence

In the US general population, the lifetime prevalence of major depression in adolescents and young adults (15–24 years of age) has been reported as 20.6% for females and 10.5% for males.[4] Lifetime rates of major depression in early- as well as late-maturing girls were even

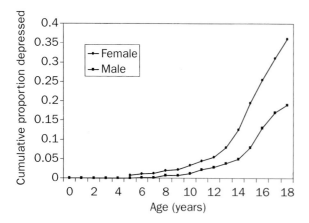

Figure 15.1 Probability of experiencing an episode of major depressive disorder as a function of age and gender.[1]

higher (30% versus 22% and 34% versus 22% respectively) when compared with 'on-time' girls. Almost three-quarters of those with major depression reported recurrent episodes.[1] The lifetime prevalence of dysthymia is also significantly greater in females than in males (estimates being 4.0–5.3% versus 1.5–2.3% respectively), with an average age of onset between 10 and 11 years of age.[5–8] The lifetime prevalence for minor depression, on the other hand, revealed a close gender prevalence ratio, with 10.4% and 9.5% for females and males respectively.[4] In community-based samples of adolescents in grades 9–12, the lifetime prevalence of bipolar disorders was about 1%, while 5.7% reported subthreshold symptoms (in particular, irritable mood) with equal sex ratios.[6,9] In one exception, Wittchen et al[8] found a significantly higher prevalence of bipolar II disorder—but not bipolar I disorder—in women 14–24 years of age compared with men. These rates are comparable with published lifetime rates of bipolar disorder in adults.[10]

Comorbidity

In the US National Comorbidity Survey (NCS), 76.7% of those with major depression and all individuals diagnosed with bipolar I disorder reported comorbid lifetime disorders.[4,11] It has been suggested that anxiety symptoms tend to predate depressive symptoms in adolescents.[12] In the NCS, more than 58% of female respondents with major depression and 36% of those with minor depression reported an anxiety disorder prior to the onset of depression.[4] Some researchers have posited that a higher rate of anxiety disorders in females compared with males prior to puberty may contribute to the higher risk in females for the onset of major depression after menarche.[13–15]

Age and gender differences

There is conflicting opinion regarding the age at which gender differences in rates of major depression emerge: researchers are divided between the 12–14-year and the 15–19-year age brackets.[13,16–21] Typically, the age of onset of bipolar I disorder is 18–19 years of age, with no significant gender difference.[10,16,22]

Cross-cultural differences

There are limited data on the prevalence of female adolescent depression in populations outside of the USA, or even among various racial or cultural groups within North America; moreover, explicit comparisons are hampered by methodological differences. Several studies, however, merit some attention.

Significantly higher levels of depressive symptoms were found in Hispanic/Latino and Asian groups compared with Caucasian and African-American groups in a nationally representative sample of 6943 US students (9–20 years of age).[23] Moreover, in another large US sampling of adolescents by this same study group, the authors noted that, among Caucasians, postmenarcheal adolescent girls had higher depression scores than did same-aged premenarcheal girls, whereas, among African-American and Hispanic groups, there were no menarche-associated differences in depressive symptoms[24] (see later). In a comparative study of Hawaiian (at least 1 parent with Hawaiian ancestry) and non-Hawaiian adolescents (mean age 16.8 years) residing in Hawaii, similar rates of major depression and dysthymic disorder in the female subjects of both groups were noted.[25]

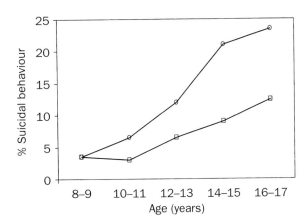

Figure 15.2 Suicide behaviour by age and gender (○) = females; (□) – males.[29]

Suicidal behaviour

Suicide ideation and attempt in female adolescents is highly associated with psychiatric morbidity. History of suicide attempt has been linked with the onset of major depression in older adolescents.[26] Conversely, being female, and having a diagnosis of affective disorder, have been identified as risk factors for suicide attempt.[27,28] In the UK, investigators have found that the frequency of suicidal behaviour (suicide ideation, attempt, or threat) in female subjects climbed sharply after age 9 years, rising from 3.6% at age 8 years to 24.6% by age 17 years (Figure 15.2).[29]

In the USA, a national school-based survey (grades 9–12) revealed that female students were significantly more likely to report suicide ideation, plan-making, or attempt. Also, a slightly higher percentage of female students reported having made a suicide attempt that required medical attention.[30] Others have delineated deliberate self-harm from 'true' suicide attempt (self-harm plus serious intent): in a survey of Australian high school students, the young women were more likely to self-harm and more frequently employed self-poisoning and self-laceration.[31]

Adolescents with bipolar disorder or subsyndromal bipolar symptomatology have higher rates of suicide attempt compared with adolescents with a history of major depression.[9]

Symptom presentation

There is general agreement that the clinical features of depression are more similar than different in adolescents and adults, with the exception of a higher frequency of irritable mood in adolescent presentation. Research suggests that women more frequently present with somatic depression (i.e. fatigue, appetite and sleep disturbance, body aches); this has been linked with the onset of major depression in early adolescence, and with the presence of a concurrent anxiety disorder.[32] A high incidence of lifetime anxiety disorder comorbid with major depression in young adult women (74.5%) was documented in a primary care sample;[13] female gender and the presence of a concurrent anxiety disorder have been significantly associated with severity of the initial depressive episode.[33]

Negative body image, low self-esteem and recent stressful events have been highly correlated with depression in samples of high school students,[23,34–36] and, compared with depressed boys, depressed girls endorsed more worthlessness, guilt feelings, and suicidal ideation.[1,37,38] Low social support has also been correlated with depression in girls.[23] Maladaptive cognitions have been significantly correlated with greater severity of depressive symptoms in depressed adolescents, although neither gender nor type of depressive illness (major depression or dysthymia) were found to contribute to this association.[39]

Bipolar disorders in adolescents can be characterized by insidious onset and a higher switch rate from mania to depression than in adults; there may only be partial remission between episodes. Mania in adolescents is often missed; accurate discrimination may be confounded by the presence of attention deficit and hyperactivity. Thus, in addition to the mood symptoms, clinicians should enquire about the presence of hypomanic behaviour, including pressured speech or activity, grandiosity, and hypersexuality.[40] Bipolar disorder is frequently comorbid with anxiety, substance use, and conduct disorders.[9,11]

Individuals with early-onset (<18 years of age) bipolar disorder demonstrate less sleep disturbance, higher levels of agitation and more suicidal behaviour than those with age of onset between 20 and 25 years of age.[41] It has been suggested that adolescent children of parents with lithium-non-responsive bipolar disorder show prodromal symptoms of mood lability and severe irritability. In comparison, children of lithium-responsive bipolar parents may manifest an episode of brief minor depression prior to the onset of bipolar disorder.[42] There is also recent evidence of neurodevelopmental antecedents of early-onset bipolar disorder: adolescents with bipolar disorder are more likely than psychiatric controls (depression without psychotic features) to have experienced delayed language, social or motor development.[43]

Aetiology

An integrative theory of depression in adolescents has been introduced,[1] although a persuasive explanation of the sharp rise in the prevalence of depression in females after menarche has yet to be elucidated.

The onset of puberty is heralded by a growth spurt, which begins with rapid increases in height and weight typically between 7.5 and 11.5 years of age. Following this initial burst, physical growth continues at a slow pace for several years. The first sign of sexual maturation in girls is breast budding at about 10.5 years, followed by growth of pubic hair, which begins at about 11.5 years, growth of the uterus and vagina, and the enlargement of the labia and clitoris. Menstruation begins after these changes occur. Finally, axillary hair appears, hips broaden, and fat deposits increase. On average, these changes take 4–5 years; however, considerable variation exists in the sequence and tempo of these events.

In North America and Europe, the age of menarche has declined by about 4 months per decade since 1850; in North America, menarche now occurs around 12.5 years of age on average.[44] This dramatic decline in the age at which girls reach puberty is one of the strongest examples of environmental factors that affect hormonal responses. The search for the particular environmental factors involved in this acceleration, however, has been only marginally helpful. It has been suggested that urbanization has a major role in this change, as well as improvements in general health, nutrition, and other socio-cultural factors. Other environmental factors, however, also seem to be implicated in the timing of menarche. Girls who are blind with some perception of light reach menarche earlier than normally sighted girls, and totally blind girls with no light perception reach puberty even earlier.[45] Moreover, fewer girls start to menstruate during spring and summer time compared with seasons with reduced amounts of daylight (autumn and winter).[46]

The relationship between psychosocial development and physical maturation has been widely examined. Girls undergoing pubertal change are thought to experience greater distress and to be more vulnerable to stress than pre- or postpubertal girls.[47] Two parameters of pubertal change in particular have received much attention: pubertal status and pubertal timing. Pubertal status is defined as the current level of physical development of an adolescent relative to the overall process of pubertal change (a biological factor), usually denoted by a series of stages from prepubertal (stage I) to adult (stage V) according to Tanner.[48] Pubertal timing, on the other hand, is defined as the maturation of an adolescent relative to her peers (a psychosocial factor).

Pubertal status

Adolescent girls are less optimistic than their prepubescent peers. It has been suggested that these attitudinal differences are a result of the co-occurrence of change in pubertal status and psychosocial stressors that impinge on youngsters—especially girls—at this developmental stage (e.g. the transition to a more senior school and the changing expectations regarding social and sexual behaviour).[49] At puberty, girls' attitudes about their physical appearance (i.e. the appearance of secondary sex characteristics) become more negative and may be closely associated with negative affect.[50,51] This

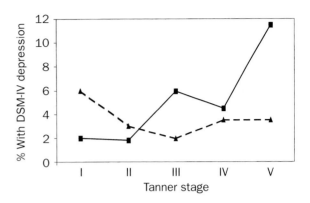

Figure 15.3 Pubertal stage and 3-month prevalence of depression in girls (■——■) and boys (▲– – –▲).[53]

contrasts sharply with the positive association in boys between increased height/muscle bulk and increased self-esteem. In addition, negative attitudes towards menstruation may be found in premenarchal girls, an association that may not decrease until several years postmenarche.[52]

There appears to be a relatively sharply demarcated period in mid-puberty when girls become more vulnerable to depression than boys. In a recent report on 1073 US children 9–13 years of age, the depression rates in girls rose significantly in mid-puberty, i.e. with the transition to Tanner stage III. In contrast, the prevalence of depression in boys declines from Tanner stage II (Figure 15.3).[53] Further, it has been determined that in girls, pubertal status (versus the age at puberty per se) better predicted the emergence of the sex ratio in depression rates. Thus, the onset of menarche may signal an increased but latent biological vulnerability to mood dysregulation in women.

Pubertal timing

Girls who mature earlier manifest more emotional and behavioural problems, specifically poorer body image,[54,55] and have poorer psychological adjustment.[51,56,57,59,60] They also initiate dating and sexual intercourse earlier, behaviours which have been associated with poor health (although this may be culturally defined).[56–58] Within this group, there is an increased likelihood of problem or delinquent behaviour,[47,61] or substance use early in adolescence.[56,62] Similarly, females who experienced later pubertal development, in particular during school transitional times, had more dysphoria and negative attitudes about menstruation compared with their peers who were not experiencing pubertal change.[63,64] Girls who perceive that they have been 'on time' have a more positive body image and feel more physically attractive than early or late maturers; this relationship has shown to be relevant to girls from diverse ethnic groups.[55]

There is some debate over whether poor psychological adjustment in precocious puberty is a magnification of pre-existing emotional/ behavioural issues during childhood, or a de novo event.[47] Early maturation affects psychological functioning when the early maturers represent a noticeable minority within a group.[65]

Psychosocial stressors

Significant changes in social functioning (e.g. peer interactions) and environment (e.g. school transitions),[66,67] as well as gender-differentiated social support concerning sexuality,[68] challenge the coping skills of young girls during the peripubertal period and beyond. For example, lack of connectedness with school, and perceived student prejudice, have been distinguished as factors associated with the onset of depression in female adolescents.[56] Exposure to violence was predictive of depression and hostility in females, but only hostility in males, in a (nonrandom) sample of inner city youth.[69] The onset of major depression in adolescence has

also been significantly related to experiencing a severe life event such as physical assault, conflicted romantic relationships, or family illness.[70,71] In a study of adult female twins, for example, the odds ratio for the onset of major depression in the month of a personal assault is significantly higher.[72] Poverty has been significantly related to serious emotional disturbance in older children/young teens; however, this relationship was not shown to be gender-specific.[73]

Similarly, there is also increasing attention to the prevalence of child physical and sexual abuse and its association with psychiatric morbidity. In a general population survey in Ontario, Canada, the prevalence of physical and/or sexual abuse in females 15–24 years of age has been estimated to be 24.3%, and the prevalence of severe physical and/or sexual abuse in this group was estimated to be 14.1%.[74] A four-times greater prevalence of sexual abuse in young females compared with males was found. The implications of these findings are heightened by the mounting evidence that childhood neglect or abuse—in particular, childhood sexual abuse—has been demarcated as a risk factor for both early- (before age 20 years) and adult-onset depression in women.[23,75–77]

Longitudinal, prospective studies of adolescents (14–18 years of age) have also shown that disease and functional impairment are risk factors for the onset of major depression, although gender differences in these factors as predictors were not detected.[78]

Family psychiatric history and genetic factors

There is indication of a strong association between parental or familial history of psychiatric disorders and onset of major depression in adolescence. Based on a study of pubertal twins, there is evidence of increased heritability for depression in adolescent girls.[71] The rate of depression in offspring categorized as being at high risk for depression (at least one depressed parent) was found to be two times higher than that among offspring regarded as being at low risk (healthy parents).[79] The presence or history of maternal depression significantly increases the likelihood of depression in female children and adolescents.[80–82] There is also some evidence of increased risk for major depression in offspring of probands with onset of major depression before 20 years of age,[83] as well as in offspring of parents with alcohol abuse or dependence,[84] and in families with a recent history of suicidality.[56] Moreover, significant associations between depression and medical problems (including hospitalization) were found for those offspring with a depressed parent.[79]

Research has shown that genetic factors contribute to the aetiology of bipolar disorder (relative risk of 10–15 : 1), although the mode of inheritance has not yet been determined.[85] There is a strong indication of intrafamilial correlation for age at onset of bipolar affective disorder among bipolar siblings, although this correlation has not been found to be gender-specific.[22]

Family support

There is accumulating evidence on the role of family dynamics and familial interpersonal relationships in adolescent health. Less supportive and more conflictual family environments are associated with greater depressive symptomatology in adolescents[35,86,87] and overall psychosocial competence.[33,88] Contrary to expectation, however, no gender differences in the association between family characteristics and adolescent depressive symptomatology have been pinpointed. Parental 'connectedness' (e.g. feelings of warmth, love and caring from parents) has been identified as a significant protective factor against health risk behaviours,[56] whereas a poor (childhood) perception of their role in the family is indicated as a (latent) risk factor for the onset of major depression in female adolescence.[36] There is some evidence (based on retrospective, population-based studies) to support an association between depression in women—but not in men—and a disturbed mother–child relationship.[15]

Sleep architecture

Studies of sleep disturbances in major depression and associated biological rhythm abnormalities suggest that they are strongly influenced by gender: an influence of gonadal hormone regulation on sleep has been posited in women of childbearing age.[89] In addition, menstrual cycle phase effects on sleep have been observed, but the impact of specific endogenous sex hormones (in particular, oestrogen and progesterone) on sleep is not yet clear. Shorter rapid eye movement (REM) latency, long known to be a neurobiological marker of depression in adults, has also been found in several studies of adolescents with major depression when compared with healthy controls.[90–92] These observations have led to two paths of investigation.

One hypothesis has focused on shorter REM latency as a potential biological predictor of major depression in female adolescents. However, it was found, in a comparison of adolescents deemed to be at risk for major depression (i.e. female; having a mother with major depression) with controls (no family psychiatric history in first-degree relatives), that baseline REM latency measures together with depressive symptom measures did not differentiate the two groups.[93] The utility of REM latency as a potential predictor of the onset of major depression is therefore doubtful.

Another postulate has centred on sleep EEG and temporal interhemispheric coherence. In a pilot study, about 25% of 21 never mentally ill offspring from families with a history of depression showed significant sleep EEG differences, suggesting a vulnerability for depression.[94] More recently, sex differences in sleep EEG were found in adolescents but not in children with major depression. Adolescent girls with major depression displayed low interhemispheric temporal coherence of EEG rhythms during sleep compared with healthy girls or depressed adolescent boys. This suggests a disruption in the fundamental brain rest–activity cycle (i.e. organization of sleep cycles, physiology, mood and behaviour) that is strongly influenced by age and gender.[95]

Hormones and neuromodulators

In general, changes in affect, mood and behaviour are considered to be related to cyclic hormonal changes, yet studies of female adolescents and premenstrual syndrome (PMS) are inconclusive, with one study reporting no relationship between menstrual cycle phase and negative affect,[96] and others showing that PMS is associated with other distress factors in this age group.[97,98] Nevertheless, relationships between changes in pubertal hormones and negative affect in female adolescents have been observed. For example, investigators have found that negative affect was significantly related to a rapid increase in oestradiol levels.[99] Negative affect in healthy girls was also associated with higher levels of testosterone and cortisol, and lower levels of dehydroepiandrosterone sulphate.[59]

There is both direct and indirect—albeit limited—evidence of the involvement of the serotonergic system in the aetiology of depressive disorders in child and adolescent depression. In a comparative study of psychiatric inpatients

and normal controls (aged 7–17 years), levels of whole-blood serotonin (5-HT) were lowest in patients with mood disorders.[100] Serotonergic dysregulation in adolescent major depression is further evidenced by a blunted prolactin response to a parenteral clomipramine challenge (a relatively selective 5-HT challenge), but no gender effects in major depression subjects were found.[101] There is some indication of the responsiveness of children and adolescents with major depression to serotonergic but not noradrenergic agents; researchers have hypothesized that, in childhood, the serotonergic systems may mature at an earlier rate than the noradrenergic systems.[102] Gonadal hormones affect the production of 5-HT receptors at the transcriptional level, and the altered distribution or function of 5-HT receptor subtypes brought on by changes in the hormonal milieu at menarche may increase vulnerability to mood disorders. On the other hand, a preliminary investigation that examined mood change in women—who were deemed to be predisposed to depression—following acute tryptophan depletion (thereby reducing brain serotonin synthesis) did not find any significant, sustained difference in mood compared with a control group.[103]

Several neurobiological variables, including other hormonal systems that might identify individuals at high risk (before they develop the depressive illness), have been examined. Unfortunately, the results of studies in this area are not very encouraging. While one study found that nocturnal hypersecretion of growth hormone significantly differentiated depressed adolescents from controls,[104] the 24-h pattern of prolactin and growth hormone secretion as well as the dexamethasone suppression test fail to differentiate between depressed and control groups.[105–107]

Altered hypothalamic–pituitary–adrenal (HPA) system function has been observed both in persons diagnosed with major depression and in their otherwise healthy first-degree relatives.[108] Also, greater susceptibility to stress-induced HPA axis dysregulation has been linked with enhanced vulnerability to depression in women.[77] Investigators have shown that early physical and emotional stress in animals is associated with altered HPA axis function and suppression of reproductive function (including delayed puberty); similar associations have been posited in young women.[109] Pituitary hyporesponsiveness is suggested by significantly decreased plasma adrenocorticotrophic hormone (ACTH) levels in response to ovine corticotrophin-releasing hormone (CRH) stimulation in childhood sexually abused girls (aged 7–15 years) compared with controls. The sexually abused group also had a significantly greater incidence of suicide ideation and attempts, and dysthymia.[110] The longer-term ramifications of HPA axis dysregulation in female children and adolescents, however, have yet to be determined.

It is nevertheless still unclear how the dramatic changes in the hormonal milieu associated with menarche and a host of psychosocial stressors combine to produce depressive symptoms. One possible unifying hypothesis suggests that disruption of biological rhythms (such as disturbed sleep patterns or irregular menstrual cycles) together with psychosocial losses causing the disruption of social rhythms (also known as 'social zeitgebers') could trigger the onset of a major depressive episode in vulnerable individuals.[111] Another complementary theory emphasizes the neurobiology of stress and the dysregulation of affect during female biological transitions such as menarche, a transition that may be associated with changes in the reactivity of the stress system.[112]

In conclusion, it is suggested that pubertal and other hormonal changes should be monitored prospectively along with individual, genetic, constitutional and psychological characteristics in our efforts to predict the development of negative affect during puberty.

The characteristics associated with the onset of mood disorders in female adolescents are summarized in Table 15.1.

Assessment

Depression and bipolar disorder are often under-recognized and undertreated in adolescents and young adults.[40,113,114] It is therefore important to emphasize that direct interview is essential and that adolescents are accurate in reporting their own feelings and emotional problems. Contrary to the long-standing practice of gathering information from multiple

---

Table 15.1 Characteristics associated with the onset of mood disorders around the time of menarche.

Caucasian ethnic group
Family psychiatric history
Prior anxiety disorder
Recent stressful events
History of emotional, physical, sexual abuse
Negative body image/low self-esteem
Negative perception of menstruation
Pubertal status/timing
Relations with family
Perceived student prejudice; lack of
    connectedness with school
Exposure to violence
Physical illness
Functional impairment
Low social support

sources, it has been observed that parent–adolescent agreement for diagnoses of emotional disturbance—including major depression, dysthymia, and anxiety—is poor;[1,115] this may be particularly relevant to females in early adolescence (12–16 years of age).[2]

A two-step process for the assessment of mood disorders in adolescents has been suggested:[1]

1. *Screening.* A depression screen to identify putative cases and specific problem areas; the Center for Epidemiological Studies Depression Scale is one example[116] (although the suitability of this particular scale to Asian groups requires further investigation).
2. *Diagnosis.* A standardized, comprehensive interview to diagnose mood as well as comorbid disorders, using instruments such as the Structured Clinical Interview for DSM-IV,[117] the Revised Diagnostic Interview Schedule for Children,[118] the Schedule for Affective Disorders and Schizophrenia for School-Age Children (K-SADS),[119] or the Diagnostic Interview for Children and Adolescents-Revised (DICA-R).[120]

As an alternative to the standardized diagnostic interviews (usually developed for research settings), the American Academy of Child and Adolescent Psychiatry (AACAP) has recommended a psychiatric symptom checklist derived from DSM-IV symptom categories.[121] The DSM-IV has been advocated as the clinical standard for the diagnosis of mood disorders in adolescents; however, as the AACAP has noted in a recent summary of practice parameters, the clinical picture of mood disorders can show wide variation across developmental stages and ethnic groups.[121] In general, *adolescents* with major depression—compared with *adults* with major depression—may manifest fewer neuro-

vegetative symptoms and more frequent irritability. High levels of depression, hopelessness, socially prescribed perfectionism and anger expression are strongly associated with suicidal ideation.[122]

The 'context' of the depression may play an important role in the assessment and treatment of adolescents: these factors can include family psychiatric history, parental–child relationship(s), familial or home environment, cultural milieu, academic functioning, social (especially peer) relationships, as well as recent stressful life events.[123,124] A summary of key questions—for parents and adolescents—pertaining to adolescent psychosocial functioning has recently been published.[125]

Treatment

Until recently, persons under the age of 18 years were excluded from clinical drug trials and mostly ignored in psychotherapy studies. This situation is now changing, but empirically based treatment options for this age group are still very scarce. The most frequently used form of treatment for adolescent depression is outpatient psychotherapy, and only a very small percentage of these young patients are prescribed antidepressants. In fact, a disturbingly high proportion of adolescents with serious mood disorders receive less than optimal treatment relative to the seriousness of their illness.[126,127]

More recently, however, researchers have advocated treatments that are informed by and address the actual characteristics of depressed youth and their environments, and which are not mere extensions of adult procedures.[123] Yet, the path to treatment planning that incorporates an adolescent's context is not clear cut. For example, although conflicted adolescent–parent relationships are thought to contribute to the persistence of major depression in adolescence,[128] little benefit of family therapy has been demonstrated.

Nevertheless, parental involvement in the treatment process is advocated to enhance communication skills between parent(s) and child, and to facilitate parental understanding of the mental health intervention(s). Parental involvement may be particularly relevant in treating youths in families in which a parent is depressed[1] or family interaction is posited to contribute to the maintenance of illness.[129]

In addition, the benefit in teaching (with 7–12 sessions of individual therapy) adult patients with bipolar disorder to recognize the symptoms of relapse and thus seek prompt treatment has been demonstrated. This method significantly prolonged the time to the next episode of mania, and reduced the frequency of subsequent manic episodes. The patients also realized significant improvement in overall social and employment role function.[130] This type of intervention might also be extended to adolescents.

Psychotherapy

Psychotherapy has been recommended as a first-line intervention for adolescents with mild to moderate depression, given sparse data from controlled studies on specific medication efficacy and long-term safety for children and adolescents. Psychotherapy for depression in adolescence is effective, albeit typically brief (seven or fewer sessions of individual psychotherapy), in particular for milder forms of depression.[21,131]

In general, the literature supports the use of cognitive-behavioural therapy (CBT), either individual or group format, for adolescents with mild to moderate depression, although sex differences in effectiveness have not yet been examined.[132–134]

The effects of both acute and maintenance CBT for adolescents with major depression or dysthymia have been examined recently in a randomized, controlled trial. Following 16 sessions (over 8 weeks) of CBT, the treatment groups (adolescent only or adolescent plus parent(s)) had a significantly greater reduction in depression scores compared with a waitlist control group. A comparable response to individual treatment was also observed in the groups. Maintenance therapy (one booster session every 4 months for 2 years) accelerated recovery among participants who were still depressed at the end of 8 weeks, but it did not reduce the rate of relapse in the 2-year follow-up period.[135]

A second controlled trial compared the efficacy of CBT with behavioural family therapy, and non-directive supportive therapy. CBT was found to have superior efficacy at the end of the 16-week acute treatment phase. Nonetheless, almost 50% of the (total) trial subjects received booster session treatment in the 2-year follow-up phase, and in this latter phase, no significant differences (in the numbers of subjects or time to additional treatment) between the treatment groups were observed.[136]

Taken together, these findings indicate the efficacy of CBT for the acute treatment of depression in adolescents; however, its effectiveness over the longer term, i.e. in the prevention of recurrent episodes, has yet to be demonstrated.

Interpersonal psychotherapy has been modified for use with adolescents (IPT-A)[137,138] and has recently demonstrated effectiveness (3 months of treatment; 1 year follow-up) in mild to moderate depression.[139] IPT-A has also demonstrated effectiveness in reducing depressive symptoms, improving social functioning as well as interpersonal problem-solving skills in adolescents with major depression.[140] The sample in this latest study consisted of female, primarily older, Latino adolescents, and the authors have noted the need for further validation of IPT-A in other adolescent populations.

Psychopharmacological treatment

In general, and compared with studies of psychopharmacotherapy in adults, controlled studies of medication for mood disorders in adolescents are few, and there are few long-term safety data. Researchers have cautioned that response to medication in adolescents should not be solely inferred from similarity in psychopathological features in adults.[141] Gender differences in pharmacokinetics may be relevant in adolescence, as girls' body fat increases more during this period, perhaps influencing drug distribution and half-lives of medication. Moreover, it is postulated that central nervous system neurotransmitter systems undergo differential development from childhood to adulthood, in part explaining age differences in response to some psychotropic medications.[141] One noticeable example of this age-related difference is the poor response of adolescents to tricyclic antidepressants.

To date, the focus of pharmacological treatment studies in childhood and adolescence has been on major depression, and there have been no (published) controlled studies of pharmacotherapy for dysthymic disorder or bipolar disorder in this age bracket. In addition, the gender differences in adolescent responses to psychopharmacological treatments have yet to be explored fully.

Major depressive disorder

There is accumulating evidence from both controlled and open studies that fluoxetine,[142–149] sertraline,[150,151] fluvoxamine[152] and venlafaxine[153] are efficacious in the treatment of major depression in adolescents. The efficacy and safety of paroxetine for the treatment of depression in children and adolescents is being explored.[154,155] It should be noted that the published controlled trials (fluoxetine[142,147] and venlafaxine[153] only) have not exceeded 8 weeks in length. The open trials (fluoxetine[144]), on the other hand, extend up to 24 weeks. Detailed descriptions (dosing, safety and tolerability, costs, drug–drug interactions, etc.) of the use of these selective serotonin reuptake inhibitors (SSRIs) in adolescents have been recently published.[156–159]

In general, the efficacy of tricyclic antidepressants has not been demonstrated in the treatment of major depression in children and adolescents,[160–163] and the evidence for the use of monoamine oxidase inhibitors is only anecdotal. While new information concerning the use of atypical and novel antidepressants (including trazodone, nefazodone, bupropion and mirtazapine) has become available,[164] the efficacy and effectiveness of these agents in youth have yet to be explored in large-scale clinical trials.

Dysthymic disorder

At present, medical opinion advocates using the principles applied in the treatment of major depression also for the treatment of dysthymia.[159]

Bipolar disorder

In children and adolescents, it is recommended that treatment for bipolar disorder be initiated with a mood stabilizer (lithium, valproic acid, or carbamazepine); if no response is observed, then an antidepressant (SSRI, monoamine oxidase inhibitor, or bupropion) should be added.[159] Special consideration should be given to the volumes of body water and rates of active renal glomerular filtration in the use of lithium in adolescents.[165] In the event of a patient presenting with a mixed manic-depressive state, valproic acid (instead of lithium) is recommended.[166,167] However, an increased risk of polycystic ovaries and elevated serum testosterone concentrations has been observed in women with epilepsy who began treatment with valproate before the age of 20 years.[168,169]

Other treatment considerations

Treatment-seeking behaviour

Research has shown that both the severity of a depressive episode and the life circumstances (e.g. conflict with family and/or social group, stressful life events, academic problems) surrounding the episode strongly influence adolescent treatment-seeking behaviour.[1] Additional factors related to treatment utilization include female gender, prior history of depression, history of suicide attempt, and current comorbid non-affective disorder.[21] Typically, compared with boys, girls report significantly more problems with poor self-esteem.[1]

Treatment response

Researchers have delineated patient characteristics that may predict poorer treatment response (Table 15.2).[1,141,170,171]

Table 15.2 Patient characteristics which may predict poor response to treatment.
Younger age
High levels of cognitive distortion and hopelessness at intake
Comorbid anxiety or conduct disorders
Family history of affective disorder
Greater externalizing problems (i.e. aggression, delinquency)
Academic problems
Non-voluntary treatment referral
Degree of cohesion with treatment group

Burden of illness

The burden of depressive illness in adolescents is potentially pervasive and disabling: 'formerly depressed adolescents continue to experience some depression symptoms, excessive interpersonal dependency, internalizing problems, depressotypic negative cognitions (pessimism) and depressotypic attributions (negative, stable internal attributions for failure) and a greater number of major life stressors' (as cited in Lewinsohn et al[1]).

Depressed children and teenagers are at high risk for recurrence. In a community-based sample of high school students, the rates of relapse for females and males with unipolar depressive disorder were estimated at 21.76% and 9.59% respectively.[6] In a comparative study of young adults with/without major depression in adolescence, 45% of the adolescents with a history of major depression developed a new episode between the ages of 19 and 24 years, and the average annual recurrence rate was 9% over a 5-year period. In this same sample, of 238 adolescents with major depression, 1.7% developed dysthymia and 0.8% developed bipolar disorder between 19 and 24 years of age. Overall, subjects with adolescent major depression were significantly more likely to develop an Axis I disorder (DSM-IV criteria) in young adulthood.[172] Opinion remains divided, however, about the influence of gender as a risk factor for future recurrence of major depression.[172,173]

Similarly, adolescents with subclinical depressive symptoms (overall symptom pattern versus any one symptom in particular) were at greater risk for an adult episode of major depression.[172] The likelihood of recurrence of a major depressive episode or the occurrence of a first episode—within 5 years—following early onset of dysthymia, regardless of treatment utilization, has been shown to be as high as

70%;[174] for this reason, dysthymia has been conceptualized as a 'gateway' to major depression and recurrent affective illness.[1,175]

Depression in young adolescent females has been strongly associated with teenage pregnancy;[176] higher rates of marriage and subsequent marital dissatisfaction,[177] increased risk for the initiation of tobacco smoking and dependence, and more medical problems.[178,179]

Conclusion

Following menarche, adolescent girls are at significantly greater risk for an episode of major depression. More than two-thirds of those with a unipolar depressive illness have a comorbid mental disorder, frequently in the form of an anxiety disorder. The aetiology of mood disorders in adolescent girls has yet to be clearly delineated. A set of characteristics associated with the onset of depression in female adolescents has been suggested. Assessment using direct interviews and a depression screen is recommended, with special attention to the context of adolescent depression, i.e. recent stressful life events, psychiatric history (personal and family), and interpersonal relationships. Treatment efficacy and long-term follow-up studies in this population are sparse; however, there is early convincing evidence of the efficacy of both psychotherapy (CBT and IPT-A) and psychopharmacotherapy (using SSRIs) in the more immediate treatment of mild and more severe unipolar depression. The burden of depressive illness with onset in adolescence is staggering, with widespread and long-lasting ramifications. The increased risk for the onset of depression in young women following menarche, therefore, reinforces the importance of early recognition and intervention.[180]

References

1. Lewinsohn PM, Rohde P, Seeley JR, Major depressive disorder in older adolescents: prevalence, risk factors and clinical implications, *Clin Psychol Rev* 1998; **18**:765–94.
2. Offord DR, Boyle MH, Fleming JE et al, Ontario Child Health Study. Summary of selected results. *Can J Psychiatry* 1989; **34**:483–91.
3. Angold A, Worthman CW, Puberty onset of gender differences in rates of depression: a developmental, epidemiologic and neuroendocrine perspective, *J Affect Disord* 1993; **29**:145–58.
4. Kessler RC, Walters EE, Epidemiology of DSM-III-R major depression and minor depression among adolescents and young adults in the National Comorbidity Survey, *Depress Anxiety* 1998; **7**:3–14.
5. Whitaker A, Johnson J, Shaffer D et al, Uncommon troubles in young people: prevalence estimates of selected psychiatric disorders in a nonreferred adolescent population, *Arch Gen Psychiatry* 1990; **47**:487–96.
6. Lewinsohn PM, Hops H, Roberts RE et al, Adolescent psychopathology: I. Prevalence and incidence of depression and other DSM-III-R disorders in high school students, *J Abnorm Psychol* 1993; **102**:133–44.
7. Klein DN, Riso LP, Donaldson SK et al, Family study of early-onset dysthymia. Mood and personality disorders in relatives of outpatients with dysthymia and episodic major depression and normal controls, *Arch Gen Psychiatry* 1995; **52**:487–96.
8. Wittchen H-U, Nelson CB, Lachner G, Prevalence of mental disorders and psychosocial impairments in adolescents and young adults, *Psychol Med* 1998; **28**:109–26.

9. Lewinsohn PM, Klein DN, Seeley JR, Bipolar disorders in a community sample of older adolescents: prevalence, phenomenology, comorbidity, and course, *J Am Acad Child Adolesc Psychiatry* 1995; **34**:454–63.

10. Weissman MM, Bland RC, Canino GJ et al, Cross-national epidemiology of major depression and bipolar disorder, *JAMA* 1996; **276**:293–9.

11. Kessler RC, Rubinow DR, Holmes C et al, The epidemiology of DSM-III-R bipolar I disorder in a general population survey, *Psychol Med* 1997; **27**:1079–89.

12. Brady EU, Kendall PC, Comorbidity of anxiety and depression in children and adolescents, *Psychol Bull* 1992; **111**:244–55.

13. Breslau N, Schultz L, Peterson E, Sex differences in depression: a role for preexisting anxiety, *Psychiatry Res* 1995; **58**:1–12.

14. Simonoff E, Pickles A, Meyer JM et al, The Virginia Twin Study of Adolescent Behavioral Development, *Arch Gen Psychiatry* 1997; **54**:801–8.

15. Veijola J, Puukka P, Lehtinen V et al, Sex differences in the association between childhood experiences and adult depression, *Psychol Med* 1998; **28**:21–7.

16. Burke KC, Burke JD Jr, Regier DA, Rae DS, Age at onset of selected mental disorders in five community populations, *Arch Gen Psychiatry* 1990; **47**:511–18.

17. Cohen P, Cohen J, Kasen S et al, An epidemiological study of disorders in late childhood and adolescence—I. Age- and gender-specific prevalence, *J Child Psychol Psychiatry* 1993; **34**:851–67.

18. Patton GC, Hibbert ME, Carlin J et al, Menarche and the onset of depression and anxiety in Victoria, Australia, *J Epidemiol Community Health* 1996; **50**:661–6.

19. Cairney J, Gender differences in the prevalence of depression among Canadian adolescents, *Can J Public Health* 1998; **89**:181–2.

20. Hankin BL, Abramson LY, Moffitt TE et al, Development of depression from preadolescence to young adulthood: emerging gender differences in a 10-year longitudinal study, *J Abnorm Psychol* 1998; **107**:128–40.

21. Lewinsohn PM, Rohde P, Seeley JR, Treatment of adolescent depression: frequency of services and impact on functioning in young adulthood, *Depress Anxiety* 1998; **7**:47–52.

22. Leboyer M, Bellivier F, McKeon P et al, Age at onset and gender resemblance in bipolar siblings, *Psychiatry Res* 1998; **81**:125–31.

23. Schraedley PK, Gotlib IH, Hayward C, Gender differences in correlates of depressive symptoms in adolescence, *J Adolesc Health* 1999; **25**:98–108.

24. Hayward C, Gotlib IH, Schraedley PK, Litt IF, Ethnic differences in the association between pubertal status and symptoms of depression in adolescent girls, *J Adolesc Health* 1999; **25**:143–9.

25. Prescott CA, McArdle JJ, Hishinuma ES et al, Prediction of major depression and dysthymia from CES-D scores among ethnic minority adolescents, *J Am Acad Child Adolesc Psychiatry* 1998; **37**:495–503.

26. Lewinsohn PM, Gotlib IH, Seeley JR, Adolescent psychopathology: IV. Specificity of psychosocial risk factors for depression and substance abuse in older adolescents, *J Am Acad Child Adolesc Psychiatry* 1995; **34**:1221–9.

27. Marttunen MJ, Henriksson MM, Aro HM et al, Suicide among female adolescents: characteristics and comparison with males in the age group 13 to 22 years, *J Am Acad Child Adolesc Psychiatry* 1995; **34**:1297–307.

28. Andrews JA, Lewinsohn PM, Suicidal attempts among older adolescents: prevalence and co-occurrence with psychiatric disorders, *J Am Acad Child Adolesc Psychiatry* 1992; **31**:655–62.

29. Wannan G, Fombonne E, Gender differences in rates and correlates of suicidal behaviour amongst child psychiatric outpatients, *J Adolesc* 1998; **21**:371–81.

30. From the Centers for Disease Control, Attempted suicide among high school students—United States, 1990, *JAMA* 1991; **266**:1911–12.

31. Patton GC, Harris R, Carlin JB et al, Adolescent suicidal behaviours: a population-based study of risk, *Psychol Med* 1997; **27**:715–24.

32. Silverstein B, Gender difference in the prevalence of clinical depression: the role played by

depression associated with somatic symptoms, *Am J Psychiatry* 1999; **156**:480–2.

33. McCauley E, Myers K, Mitchell J et al, Depression in young people: initial presentation and clinical course, *J Am Acad Child Adolesc Psychiatry* 1993; **32**:714–22.

34. Allgood-Merten B, Lewinsohn PM, Hops H, Sex differences and adolescent depression, *J Abnorm Psychol* 1990; **99**:55–63.

35. Fleming JE, Offord DR, Epidemiology of childhood depressive disorders: a critical review, *J Am Acad Child Adolesc Psychiatry* 1990; **29**:571–80.

36. Reinherz HZ, Giaconia RM, Pakiz B et al, Psychosocial risks for major depression in late adolescence: a longitudinal community study, *J Am Acad Child Adolesc Psychiatry* 1993; **32**:1155–63.

37. Kashani JH, Orvaschel H, Rosenberg TK, Reid JC, Psychopathology in a community sample of children and adolescents: a developmental perspective, *J Am Acad Child Adolesc Psychiatry* 1989; **28**:701–6.

38. Olsson G, von Knorring A-L, Beck's Depression Inventory as a screening instrument for adolescent depression in Sweden: gender differences, *Acta Psychiatr Scand* 1997; **95**:277–82.

39. Marton P, Kutcher S, The prevalence of cognitive distortion in depressed adolescents, *J Psychiatry Neurosci* 1995; **20**:33–8.

40. Berenson CK, Frequently missed diagnoses in adolescent psychiatry, *Psychiatr Clin North Am* 1998; **21**:917–26.

41. Sax KW, Strakowski SM, Keck PE et al, Comparison of patients with early-, typical-, and late-onset affective psychosis, *Am J Psychiatry* 1997; **154**:1299–301.

42. Duffy A, Alda M, Kutcher S et al, Psychiatric symptoms and syndromes among adolescent children of parents with lithium-responsive or lithium nonresponsive bipolar disorder, *Am J Psychiatry* 1998; **155**:431–3.

43. Sigurdsson E, Fombonne E, Sayal K, Checkley S, Neurodevelopmental antecedents of early-onset bipolar affective disorder, *Br J Psychiatry* 1999; **174**:121–7.

44. Tanner JM, Earlier maturation in man, *Sci Am* 1968; **218**:21–7.

45. Zacharias L, Wurtman RJ, Blindness: its relation to age of menarche, *Science* 1964; **144**:1154–5.

46. Bojlen K, Bentzon MW, Seasonal variation in the occurrence of menarche, *Dan Med Bull* 1974; **21**:161–8.

47. Caspi A, Moffitt TE, Individual differences are accentuated during periods of social change: the sample case of girls at puberty, *J Pers Soc Psychol* 1991; **61**:157–68.

48. Tanner JM, *Growth at Adolescence*, 2nd edn (Blackwell Scientific Publications: Oxford, 1962).

49. Nolen-Hoeksema S, Girgus JS, The emergence of gender differences in depression during adolescence, *Psychol Bull* 1994; **115**:424–43.

50. Brooks-Gunn J, Antecedents and consequences of variations in girls' maturational timing, *J Adolesc Health Care* 1988; **9**:365–73.

51. Hayward C, Killen JD, Wilson DM et al, Psychiatric risk associated with early puberty in adolescent girls, *J Am Acad Child Adolesc Psychiatry* 1997; **36**:255–62.

52. Brooks-Gunn J, Ruble D, Menarche: the interaction of physiological, cultural and social factors. In: Dan AJ, Beecher CP, Graham EA, eds, *The Menstrual Cycle: A Synthesis of Interdisciplinary Research* (Springer: New York, 1980) 141–59.

53. Angold A, Costello EJ, Worthman CM, Puberty and depression: the roles of age, pubertal status and pubertal timing, *Psychol Med* 1998; **28**:51–61.

54. Dubas J, Graber J, Petersen A, A longitudinal investigation of adolescents' changing perceptions of pubertal status, *Dev Psychol* 1991; **27**:580–6.

55. Siegel JM, Yancey AK, Aneshensel CS, Schuler R, Body image, perceived pubertal timing, and adolescent mental health, *J Adolesc Health* 1999; **25**:155–65.

56. Resnick MD, Bearman PS, Blum RW et al, Protecting adolescents from harm. Findings from the National Longitudinal Study on Adolescent Health, *JAMA* 1997; **278**:823–32.

57. Simmons R, Blyth D, *Moving into Adolescence: The Impact of Pubertal Change on School Context* (Plenum Press: New York, 1987).

58. Kim K, Smith PK, Childhood stress, behav-

ioural symptoms and mother–daughter pubertal development, *J Adolesc* 1998; **21:**231–40.

59. Sussman EJ, Dorn LD, Chrousos G, Negative affect and hormone level in young adolescents: concurrent and longitudinal perspectives, *J Youth Adolesc* 1991; **121:**167–90.

60. Ge X, Conger RD, Elder GH, Coming of age too early: pubertal influences on girls' vulnerability to psychological distress, *Child Dev* 1996; **67:**3386–400.

61. Stattin H, Magnusson D, *Paths through Life; Pubertal Maturation in Female Development* (Erlbaum Press: Hillsdale, NJ, 1990).

62. Tschann JM, Adler NE, Irwin CE et al, Initiation of substance use in early adolescence: the roles of pubertal timing and emotional distress, *Health Psychol* 1994; **13:**326–33.

63. Graber JA, Lewinsohn PM, Seeley JR, Brooks-Gunn J, Is psychopathology associated with the timing of pubertal development? *J Am Acad Child Adolesc Psychiatry* 1997; **36:**1768–76.

64. Koenig LJ, Gladstone TRG, Pubertal development and school transition, *Behav Modif* 1998; **22:**335–57.

65. Rierdan J, Koff E, Depressive symptomatology among very early maturing girls, *J Youth Adolesc* 1991; **20:**415–25.

66. Hartup W, Peer relations. In: Mussen PH, ed., *Handbook of Child Psychology*, Vol IV (Wiley: New York, 1983) 103–96.

67. Petersen A, Hamburg B, Adolescence: a developmental approach to problems and psychopathology, *Behav Ther* 1986; **17:**480–99.

68. Henriques-Mueller MH, Yunes J, Adolescence: misunderstandings and hopes. In: Gomez EG, ed., *Gender, Women, and Health in the Americas* (World Health Organization, Scientific Publication No. 541: Washington, DC, 1993) 43–61.

69. Moses A, Exposure to violence, depression, and hostility in a sample of inner city high school youth, *J Adolesc* 1999; **22:**21–32.

70. Williamson DE, Birmaher B, Frank E et al, Nature of life events and difficulties in depressed adolescents, *J Am Acad Child Adolesc Psychiatry* 1998; **37:**1049–57.

71. Silberg J, Pickles A, Rutter M et al, The influence of genetic factors and life stress on depression among adolescent girls, *Arch Gen Psychiatry* 1999; **56:**225–32.

72. Kendler KS, Karkowski LM, Prescott CA, Causal relationship between stressful events and the onset of major depression, *Am J Psychiatry* 1999; **156:**837–41.

73. Costello EJ, Angold A, Burns BJ et al, The Great Smoky Mountains Study of Youth. Functional impairment and serious emotional disturbance, *Arch Gen Psychiatry* 1996; **53:**1137–43.

74. MacMillan HL, Fleming JE, Trocmé N et al, Prevalence of child physical and sexual abuse in the community. Results from the Ontario Health Supplement. *JAMA* 1997; **278:**131–5.

75. Bifulco A, Brown GW, Moran P et al, Predicting depression in women: the role of past and present vulnerability, *Psychol Med* 1998; **28:**39–50.

76. Levitan RD, Parikh SV, Lesage AD et al, Major depression in individuals with a history of childhood physical or sexual abuse: relationship to neurovegetative features, mania, and gender, *Am J Psychiatry* 1998; **155:** 1746–52.

77. Weiss EL, Longhurst JG, Mazure CM, Childhood sexual abuse as a risk factor for depression in women: psychosocial and neurobiological correlates, *Am J Psychiatry* 1999; **156:**816–28.

78. Lewinsohn PM, Seeley JR, Hibbard J et al, Cross-sectional and prospective relationships between physical morbidity and depression in older adolescents, *J Am Acad Child Adolesc Psychiatry* 1996; **35:**1120–9.

79. Kramer RA, Warner V, Olfson M et al, General medical problems among the offspring of depressed parents, *J Am Acad Child Adolesc Psychiatry* 1998; **37:**602–11.

80. Goodyer IM, Cooper PJ, Vize CM, Ashby L, Depression in 11- to 16-year old girls: the role of past parental psychopathology and exposure to recent life events, *J Child Psychol Psychiatry* 1993; **34:**1103–15.

81. Boyle MH, Pickles A, Maternal depressive symptoms and ratings of emotional disorder symptoms in children and adolescents, *J Child Psychol Psychiatry* 1997; **38:**981–92.

82. Shiner RL, Marmorstein NR, Family environments of adolescents with lifetime depression:

associations with maternal depression history, *J Am Acad Child Adolesc Psychiatry* 1998; **37**:1152–60.

83. Weissman MM, Wickramaratne P, Merikangas KR et al, Onset of major depression in early adulthood. Increased familial loading and specificity, *Arch Gen Psychiatry* 1984; **41**:1136–43.

84. Chassin L, Pitts SC, DeLucia C, Todd M, A longitudinal study of children of alcoholics: predicting young adult substance use disorders, anxiety, and depression, *J Abnorm Psychol* 1999; **108**:106–19.

85. Alda M, Bipolar disorder: from families to genes, *Can J Psychiatry* 1997; **42**:378–87.

86. Cohen P, Brook J, Family factors related to the persistence of psychopathology in childhood and adolescence, *Psychiatry* 1987; **50**:332–45.

87. Sheeber L, Hops H, Alpert A et al, Family support and conflict: prospective relations to adolescent depression, *J Abnorm Child Psychol* 1997; **25**:333–44.

88. Puig-Antich J, Kaufman J, Ryan ND et al, The psychosocial functioning and family environment of depressed adolescents, *J Am Acad Child Adolesc Psychiatry* 1993; **32**:244–53.

89. Manber R, Armitage R, Sex steroids and sleep: a review, *Sleep* 1999; **22**:540–55.

90. Kutcher S, Williamson P, Marton P, Szalai J, REM latency in endogenously depressed adolescents, *Br J Psychiatry* 1992; **161**:399–402.

91. Lahmeyer HW, Poznanski EO, Bellur SN, EEG Sleep in depressed adolescents, *Am J Psychiatry* 1983; **140**:1150–3.

92. Emslie GJ, Rush AJ, Weinberg WA et al, Sleep EEG features of adolescents with major depression, *Biol Psychiatry* 1994; **36**:573–81.

93. Kutcher S, Kusumakar V, LeBlanc J et al, Baseline depressive symptoms in adolescent girls at high and at usual risk for major depressive disorder, *Biol Psychiatry* 1999; **45**:78S.

94. Armitage R, Microarchitectural findings in sleep EEG in depression: diagnostic implications, *Biol Psychiatry* 1995; **37**:72–84.

95. Armitage R, Emslie GJ, Hoffmann RF et al, Ultradian rhythms and temporal coherence in sleep EEG in depressed children and adolescents, *Biol Psychiatry* 2000; **47**:338–50.

96. Golub S, Harrington D, Premenstrual and menstrual mood changes in adolescent women, *J Person Soc Psychol* 1981; **41**:1961–5.

97. Raja SN, Feehan M, Stanton WR, McGee R, Prevalence and correlates of the premenstrual syndrome in adolescence, *J Am Acad Child Adolesc Psychiatry* 1992; **31**:783–9.

98. Freeman EW, Rickels K, Sondheimer SJ, Premenstrual symptoms and dysmenorrhea in relation to emotional distress factors in adolescents, *J Psychosom Obstet Gynaecol* 1993; **14**:41–50.

99. Warren MP, Brooks-Gunn J, Mood and behavior at adolescence: evidence for hormonal factors, *J Clin Endocrinol Metab* 1989; **69**:77–83.

100. Hughes CW, Petty F, Sheikha S, Kramer GL, Whole-blood serotonin in children and adolescents with mood and behavior disorders, *Psychiatry Res* 1996; **65**:79–95.

101. Sallee FR, Vrindavanam NS, Deas-Nesmith D et al, Parenteral clomipramine challenge in depressed adolescents: mood and neuroendocrine response, *Biol Psychiatry* 1998; **44**:562–7.

102. Ryan ND, Varma D, Child and adolescent mood disorders—experience with serotonin-based therapies, *Biol Psychiatry* 1998; **44**:336–40.

103. Ellenbogen MA, Young SN, Dean P et al, Acute tryptophan depletion in healthy young women with a family history of major affective disorder, *Psychol Med* 1999; **29**:35–46.

104. Kutcher S, Malkin D, Silverberg J et al, Nocturnal cortisol, thyroid stimulating hormone, and growth hormone secretory profiles in depressed adolescents, *J Am Acad Child Adolesc Psychiatry* 1991; **30**:407–14.

105. Waterman GS, Dahl RE, Birmaher B et al, The 24-hour pattern of prolactin secretion in depressed and normal adolescents, *Biol Psychiatry* 1994; **35**:440–5.

106. Dahl RE, Ryan ND, Williamson DE et al, Regulation of sleep and growth hormone in adolescent depression, *J Am Acad Child Adolesc Psychiatry* 1992; **31**:615–21.

107. Dahl RE, Kaufman J, Ryan ND et al, The dexamethasone suppression test in children and adolescents: a review and a controlled

study, *Biol Psychiatry* 1992; **32**:109–26.

108. Holsboer F, Lauer CJ, Schreiber W, Krieg JC, Altered hypothalamic–pituitary–adrenocortical regulation in healthy subjects at high familial risk for affective disorders, *Neuroendocrinology* 1995; **62**:340–7.

109. De Bellis MD, Putnam FW, The psychobiology of childhood maltreatment, *Child Adolesc Psychiatric Clin North Am* 1994; **3**:663–77.

110. De Bellis MD, Chrousos GP, Dorn LD et al, Hypothalamic–pituitary–adrenal axis dysregulation in sexually abused girls, *J Clin Endocrinol Metab* 1994; **78**:249–55.

111. Ehlers CL, Frank E, Kupfer DJ, Social zeitgebers and biological rhythms, *Arch Gen Psychiatry* 1988; **45**:948–52.

112. Dorn LD, Chrousos GP, The neurobiology of stress: understanding regulation of affect during female biological transitions, *Semin Reprod Endocrinol* 1997; **15**:19–35.

113. Kramer T, Garralda ME, Psychiatric disorders in adolescents in primary care, *Br J Psychiatry* 1998; **173**:508–13.

114. Lecrubier Y, Is depression under-recognized and undertreated? *Int Clin Psychopharmacol* 1998; **13** (suppl):S3–6.

115. Boyle MH, Offord DR, Racine Y et al, Evaluation of the Diagnostic Interview for Children and Adolescents for use in general population samples, *J Abnorm Child Psychol* 1993; **21**:663–81.

116. Radloss LS, The CES-D Scale: A self-report depression scale for research in the general population, *Appl Psychol Meas* 1977; **1**:385–401.

117. First MB, Spitzer RL, Gibson M et al, *Structured Clinical Interview for DSM-IV Axis I Disorders—Patient Edition* (Biometrics Research Department, New York State Psychiatric Institute: New York, 1996).

118. Schwab-Stone M, Fisher P, Piacentini J et al, The Diagnostic Interview Schedule of Children—Revised Version (DISC-R): II. Test-retest reliability, *J Am Acad Child Adolesc Psychiatry* 1993; **32**:651–7.

119. Orvaschel H, Puig-Antich J, Chambers W et al, Retrospective assessment of prepubertal major depression with the Kiddie-SADS-E, *J Am Acad Child Psychiatry* 1982; **21**:392–7.

120. Reich W, Cottler L, McCallum K et al, Computerized interviews as a method of assessing psychopathology in children, *Compr Psychiatry* 1995; **36**:40–5.

121. Birmaher B, Brent DA, Benson RS, Summary of the practice parameters for the assessment and treatment of children and adolescents with depressive disorders, *J Am Acad Child Adolesc Psychiatry* 1998; **37**:1234–8.

122. Boergers J, Spirito A, Donaldson D, Reasons for adolescent suicide attempts: associations with psychological functioning, *J Am Acad Child Adolesc Psychiatry* 1998; **37**:1287–93.

123. Hammen C, Rudolph K, Weisz J et al, The context of depression in clinic-referred youth: neglected areas in treatment, *J Am Acad Child Adolesc Psychiatry* 1999; **38**:64–71.

124. Pfefferbaum B, Pfefferbaum RL, Strickland RJ, Brandt EN, Juvenile delinquency in American Indian youths: historical and cultural factors, *J Okla State Med Assoc* 1999; **92**:121–5.

125. Cassidy LJ, Jellinek MS, Approaches to recognition and management of childhood psychiatric disorders in pediatric primary care, *Pediatr Clin North Am* 1998; **45**:1037–52.

126. Strober M, DeAntonio M, Lampert C, Diamond J, Intensity and predictors of treatment received by adolescents with unipolar major depression prior to hospital admission, *Depression Anxiety* 1998; **7**:40–6.

127. Sclar DA, Robison LM, Skaer TL et al, Prescribing pattern for antidepressant pharmacotherapy, diagnosis of depression, and receipt of psychotherapy among children and adolescents: 1990–1995. In: *New Clinical Drug Evaluation Unit Program* (Boca Raton, FL: 1999) Poster No. 178.

128. Sanford M, Szatmari P, Spinner M et al, Predicting the one-year course of adolescent major depression, *J Am Acad Child Adolesc Psychiatry* 1995; **34**:1618–28.

129. Marton P, Maharaj S, Family factors in adolescent unipolar depression, *Can J Psychiatry* 1993; **38**:373–82.

130. Perry A, Tarrier N, Morriss R et al, Randomised controlled trial of efficacy of teaching patients with bipolar disorder to identify early symptoms of relapse and obtain treatment, *Br Med J* 1999; **318**:149–53.

131. Renaud J, Brent DA, Baugher M et al, Rapid response to psychosocial treatment for adoles-

cent depression: a two-year follow-up, *J Am Acad Child Adolesc Psychiatry* 1998; 37:1184–90.

132. Lewinsohn PM, Clarke GN, Psychosocial treatments for adolescent depression, *Clin Psychol Rev* 1999; 19:329–42.

133. Harrington R, Whittaker J, Shoebridge P, Psychological treatment of depression in children and adolescents. A review of treatment research, *Br J Psychiatry* 1998; 173:291–8.

134. Harrington R, Whittaker J, Shoebridge P, Campbell F, Systematic review of efficacy of cognitive behaviour therapies in childhood and adolescent depressive disorder, *Br Med J* 1998; 316:1559–63.

135. Clarke GN, Rohde P, Lewinsohn PM et al, Cognitive-behavioural treatment of adolescent depression: efficacy of acute group treatment and booster sessions, *J Am Acad Child Adolesc Psychiatry* 1999; 38:272–9.

136. Brent DA, Kolko DJ, Birmaher B et al, A clinical trial for adolescent depression: predictors of additional treatment in the acute and follow-up phases of the trial, *J Am Acad Child Adolesc Psychiatry* 1999; 38:263–70.

137. Moreau D, Mufson L, Weissman MM, Klerman GL, Interpersonal psychotherapy for adolescent depression: description of modification and preliminary application, *J Am Acad Child Adolesc Psychiatry* 1991; 30:642–51.

138. Mufson L, Moreau D, Weissman MM et al, Modification of interpersonal psychotherapy with depressed adolescents (IPT-A): phase I and II studies, *J Am Acad Child Adolesc Psychiatry* 1994; 33:695–705.

139. Mufson L, Fairbanks J, Interpersonal psychotherapy for depressed adolescents: a one-year naturalistic follow-up study, *J Am Acad Child Adolesc Psychiatry* 1996; 35:1145–55.

140. Mufson L, Weissman MM, Moreau D, Garfinkel R, Efficacy of interpersonal psychotherapy for depressed adolescents, *Arch Gen Psychiatry* 1999; 56:573–9.

141. Tosyali MC, Greenhill LL, Child and adolescent psychopharmacology. Important developmental issues, *Pediatr Clin North Am* 1998; 45:1021–35.

142. Simeon J, Dinicola VF, Ferguson HB, Copping W, Adolescent depression: a placebo-controlled fluoxetine treatment study and fol-

low-up, *Prog Neuropsychopharmacol Biol Psychiatry* 1990; 14:791–5.

143. Boulos C, Kutcher S, Gardner D, Young E, An open naturalistic trial of fluoxetine in adolescents and young adults with treatment resistant depression, *J Child Adolesc Psychopharmacol* 1992; 2:103–11.

144. Colle LM, Belair JF, DiFeo M et al, Extended open-label fluoxetine treatment of adolescents with major depression, *J Child Adolesc Psychopharmacol* 1994; 4:225–32.

145. Ghaziuddin N, Naylor MW, King CA, Fluoxetine in tricyclic refractory depression in adolescents, *Depression* 1995; 2:287–91.

146. Nguyen N, Bui B, Whittlesey S et al, A plot study: pattern analysis of fluoxetine in childhood depression, *Psychopharm Bull* 1995; 31:602.

147. Emslie GJ, Rush AJ, Weinberg WA et al, A double-blind, randomized, placebo-controlled trial of fluoxetine in children and adolescents with depression, *Arch Gen Psychiatry* 1997; 54:1031–7.

148. Emslie GJ, Rush AJ, Weinberg WA et al, Fluoxetine in child and adolescent depression: acute and maintenance treatment, *Depress Anxiety* 1998; 7:32–9.

149. Strober M, DeAntonio M, Schmidt-Lackner S et al, The pharmacotherapy of depressive illness in adolescents: an open-label comparison of fluoxetine with imipramine-treated historical controls, *J Clin Psychiatry* 1999; 60:164–9.

150. McConville BJ, Minnery KL, Sorter MT et al, An open study of the effects of sertraline on adolescent major depression, *J Child Adolesc Psychopharmacol* 1996; 6:41–51.

151. Alderman J, Wolkow R, Chung M, Johnston HF, Sertraline treatment of children and adolescents with obsessive-compulsive disorder or depression: pharmacokinetics, tolerability, and efficacy, *J Am Acad Child Adolesc Psychiatry* 1998; 37:386–94.

152. Apter A, Ratzoni G, King RA et al, Fluvoxamine open-label treatment of adolescent inpatients with obsessive-compulsive disorder or depression, *J Am Acad Child Adolesc Psychiatry* 1994; 33:342–8.

153. Mandoki MW, Tapia MR, Tapia MA et al, Venlafaxine in the treatment of children and

adolescents with major depression, *Psycho-pharmacol Bull* 1997; **33**:149–54.

154. Rey-Sanchez F, Gutierrez-Casares JR, Paroxetine in children with major depressive disorder: an open trial, *J Am Acad Child Adolesc Psychiatry* 1997; **36**:1443–7.

155. Findling RL, Reed MD, Myers C et al, Paroxetine pharmacokinetics in depressed children and adolescents, *J Am Acad Child Adolesc Psychiatry* 1999; **38**:952–9.

156. Labellarte MJ, Walkup JT, Riddle MA, The new antidepressants. Selective serotonin reuptake inhibitors, *Pediatr Clin North Am* 1998; **45**:1137–55.

157. Ten-Eick AP, Nakamura H, Reed MD, Drug–drug interactions in pediatric psycho-pharmacology, *Pediatr Clin North Am* 1998; **45**:1233–64.

158. Bostic JQ, Wilens TE, Spencer T, Biederman J, Antidepressant treatment of juvenile depression, *Int J Psych Clin Pract* 1999; **3**:171–9.

159. Renaud J, Axelson D, Birmaher B, A risk–benefit assessment of pharmacotherapies for clinical depression in children and adolescents, *Drug Safety* 1999; **20**:59–75.

160. Anderson I, Place of tricyclics in depression of young people is not proved, *Br Med J* 1995; **311**:390.

161. Hazell P, O'Connell D, Heathcote D et al, Efficacy of tricyclic drugs in treating child and adolescent depression: a meta-analysis, *Br Med J* 1995; **310**:897–901.

162. Birmaher B, Waterman GS, Ryan ND et al, Randomized, controlled trial of amitriptyline versus placebo for adolescents with 'treatment resistant' major depression, *J Am Acad Child Adolesc Psychiatry* 1998; **37**:527–35.

163. Daly JM, Wilens T, The use of tricyclic antidepressants in children and adolescents, *Pediatr Clin North Am* 1998; **45**:1123–35.

164. McConville BJ, Chaney RO, Browne KL et al, Newer antidepressants. Beyond selective serotonin reuptake inhibitor antidepressants, *Pediatr Clin North Am* 1998; **45**:1157–71.

165. Tueth MJ, Murphy TK, Evans DL, Special considerations: use of lithium in children, adolescents and elderly populations, *J Clin Psychiatry* 1998; **59** (suppl 6):66–73.

166. Swann AC, Bowden CL, Morris D et al, Depression during mania. Treatment response to lithium or divalproex, *Arch Gen Psychiatry* 1997; **54**:37–42.

167. Deltito JA, Levitan J, Damore J et al, Naturalistic experience with the use of divalproex sodium on an in-patient unit for adolescent psychiatric patients, *Acta Psychiatr Scand* 1998; **97**:236–40.

168. Isojarvi JIT, Laatikainen TJ, Pakarinen AJ et al, Polycystic ovaries and hyperandrogenism in women taking valproate for epilepsy, *N Engl J Med* 1993; **329**:1383–88.

169. Isojarvi JI, Rattya J, Myllyla VV et al, Valproate, lamotrigine, and insulin-mediated risks in women with epilepsy, *Ann Neurol* 1998; **43**:446–51.

170. Baruch G, Gerber A, Fearon P, Adolescents who drop out of psychotherapy at a community-based psychotherapy centre: a preliminary investigation of the characteristics of early drop-outs, late drop-outs and those who continue treatment, *Br J Med Psychol* 1998; **71**:233–45.

171. Brent DA, Kolko DJ, Birmaher B et al, Predictors of treatment efficacy in a clinical trial of three psychosocial treatments for adolescent depression, *J Am Acad Child Adolesc Psychiatry* 1998; **37**:906–14.

172. Pine DS, Cohen E, Cohen P, Brook J, Adolescent depressive symptoms as predictors of adult depression: moodiness or mood disorder? *Am J Psychiatry* 1999; **156**:133–5.

173. Lewinsohn PM, Rohde P, Klein DN, Seeley JR, Natural course of adolescent major depressive disorder: I. Continuity into young adulthood, *J Am Acad Child Adolesc Psychiatry* 1999; **38**:56–63.

174. Kovacs M, Feinberg TL, Crouse-Novak M et al, Depressive disorders in childhood. II. A longitudinal study of the risk for a subsequent major depression, *Arch Gen Psychiatry* 1984; **41**:643–9.

175. Kovacs M, Akiskal HS, Gatsonis C, Parrone PL, Childhood-onset dysthymic disorder. Clinical features and prospective naturalistic outcome, *Arch Gen Psychiatry* 1994; **51**:365–74.

176. Kessler RC, Berglund PA, Foster CL et al, Social consequences of psychiatric disorders, II: Teenage parenthood, *Am J Psychiatry* 1997; **154**:1405–11.

177. Gotlib IH, Lewinsohn PM, Seeley JR, Consequences of depression during adolescence: marital status and marital functioning in early adulthood, *J Abnorm Psychol* 1998; **107**:686–90.

178. Bardone AM, Moffitt TE, Caspi A et al, Adult physical health outcomes of adolescent girls with conduct disorder, depression, and anxiety, *J Am Acad Child Adolesc Psychiatry* 1998; **37**:594–601.

179. Patton GC, Carlin JB, Coffey C et al, Depression, anxiety, and smoking initiation: a prospective study over 3 years, *Am J Public Health* 1998; **88**:1518–22.

180. Beardslee WR, Versage EM, Gladstone JR, Children of affectively ill parents: a review of the past 10 years, *J Am Acad Child Adolesc Psychiatry* 1998; **37**:1134–41.

16

Premenstrual dysphoria and related conditions: symptoms, pathophysiology and treatment

Elias Eriksson, Charlotta Sundblad, Kimberly A Yonkers and Meir Steiner

Introduction

The majority of women of fertile age experience symptoms such as irritability and depressed mood during the luteal phase of the menstrual cycle; often these symptoms are accompanied by various somatic complaints, such as breast tenderness and a sense of bloating. In most women, these cycle-related symptoms are mild and can be easily mastered without pharmacological treatment. The very high prevalence of subtle premenstrual complaints must not, however, conceal the fact that approximately 5% of all women of reproductive age suffer from a severe variant of this condition, leading to a drastic reduction in life quality and probably to an increased risk of developing other mood disorders. This form of premenstrual distress constitutes a serious condition that must be neither trivialized nor neglected.

The terms 'premenstrual syndrome' (PMS) and 'premenstrual tension' (PMT) have been frequently used but are poorly defined; a woman given the diagnosis of PMS (or PMT) may thus suffer from somatic or mental symp-

toms only, or a mixture of somatic and mental complaints. Also, the PMS concept does not discriminate between mild symptoms and severe complaints. In contrast, the term 'premenstrual dysphoria' (PMD) usually implies that mood symptoms—such as irritability, depressed mood, and affect lability—are prominent, and that the condition is of such severity that it markedly influences work, social activities, or relationships with others. The term 'premenstrual dysphoric disorder' (PMDD) is equivalent to PMD, but should be used only when the condition has been diagnosed using certain criteria listed in the DSM-IV[1] (Table 16.1). In this review, the term PMD will be used to describe a disorder fulfilling either the criteria of PMDD or other, similar criteria.

Until recently, research on the clinical presentation, pathophysiology and treatment of PMD has been remarkably sparse as compared to that devoted to other psychiatric disorders. During the past 10 years, there has, however, been a marked increase in the scientific efforts in this area, and significant progress has been

Table 16.1 Diagnostic criteria for premenstrual dysphoric disorder (modified).[1]

A. Symptoms must occur during the week before menses and remit a few days after onset of menses in most menstrual cycles during the past year

Five of the following symptoms must be present and at least one must be 1, 2, 3 or 4
 1. Depressed mood or dysphoria
 2. Anxiety or tension
 3. Affective lability
 4. Irritability
 5. Decreased interest in usual activities
 6. Concentration difficulties
 7. Marked lack of energy
 8. Marked change in appetite, overeating or food cravings
 9. Hypersomnia or insomnia
 10. Feeling overwhelmed
 11. Other physical symptoms, i.e. breast tenderness, bloating

B. Symptoms must interfere with work, school, usual activities or relationships

C. Symptoms must not merely be an exacerbation of another disorder

D. Criteria A, B, or C must be confirmed by prospective daily ratings for at least two consecutive symptomatic menstrual cycles

made both with respect to the diagnosis and classification of different forms of premenstrual distress, and with respect to how these conditions can be effectively mastered by means of pharmacotherapy. In this chapter, the recent achievements in this area will be summarized and discussed.

Symptom cyclicity

To be defined as PMD (or PMS), the symptoms should appear regularly after ovulation or within the 2 weeks prior to the menstruation;[2,3] notably, some women experience a brief episode of symptoms around ovulation, followed by a few symptom-free days, and a recurrence of symptoms in the late luteal phase.

Often, the complaints reach a maximum during the last days before the bleeding. From days 4–5 of the cycle, and until the next ovulation, the symptoms should be absent; if they are not, other diagnoses should be considered.

Many psychiatric and somatic disorders may get worse during the luteal phase;[4–9] this phenomenon—which has been referred to as premenstrual magnification,[5] premenstrual exacerbation,[6] premenstrual aggravation,[8] or secondary PMS[9]—should be separated from genuine PMD (or PMS). The presence of symptoms during luteal phases that are completely absent during follicular phases ('on-offness') hence constitutes the cardinal pathognomonic feature of PMD (and PMS), and should always serve as a diagnostic criterion.

In some women who are convinced that they

suffer from PMS (or PMD), daily self-assessment of symptom severity during a number of consecutive menstrual cycles reveals that the symptoms are in fact unrelated to cycle phase. Thus, for a definite diagnosis, prospective symptom rating during at least two consecutive cycles is warranted.[2,5,10] There is agreement that such prospective confirmation of the diagnosis should be required in drug trials (see below); to what extent it should be applied also in the clinical setting—before treatment is initiated—is a matter of debate. According to the DSM-IV criteria of PMDD, the diagnosis must be confirmed by means of daily symptom rating for two symptomatic menstrual cycles.[1]

Symptom clusters

Many premenstrual symptoms have been described. Whereas irritability, anger, depressed mood, mood swings, affect lability, tension, anxiety, fatigue and food craving are frequently reported mental symptoms, a sense of bloating, breast tenderness, headache, cramps and acne seem to be the most common somatic complaints.[11-16]

Epidemiological studies have provided some support for the concept that all premenstrual complaints—mental as well as somatic—should be regarded as different manifestations of one disorder.[13,16] However, the fact that mood symptoms and somatic symptoms may correlate in epidemiological studies does not necessarily indicate that they should be regarded as parts of the same syndrome; rather, such a correlation may reflect merely a reduced tolerability to somatic symptoms in patients with dysphoria, and vice versa. Some authors have indeed suggested that disparate premenstrual complaints should be regarded as independent epiphenomena, each of them probably related to the hormonal cyclicity, but otherwise

unrelated to each other.[17,18] Supporting this point of view is the clinical observation that many patients with severe mental symptoms in the luteal phase are completely devoid of somatic complaints, whereas many subjects with symptoms such as breast tenderness or headache may experience no premenstrual changes in mood.

If indeed the biological mechanisms underlying somatic symptoms such as breast tenderness, headache, bloating and acne are different from those causing irritability, affect lability, and depressed mood, the search for biological markers and effective treatment may be marred by selecting subjects for these studies by means of the poorly defined PMS concept, or by using the sum of the ratings of many heterogeneous symptoms as a measure of severity. Until the putative interrelationship between different premenstrual complaints has been clarified, it is probably sensible not to regard all the disparate symptoms that may occur premenstrually as parts of the same disorder. In line with this reasoning, the PMDD diagnosis in DSM-IV is based on the assumption that a condition in which the premenstrual symptoms are mainly psychiatric in nature should be separated from a condition with merely somatic complaints; to fulfil the diagnostic criteria of PMDD, the patient thus must report at least one of the core mental symptoms, namely depressed mood, tension, affect lability, and anger/irritability.[1]

The relative clinical significance of the different mood symptoms characterizing PMD (and PMDD) remains to be established. Needless to say, the fact that a certain symptom is more frequently reported than others in epidemiological surveys does not imply that this symptom is the one that is most distressing in subjects with severe PMD. Whereas many researchers regard irritability as the cardinal symptom of PMD,[5,19] others have emphasized the importance of depressed mood, anxiety, affect lability and food craving.

It is important to underline that severe PMD is a condition that profoundly influences the life of the afflicted woman and her family.[20-22] An association between premenstrual complaints and suicidal ideation was recently reported.[23,24]

Epidemiology and aetiology

Premenstrual complaints have sometimes been regarded as a modern phenomenon, closely related to various cultural and social factors.[25,26] The suffering from mental and somatic complaints during the luteal phase of the menstrual cycle is, however, by no means unique to the Western civilization of today. Hippocrates (ancient Greece) noticed that women experience a feeling of 'heaviness' prior to menstruation,[27] Trotula of Salerno (11th-century Italy) noted that 'There are young women who suffer in the same manner who are relieved when the menses are called forth,'[28] and von Feuchtersleben (late 19th century) wrote that 'menstruation is always attended, in sensitive individuals, with mental uneasiness, which manifests itself according to the temperament, as irritability or sadness'.[29] The first modern-day description of a detailed premenstrual tension syndrome appeared in 1931, in which Frank reported that many women in the latter part of their menstrual cycle experience a state of 'indescribable tension'.[11] Moreover, epidemiological studies have revealed that premenstrual complaints are common in non-Western societies[30-36] unless the fertile women are 'protected' from such symptoms by being more or less constantly in a state of pregnancy or lactation.

Although sociological and cultural factors may influence the ability to cope with premenstrual symptoms, PMD should rather be regarded as a manifestation of the female biology than merely a cultural phenomenon. This assumption is supported also by studies suggesting PMD to be hereditary to a great extent,[37-39] and by the observation that premenstrual complaints can be abolished by inhibition of ovarian activity, and revived by the administration of sex steroids.[40] Moreover, cycle-related changes in behaviour have also been observed in non-human primates.[41,42]

Approximately 80% of all women report that they have experienced at least occasional psychological or somatic symptoms in association with the luteal phase of the menstrual cycle. In the vast majority of these women, the symptoms are, however, mild and insignificant; some women may even report positive changes during the luteal phase.[43] Severe symptoms and symptoms of such intensity that require medical attention have been reported in most epidemiological surveys to be in the range of 3–10% of all women of fertile age.[12,15,21,44-53]

However, most of these epidemiological studies have not used the DSM-IV definition of PMDD (or the DSM-III-R definition of late luteal phase dysphoric disorder, LLPDD[54]), nor have they used prospective confirmation of the diagnosis by means of daily symptom rating. In two studies that did use prospective ratings and DSM criteria, the prevalence of LLPDD was found to be 3.4% and 4.6%, respectively.[47,51]

Premenstrual complaints can make their debut at any time after menarche. A common clinical impression is that PMD and PMS tend to worsen with age until menopause; this impression has been confirmed by some workers[15] but not by others.[12,55,56] The average age of onset is believed to be 26.[56]

Relationship between PMD and other disorders

The lifetime prevalence of depression is higher in women with PMD than in controls.[7] This high comorbidity between PMD and depression, the notion that depressed mood is an important symptom in patients with PMD, and the observation that some antidepressant drugs are effective in the treatment of PMD, have led to the suggestion that the two conditions are different expressions of similar pathophysiological mechanisms.[46] However, it should be underlined that irritability and affect lability are cardinal symptoms of PMD but not of depression. Depression and PMD also clearly differ from each other with respect to biological markers[57] and genetics.[38] In addition, not all antidepressant drugs are effective in PMD, and those that are effective display a different clinical profile with respect to dosage and onset of action when they are used for PMD as compared to when they are used for depression (see below). Most researchers in this field tend to agree by now that PMD should not be regarded merely as a variant of depression.[58]

Some of the cardinal symptoms of PMD—such as irritability and food craving—are often reported by patients with seasonal affective disorder (SAD). The hypothesis that SAD and PMD may be related gains support from the observation that both conditions—in contrast to depression—are acutely relieved by administration of either of the two serotonin-releasing agents fenfluramine[59,60] or m-CPP.[61–64] Light therapy has been shown to be effective in SAD[65] and may tentatively also be of some benefit in PMD.[66]

The possible relationship between PMD and panic disorder is also of considerable interest.[6,67,68] Panic disorder may improve during pregnancy,[69] and some studies suggest that panic attacks may display a certain premenstrual aggravation.[6] Intravenous infusion of lactate or CCK-4 or inhalation of CO_2 elicits anxiety attacks not only in panic disorder subjects, but also in women with PMD;[70–73] moreover, a blunted benzodiazepine-induced reduction in saccadic eye movement has been reported both in patients with panic disorder[74] and in subjects with PMD.[75] Finally, both conditions respond to strikingly low doses of the non-selective but forceful serotonin reuptake inhibitor (SRI) clomipramine, to selective SRIs, and—to some extent—to the triazolobenzodiazepine alprazolam (see below).

Craving for carbohydrates, poor impulse control and depressed mood are prominent symptoms in some PMD subjects, and also in patients with bulimia nervosa. Further support for a relationship between PMD and bulimia nervosa is provided by the fact that bulimia is much more common in women than in men, by the observation that the symptoms of bulimia nervosa tend to aggravate premenstrually,[76] and by the finding that both conditions respond to SRIs.[77] Moreover, as discussed in Chapter 14, preliminary data suggest that some women with PMD as well as women with bulimia nervosa display relatively high levels of testosterone (see below).[78–80]

Pathophysiology
Sex steroids

Since the symptoms of PMS and PMD, by definition, are related to the menstrual cycle, the assumption that they are due to the influence of female sex steroids on the brain and on other organs is not farfetched[11,81] (see Chapters 5 and 13). As discussed below, the hypothesis that ovarian steroids are of importance for the pathophysiology of PMD is supported by the findings that premenstrual complaints are reduced by surgical ovariectomy as well as by drug-induced inhibition of ovulation; also, in subjects normally experiencing premenstrual distress, the symptoms are reported to be more intense in cycles with high peak levels of oestradiol and progesterone,[82] and absent during non-ovulatory cycles.[83]

It was previously assumed that premenstrual complaints were triggered by the reduction in serum levels of progesterone and/or oestradiol in the late luteal phase; PMD was regarded as a manifestation of 'steroid withdrawal'. This hypothesis is, however, challenged by the observation that administration of a progesterone antagonist during the late luteal phase neither reduces nor aggravates the symptoms;[84,85] likewise, luteal administration of oestrogen[86] or progesterone[87] is not an effective treatment for PMD. These and other observations suggest that the hormonal changes occurring during the late luteal phase are in fact irrelevant to the onset of premenstrual distress; rather, it may be assumed that premenstrual symptoms are initiated by the high mid-cycle peak of progesterone and/or oestradiol, and expressed with a delay of a few days or a week, independently of the subsequent changes in serum hormonal levels[88,89] (see Chapter 13).

Some authors have observed differences between PMD subjects and controls with respect to serum levels of gonadotrophins, oestradiol, and progesterone; however, other groups have failed to replicate these findings.[5,81,87,90] The assumption that PMD is not due to abnormal ovarian activity, but to an enhanced responsiveness to changes in hormonal levels, is supported by the observation that symptoms often persist in women treated with oral contraceptives.[91] Moreover, according to some[40] but not all[92,93,94] studies, a relapse in symptoms may be observed after administra-

tion of oestrogen or progesterone to women with PMD in whom the symptoms have first been abolished by means of an ovulation inhibitor. Also of interest in this context is the observation that sequential administration of oestrogen and progesterone may elicit PMD-like symptoms in menopausal women.[88,89]

Both animal experiments and clinical studies indicate that androgens may increase irritability and aggression in both males and females (see Chapter 14). In some[78,79] but not all[95,96] studies addressing this issue, androgen levels were found to be slightly higher in PMD subjects than in controls; moreover, in PMD women, serum levels of testosterone have been shown to correlate with the rating of irritability.[97] Supporting the assumption that an increased androgenicity may contribute to the pathophysiology of PMD, the combined androgen and aldosterone antagonist spironolactone may reduce the symptoms, particularly in subjects with elevated serum androgen levels in the luteal phase[98,99] (see below). The possible role of androgens in PMD is further discussed in Chapter 14.

Neurotransmitters

Animal experiments and clinical studies suggest that the brain neurotransmitter serotonin is of critical importance for the regulation of several of the symptoms characterizing PMD. Among the most striking behavioural effects of serotonin depletion in animals is an increase in irritability and aggression; conversely, drugs facilitating brain serotonergic neurotransmission (administered systemically or in discrete areas of the brain) have been shown to reduce aggressive behaviour in rats and mice.[100] An effect of serotonin on mood is also supported by the numerous studies showing that drugs facilitating brain serotonin neurotransmission have antidepressant effects, and that treatments reducing the serotonergic activity may induce or aggravate depression[100] (see Chapters 5, 13 and 29). Serotonin also seems to exert an inhibitory influence on food intake in general, and on carbohydrate craving in particular (see Chapter 25).

In line with the assumption that PMD may be related to serotonin, a number of biological abnormalities putatively related to brain serotonergic neurotransmission have been observed in women with PMD. The increase in serum levels of prolactin and/or cortisol after administration of the $5-HT_{1A}$ agonist buspirone,[101] the serotonin precursor tryptophan,[102] the serotonin-releasing agent fenfluramine[103] (but see also the study by Bancroft and Cook[104]) and the combined serotonin releaser and $5-HT_2$ agonist m-CPP[105,106] thus appear to be reduced in patients with PMD when compared to symptom-free controls. Also, studies using platelets from PMD subjects have revealed a reduced number of serotonin transporters, a reduction in serotonin uptake, and a reduced monoamine oxidase (MAO) activity; however, these findings have not been unanimous.[7,106] Cerebrospinal fluid (CSF) concentrations of the serotonin metabolite 5-hydroxyindoleacetic acid (5-HIAA) are not subnormal in women with PMD; rather, similarly to patients with depression, women with PMD may display a reduced ratio between the dopamine metabolite homovanillic acid (HVA) and 5-HIAA in CSF.[79] Both platelet paroxetine binding[97] and the CSF HVA/HIAA ratio[79] have been shown to correlate with serum levels of sex steroids.

Although the relationship between these putative markers of serotonergic function and the actual serotonergic activity in areas of the brain that regulate mood and irritability may be questioned, the large number of independent observations suggesting that women with PMD display serotonin-related abnormalities do indicate that PMD may indeed be related to a dysfunctional serotonergic neurotransmission; in particular, the findings of blunted hormonal responses to serotonergic probes in women with PMD seem relatively consistent. The major argument for the assumption that serotonin may be involved in the control of luteal dysphoria is however the fact that drugs facilitating serotonergic neurotransmission, such as the SRIs, are very effective in reducing the symptoms (Table 16.2) (see below). Also of considerable interest in this context is a report by Menkes et al[107] showing aggravation of irritability in PMD subjects exposed to a diet devoid of the serotonin precursor tryptophan.

The hypothesis that brain serotonin is of importance for the pathophysiology of PMD is by no means incompatible with the assumption that the symptoms are triggered by sex steroids. In animals, oestradiol, progesterone and testosterone have all been reported to influence serotonergic function and behaviours that are regulated by serotonin, such as sexual behaviour and aggression[108,109] (see Chapters 5, 12 and 13).

Apart from serotonin, several other brain neurotransmitters have been attributed importance for the pathophysiology of PMD. The anxiolytic effects of benzodiazepines appear to be mediated by an interaction with GABA receptors of the GABA A subtype, and a number of progesterone derivatives have also been shown to interact with the GABA A receptor complex in an anxiolytic-like manner.[8] Recent studies suggest that the levels of such putatively anxiolytic progesterone derivatives in the serum of PMD patients may be related to symptom severity;[110–113] also, the responsiveness of the GABA A receptor complex may be reduced in women with PMD[75] (see Chapter 5). Albeit difficult to interpret in terms of brain neurotransmission, it is noteworthy that PMD women may display reduced plasma levels of GABA in the luteal phase.[113] The potent benzodiazepine receptor agonist alprazolam has been shown to

Table 16.2 Effect of modulating brain serotonergic neurotransmission on the symptoms of premenstrual dysphoria (data from controlled trials).

Treatment	Mechanism of action	Effect in women with premenstrual dysphoria
Citalopram Clomipramine Fluoxetine Paroxetine Sertraline	Serotonin reuptake inhibition	Symptom reduction
Fenfluramine m-CPP	Serotonin release	Symptom reduction
Buspirone	5-HT$_{1A}$ receptor agonism	Symptom reduction
Tryptophan	Enhanced serotonin synthesis	Symptom reduction
Tryptophan-free diet	Impaired serotonin synthesis	Symptom aggravation

m-CPP; *m*-chlorophenylpiperazine

induce a reduction in PMD symptoms in some studies but not in others (see below).

A hypothesis suggesting that endogenous opioids are involved in the pathophysiology of PMD[114] inspired the use of naltrexone in a preliminary trial;[115] however, to our knowledge, no subsequent reports on the effect of opiate antagonism in PMD have been published.

The putative importance of noradrenaline for the regulation of depressed mood in the luteal phase is discussed below.

PMD drug trials: methodological aspects

Early drug trials in PMS research were often marred by methodological shortcomings such as imprecise inclusion criteria, heterogeneous patient populations, and questionable techniques for symptom registration. Today, most researchers in this field appear to have reached at least partial consensus as to how to evaluate treatment effects in PMD.[116]

Although various retrospective rating scales,[117,118] as well as the A–C criteria of PMDD in DSM-IV,[1] may be useful to obtain a preliminary diagnosis, the necessity for daily symptom rating in PMS/PMD research is now generally acknowledged; thus, only subjects displaying a clear menstruation-related cyclicity in symptomatology during at least two cycles of baseline symptom rating should be included in a PMD drug trial.[5] The required number of symptoms displaying cyclicity during the pretreatment reference cycles, the required magnitude of luteal worsening and the maximal symptom severity allowed in the follicular phase remain matters of debate.

Visual analogue scales (VAS) are easy to use and may increase rating compliance; they have also been found feasible for measuring changes in symptom severity over time.[2,67,119–123] Alternatively, one may use one of the several PMD rating scales that are designed to be used on a daily basis.[22,124,125]

Premenstrual complaints are probably more accurately assessed by the patient than by an independent observer. In most recent drug trials, self-rating of symptom severity has thus constituted the primary outcome measure. That an independent assessment of symptom severity should add useful information to the data registered by the patient herself remains to be demonstrated.

In most early drug trials, the total score of both mental and somatic symptoms was used as the primary outcome measure. This way of assessing efficacy would be appropriate if all symptoms occurring in the premenstrual phase were part of the same disorder, but is questionable when the different symptoms are not necessarily related to each other. Thus, a marked effect of a particular drug on one important premenstrual symptom may be masked by its lack of effect on other symptoms. For example, the dopamine receptor agonist bromocriptine, known as an effective treatment for patients in whom breast tenderness is the cardinal symptom,[126] will appear ineffective if only a minority of the patients investigated display this particular symptom, and if response is defined as the total reduction of a combination of somatic and mental complaints. It is therefore probably advisable when investigating the possible efficacy of a novel treatment to examine each symptom separately rather than using the sum of many disparate symptoms as the primary measure of outcome.

The possibility that even different mental symptoms characterizing patients with PMD do not respond uniformly to a certain treatment should be taken into consideration. Indeed, a selective noradrenaline reuptake inhibitor has been found to be considerably less effective than an SRI in reducing premenstrual irritability (and no better than placebo), but equally effective as the SRI in reducing premenstrual dysphoria.[121]

A definition of 'responder' allowing a comparison of the outcomes of independent PMD drug trials is warranted. According to a suggestion by Steiner et al,[122] 'moderate improvement' should be defined as a 50% reduction in the severity of one or several target symptoms (as measured by VAS), and 'marked improvement' as a 75% symptom reduction. In addition, a retrospective self-rating of improvement or deterioration is often useful as a measure of global efficacy.[67,120,121]

Treatment of PMD: hormones and antihormonal treatments

Inhibition of ovulation

Most (but not all) studies suggest that the symptoms of PMD are effectively reduced by inhibition of ovulation by gonadotrophin-releasing hormone (GnRH) analogues,[127–134] oestradiol implants or patches,[135–137] or danazol.[138] Likewise, surgical ovariectomy[139,140] appears to be effective. However, for the long-term management of PMD all these strategies are somewhat problematic. Treatments causing reduced levels of oestradiol, such as GnRH analogues or ovariectomy, may induce a variety of negative effects, including an enhanced risk of osteoporosis and cardiovascular disease, and therefore are not feasible for long-term treatment. To avoid these side-effects, the ovulation inhibitor may be combined with hormonal replacement ('add-back');[92,93,141] however, in some but not all patients, the administration of oestrogen and progesterone to GnRH-treated patients may lead to a relapse of symptoms.[40] Likewise, when ovulation is prevented by means of oestradiol implants or transdermal oestradiol patches, the cyclical addition of a progesterone analogue required to induce endometrial shedding may lead to a relapse of PMD-like complaints.[89,136] The combination of oestradiol patches and a progesterone-releasing intrauterine device as a treatment for PMD has been suggested by O'Brien et al;[9] this strategy appears attractive but remains to be evaluated.

Progesterone

For decades, administration of progesterone during the luteal phase was suggested to be the treatment of choice for PMS.[142] Well-designed, controlled investigations, however, challenge this assumption; progesterone seems no better than placebo for the treatment of premenstrual irritability and depressed mood, but may exert some effect on the somatic complaints.[87,143]

Oral contraceptives

The possible effect of oral contraceptives on the symptoms of PMS and PMD is a matter of debate; thus, symptom reduction and symptom aggravation, and lack of effect have all been reported. Oral contraceptives may reduce breast tenderness, but they probably have no beneficial effects on mood symptoms.[91]

Spironolactone

Spironolactone, an antagonist of aldosterone but also of testosterone, has been reported to induce a modest but significant reduction in premenstrual complaints.[144,145] Given the possibility that PMD is related to enhanced androgenicity (see Chapter 14), it is tempting to suggest that the beneficial effect of spironolactone observed in some patients may at least partly be due to the antiandrogenic properties of the drug.[98,99]

Treatment of PMD: serotonin reuptake inhibitors

Efficacy

As discussed above, the role of serotonin in the regulation of irritability/aggression, mood and food intake is well established.[100] Since depressed mood, irritability and food craving are all prominent symptoms of PMD, the suggestion that women with this disorder may benefit from treatment with drugs facilitating serotonergic neurotransmission, such as the SRIs, is by no means farfetched.

The first potent SRIs reported to be effective for the treatment of PMD were the non-selective, tricyclic antidepressant clomipramine[146] and the selective SRI fluoxetine;[147,148] subsequently, a large number of trials have almost unanimously confirmed that PMD can be effectively treated with SRIs.[124,149] Placebo-controlled trials have thus confirmed the efficacy not only of clomipramine[67] and fluoxetine,[64,148,150–154] but also of the selective SRIs paroxetine,[121] sertraline,[22,155] and citalopram.[19] In addition, the efficacy of fluoxetine,[156–160] paroxetine,[161,162] sertraline[163,164] the combined SRI and 5-HT$_2$ antagonist nefazodone,[165] and the combined serotonin + noradrenaline reuptake inhibitor venlafaxin (Yonkers et al, unpublished observation), is underpinned by numerous open trials. Only one controlled trial[166] has failed to demonstrate superiority of an SRI (fluvoxamine) over placebo; this study was, however, relatively small, and a more recent open trial suggests that fluvoxamine may indeed be effective.[167]

Most trials exploring the usefulness of SRIs for the treatment of PMD have been relatively small; however, as a definite confirmation of efficacy, two multicentre trials—each comprising about 100 patients per treatment group—demonstrated a clearcut superiority of fluoxetine[122] and sertraline,[22] respectively, over placebo. The latter of these trials also showed that treatment with an SRI not only reduces the symptoms of PMD, but also leads to an improvement in psychosocial functioning.

The response rate in most controlled trials using selective SRIs for PMD has been around 60% or higher. When selective SRIs have been tested in clinical trials for other disorders, such as depression, panic disorder, obsessive-compulsive disorder (OCD), social phobia, or bulimia nervosa, the response rate has usually been of the same magnitude, or lower. The SRIs are thus at least as effective for PMD as they are for other, more well-established indications.

In two small but placebo-controlled trials using low doses of the potent but non-selective SRI clomipramine, the response rate was higher than that usually reported for selective SRIs: all patients receiving clomipramine reported at least a moderate improvement, and 90% reported marked or enormous improvement.[67,120] One explanation of the high response rate in these studies could be that the patients were all characterized by marked irritability; possibly, irritability is one of the symptoms that responds most reliably to SRIs.[19] However, the possibility cannot be excluded that clomipramine is in fact somewhat superior to selective SRIs with respect to efficacy. Indeed, a superiority of clomipramine over selective SRIs for the treatment of depression[168] and OCD[169] has previously been suggested; a very high response rate has also been reported

when clomipramine has been administered to patients with panic disorder.[170] In order to confirm or reject the impression that clomipramine may be somewhat superior to the selective SRIs for the treatment of PMD, head-to-head comparisons are clearly warranted.

Potency

Like patients with panic disorder,[171,172] women with PMD[67,120,146] respond to considerably lower doses of clomipramine (10–50 mg/day) than those usually needed to achieve a maximal response in depression or OCD (i.e. 150–200 mg/day). Whether selective SRIs may also be given in lower doses when used for PMD than for depression or OCD remains to be established. To date, the only dose–response study undertaken with SRIs in PMD is the fluoxetine multicentre trial by Steiner et al,[122] showing that a daily dose of 60 mg fluoxetine had no advantage over a dose of 20 mg/day, and that patients on 60 mg/day had a higher incidence of side-effects.

Onset of action/intermittent administration

When used for the treatment of depression, panic disorder and OCD, SRIs are characterized by a lag phase of 1–4 weeks before inducing any marked improvement. In contrast, as shown in a trial in which clomipramine was administered intermittently (i.e. during luteal phases only) to women with PMD, the onset of action is much shorter (i.e. 1–2 days) for this condition.[120] The feasibility of intermittent administration of SRIs for PMD—supporting a short onset of action—has recently been confirmed in trials using sertraline,[163,164] fluoxetine[160] and citalopram[19] (Figure 16.1).

The difference between PMD and other indications with respect to onset of action of SRIs

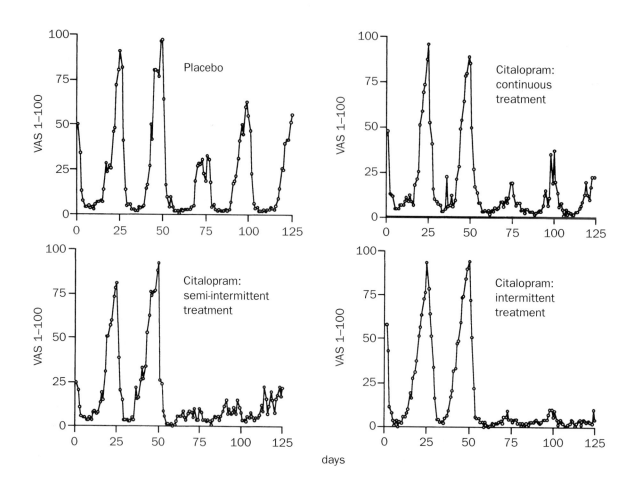

Figure 16.1 The effect of serotonin reuptake inhibitors in PMD is short in onset and probably the subject of some development of tolerance. Shown is daily self-rated irritability (VAS 1–100 mm; medians) during two reference cycles and three treatment cycles in subjects with premenstrual dysphoria treated with the selective SRI citalopram continuously (20 ± 10 mg/day throughout the cycle; n = 17)), semi-intermittently (20 ± 10 mg/day during luteal phases and 5 mg/day during follicular phases; n = 17), or intermittently (20 ± 10 mg/day during luteal phases and placebo during follicular phases; n = 18), or with placebo (n = 17). First day of menstruation occurred at days 1, 26, 51, 76 and 101. Supporting the assumption that intermittent administration during luteal phases only is more effective than continuous or semi-intermittent administration, the rating in the luteal phase of the last treatment cycle was significantly lower in the group given citalopram intermittently than in any of the other treatment groups (p < 0.01).[19]

is intriguing. As mentioned, the serotonin-releasing agents fenfluramine[60] and m-CPP[63,64] have both been reported to induce a rapid reduction in PMD symptomatology; in contrast, neither of these substances appears to induce an immediate symptom reduction in patients with depression, panic disorder or OCD. A rapid increase in synaptic concentrations of serotonin therefore seems to effectively reduce the symptoms of PMD, especially irritability, almost instantly, whereas a more prolonged facilitation of serotonergic neurotransmission is required to reduce the symptoms of depression, panic disorder, or OCD. That SRIs indeed cause a prompt increase in the synaptic levels of serotonin has been shown in animal experiments[173] and is also evident from the fact that in humans certain serotonin-related side-effects—such as nausea—are immediate in onset.

Tolerance

In a recent trial, intermittent administration of citalopram to women with PMD was found to be not only more effective than placebo, but also more effective than continuous administration of the drug (Figure 16.1).[19] This superiority in terms of efficacy of intermittent over continuous medication may lead to the suggestion that the beneficial effect of citalopram in PMD is characterized by a slight but rapid development of tolerance that can be avoided by repeated drug-free intervals.

It is possible that some SRIs are more inclined to display tolerance than others, and/or that the likelihood of tolerance development is related to dose. In the study showing intermittent administration of citalopram (20 ± 10 mg/day) to be superior to continuous administration, not only the symptom-reducing effect of continuous administration of citalopram, but also the sexual side-effects, were less pronounced in the third treatment cycle as compared to the first. In contrast, when another selective SRI, paroxetine, was given continuously (20 ± 10 mg/day), in a trial using identical design, both the symptom-reducing effect and the sexual side-effects were unabated

throughout the three cycles of treatment.[121] The two large-scale studies evaluating continuous fixed dosing of fluoxetine[122] and continuous flexible dosing of sertraline[22] were not designed to address this issue.

In most PMD trials, the treatment period has been six cycles or shorter; to clarify the issue of tolerance, longer trials are required. Three open trials using fluoxetine for ≥1 year (continuous treatment),[157–159] and one open 10-cycle trial using paroxetine (continuous or intermittent treatment),[162] suggest that the effect does not decline with time.

Effect on somatic symptoms

Given the well-established influence of serotonin on aggression and depressed mood, the observation that SRIs reduce symptoms such as irritability and dysphoria in women with PMD is not surprising. In contrast, an effect of SRIs on somatic premenstrual complaints, such as breast tenderness and bloating, would be less expected. Nevertheless, in most controlled trials, the SRI investigated has been more effective than placebo not only for psychological and behavioural symptoms, but also for somatic complaints.[67,121,123] Whether this effect is due to the fact that the somatic symptoms are perceived as less bothersome because of the SRI-induced reduction in irritability and depressed mood, or if the SRIs have a primary effect on somatic symptoms has yet to be determined.

Side-effects

In most PMD trials using selective SRIs, side-effects have been relatively mild and not different from those described for SRIs when used for other indications, i.e. nausea, sweating, sedation and sexual dysfunction. Whereas nausea and sedation usually decline during the course of treatment, anorgasmia and reduced libido appear to be more persistent[121,162] (but see also Wikander et al[19]). Thus, during continuous, long-term treatment of PMD with an SRI, sexual dysfunction is often a bothersome side-effect. In one open trial, the combined SRI and 5-HT$_2$ receptor antagonist nefazodone was shown to reduce the symptoms of PMD without causing sexual dysfunction;[165] in order to confirm these results, controlled trials evaluating the possible efficacy of nefazodone in PMD are warranted.

Like other tricyclic antidepressants, clomipramine displays affinity not only for the serotonin and noradrenaline transporters, but also for postsynaptic receptors for acetylcholine, histamine, serotonin (5-HT$_2$), and noradrenaline (alpha-1).[100] Clomipramine may therefore induce side-effects such as dry mouth, sedation and weight gain to a greater extent than do the selective SRIs. With the very low doses of clomipramine sufficient for the treatment of PMD, these side-effects, however, are usually tolerable.[67,120]

Further underlining the similarities between PMD and panic disorder (see above), some PMD subjects, like patients with panic disorder,[170] appear to be more sensitive to the initial anxiety-provoking effects of clomipramine than depressed patients. Consequently, when prescribing clomipramine for the treatment of PMD to a woman with no previous experience of this compound, it is advisable to start with a very low dose (5–10 mg/day). Initial anxiety provocation—which is always a transient side-effect—may be less common with selective SRIs than with clomipramine.

All SRI-induced side-effects vanish quickly when medication is stopped. For patients with SRI-induced sexual dysfunction—or any other bothersome side-effect—intermittent treatment during the luteal phase only may consequently be more acceptable than continuous administration. However, some patients on intermittent medication with an SRI may experience initial side-effects each time they start taking the drug, and others may display withdrawal symptoms when quickly tapering the drug after the onset of menstruation. Thus, when using SRIs for PMD, the treatment regimen should be individualized; whereas for some patients intermittent treatment is preferable, others may experience less side-effects when the compound is given continuously throughout the menstrual cycle. A third alternative is to give the drug in a semi-intermittent fashion, i.e. to give a very low dose during the follicular phase, and a higher dose from ovulation until the onset of menstruation.[19,162]

Treatment with SRIs does not usually have any major effects on the menstrual cyclicity. However, a high dose of fluoxetine (continuous treatment) has been reported to increase the cycle length variability significantly more than placebo.[174]

SRIs versus non-serotonergic antidepressants

In a controlled trial, a selective SRI, paroxetine, was shown to be significantly better than a selective noradrenaline reuptake inhibitor, maprotiline, in reducing premenstrual irritability, food craving, bloating, and breast tenderness; in addition, patients in the paroxetine group reported significantly greater global improvement than patients in the maprotiline group.[121] This clearcut superiority of paroxetine over maprotiline indicates that all antidepressants are not equally effective for the treatment of PMD. However, it should be noted that the maprotiline-treated group did not differ from the paroxetine-treated group with respect to reduction in depressed mood; thus, the possibility that noradrenaline reuptake inhibitors may selectively influence some of the symptoms of PMD, but not others, should not be excluded. The impression that the combined serotonin and noradrenaline reuptake inhibitor clomipramine may be somewhat more effective than selective SRIs lends further support for this assumption.

The assumption that serotonin reuptake inhibitors are more effective than antidepressants with a noradrenergic profile for the treatment of PMD was recently confirmed by a controlled trial showing a selective SRI, sertraline, to be clearly superior to a preferential noradrenaline reuptake inhibitor, desipramine.[163] Moreover, in another recent trial, desipramine was shown to be no more effective than an anticholinergic drug (methylscopolamine—used as placebo) for the treatment of PMD;[175] in a separate trial using similar design, the same investigators observed a marked symptom reduction when using fluoxetine.[151] Nortriptyline, a preferential noradrenaline reuptake inhibitor, has been shown to reduce premenstrual complaints; however, as judged by the data presented, the effect was less impressive than that usually obtained with SRIs.[176] Notably, desipramine and nortriptyline are preferential but—in contrast to maprotiline—not selective noradrenaline reuptake inhibitors; thus, to some extent, both also inhibit the uptake of serotonin.[100]

A superiority of SRIs over noradrenaline reuptake inhibitors has previously been reported for panic disorder, OCD, and OCD-related conditions such as trichotillomania and compulsive nail biting.[100] Of particular interest in this context is the observation by Gordon et al[177] that clomipramine is more effective than desipramine in reducing the symptom of anger in autistic patients. On the other hand, when used for the treatment of depression, strong SRIs are not superior to antidepressants with a noradrenergic profile.[100]

The notion that not all antidepressants are equally effective for PMD is supported by a recent small, but controlled trial showing fluoxetine to be more effective than bupropion, an antidepressant drug with an atypical profile preferentially interacting with noradrenaline and dopamine synapses.[153]

Mechanism of action of SRIs when used for PMD

The assumption that the SRI-induced reduction in premenstrual complaints is indeed due to inhibition of the serotonin transporter is based on the finding that all SRIs—regardless of molecular structure—appear to be effective. The observations that the serotonin-releasing agents fenfluramine and m-CPP,[60,63,64] and the serotonin precursor tryptophan,[178] may also reduce premenstrual complaints—and that tryptophan depletion may aggravate irritability in PMD women[107]— lend further support to the concept that serotonergic activity is indeed closely associated with the expression of PMD symptoms (Table 16.2).

The first reports regarding the efficacy of SRIs for the treatment of PMD were also the first to show that, in humans, symptoms such as irritability and affect lability may be reduced by serotonergic drugs. More recently, SRIs have, however, been reported to reduce symptoms such as irritability, aggression, anger, hostility, affect lability and pathological crying in patients with depression, personality disorders, schizophrenia, dementia disorders, autism, mental retardation, brain injury or stroke (for references, see Eriksson et al[121]). Although the majority of these trials have been open and thus need to be replicated under placebo-controlled conditions, taken together they strongly support the assumption that SRIs may reduce irritability, aggression and affect lability not only in women with PMD, but in a large variety of conditions. Of particular interest in this context is the preliminary observation that the effect of SRIs on symptoms such as irritability and affect lability seem to be characterized by a very short onset of action, not only in women with PMD, but also in patients with other diagnoses.[179–182]

In animal experiments, as well as in clinical studies, the 5-HT$_{1A}$ receptor agonist buspirone has been shown to reduce various forms of aggression and affect lability.[183] The preliminary finding that buspirone may also be effective for PMD[184] suggests that the influence of serotonin on PMD is at least partly mediated by postsynaptic 5-HT$_{1A}$ receptors. The putative involvement of the many other subtypes of postsynaptic serotonin receptors[100] in mediating the beneficial effects of SRIs in PMD remains to be explored.

To conclude, there are several arguments supporting the notion that the effect of SRIs in PMD is not equivalent to the antidepressant effects of these compounds: (1) not all antidepressants are effective for PMD; (2) the doses of clomipramine required for the treatment of PMD are much lower than those usually required for the treatment of depression; (3) the onset of action is entirely different when SRIs are used for PMD and depression, respectively; and (4) buspirone, fenfluramine and m-CPP are effective for PMD, but not for depression. Thus, although inhibition of the serotonin transporter is probably the mode of action of SRIs when used for both depression and for PMD, the antidepressant effect and the effect in PMD are probably mediated by different synapses and by different postsynaptic serotonin receptors. The impressive efficacy of SRIs in PMD should thus not be taken as support for the concept that PMD is to be regarded as a variant of depression. With respect to the fast onset of action of SRIs, the superiority of SRIs over noradrenergic antidepressants, and the efficacy of buspirone, PMD appears in fact to

be more related to other conditions characterized by irritability or affect lability than to major depressive disorder.

Other treatments

A variety of pharmacological treatments have been claimed to have efficacy in PMS and/or PMD. However, for severe PMD, no drugs apart from those inhibiting ovulation and those facilitating serotonin transmission have been shown to be clearly effective.

The triazolobenzodiazepine alprazolam has been shown to be effective in some controlled trials; however, two trials failed to detect any superiority of alprazolam over placebo.[87] Due to the risk of physical dependence, benzodiazepines should be used for PMD only by way of exception.

The possible efficacy of the dopamine receptor agonist bromocriptine for the treatment of PMS or PMD has been evaluated in a large number of trials. The drug does seem to reduce breast tenderness—probably by inhibiting the release of prolactin—but appears to be ineffective for other premenstrual complaints.[126]

Preliminary data suggested that the alpha-2 receptor agonist clonidine may reduce premenstrual complaints;[185] however, in a controlled trial, no difference between clonidine and placebo could be demonstrated (Eriksson et al, unpublished). Likewise, the suggestion that lithium is effective for PMD has not been verified.[186]

The efficacy of pyridoxine (vitamin B$_6$) for the treatment of PMD is not impressive but probably slightly better than that of placebo.[187] Notably, pyridoxine is a cofactor for an enzyme of importance for the synthesis of serotonin (tryptophan hydroxylase).[100]

The naturopathic drug evening primrose oil is marketed for PMD in many countries, but is no more effective than placebo.[188]

Conclusion

PMD (PMDD, LLPDD) afflicts approximately 5% of all women of fertile age and is characterized by symptoms such as irritability, depressed mood and affect lability that are of such severity that they markedly influence work, social activities, or relationships with others. The symptoms surface regularly in the luteal phase and disappear within a few days after the onset of menstruation, and may or may not be accompanied by somatic complaints such as breast tenderness and bloating. PMD should not be confused with a condition in which the premenstrual complaints are mild and clinically insignificant; also, it should be separated from a condition in which somatic complaints are predominant. Although PMD is probably related to the influence of sex steroids on brain neurotransmission, the reason why some women are afflicted by PMD while others are not is still unknown. Drugs of choice for the treatment of severe PMD are the SRIs; these compounds induce a satisfying reduction in mood symptoms in a majority of patients, and have a beneficial effect on the somatic complaints as well. SRIs can be administered either continuously throughout the menstrual cycle or intermittently during the luteal phase only. Side-effects are usually mild, reduced libido and anorgasmia being the most bothersome. For patients not responding to the SRIs, various pharmacological strategies leading to an inhibition of ovulation may be considered.

References

1. American Psychiatric Association, *Diagnostic and Statistical Manual of Mental Disorders*, 4th edn (APA Press: Washington DC, 1994) 715–18.
2. Rubinow DR, Roy-Byrne P, Hoban MC et al, Premenstrual mood changes. Characteristic patterns in women with and without premenstrual syndrome, *J Affect Disord* 1986; **10**:85–90.
3. Severino SK, Hurt SW, Schindledecker RD, Spectral analysis of cyclic symptoms in late luteal phase dysphoric disorder, *Am J Psychiatry* 1989; **146**:1155–60.
4. Endicott J, The menstrual cycle and mood disorders, *J Affect Disord* 1993; **29**:193–200.
5. Korzekwa MI, Steiner M, Premenstrual syndromes, *Clin Obstet Gynecol* 1997; **40**:564–76.
6. Yonkers KA, Anxiety symptoms and anxiety disorders: how are they related to premenstrual disorders? *J Clin Psychiatry* 1997; **58** (suppl 3):62–7.
7. Yonkers KA, The association between premenstrual dysphoric disorder and other mood disorders, *J Clin Psychiatry* 1997; **58** (suppl 15):19–25.
8. Bäckström T, Hammarbäck S, Premenstrual syndrome—psychiatric or gynaecological disorder, *Ann Med* 1991; **23**:625–33.
9. O'Brien PMS, Abukhalil IEH, Henshaw C, Premenstrual syndrome, *Curr Obstet Gynaecol* 1995; **5**:30–5.
10. Endicott J, Halbreich U, Retrospective report of premenstrual depressive changes: factors affecting confirmation by daily ratings, *Psychopharmacol Bull* 1982; **18**:109–23.
11. Frank RT, Hormonal causes of premenstrual tension, *Arch Neurol Psychiatry* 1931; **26**:1053–7.
12. Andersch B, Wendestam C, Hahn L, Öhman R, Premenstrual complaints. I. Prevalence of premenstrual symptoms in a Swedish urban population, *J Psychosom Obstet Gynaecol* 1986; **5**:39–49.
13. Magos AL, Brincat M, Studd JW, Trend analysis of the symptoms of 150 women with a history of the premenstrual syndrome, *Am J Obstet Gynecol* 1986; **155**:277–82.

14. Hurt SW, Schnurr PP, Severino SK, Late luteal phase dysphoric disorder in 670 women evaluated for premenstrual complaints, *Am J Psychiatry* 1992; **149**:525–30.

15. Merikangas KR, Foeldenyi M, Angst J, The Zurich Study. XIX. Patterns of menstrual disturbances in the community: results of the Zurich Cohort Study, *Eur Arch Psychiatry Clin Neurosci* 1993; **243**:23–32.

16. Jorgensen J, Rossignol AM, Bonnlander H, Evidence against multiple premenstrual syndromes: results of a multivariate profile analysis of premenstrual symptomatology, *J Psychosom Res* 1993; **37**:257–63.

17. Endicott J, Nee J, Cohen J, Halbreich U, Premenstrual changes: patterns and correlates of daily ratings, *J Affect Disord* 1986; **10**: 127–35.

18. Brown WA, Commentary on 'Menstrually related disorders: point of consensus, debate, and disagreement', *Neuropsychopharmacology* 1993; **9**:23–4.

19. Wikander I, Sundblad C, Andersch B et al, Citalopram in premenstrual dysphoria: is intermittent treatment during luteal phases more effective than continuous medication throughout the menstrual cycle? *J Clin Psychopharmacol* 1998; **18**:390–8.

20. Kuczmierczyk AR, Labrum AH, Johnson CC, Perception of family and work environments in women with premenstrual syndrome, *J Psychosom Res* 1992; **36**:787–95.

21. Brown WJ, Doran FM, Women's health: consumer views for planning local health promotion and health care priorities, *Aust NZ J Public Health* 1996; **20**:149–54.

22. Yonkers KA, Halbreich U, Freeman E et al, Symptomatic improvement of premenstrual dysphoric disorder with sertraline treatment. A randomized controlled trial, *JAMA* 1997; **278**:983–8.

23. Chaturvedi SK, Chandra PS, Gururaj G et al, Suicidal ideas during premenstrual phase, *J Affect Disord* 1995; **34**:193–9.

24. Endicott J, Halbreich U, Clinical significance of premenstrual dysphoric changes, *J Clin Psychiatry* 1988; **49**:486–9.

25. Johnson TM, Premenstrual syndrome as a western culture-specific disorder, *Cult Med Psychiatry* 1987; **11**:337–56.

26. Gurevich M, Rethinking the label: who benefits from the PMS construct? *Women Health* 1995; **23**:67–98.

27. Simon B, *Mind and Madness in Ancient Greek* (Cornell University Press: Ithaca, NY, 1978) 273.

28. Mason-Hohl E, *The Diseases of Women by Trotula of Salerno*, (The Ward Ritchie Press: Los Angeles, 1940).

29. von Feuchtersleben E, *The Principles of Medical Psychology* (Sydenham Society: London, 1847) 182.

30. Janiger O, Riffenburgh R, Kersh R, Cross cultural study of premenstrual symptoms, *Psychosomatics* 1972; **13**:226–35.

31. Mao K, Chang A, The premenstrual syndrome in Chinese, *Aust NZ J Obstet Gynaecol* 1985; **25**:118–20.

32. Cenac A, Maikibi DK, Develoux M, Premenstrual syndrome in Sahelian Africa. A comparative study of 400 literate and illiterate women in Niger, *Trans R Soc Trop Med Hyg* 1987; **81**:544–7.

33. Rupani NP, Lema VM, Premenstrual tension among nurses in Nairobi, Kenya, *East Afr Med J* 1993; **70**:310–13.

34. Fakeye O, Adegoke A, The characteristics of the menstrual cycle in Nigerian schoolgirls and the implications for school health programmes, *Afr J Med Sci* 1994; **23**:13–17.

35. Chang AM, Holroyd E, Chau JP, Premenstrual syndrome in employed Chinese women in Hong Kong, *Health Care Women Int* 1995; **16**:551–61.

36. Yu M, Zhu X, Li J et al, Perimenstrual symptoms among Chinese women in an urban area of China, *Health Care Women Int* 1996; **17**:161–72.

37. Kendler KS, Silberg JL, Neale MC et al, Genetic and environmental factors in the aetiology of menstrual, premenstrual and neurotic symptoms: a population-based twin study, *Psychol Med* 1992; **22**:85–100.

38. Condon JT, The premenstrual syndrome: a twin study, *Br J Psychiatry* 1993; **162**:481–6.

39. Kendler KS, Karkowski LM, Corey LA, Neale MC, Longitudinal population-based twin study of retrospectively reported premenstrual symptoms and lifetime major depression, *Am J Psychiatry* 1998; **155**:1234–40.

40. Schmidt PJ, Nieman LK, Danaceau MA et al, Differential behavioral effects of gonadal steroids in women with and in those without premenstrual syndrome, *N Engl J Med* 1998; **338**:209–16.

41. Rapkin AJ, Pollack DB, Raleigh MJ et al, Menstrual cycle and social behavior in vervet monkeys, *Psychoneuroendocrinology* 1995; **20**:289–97.

42. Haufstater G, Skoblick B, Perimenstrual behaviour changes among female yellow baboons: some similarities to premenstrual syndrome (PMS) in women, *Am J Primatol* 1985; **9**:165–72.

43. Stewart DE, Positive changes in the premenstrual period, *Acta Psychiatr Scand* 1989; **79**:400–5.

44. Woods NF, Most A, Dery GK, Prevalence of perimenstrual symptoms, *Am J Public Health* 1982; **72**:1257–64.

45. Logue CM, Moos RH, Perimenstrual symptoms: prevalence and risk factors, *Psychosom Med* 1986; **48**:388–414.

46. Hallman J, The premenstrual syndrome—an equivalent of depression? *Acta Psychiatr Scand* 1986; **73**:403–11.

47. Haskett RF, DeLongis A, Kessler RC, Premenstrual dysphoria: a Community survey, *Annual American Psychiatric Association Meeting* 1987, Chicago, Illinois.

48. Johnson SR, The epidemiology and social impact of premenstrual symptoms, *Clin Obstet Gynecol* 1987; **30**:367–76.

49. Busch CM, Costa PT Jr, Whitehead WE, Heller BR, Severe perimenstrual symptoms: prevalence and effects on absenteeism and health care seeking in a non-clinical sample, *Women Health* 1988; **14**:59–74.

50. Johnson SR, McChesney C, Bean JA, Epidemiology of premenstrual symptoms in a nonclinical sample. I. Prevalence, natural history and help-seeking behavior, *J Reprod Med* 1988; **33**:340–6.

51. Rivera-Tovar AD, Frank E, Late luteal phase dysphoric disorder in young women, *Am J Psychiatry* 1990; **147**:1634–6.

52. Ramcharan S, Love EJ, Fick GH, Goldfien A, The epidemiology of premenstrual symptoms in a population based sample of 2650 urban women. Attributable risk and risk factors, *J Clin Epidemiol* 1992; **45**:377–92.

53. Campbell EM, Peterkin D, O'Grady K, Sanson-Fisher R, Premenstrual symptoms in general practice patients. Prevalence and treatment, *J Reprod Med* 1997; **42**:637–46.

54. American Psychiatric Association, *Diagnostic and Statistical Manual of Mental Disorders*, 3rd edn, revised (APA Press: Washington DC, 1987) 367–9.

55. Metcalf MG, Braiden V, Livesey JH, Symptom cyclicity in women with the premenstrual syndrome: an 8-year follow-up study, *J Psychosom Res* 1992; **36**:237–41.

56. Freeman EW, Rickels K, Schweizer E, Ting T, Relationships between age and symptom severity among women seeking medical treatment for premenstrual symptoms, *Psychol Med* 1995; **25**:309–15.

57. Haskett RF, Steiner M, Carroll BJ, A psychoendocrine study of premenstrual tension syndrome. A model for endogenous depression? *J Affect Disord* 1984; **6**:191–9.

58. Endicott J, Amsterdam J, Eriksson E et al, Is premenstrual dysphoric disorder a distinct clinical entity? *J Women's Health* 1999; **8**:663–79.

59. O'Rourke D, Wurtman JJ, Wurtman RJ et al, Treatment of seasonal depression with d-fenfluramine, *Clin Psychiatry* 1989; **50**:343–7.

60. Brzezinski AA, Wurtman JJ, Wurtman RJ et al, d-Fenfluramine suppresses the increased calorie and carbohydrate intake and improves the mood of women with premenstrual depression, *Obstet Gynecol* 1990; **76**:296–301.

61 Schwartz PJ, Murphy DL, Wehr TA et al, Effects of meta-chlorophenylpiperazine infusions in patients with seasonal affective disorder and healthy control subjects. Diurnal responses and nocturnal regulatory mechanisms, *Arch Gen Psychiatry* 1997; **54**:375–85.

62. Jacobsen FM, Mueller EA, Rosenthal NE et al, Behavioral responses to intravenous metachlorophenylpiperazine in patients with seasonal affective disorder and control subjects before and after phototherapy, *Psychiatry Res* 1994; **52**:181–97.

63. Su T-P, Schmidt PJ, Danaceau M et al, Effect of menstrual cycle phase on neuroendocrine and behavioral responses to the serotonin agonist m-chlorophenylalanine in women with premenstrual syndrome and controls, *J Clin Endocrin Metab* 1997; **82**:1220–8.

64. Su T-P, Schmidt P, Danaceau M et al, Fluoxetine in the treatment of premenstrual dysphoria, *Neuropsychopharmacology* 1997; 16:346–56.

65. Rosenthal NE, Sack DA, Carpenter CJ et al, Antidepressant effects of light in seasonal affective disorder, *Am J Psychiatry* 1985; 142:163–70.

66. Parry BL, Mahan AM, Mostofi N et al, Light therapy of late luteal phase dysphoric disorder: an extended study, *Am J Psychiatry* 1993; 150:1417–19.

67. Sundblad C, Modigh K, Andersch B, Eriksson E, Clomipramine effectively reduces premenstrual irritability and dysphoria: a placebo-controlled trial, *Acta Psychiatr Scand* 1992; 85:39–47.

68. Klein DF, False suffocation alarms, spontaneous panics, and related conditions. An integrative hypothesis, *Arch Gen Psychiatry* 1993; 50:306–17.

69. George DT, Ladenheim JA, Nuff DJ, Effect of pregnancy on panic attacks, *Am J Psychiatry* 1987; 144:1078–9.

70. Harrison WM, Sandberg D, Gorman JM et al, Provocation of panic with carbon dioxide inhalation in patients with premenstrual dysphoria, *Psychiatry Res* 1989; 27:183–92.

71. Facchinetti F, Romano G, Fava M, Genazzani AR, Lactate infusion induces panic attacks in patients with premenstrual syndrome, *Psychosom Med* 1992; 54:288–96.

72. Sandberg D, Endicott J, Harrison W et al, Sodium lactate infusion in late luteal phase dysphoric disorder, *Psychiatry Res* 1993; 46:79–88.

73. Le Melledo JM, Bradwejn J, Koszycki D, Bichet D, Premenstrual dysphoric disorder and response to cholecystokinin-tetrapeptide, *Arch Gen Psychiatry* 1995; 52:605–6.

74. Roy-Byrne P, Wingerson DK, Radant A et al, Reduced benzodiazepine sensitivity in patients with panic disorder: comparison with patients with obsessive-compulsive disorder and normal subjects, *Am J Psychiatry* 1996; 153:1444–9.

75. Sundström I, Nyberg S, Bäckström T, Patients with premenstrual syndrome have reduced sensitivity to midazolam compared to control subjects, *Neuropsychopharmacology* 1997; 17: 370–81.

76. Gladis MM, Walsh BT, Premenstrual exacerbation of binge eating in bulimia, *Am J Psychiatry* 1987; 144:1592–5.

77. Fluoxetine Bulimia Nervosa Collaborative Study Group, Fluoxetine in the treatment of bulimia nervosa. A multicenter, placebo-controlled, double-blind trial, *Arch Gen Psychiatry* 1992; 49:139–47.

78. Eriksson E, Sundblad C, Lisjö P et al, Serum levels of androgens are higher in women with premenstrual irritability and dysphoria than in controls, *Psychoneuroendocrinology* 1992; 17: 195–204.

79. Eriksson E, Alling C, Andersch B et al, Cerebrospinal fluid levels of monoamine metabolites, *Neuropsychopharmacology* 1994; 11:201–13.

80. Sundblad C, Bergman L, Eriksson E, High levels of free testosterone in women with bulimia nervosa, *Acta Psychiatr Scand* 1994; 90:397–8.

81. Rubinow DR, Schmidt PJ, The neuroendocrinology of menstrual cycle mood disorders, *Ann NY Acad Sci* 1995; 771:648–59.

82. Hammarbäck S, Damber JE, Bäckström T, Relationship between symptom severity and hormone changes in women with premenstrual syndrome, *J Clin Endocrinol Metab* 1989; 68:125–30.

83. Hammarbäck S, Ekholm UB, Bäckström T, Spontaneous anovulation causing disappearance of cyclical symptoms in women with the premenstrual syndrome, *Acta Endocrinol* 1991; 125:132–7.

84. Schmidt PJ, Nieman LK, Grover GN et al, Lack of effect of induced menses on symptoms in women with premenstrual syndrome, *N Engl J Med* 1991; 324:1174–9.

85. Chan AF, Mortola JF, Wood SH, Yen SS, Persistence of premenstrual syndrome during low-dose administration of the progesterone antagonist RU 486, *Obstet Gynecol* 1994; 84:1001–5.

86. Dhar V, Murphy BE, Double-blind randomized crossover trial of luteal phase oestrogens (Premarin®) in the premenstrual syndrome (PMS), *Psychoneuroendocrinology* 1990; 15:489–93.

87. Freeman EW, Rickels K, Sondheimer SJ, Polansky M, Ineffectiveness of progesterone suppository treatment for premenstrual syndrome, *JAMA* 1990; 264:349–53.

88. Hammarbäck S, Bäckström T, Holst J et al, Cyclical mood changes as in the premenstrual tension syndrome during sequential oestrogen–progestagen postmenopausal replacement therapy, *Acta Obstet Gynecol Scand* 1985; **64**:393–7.

89. Magos AL, Brewster E, Singh R et al, The effects of norethisterone in postmenopausal women on oestrogen replacement therapy: a model for the premenstrual syndrome, *Br J Obstet Gynaecol* 1986; **93**:1290–6.

90. Bancroft J, The premenstrual syndrome—a reappraisal of the concept and the evidence, *Psychol Med* 1993; (suppl 24):1–47.

91. Bancroft J, Rennie D, The impact of oral contraceptives on the experience of perimenstrual mood, clumsiness, food craving and other symptoms, *J Psychosom Res* 1993; **37**: 195–202.

92. Leather AT, Studd JW, Watson NR, Holland EF, The treatment of severe premenstrual syndrome with goserelin with and without 'add-back' estrogen therapy: a placebo-controlled study, *Gynecol Endocrinol* 1999; **13**:48–55.

93. Mortola JF, Girton L, Fischer U, Successful treatment of severe premenstrual syndrome by combined use of gonadotropin-releasing hormone agonist and estrogen/progestin, *J Clin Endocrinol Metab* 1991; **72**:252A–F.

94. Henshaw C, Foreman D, Belcher J et al, Can one induce premenstrual symptomatology in women with prior hysterectomy and bilateral oophorectomy? *J Psychosom Obstet Gynaecol* 1996; **17**:21–8.

95. Bäckström T, Aakvaagt A, Plasma prolactin and testosterone during the luteal phase in women with premenstrual tension syndrome, *Psychoneuroendocrinology* 1981; **6**:245–51.

96. Bloch M, Schmidt PJ, Su TP et al, Pituitary-adrenal hormones and testosterone across the menstrual cycle in women with premenstrual syndrome and controls, *Biol Psychiatry* 1998; **43**:897–903.

97. Steiner M, Coote M, Wilkins A, Dunn E, Biological correlates of irritability in women with premenstrual dysphoria, *Eur Neuropsychopharmacol* 1997; 7 (suppl 2): S172.

98. Burnet RB, Radden HS, Easterbrook EG, McKinnon RA, Premenstrual syndrome and spironolactone, *Aust NZ J Obstet Gynaecol* 1991; **31**:366–8.

99. Rowe T, Sasse V, Androgens and premenstrual symptoms—the response to therapy. In: Deneerstein L, Frazer I, eds, *Hormones and Behaviour* (Elsevier: Amsterdam, 1986) 160–5.

100. Eriksson E, Humble M, Serotonin in psychiatric pathophysiology. A review of data from experimental and clinical research. In: Pohl R, Gershon S, eds, *The Biological Basis of Psychiatric Treatment* (Karger: Basel, 1990) 66–119.

101. Yatham LN, Is 5HT1A receptor subsensitivity a trait marker for late luteal phase dysphoric disorder? A pilot study, *Can J Psychiatry* 1993; **38**:662–4.

102. Bancroft J, Cook A, Davidson D et al, Blunting of neuroendocrine responses to infusion of L-tryptophan in women with perimenstrual mood change, *Psychol Med* 1991; **21**: 305–12.

103. FitzGerald M, Malone KM, Li S et al, Blunted serotonin response to fenfluramine challenge in premenstrual dysphoric disorder, *Am J Psychiatry* 1997; **154**:556–8.

104. Bancroft J, Cook A, The neuroendocrine response to d-fenfluramine in women with premenstrual depression, *J Affect Disord* 1995; **36**:57–64.

105. Halbreich U, Gonadal hormones and antihormones, serotonin and mood, *Psychopharmacol Bulletin* 1990; **26**:291–5.

106. Rapkin AJ, The role of serotonin in premenstrual syndrome, *Clin Obstet Gynecol* 1992; **35**:629–36.

107. Menkes DB, Coates DC, Fawcett JP, Acute tryptophan depletion aggravates premenstrual syndrome, *J Affect Disord* 1994; **32**:37–44.

108. Steiner M, The effects of gonadal hormones on brain and behavior, *Prog Neuropsychopharmacol Biol Psychiatry* 1987; **11**:115–19.

109. Sundblad C, Eriksson E, Reduced extracellular levels of serotonin in the amygdala of androgenized female rats, *Eur Neuropsychopharmacol* 1997; **7**:253–9.

110. Wang M, Seippel L, Purdy RH, Bäckström T, Relationship between symptom severity and steroid variation in women with premenstrual syndrome, *J Clin Endocrinol Metab* 1996; **81**:1076–82.

111. Rapkin AJ, Morgan M, Goldman L et al,

Progesterone metabolite allopregnanolone in women with premenstrual syndrome, *Obstet Gynecol* 1997; **90**:709–14.

112. Schmidt PJ, Purdy RH, Moore PH Jr et al, Circulating levels of anxiolytic steroids in the luteal phase in women with premenstrual syndrome and in control subjects, *J Clin Endocrinol Metab* 1994; **79**:1256–60.

113. Halbreich U, Petty F, Yonkers K et al, Low plasma gamma-aminobutyric acid levels during the late luteal phase of women with premenstrual dysphoric disorder, *Am J Psychiatry* 1996; **153**:718–20.

114. Rapkin AJ, Shoupe D, Reading A et al, Decreased central opioid activity in premenstrual syndrome: luteinizing hormone response to naloxone, *J Soc Gynecol Invest* 1996; **3**:93–8.

115. Chuong CJ, Coulam CB, Bergstralh EJ et al, Clinical trial of naltrexone in premenstrual syndrome, *Obstet Gynecol* 1988; **72**:332–6.

116. Steiner M, Wilkins A, Diagnosis and assessment of premenstrual dysphoria, *Psychiatr Ann* 1996; **26**:571–5.

117. Steiner M, Haskett RF, Carroll BJ, Premenstrual tension syndrome: the development of research diagnostic criteria and new rating scales, *Acta Psychiatr Scand* 1980; **62**:177–90.

118. Halbreich U, Endicott J, Schacht S, Nee J, The diversity of premenstrual changes as reflected in the premenstrual assessment form, *Acta Psychiatr Scand* 1982; **65**:46–65.

119. Steiner M, Streiner DL, Steinberg S et al, The measurement of premenstrual mood symptoms, *J Affective Dis* 1999; **53**:269–73.

120. Sundblad C, Hedberg MA, Eriksson E, Clomipramine administered during the luteal phase reduces the symptoms of premenstrual syndrome: a placebo-controlled trial, *Neuropsychopharmacology* 1993; **9**:133–45.

121. Eriksson E, Hedberg MAA, Andersch B, Sundblad C, The serotonin reuptake inhibitor paroxetine is superior to the noradrenaline reuptake inhibitor maprotiline in the treatment of premenstrual syndrome: a placebo-controlled trial, *Neuropsychopharmacology* 1995; **12**: 167–76.

122. Steiner M, Steinberg S, Stewart D et al, Fluoxetine in the treatment of premenstrual dysphoria. Canadian Fluoxetine/Premenstrual Dysphoria Collaborative Study Group, *N Engl J Med* 1995; **332**:1529–34.

123. Steiner M, Romano S, Babcock S, Fluoxetine's efficacy in improving physical symptoms associated with PMDD, *Eur Neuropsychopharmacol* 1999; **9**:S208.

124. Yonkers KA, Antidepressants in the treatment of premenstrual dysphoric disorder, *J Clin Psychiatry* 1997; **58** (suppl 14):4–10.

125. Thys-Jacobs S, Alvir JM, Fratarcangelo P, Comparative analysis of three PMS assessment instruments – the identification of premenstrual syndrome with core symptoms, *Psychopharmacol Bull* 1995; **31**:389–96.

126. Andersch B, Bromocriptine and premenstrual symptoms: a survey of double blind trials, *Obstet Gynecol Surv* 1983; **38**:643–6.

127. Muse KN, Cetel NS, Futterman LA, Yen SC, The premenstrual syndrome. Effects of 'medical ovariectomy', *N Engl J Med* 1984; **311**:1345–9.

128. Bancroft J, Boyle H, Warner P, Fraser HM, The use of an LHRH agonist, buserelin, in the long-term management of premenstrual syndromes, *Clin Endocrinol* 1987; **27**:171–82.

129. Hammarbäck S, Bäckström T, Induced anovulation as treatment of premenstrual tension syndrome. A double-blind cross-over study with GnRH agonist versus placebo, *Acta Obstet Gynecol Scand* 1988; **67**:159–62.

130. Helvacioglu A, Yeoman RR, Hazelton JM, Aksel S, Premenstrual syndrome and related hormonal changes: long-acting gonadotropin releasing hormone agonist treatment, *J Reprod Med* 1993; **38**:864–70.

131. Hussain SY, Massil JH, Matta WH et al, Buserelin in premenstrual syndrome, *Gynecol Endocrinol* 1992; **6**:57–64.

132. Freeman EW, Sondheimer SJ, Rickels K, Albert J, Gonadotropin-releasing hormone agonist in treatment of premenstrual symptoms with and without comorbidity of depression: a pilot study, *J Clin Psychiatry* 1993; **54**:192–5.

133. West CP, Hillier H, Ovarian suppression with the gonadotrophin-releasing hormone agonist goserelin (Zoladex) in management of the premenstrual tension syndrome, *Hum Reprod* 1994; **9**:1058–63.

134. Brown CS, Ling FW, Andersen RN et al,

Efficacy of depot leuprolide in premenstrual syndrome: effect of symptom severity and type in a controlled trial, *Obstet Gynecol* 1994; 84:779–86.

135. Magos AL, Brincat M, Studd JW, Treatment of the premenstrual syndrome by subcutaneous oestradiol implants and cyclical oral norethisterone: placebo controlled study, *Br Med J* 1986; 292:1629–33.

136. Watson NR, Studd JW, Savvas M et al, Treatment of severe premenstrual syndrome with oestradiol patches and cyclical oral norethisterone, *Lancet* 1989; 23:730–2.

137. Smith RN, Studd JW, Zamblera D, Holland EFN, A randomized comparison over 8 months of 100 μg and 200 μg twice weekly doses of transdermal oestradiol in the treatment of severe premenstrual syndrome, *Br J Obstet Gynaecol* 1995; 102:475–84.

138. Hahn PM, Van Vugt DA, Reid RL, A randomized, placebo-controlled, crossover trial of danazol for the treatment of premenstrual syndrome, *Psychoneuroendocrinology* 1995; 20: 193–209.

139. Casper RF, Hearn MT, The effect of hysterectomy and bilateral oophorectomy in women with severe premenstrual syndrome, *Am J Obstet Gynecol* 1990; 162:105–9.

140. Casson P, Hahn PM, Van Vugt DA, Reid RL, Lasting response to ovariectomy in severe intractable premenstrual syndrome, *Am J Obstet Gynecol* 1990; 162:99–105.

141. Mezrow G, Shoupe D, Spicer D et al, Depot leuprolide acetate with oestrogen and progestin add-back for long-term treatment of premenstrual syndrome, *Fertil Steril* 1994; 62:932–7.

142. Dalton K, The aetiology of premenstrual syndrome stays as is with the progesterone receptors, *Med Hypotheses* 1990; 31:323–7.

143. Freeman EW, Rickels K, Sondheimer SJ, Polansky M, A double-blind trial of oral progesterone, alprazolam and placebo in treatment of severe premenstrual syndrome, *JAMA* 1995; 274:51–7.

144. O'Brien PMS, Craven D, Selby C, Symonds EM, Treatment of premenstrual syndrome by spironolactone, *Br J Obstet Gynaecol* 1979; 86:142–7.

145. Wang M, Hammarbäck S, Lindhe BÅ, Bäckström T, Treatment of premenstrual syndrome by spironolactone: a double-blind, placebo-controlled study, *Acta Obstet Gynecol Scand* 1995; 74:803–8.

146. Eriksson E, Lisjö P, Sundblad C et al, Effect of clomipramine in the premenstrual syndrome, *Acta Psychiatr Scand* 1990; 81:87–8.

147. Rickels K, Freeman EW, Sondheimer SJ, Albert J, Fluoxetine in the treatment of premenstrual syndrome, *Curr Ther Res* 1990; 48:161–6.

148. Stone AB, Pearlstein TB, Brown WA, Fluoxetine in the treatment of late luteal phase dysphoric disorder, *J Clin Psychiatry* 1991; 52:290–3.

149. Steiner M, Judge R, Kumar R, Serotonin reuptake inhibitors in the treatment of premenstrual dysphoria: current state of knowledge, *Int J Psychiatry Clin Pract* 1997; 1:241–7.

150. Wood SH, Mortola JF, Chan YF et al, Treatment of premenstrual syndrome with fluoxetine: a double-blind, placebo-controlled, crossover study, *Obstet Gynecol* 1992; 80: 339–44.

151. Menkes DB, Taghavi E, Mason PA et al, Fluoxetine treatment of severe premenstrual syndrome, *Br Med J* 1992; 305:346–7.

152. Menkes DB, Taghavi E, Mason PA et al, Howard RC, Fluoxetine's spectrum of action in premenstrual syndrome, *Int Clin Psychopharmacol* 1993; 8:95–102.

153. Pearlstein TB, Stone AB, Lund SA et al, Comparison of fluoxetine, bupropion, and placebo in the treatment of premenstrual dysphoric disorder, *J Clin Psychopharmacol* 1997; 17:261–6.

154. Ozeren S, Corakci A, Yucesoy I et al, Fluoxetine in the treatment of premenstrual syndrome, *Eur J Obstet Gynecol Reprod Biol* 1997; 73:167–70.

155. Young SA, Hurt PH, Benedek DM, Howard RS, Treatment of premenstrual dysphoric disorder with sertraline during the luteal phase: a randomized, double-blind, placebo-controlled crossover trial, *J Clin Psychiatry* 1998; 59:76–80.

156. Brandenburg S, Tuynman-Qua H, Verheij R, Pepplinkhuizen L, Treatment of premenstrual syndrome with fluoxetine: an open study, *Int Clin Psychopharmacol* 1993; 8:315–17.

157. Elks ML, Open trial of fluoxetine therapy for

premenstrual syndrome, *South Med J* 1993; **86**:503–7.

158. Pearlstein T, Stone AB, Long-term fluoxetine treatment of late luteal phase dysphoric disorder, *J Clin Psychiatry* 1994; **55**:332–5.

159. de la Gandara Martin JJ, Premenstrual dysphoric disorder: long-term treatment with fluoxetine and discontinuation, *Actas Luso Esp Neurol Psiquiatr Cienc Afines* 1997; **25**:235–42.

160. Steiner M, Korzekwa M, Lamont J, Wilkins A, Intermittent fluoxetine dosing in the treatment of women with premenstrual dysphoria, *Psychopharmacol Bull* 1997; **33**:771–4.

161. Yonkers KA, Gullion C, Williams A et al, Paroxetine as a treatment for premenstrual dysphoric disorder, *J Clin Psychopharmacol* 1996; **16**:3–8.

162. Sundblad C, Wikander I, Andersch B, Eriksson E, A naturalistic study of paroxetine in premenstrual syndrome: efficacy and side-effects during 10 cycles of treatment, *Eur Neuropsychopharmacol* 1997; **7**:201–6.

163. Freeman EW, Rickels K, Sondheimer SJ, Polansky M, Differential response to antidepressants in women with premenstrual syndrome/premenstrual dysphoric disorder, *Arch Gen Psychiatry* 1999; **56**:932–9.

164. Halbreich U, Smoller JW, Intermittent luteal phase sertraline treatment of dysphoric premenstrual syndrome, *J Clin Psychiatry* 1997; **58**:399–402.

165. Freeman EW, Rickels K, Sondheimer SJ et al, Nefazodone in the treatment of premenstrual syndrome: a preliminary study, *J Clin Psychopharmacol* 1994; **14**:180–6.

166. Veeninga AT, Westenberg HGM, Weusten JT, Fluvoxamine in the treatment of menstrually related mood disorders, *Psychopharmacology* 1990; **102**:414–16.

167. Freeman EW, Rickels K, Sondheimer SJ, Fluvoxamine for premenstrual dysphoric disorder: a pilot study, *J Clin Psychiatry* 1996; **57** (suppl 8):56–9.

168. Danish University Antidepressant Group, Paroxetine: a selective serotonin reuptake inhibitor showing better tolerance, but weaker antidepressant effect than clomipramine in a controlled multicenter study, *J Affect Disord* 1990; **18**:289–99.

169. Greist JH, Jefferson JW, Kobak KA et al, Efficacy and tolerability of serotonin transport inhibitors in obsessive-compulsive disorder. A meta-analysis, *Arch Gen Psychiatry* 1995; **52**:53–60.

170. Modigh K, Westberg P, Eriksson E, Superiority of clomipramine over imipramine in the treatment of panic disorder: a placebo-controlled trial. *J Clin Psychopharmacol* 1992; **12**:251–6.

171. Gloger S, Grunhaus BL, Birmacher B, Troudart T, Treatment of spontaneous panic attacks with clomipramine, *Am J Psychiatry* 1981; **138**:1215–17.

172. Modigh K, Eriksson E, Lisjö P, Westberg P, Follow-up study of clomipramine in the treatment of panic disorder, *Psychiatr Fennica (Suppl)* 1989; 145–53.

173. Rutter JJ, Auerbach SB, Acute uptake inhibition increases extracellular serotonin in the rat forebrain, *J Pharmacol Exp Ther* 1993; **265**:1319–24.

174. Steiner M, Lamont J, Steinberg S et al, Effect of fluoxetine on menstrual cycle length in women with premenstrual dysphoria, *Obstet Gynecol* 1997; **90**:590–5.

175. Taghavi E, Menkes DB, Howard RC et al, Premenstrual syndrome: a double-blind controlled trial of desipramine and methylscopolamine, *Int Clin Psychopharmacol* 1995; **10**:119–22.

176. Harrison WM, Endicott J, Nee J, Treatment of premenstrual depression with nortriptyline: a pilot study, *J Clin Psychiatry* 1989; **50**:136–9.

177. Gordon CT, State RC, Nelson JE et al, A double-blind comparison of clomipramine, desipramine, and placebo in the treatment of autistic disorder, *Arch Gen Psychiatry* 1993; **50**:441–7.

178. Steinberg S, Annable L, Young SN, Liyanage N, A placebo-controlled clinical trial of L-tryptophan in premenstrual dysphoria, *Biol Psychiatry* 1999; **45**:313–20.

179. Seliger GM, Hornstein A, Flax J et al, Fluoxetine improves emotional incontinence, *Brain Inj* 1992; **6**:267–70.

180. Andersen G, Vestergaard K, Roos JO, Citalopram for post-stroke pathological crying, *Lancet* 1993; **342**:837–9.

181. Sloan RL, Brown KW, Pentland B, Fluoxetine as a treatment for emotional lability after brain injury, *Brain Inj* 1992; **6**:315–19.

182. van Praag HM, Kahn R, Asnis GM et al, Therapeutic indications for serotonin potentiating compounds: a hypothesis, *Biol Psychiatry* 1987; **22**:205–12.

183. Kavoussi R, Armstead P, Coccaro E, The neurobiology of impulsive aggression, *Psychiatr Clin North Am* 1997; **20**:395–403.

184. Rickels K, Freeman E, Sondheimer S, Buspirone in treatment of premenstrual syndrome, *Lancet* 1989; **1**:777.

185. Giannini AJ, Sullivan B, Sarachene J, Loiselle RH, Clonidine in the treatment of premenstrual syndrome: a subgroup study, *J Clin Psychiatry* 1988; **49**:62–3.

186. Steiner M, Haskett RF, Osmun JN, Carroll BJ, Treatment of premenstrual tension with lithium carbonate. A pilot study, *Acta Psychiatr Scand* 1980; **61**:96–102.

187. Kleijnen J, Ter Riet G, Knipschild P, Vitamin B6 in the treatment of the premenstrual syndrome—a review, *Br J Obstet Gynaecol* 1990; **97**:847–52.

188. Collins A, Cerin A, Coleman G, Landgren BM, Essential fatty acids in the treatment of premenstrual syndrome, *Obstet Gynecol* 1993; **81**:93–8.

17

Psychopharmacological treatment of mood and anxiety disorders during pregnancy

Eva M Szigethy and Katherine L Wisner

Introduction

Pregnancy is a complex developmental process. An interplay between physiological changes and psychological maturation towards motherhood occurs through gestation. Many theoretical constructs have been proposed to understand motivation for motherhood.[1] These include: the satisfaction of a narcissistic need to create another being, as an extension of the self; a compensatory process by which the baby is a substitute for the unconscious wish for a penis;[2] primary gratification from a woman's biological role;[3] the wish for a child as a manifestation of the woman's ambitions and ideals; and consolidation of a mature female identity.[4]

Pregnancy is an evolving process. Hormonal changes produce unaccustomed mood swings and physical discomforts. These fluctuations contribute to the revival of past conflicts and anxieties, particularly early childhood identifications with maternal figures.[5,6] How a woman responds to pregnancy is related to her early childhood experiences, coping mechanisms, personality style, life situation, emotional supports

and physical problems.[7] For some women, the stress of pregnancy leads to severe behavioural regression, unmasks psychiatric illness, or leads to difficult early mother–child relationships.[5,7,8] A first pregnancy is a stressful time, as the expectant mother attempts to deal with the perceived demands of a helpless, dependent human being. Motherhood has been described as the transition from investing in a developing fetus as an extension of the self to the child becoming a separate part of the external world.[6] Regardless of the outcome, pregnancy represents the 'end of the woman as an independent single unit and the beginning of an unalterable irrevocable mother–child relationship'.[8]

This chapter will summarize theoretical and clinical aspects of pharmacological treatment of mood and anxiety disorders during pregnancy. The objectives are:

(1) To describe the developmental tasks of pregnancy. Normal emotional responses must be understood and integrated into treatment. They must also be differentiated from pathological mood states.

(2) To present principles of drug therapy during pregnancy.

(3) To review current literature on the natural history of mood and anxiety disorders during pregnancy.

(4) To discuss the risk–benefit assessment for psychotropic drugs. The benefits of treating maternal psychiatric disorder must be weighed against potential teratogenic risks to the fetus. Treatment guidelines for these disorders during gestation will be summarized.

General principles of psychopharmacology during gestation

Competent psychiatric treatment entails educating patients about the risks and benefits of treatments for their specific psychiatric condition. The psychiatrist must discuss the influence of the pregnancy on the treatment choices and include risk–benefit information pertaining to the expectant mother and to the fetus. Most mental health clinicians would agree that psychiatric symptoms during pregnancy should be treated with non-pharmacological interventions when possible. No psychotropic medication has been approved by the US Food and Drug Administration for use during pregnancy. However, because of the growing numbers of studies that demonstrate a high rate of recurrence when medications are discontinued in patients suffering from mood or anxiety disorders,[10–12] the decision to stop psychopharmacological treatment during pregnancy must be carefully reviewed.

There are several clinical situations in which the risks associated with failing to treat psychiatric conditions are greater than the risks associated with drug therapy. These include suicidality or failure to eat, mania with impulsive risk-taking behaviours, and obsessive-compulsive disorder (OCD) with obsessions about killing the fetus or inability to attend prenatal appointments because of compulsions. Untreated psychiatric illness may lead to violent behaviour, fetal abuse or neonaticide, failure to seek appropriate neonatal care, and attempts at premature self-delivery.[13,14] In addition to the immediate risks to the expectant mother and fetus, there are psychosocial consequences of failing to treat these patients. The need for prolonged hospitalization, marital discord and divorce, inability to care for other children, and loss of employment, are consequences of maternal psychiatric illness.

Consideration of the following factors is useful in assessing psychiatric symptoms and developing an appropriate treatment plan during gestation:[7,14]

(1) the specific psychiatric symptoms or disorders being treated and their natural course during pregnancy;

(2) prior psychiatric history with attention to episodes during childbearing;

(3) history of recurrences and remissions of the psychiatric illness during previous medication-free periods;

(4) previous response to psychotropic medications as well as non-pharmacological treatments;

(5) past history of psychological problems at times of maturational crisis and conflicts about sexual identity;

(6) presence of early parental deprivation and abuse, difficulties in separating from parents, and conflicts about mothering;

(7) the woman's psychosocial stability in managing stresses associated with pregnancy;

(8) social support system and interactional capabilities with her family;

(9) her thoughts about continuing the pregnancy;
(10) history of miscarriages and abortions;
(11) known familial congenital disorders or previous birth of a handicapped/challenged child; and
(12) family history of psychiatric as well as pregnancy-related problems.

Therapeutic benefits gained from psychopharmacological treatment must be weighed against potential risks to the fetus. All commonly used psychotropic medications cross the placenta.[15] The most common mechanism of placental transfer is simple diffusion, which depends on multiple drug characteristics such as molecular weight, degree of ionization, lipid solubility, and protein binding (see Wisner and Perel[14] for a review). In addition, the degree of placental maturation and metabolism also alters fetal drug effect, given that fetoplacental circulation is established between 8 and 21 days after ovulation.[16]

The fetus can oxidatively metabolize drugs through its own hepatic enzyme system, which appears as early as 8 weeks of gestation and reaches a plateau by mid-pregnancy.[17] However, fetal drug metabolism is unlikely to change steady-state plasma drug levels in the mother. When a woman takes repeated doses of a drug to sustain plasma level concentrations, the drug distribution will be approximately equal in the mother and fetus.[15] Factors that may be associated with adverse effects of a drug in utero include: dosage; duration of exposure; administration route; active or toxic metabolites; and genetic susceptibility of the target organism.[18] Fetal risks from exposure include intrauterine fetal death, identifiable anatomical anomalies, abnormal fetal growth, behavioural teratogenicity, acute fetal or neonatal toxicity, and fetal or neonatal withdrawal.

Substantiation of a claim that a pharmacological agent is completely without teratogenic effects is difficult, because low teratogenic rates are indistinguishable from the spontaneous occurrence of anomalies. The incidence of major birth defects in the USA is about 2–4%, and the cause of 65–70% of these defects is unknown.[19] A bias in the literature against publication of studies that show no or insignificant differences among comparison groups may lead to exaggerated estimates of teratogenic risks.[20]

Behavioural teratogenicity describes postbirth abnormalities in the behaviour of offspring exposed to teratogens in utero. Exposure induces prenatal changes in neurobiological systems which then result in behavioural abnormalities later in development. Examples of behaviours include delayed maturation, impaired rates of learning and problem-solving, abnormal activity, and pathological arousal states. Behavioural teratogenesis can occur throughout pregnancy because brain development continues into infancy.

Data on behavioural teratogenicity have been derived primarily from animal studies. To date, no behavioural teratogenicity has been published or proven unequivocally for antidepressants, benzodiazepines, lithium, or antipsychotic agents in humans. Medication-induced effects from psychoteratogens are difficult to isolate from environmental influences on behaviour. Because of the need for research in behavioural teratogenicity in humans, it is premature to label psychotropic agents as safe during pregnancy.

In addition to fetal risks, the pregnant woman is at increased risk from pharmacological treatment, due to physiological changes during pregnancy. Somatic symptoms of pregnancy can be intensified by medication effects. For example, decreased gastrointestinal emptying can aggravate constipation,[18] a common problem in pregnancy for many women.

Physiological changes that contribute to progressive increases in dose requirements during pregnancy include increased volume of distribution, decreased protein-binding capacity, progesterone-induced decrease in gastrointestinal motility, which reduces and/or delays absorption, increased uterine bloodflow during gestation, increased renal elimination of drugs owing to increased glomerular filtration, and enhancement of hepatic metabolism (although the effect on first-pass metabolism is minimal).[18,21] Proliferation of the hepatic endoplasmic reticulum during the last 3 months of pregnancy has been demonstrated.[22] The activity of the cytochrome P4502D6 isoenzyme is also increased during pregnancy.[23]

The American Medical Association[19] has defined the following physician responsibilities in prescribing drugs for pregnant women: select the drug with the most favourable risk–benefit profile, inform patients about the implications of drug exposures and on the priority of birth-control measures in the case of inadvertent drug exposures, and determine the exposures and report them if birth defects are observed.

Careful documentation of clinical decision-making during pregnancy is essential. In legal proceedings, the plaintiff must show that the physician deviated from the standard of care by either an error of omission (failure to treat or to inform) or an error of commission (failure to treat in accordance with the standard of care).[24] The psychiatrist is not a guarantor of a good result for the patient, and an adverse clinical outcome does not presume malpractice. It is impossible to determine and present a complete risk–benefit profile. Behavioural teratogenicity remains a theoretical risk that cannot be quantified. The lack of data in the field[24] can be discussed with mothers directly. Ideally, the patient should agree in advance about the course of action to be taken if symptoms recur during pregnancy, and she should provide informed consent for medications or alternative treatments. If the practitioner is uncomfortable with the risk–benefit analysis, expert consultation is advisable.

The choice of psychiatric treatment will be dictated by the patient's past response to treatment, severity of symptoms, and patient choice. Provide a discussion of treatment choices appropriate for non-pregnant patients with similar clinical presentations, and explain how pregnancy influences our recommendations. Specific psychotherapies, light therapy and electroconvulsive therapy are considered in the discussion if appropriate. The woman's response to treatment should be carefully monitored, and more aggressive interventions can be considered if the response is not optimal. Monitoring symptom response is vital, since pharmacological intervention cannot be justified if the response that defined its benefit did not occur. Monitoring instruments such as self-report inventories (e.g. Inventory to Diagnose Depression[25]) or clinician-rated scales (e.g. Hamilton Rating Scale for Depression[26] or the Montgomery-Åsberg Depression Rating Scale[27]) are useful for documenting not only level of initial symptom severity but also treatment response. Regardless of the treatment intervention chosen, coordination of the treatment plan with the obstetrician is essential.

Natural course of mood and anxiety disorders during pregnancy

Women of childbearing age are at high risk for major depression, with a lifetime risk in community samples varying between 10% and 25% (see Chapter 1). This is similar to the incidence of clinical depression in pregnant women, which has been estimated at

9–10%.[28,29] These data indicate that pregnancy does not protect women from the development of depression.

Bipolar disorder occurs in 0.4–1.2% of the adult population. Rates of bipolar I disorder are equal in men and women, but bipolar II disorder may be more common in women.[30] In one study of three women with bipolar disorder who were withdrawn from long-term, efficacious lithium therapy prior to pregnancy, all three remained in remission during gestation, but two of three developed a manic episode within 2 weeks postpartum.[31] Suppes et al[11] summarized data from 14 studies regarding episode recurrence rate in patients with bipolar disorder who were rapidly discontinued from maintenance treatment with lithium. An overall 50% recurrence risk by 5 months off lithium treatment with 50% of new manic episodes occurring within 3 months was reported. Thus, rapid discontinuation of treatment in lithium-responsive women during pregnancy may increase the risk for recurrence during gestation.

More recent data suggest that recurrence risk in pregnant women differed little from that of non-pregnant women after discontinuing lithium, whereas no recurrence of mania or depression was observed in patients who continued lithium. The risk of recurrence, however, rose sharply during the postpartum period.[32] A hospital-based epidemiological study has suggested that pregnancy does not alter the natural course of bipolar disorder until the postpartum period, which is a time of dramatically increased risk for a new episode.[33]

Anxiety disorders are common in childbearing women. The natural history of panic disorder during pregnancy is variable (see Chapter 18). Some studies have suggested a trend towards decreased panic attacks during pregnancy, while others describe increased symptoms. Villeponteaux et al[34] studied 22 women

who had a combined total of 44 pregnancies after the onset of panic disorder. Out of 22 women, 14 reported a decrease in panic attack frequency or remission during pregnancy, three reported an increase, two reported no change, and three reported variable changes during different pregnancies. Cohen et al[35] found a similar variable impact of pregnancy on panic disorder in 48 non-depressed pregnant women, but the results were confounded by pharmacological treatment in the majority of cases.

In a study of 46 women with 67 pregnancies, Northcott and Stein[36] reported approximately equal proportions of pregnancies during which improvement (43%), no change (23%) or worsening (33%) of panic symptoms occurred. Wisner et al[37] explored the effects of childbearing on the natural history of panic disorder in 31 women with 45 pregnancies. They found that 31 pregnancies (69%) had no change in panic symptoms, 12 had decreased symptoms and two had recurrence of panic attacks during pregnancy. Interestingly, 13 out of 22 women had major depression in addition to panic disorder that pre-dated or was associated with 32 out of 45 pregnancies. Of these 32 pregnancies, 94% were associated with no changes in depressive symptoms, while the remaining 6% showed an increase or onset of depressive symptoms. These results suggested that pregnancy has a differential effect on anxiety versus depressive symptoms. In both of these studies,[36,37] there was a lack of consistency of panic symptom course across multiple pregnancies for the same woman.

Recent reports suggest that there is an increased risk for the onset of OCD during pregnancy and the puerperium.[38–40] Neziroglu et al[38] found that 23 out of 59 (39%) women with children had onset of OCD during pregnancy. Buttolph and Holland[39] reported that 15% of 29 women with OCD had onset during pregnancy and 8% had worsening of pre-existing OCD. In a retrospective analysis of ever-pregnant women with OCD, pregnancy was associated with the onset of OCD in five (13%).[40] Of the remaining 29 women with pre-existing OCD who experienced a pregnancy, 17% had worsening, 14% had improvement, and 69% described no change in symptoms during pregnancy. One hypothesis for the increased risk of OCD onset during pregnancy is gonadal steroid-induced changes in serotonin neurotransmission.[41]

Risk assessment for the use of pharmacological agents during pregnancy

Tricyclic antidepressants

Metabolism during pregnancy

Tricyclic antidepressants (TCAs) have been studied during pregnancy. Physiological changes that contribute to progressive increases in TCA dose requirements during pregnancy are primarily enhanced hepatic metabolism and increased volume of distribution, although changes in protein binding and gastrointestinal absorption also occur.[21] In our investigation,[42] TCA dosage requirements increased across gestation. During the final trimester, the dose required to sustain remission from depression and provide adequate serum drug levels ranged from 1.3 to 2 times the non-pregnant dose, with the average increase being 1.6. Therefore, breakthrough depressive symptoms during pregnancy may be due to subtherapeutic serum levels, and a serum level should be obtained in this situation. Fluctuations in the processing of TCA are particularly problematic for women who are at the extremes of genetically controlled cytochrome P450 metabolic capacity.[23,43] During pregnancy, women with rapid metabolism will require high doses to sustain

therapeutic levels. If clinically feasible, doses should be tapered and discontinued during the 2-week period prior to the due date to reduce the fetal drug load at birth.[14]

Morphological teratogenicity

Studies conducted to date have shown no increased risk of major malformations after in utero exposure to TCAs. Using a meta-analytic approach, Altshuler et al[44] identified 414 cases of first-trimester exposure to TCA. There was no significant association between fetal exposure to TCA and increased risk for congenital malformations.

Behavioural teratogenicity

Misri et al[45] examined the behavioural development in children exposed in utero to TCA. They found normal motor skills and behaviour 3 years after birth. Nulman et al[46] performed a study of the development of children exposed prenatally to TCA ($n = 80$) or the selective serotonin reuptake inhibitor (SSRI) fluoxetine ($n = 55$) compared with a control group ($n = 84$). At birth and at the time of testing, the percentiles of weight, height and head circumference of the children in the three groups were similar, as was the incidence of major malformations. There was no difference between the three groups with respect to global intelligence, language development, or behavioural development (temperament, mood, arousability, activity levels, distractibility and behaviour problems). The age at assessment was between 16 and 86 months. Timing of antidepressant therapy (first trimester versus the entire pregnancy) did not affect the neurobehavioural outcomes.

Effects on the newborn

A neonatal behavioural syndrome has been reported in the offspring of women treated with TCA until delivery. Symptoms include cyanosis, tachypnoea, tachycardia, irritability, hypotonia, tremor, feeding difficulties, urinary retention, bowel obstruction and profuse sweating.[47] These symptoms represent either direct effects of the TCA or withdrawal secondary to rebound cholinergic hyperactivity.

Selective serotonin reuptake inhibitors

Morphological teratogenicity

Prenatal exposure to the SSRIs such as fluoxetine is not associated with increased risk for major birth defects. Pastuszak et al[48] compared prospectively pregnancy outcomes after first-trimester exposure to fluoxetine ($n = 128$) with two matched control groups: one exposed to TCA ($n = 74$) and the other to non-teratogens ($n = 128$). The mean daily dose of fluoxetine was 25.8 ± 13.1 mg/day. Rates of major malformations were comparable across the three groups and did not exceed the expected rate in the general population. Note that the results of this study are in agreement with those of Altshuler et al[44] with regard to prenatal exposure to TCA.

Chambers et al[49] compared prospectively 228 pregnant women taking fluoxetine with 254 controls and found no increased risk of major fetal anomalies. However, they found a significantly higher rate of three or more minor anomalies, which was not explained by concomitant use of other psychotropic medications. The authors suggested that a teratrogenic effect may become evident in later development. Kulin et al[50] reported pregnancy outcomes following maternal use of the newer SSRIs fluvoxamine, paroxetine, and sertraline. The study was a prospective, multicentre, controlled investigation. In total, 267 women exposed to an SSRI and 267 controls were studied. Exposure to SSRI was not associated with increased risk for major malformations or higher rates of miscarriage, stillbirth, or prematurity. Birth weights of infants and gestational ages were similar in cases and controls.

Effects on the newborn

Spencer[51] described a case of fluoxetine toxicity in a newborn delivered at 38 weeks of gestation. The infant had agitation and tachycardia. Hypotonia and bleeding abnormalities in a newborn exposed to fluoxetine in utero have also been described.[52] Chambers et al[49] reported that women who took fluoxetine during the third trimester had an increased risk of perinatal complications compared with women who discontinued fluoxetine prior to 25 weeks of gestation. Premature delivery and poor neonatal adaptation, as evidenced by respiratory difficulties, cyanosis with feeding, and jitteriness, were more common in the third-trimester-exposed newborns. Lower birth-weight and length were also observed. Lower birthweights were associated with poor maternal weight gain.

Monoamine oxidase inhibitors

Monoamine oxidase inhibitors (MAOIs) are not typically chosen for treatment of the pregnant patient, unless the woman has failed all other treatments. The Collaborative Perinatal Project monitored 21 children exposed in utero to MAOI and observed three congenital malformations.[53] Two reports provided guidelines for MAOI use during pregnancy, with particular attention to safe obstetrical anaesthesia and postpartum pain management.[54,55]

Electroconvulsive therapy (ECT)

ECT is useful during pregnancy in situations that require aggressive treatment. Few complications of treatment have been described.[14,56,57]

ECT-induced premature labour, with successful tocolysis and subsequent ECT treatment without further complication, has been described.[58]

Guidelines for treatment of pregnant depressed women

For ethical reasons, the literature on psychotropic medication use during pregnancy consists of non-randomized epidemiological studies. In reports about the effects of antidepressants during pregnancy, drug use is coupled with maternal psychiatric illness. The role of depression and its psychosocial sequelae must be considered when interpreting these studies. Independent of biomedical risk, maternal prenatal stress is associated significantly with infant birthweight and age at birth.[59]

The following general guidelines are provided for depressed patients who are or wish to become pregnant:

(1) Ideally, antidepressant medication should be tapered prior to attempts at conception if depressive symptoms have not been severe, or the woman has not had multiple episodes. Careful monitoring for symptom recurrence is essential. Non-pharmacological alternatives such as maintenance psychotherapy should be considered. Spinelli[60] has developed a modification of interpersonal therapy for antepartum depression.

(2) Drug therapy should be avoided during the first 10 weeks after conception unless the risk–benefit analysis shows greater risk in not treating the mother pharmacologically.

(3) ECT is a viable option for depression that poses serious risk to the mother and fetus, such as suicidality, inability to care for self, severe neurovegetative symptoms or psychosis.

(4) If a TCA is appropriate, nortriptyline is the preferable TCA because it has been used successfully for decades, has low relative anticholinergic activity, and has a relationship between plasma concentration and therapeutic effect,[14,43] However, full response to an alternative TCA dictates use of the effective agent.

(5) Fluoxetine is also well studied and does not produce increased risk for major birth defects or neurodevelopmental delay. Although not as extensively studied, other SSRIs, such as paroxetine and sertraline, appear to be reasonable alternatives for women who cannot tolerate fluoxetine or are non-responders.

Bipolar disorders

Lithium

Metabolism during pregnancy

Lithium clearance gradually increases by 30–50% during the second half of pregnancy. The dose must be increased to maintain the therapeutic level as pregnancy progresses.[61] To avoid dose pulses, lithium carbonate should be divided into three to five equal doses throughout the day. At labour onset, lithium should be discontinued. With the rapid fall in lithium clearance at delivery, toxic maternal concentrations can occur if the dose is not rapidly decreased. In the immediate postpartum period, pre-pregnancy doses should be resumed to prevent recurrence of mood disorder.

Weinstein[62] warned that signs of lithium toxicity may be attributed to somatic symptoms of pregnancy. Typical corrective measures may worsen the toxic state (for example, sodium restriction for fluid retention associated with mild lithium toxicity). Assessment of lithium levels at least once a month in the first half of pregnancy and once weekly later in gestation was recommended.

Morphological teratogenicity

Weinstein and Goldfield[63] summarized data from 225 cases reported to the Lithium Registry and found 25 (11%) with congenital malformations. Cardiovascular anomalies were present in 8%, including Ebstein's anomaly. A reporting bias exists for voluntary registries because physicians are more likely to report drug-associated pathology rather than normality. Two subsequent case-control studies suggested that the association between lithium and Ebstein's anomaly was weak. Zalzstein et al[64] compared 59 children born with Ebstein's anomaly to 168 children born with neuroblastoma and found that none in the former group and only one in the latter group had lithium exposure during the first trimester, thus establishing that the potential risk is much lower than previously suggested.

Jacobsen et al[65] studied prospectively 138 first-trimester lithium-treated women and 148 age-matched control subjects. The mean dose of lithium was 927 mg/day. Rates of major congenital malformations did not differ between the lithium-treated and the control groups. Although the rate of lithium-induced cardiac anomalies is lower than previously thought, it is higher than the spontaneous rate. Cohen et al[66] concluded that the risk of major congenital anomalies among the children of women treated with lithium during early pregnancy was between 4% and 12%, compared with the general population rate of 2–4%.

Behavioural teratogenicity

Schou[67] studied 50 normal children of at least 5 years of age reported to the Lithium Registry and their 57 non-exposed siblings with parent reports of development. The difference in the number of developmental difficulties between the lithium-exposed children and control siblings was not statistically significant. Jacobsen et al[65] reported that the attainment of major motor and language milestones in 22 children exposed prenatally to lithium did not differ from that of control subjects.

Effects on the newborn

There are many case reports of transplacental fetal lithium exposure with adverse effects for the newborn. Neonatal lithium toxicity may result in poor sucking, abnormal respiratory patterns, cyanosis, hypotonia, cardiac arrhythmias, poor myocardial contractility and hypoglycaemia.[68,69] Neonatal hypothyroidism appears to be transient and not associated with developmental delays.[61]

Birthweight was significantly higher in lithium-exposed infants than in control infants, despite identical gestational ages (3475 versus 3383 g).[65] When reviewing the records from the International Registry of Lithium Babies, Troyer et al[70] found that 36% were delivered prematurely and 37% of the premature infants were large for gestational age.

Anticonvulsants

Metabolism during pregnancy

Anticonvulsants, particularly carbamazepine and valproate, are widely used to treat bipolar disorder. Women who respond to these agents present a clinical challenge during gestation, because fetal toxicity has been described for both.

Battino et al[71] reported no change in plasma carbamazepine concentration during pregnancy in nine epileptic patients treated with constant doses of medication. In contrast, Dam et al[72] found that the clearance of carbazamepine increased markedly during pregnancy and reached its maximum 3 weeks before to 1 week after delivery. The ratio of the plasma concentration of the metabolite, carbamazepine-10, 11-epoxide, to carbamazepine also increased during pregnancy. These findings were explained by a higher rate of hepatic drug metabolism.

Philbert et al[73] studied the serum valproate levels of women with epilepsy. Three patients with full-term deliveries had a decrease in serum levels during the last 2–4 weeks of pregnancy due to an increase in valproate clearance. Omtzigt et al[74] suggested that clearance of valproate and its metabolites from the fetal compartment lagged behind that of the maternal compartment. Therefore, chronic valproate treatment resulted in fetal accumulation. Dickenson et al[75] also found that valproic acid crossed the placenta to achieve fetal serum concentrations 1.4 times maternal serum levels. The half-life of the drug in the newborn is increased to 45 h because of reduced glucuronidation.

Monitoring of serum levels and adjustment of dosage during pregnancy, particularly later in gestation, is clinically prudent.

Morphological teratogenicity
Studies of rates of anomalies in children exposed to anticonvulsants during pregnancy have included patients treated for epilepsy. Women with epilepsy account for approximately one in 200 pregnancies (0.5%). The incidence of malformations associated with anticonvulsant exposure remains higher than the rates for comparison groups, even after the effects of epilepsy are controlled.[76]

First-trimester exposure to either carbamazepine or valproic acid has been linked to spina bifida. Exposure to carbamazepine has been associated with a 0.5–1.0% estimated risk for this defect.[77] Prenatal exposure to valproic acid has been associated with a dose-related risk of spina bifida of 1–5% if used between 15 and 30 days post-fertilization.[74,78] Since the risk of spina bifida in the general population is 3 in 10 000 (0.03%), anticonvulsants increase the risk by 15-fold or greater. Risk increases with

the use of multiple anticonvulsants and probably with higher maternal plasma levels.[73,74,79]

Orofacial clefts have also been associated with first-trimester exposure to anticonvulsants.[80] Minor malformations such as rotated ears, depressed nasal bridge, short nose, elongated upper lip and fingernail hypoplasia have been described in infants exposed prenatally to anticonvulsants.[76] First-trimester use of carbamazepine has been associated with meningomyelocele, anal atresia, ambiguous genitalia, congenital heart disease and torticollis. Valproic acid exposure has been associated with developmental anomalies such as craniofacial and congenital heart defects, polydactyly, hypospadias and low birthweight.

According to the Neurology Consensus Statement about treatment of women with epilepsy during pregnancy,[76] adequate daily folate intake is recommended prior to and following conception to decrease the risk of neural tube defects. However, a specific protective effect from folate during teratogenic drug therapy has not been demonstrated in humans.

Behavioural teratogenicity
The data regarding the neurobiological effects of prenatal exposure to anticonvulsants are contradictory. Studies that describe intellectual and motor development in exposed children are difficult to interpret, in part because of a failure to control for factors such as parental intelligence, seizures during pregnancy, and psychosocial factors. Scolnik et al[81] did not find a change in global intelligence or language development in children exposed to carbamazepine in utero, whereas both were lower in children exposed to phenytoin. Similarly, children exposed to valproate prenatally showed normal psychomotor development in assessments completed up to 4 years later.[82]

Effects on the newborn

Mean head circumference was significantly lower in carbamazepine-exposed babies compared with controls, and no catch-up growth had occurred by 18 months of age.[83] Growth variables did not correlate with maternal serum drug levels, aetiology, duration of maternal epilepsy, or number and distribution of seizures during pregnancy. Transient hepatic dysfunction has occurred in a carbamazepine-exposed neonate.[84] Acute liver failure and hyperbilirubinaemia have been reported in infants exposed prenatally to valproic acid.[85]

In summary, women with bipolar disorder may exhibit significant affective symptoms while pregnant or during the postpartum period. However, first-trimester exposure to any of the mood stabilizers is associated with increased risk of birth defects and should be avoided if possible. In pregnant women who are manic, severely depressed, or psychotic, the safest and most effective treatment is often ECT. In women for whom discontinuation of mood stabilizers poses an unacceptable risk of increased morbidity, the following should be considered:

(1) Provide reproductive risk counselling prior to or as early as possible in pregnancy, particularly regarding first-trimester risks. This discussion must be balanced against the risks of active maternal mood disorder.
(2) In collaboration with the obstetrician, monitor fetal development. Fetal echocardiography and high-resolution ultrasound examinations can be performed at 16–18 weeks of gestation, along with serum or amniotic fluid α-fetoprotein levels.[66]
(3) Throughout pregnancy, monitor serum concentrations and adjust doses of mood stabilizers carefully.
(4) Decrease or taper anticonvulsants about a week before delivery to minimize neonatal toxic effects; stop lithium with labour onset. Resume treatment immediately post-birth to reduce the risk of a postpartum episode and monitor plasma levels carefully.[61]
(5) If lithium is discontinued in early pregnancy, consider tapering over at least 2 weeks to avoid the high rate of recurrence observed in patients who discontinued it abruptly.[11,31]

Antipsychotics

Antipsychotics are commonly used in the management of acute mania. Neither animal nor human studies have established consistently a causal relationship between maternal ingestion of typical antipsychotic drugs and fetal malformations. However, anomalies associated with phenothiazine use during the first trimester have been reported in several organ systems, including the cardiovascular, skeletal and central nervous systems.[44,68] Antipsychotics administered in the third trimester are unlikely to be teratogenic but can produce other adverse effects in the neonate such as hyperbilirubinaemia, impaired temperature regulation, agitation, hypertonicity, tremor, primitive reflexes and poor sucking.

When manic symptoms resolve, antipsychotics should be discontinued or decreased to the lowest effective dose. In cases in which continued use is necessary, tapering and discontinuation before delivery is desirable. Extrapyramidal symptoms in neonates have been treated with diphenhydramine; however, this has precipitated seizures in infants[86] and should be used cautiously.

The National Institute of Mental Health has organized a multicentre study to determine the efficacy of the calcium channel blocker verapamil in childbearing-aged women with bipolar disorder. If effective, verapamil may allow a less teratogenic choice during pregnancy.[87]

Anxiety disorders

Benzodiazepines

Metabolism during pregnancy

Kanto[88] reviewed the pharmacokinetics of benzodiazepines (BNZ) during pregnancy. Fetal levels of lipophilic BNZ that rapidly cross the placental barrier may initially be higher than maternal concentrations, until a steady state is reached. If BNZ use is necessary, a clear time-limited indication should be determined (such as vomiting secondary to anxiety or agitation secondary to mania). Other drugs that require a longer period of treatment before symptom reduction should be introduced with the plan to eventually taper the BNZ.

Morphological teratogenicity

There are many studies in which the relationship between the first-trimester BNZ and congenital anomalies has been assessed.[44,68] On average, about 0.4% of infants exposed prenatally to BNZ will have oral clefts, and many of these are surgically correctable.[89] Oral clefts develop in the first trimester, with closure being complete by week 10 of gestation. The risk for cleft palate in the general population is 6 per 10 000. Although there appears to be a positive association between first-trimester exposure to BNZ and oral cleft formation, the extent to which BNZ heightens the risk for oral cleft or other anomalies in humans remains controversial.

Milkovich and van den Berg[90] suggested that chlordiazepoxide may be teratogenic during the first 42 days of pregnancy, because the rate of severe malformations was three times as great during this period as in later pregnancy. In a case-control study by Bracken and Holdford,[91] mothers of congenitally malformed infants were more likely than mothers of normally developed infants to have used a tranquillizer (usually chlordiazepoxide) in the first trimester.

In contrast, data from the Collaborative Perinatal Project[92] did not demonstrate a relationship between chlordiazepoxide exposure and congenital anomalies.

In a case-control study, Laegreid et al[93] evaluated whether infants exposed to BNZ were more frequently affected by the following four problems assessed in the neonatal period: congenital malformations of the nervous system, dysmorphic features, cleft lip/palate, and congenital malformations of the urinary tract. Maternal serum samples drawn at gestational week 12 showed that 8 out of 18 maternal case samples and 2 out of 60 control samples were positive for BNZ. The association between one or more of the problems evaluated and BNZ-positive maternal serum samples was highly significant. These findings are important because they did not depend on maternal report of BNZ use.

St Clair and Schirmer[94] assessed prospectively pregnancy outcome associated with first-trimester exposure to alprazolam in 411 pregnancies and found that the rates of spontaneous abortion and stillbirth were similar to those in the general population.

Behavioural teratogenicity

Viggeda et al[95] found delays in mental and motor development in prenatally exposed toddlers. However, other studies have failed to show a link between in utero BNZ exposure and lower intelligence or motor score differences as assessed up to 4 years post-exposure.[13,92]

Effects on the newborn

Two syndromes of neonatal toxicity are associated with BNZ, the floppy infant syndrome and a withdrawal syndrome. The floppy infant syndrome occurs after prolonged maternal therapy with BNZ.[95] Neonates exposed to high-dose (at least 30 mg diazepam equivalent)

BNZ in late pregnancy showed signs of toxicity including lethargy, irritability, abnormal sleep patterns, difficulty in sucking, poor respiratory efforts, hypotonia or hypertonia, hyporeflexia or hyperreflexia, hypothermia, and bradycardia or tachycardia.[13] Fetal toxicity manifests itself primarily in decreased cardiac variability and absence of accelerations. In one such study involving clonazepam, the infant had excessive apnoeic episodes until age 10 weeks. The neuro-developmental examination was normal at 5 months.[96] Passive addiction of the newborn also occurs. Neonatal BNZ withdrawal can include tremors, irritability, muscular hyper tonicity, impaired temperature regulation, apnoea, low Apgar scores and vigorous sucking 2–6 h after birth.[44,68] The symptom picture depends upon whether the infant is intoxicated or in a withdrawal state.

Guidelines for use during pregnancy

Antidepressants are the first-line treatment choices for anxiety disorders; however, adjunctive use of BNZ is common in clinical practice for non-pregnant patients. BNZ are indicated when target symptoms are severe and immediate relief is required. Duration of use should be as brief as possible and doses should be as low as possible. If fetal or neonatal toxicity occurs, it can be reversed with flumazenil, an α-aminobutyric acid (GABA) antagonist.[97] Because of the short half-life of flumazenil, close observation is warranted for at least 24 h to determine the need for repeat doses.

Wisner and Perel[14] selected lorazepam as the drug of choice during gestation because it is associated with a slower rate of placental transfer than diazepam, has no active metabolites and has high potency with good absorption. Among the non-BNZ anxiolytics, the teratogenic potential and adverse effects of buspirone resulting from prenatal exposure are unknown.

Clomipramine

Clomipramine is indicated for treatment of OCD. Its use during pregnancy is subject to the same fetal and neonatal risks as those described for TCAs. As with other TCAs, neonatal withdrawal from clomipramine has been described.[98] Symptoms began in utero, with premature contraction and delivery occurring 4 days after the mother abruptly discontinued clomipramine 150 mg/day. The infant suffered respiratory distress, and 10 min after birth had seizures refractory to phenobarbitone and phenytoin for 3 days. The seizures remitted after clomipramine was given. Clomipramine was tapered over 30 days with no evidence of neurological sequelae.

For patients with OCD, behavioural strategies (cognitive therapy) can be considered as an alternative to medication. Patients who suffer from OCD may benefit from treatment with SSRIs. Alternatively, clomipramine can be used if it has previously been successful, with the same gradual taper recommendations prior to delivery as for the other TCAs.

Conclusions

The physician must assist the expectant mother in understanding and processing the many factors that affect her decision about treatment choices. Her assessment of the need for pharmacotherapy, her perception of teratogenic risk, and her likelihood to terminate the pregnancy for fear of drug toxicity, are affected by a number of factors. These include the severity of her psychiatric symptoms, her feelings about the pregnancy, her trust in the treating physician, and the degree to which she feels like an informed participant in the decision-making process. The physician's role in this process is to educate the patient (and partners) about the risks and benefits of the various treatment options in the context of a collaborative doctor–patient relationship. Because pregnancy represents a complex and ever-changing interplay between physiological and psychological factors, both psychiatric symptoms and treatment response must be re-assessed throughout the pregnancy. Pharmacological treatment during gestation must be integrated with psychosocial interventions to ensure optimal outcome for both the mother and her baby not only during pregnancy but also into the postpartum period. Few endeavours are as rewarding as facilitating a healthy mother–infant attachment that allows the family to experience the joys of childbearing.

References

1. Robinson GE, Stewart DE, Motivation for motherhood and the experience of pregnancy, *Can J Psychiatry* 1989; **34**:861–5.
2. Freud S, Femininity, new introductory lectures. In: London JS, ed., *Standard Edition of the Complete Works of Sigmund Freud* (Hogarth Press: London, 1933) 112–35.
3. Horney K, The flight from womenhood, *Int J Psychoanal* 1926; **12**:360–74.
4. Erikson E, Womanhood and the inner space. In: Erikson E, ed., *Identity, Youth and Crisis* (Norton: New York, 1968) 261–94.
5. Bibring G, Some considerations of the psychological processes in pregnancy, *Psychoanalytic Study Child* 1959; **14**:113–21.
6. Deutch H, *Psychology of Women*, Vol. II (Grund and Stratton: New York, 1952).
7. Rosenthal MB, Benson RC, Psychologic aspects of obstetrics and gynecology. In: Pernoll ML, ed., *Current Obstetric and Gynecologic Diagnosis and Treatment* (Appelton & Lange: Norwell, CT, 1991) 1121–41.
8. Pines D, *A Woman's Unconscious Use of Her Body* (Yale University Press: New Haven, 1993).
9. Caplan G, Insley V, *Concepts of Mental Health and Consultation* (US Children's Bureau: Washington DC, 1959).
10. Kupfer DJ, Frank E, Perel JM et al, Five-year outcome for maintenance therapies in recurrent depression, *Arch Gen Psychiatry* 1992; **49**:769–73.
11. Suppes T, Baldessarini RJ, Faedda GL, Tohen M, Risk of recurrence following discontinuation of lithium treatment in bipolar disorder, *Arch Gen Psychiatry* 1991; **48**:1082–8.
12. Pollack MH, Smoller JW, The longitudinal course and outcome of panic disorder, *Psychiatr Clin North Am* 1995; **18**:785–801.
13. Miller LJ, Clinical strategies for the use of psychotropic drugs during pregnancy, *Psychiatr Med* 1991; **9**:275–98.
14. Wisner KL, Perel JM, Psychopharmacologic agents and ECT during pregnancy and the puerperium. In: Cohen RL, ed. *Psychiatric Consultations in Childbirth Settings* (Plenum: New York, 1988) 165–74.
15. Levy G, Pharmacokinetics of fetal and neonatal exposure to drugs, *Obstet Gynecol* 1981; **58** (suppl):9S–16S.
16. Mirkin BL, Drug disposition and therapy in the developing human being, *Pediatr Ann* 1976; **5**:542–57.
17. Soyka LF, Bigelow SW, Drug metabolizing enzymes and their activity in the human fetus. In: Stern L, ed., *Drug Use in Pregnancy* (Adis Health Sciences Press: Sydney, 1984) 17–44.
18. Cupit GC, Rotmensch HH, Principles of drug therapy in pregnancy. In: Gleicher N, ed. *Principles of Medical Therapy in Pregnancy* (Plenum Press: New York, 1985) 77–90.
19. American Medical Association, Drug interactions and adverse drug reactions. In: *AMA Drug Evaluations* (AMA: Chicago, 1983) 31–44.
20. Koren G, Bias against the null hypothesis in maternal fetal pharmacology and toxicology, *Clin Pharmacol Ther* 1997; **62**:1–5.
21. Livezey GT, Rayburn WF, Principles of perinatal pharmacology. In: Rayburn WF, Zuspan FP,

eds, *Drug Therapy in Obstetrics and Gynecology*, 3rd edn (Mosby-Year Book Inc.: St Louis, 1992) 3–12.

22. Perez V, Gorodisch S, Casavilla F, Maruffo C, Ultrastructure of human liver at the end of normal pregnancy, *Am J Obstet Gynecol* 1971; **110**:428–31.

23. Wadelius M, Darj E, Frenne G, Rane A, Induction of CYP2D6 in pregnancy, *Clin Pharmacol Ther* 1997; **62**:400–7.

24. Wettstein RM, Psychiatric malpractice. In: Tasman A, Hales RE, Frances AJ, eds, *American Psychiatric Press Review of Psychiatry*, Vol. 8 (American Psychiatric Press: Washington DC, 1989) 390–408.

25. Zimmerman M, Coryell W, Corenthal C, Wilson S, A self-report scale to diagnose major depressive disorder, *Arch Gen Psychiatry* 1986; **43**:1076–81.

26. Hamilton M, A rating scale for depression, *J Neurol Neurosurg Psychiatry* 1960; **23**:56–62.

27. Montgomery SA, Åsberg M, A new depression scale designed to be sensitive to change, *Br J Psychiatry* 1979; **134**:382–9.

28. O'Hara MW, Social support, life events, and depression during pregnancy and the puerperium, *Arch Gen Psychiatry* 1986; **43**:569–73.

29. Gotlib IH, Whiffen VE, Mount JH et al, Prevalence rates and demographic characteristics associated with depression in pregnancy and the postpartum, *J Consult Clin Psychol* 1989; **57**:269–74.

30. American Psychiatric Association, *Diagnostic and Statistical Manual of Mental Disorders*, 4th edn (American Psychiatric Association: Washington DC, 1994) 360.

31. Targum SD, Davenport YB, Webster MJ, Postpartum mania in bipolar manic-depressive patients withdrawn from lithium carbonate, *J Nerv Ment Dis* 1979; **167**:572–4.

32. Viguera AC, Cohen LS, The course and management of bipolar disorder during pregnancy, *Psychopharmacol Bull* 1998; **34**:339–46.

33. Wisner KL, Peindl K, Hanusa BH, Relationship of psychiatric illness to childbearing status: a hospital-based epidemiologic study, *J Affect Disord* 1993; **28**:39–50.

34. Villeponteaux VA, Lydiard RB, Laraia MT, The effects of pregnancy on preexisting panic disorder, *J Clin Psychiatry* 1992; **53**:201–3.

35. Cohen LS, Sichel DA, Dimmock JA, Rosenbaum JF, Impact of pregnancy on panic disorder: a case series, *J Clin Psychiatry* 1994; **55**:284–8.

36. Northcott CJ, Stein MB, Panic disorder in pregnancy, *J Clin Psychiatry* 1994; **55**:539–42.

37. Wisner KL, Peindl KS, Hanusa BH, Effects of childbearing on the natural history of panic disorder with comorbid mood disorder, *J Affect Disord* 1996; **41**:173–88.

38. Neziroglu F, Anemone R, Yaryura-Tobias JA, Onset of obsessive-compulsive disorder in pregnancy, *Am J Psychiatry* 1992; **149**:947–50.

39. Buttolph ML, Holland A, Obsessive compulsive disorders in pregnancy and childbirth. In: Jenike MA, Baer L, Minichiello WE, eds, *Obsessive Compulsive Disorders, Theory and Management*, 2nd edn (Yearbook Medical Publishers: Chicago, 1990).

40. Williams KE, Koran LM, Obsessive-compulsive disorder in pregnancy, the puerperium, and the premenstruum, *J Clin Psychiatry* 1997; **58**:330–4.

41. Wisner KL, Stowe ZN, Psychobiology of postpartum mood disorders. *Semin Reprod Endocrinol* 1997; **15**:77–89.

42. Wisner KL, Perel JM, Wheeler SB, Tricyclic dose requirements across pregnancy, *Am J Psychiatry* 1993; **150**:1541–2.

43. Wisner KL, Perel JM, Peindl KS et al, Effects of the postpartum period on nortriptyline pharmacokinetics, *Psychopharmacol Bull* 1997; **33**:243–8.

44. Altshuler LL, Cohen L, Szuba MP et al, Pharmacologic management of psychiatric illness during pregnancy: dilemmas and guidelines, *Am J Psychiatry* 1996; **153**:592–606.

45. Misri S, Sivertz K, Tricyclic drugs in pregnancy and lactation: a preliminary report, *Int J Psychiatry Med* 1991; **21**:157–71.

46. Nulman I, Rovet J, Stewart DE et al, Neurodevelopment of children exposed in utero to antidepressant drugs, *N Engl J Med* 1997; **336**:258–62.

47. Webster PA, Withdrawal symptoms in neonates associated with maternal antidepressant therapy, *Lancet* 1973; **ii**:318–19.

48. Pastuszak A, Schick-Boschetto B, Zuber C et al, Pregnancy outcome following first-trimester exposure to fluoxetine, *JAMA* 1993; **269**:2246–8.

49. Chambers CD, Johnson KA, Dick LM et al, Birth outcomes in pregnant women taking fluoxetine, *N Engl J Med* 1996; **335**:1010–15.

50. Kulin NA, Pastuszak A, Sage SR et al, Pregnancy outcome following maternal use of the new selective serotonin reuptake inhibitors, *JAMA* 1998; **279**:609–10.

51. Spencer MJ, Fluoxetine hydrochloride (Prozac) toxicity in a neonate, *Pediatrics* 1993; **92**:721–2.

52. Mhanna MJ, Bennet JB 2nd, Izatt SD, Potential fluoxetine chloride (Prozac) toxicity in a newborn, *Pediatrics* 1997; **100**:158–9.

53. Heinonen OP, Slone D, Shapiro S, *Birth Defects in Pregnancy* (Publishing Sciences Group: Littleton, 1977).

54. Pavy TJ, Kliffer AP, Douglas MJ, Anaesthetic management of labour and delivery in a woman taking long-term MAOI, *Can J Anaesth* 1995; **42**:618–20.

55. Gracious BL, Wisner KL, Phenelzine use throughout pregnancy and the puerperium: case report, review of the literature, and management recommendations, *Depress Anxiety* 1997; **6**:124–8.

56. Repke JT, Berger NG, Electroconvulsive therapy during pregnancy, *Obstet Gynecol* 1984; **63** (suppl):39S–41S.

57. American Psychiatric Association, *The Practice of Electroconvulsive Therapy, Recommendations for Treatment, Training, and Privileging* (APA: Washington DC, 1990).

58. Polster DS, Wisner KL, ECT-induced premature labor: a case report, *J Clin Psychiatry* 1999; **60**:53–4.

59. Wadhwa PD, Sandman CA, Porto M et al, The association between prenatal stress and infant birth weight and gestational age at birth: a prospective investigation, *Am J Obstet Gynecol* 1993; **169**:858–65.

60. Spinelli MG, Interpersonal psychotherapy for depressed antepartum women: a pilot study, *Am J Psychiatry* 1997; **154**:1028–30.

61. Schou M, Amdisen A, Steenstrup OR, Lithium and pregnancy. II. Hazards to women given lithium during pregnancy and delivery, *Br Med J* 1973; **2**:137–8.

62. Weinstein MR, Lithium treatment of women during pregnancy and in the post-delivery period. In: Johnson FN, ed., *Handbook of Lithium Therapy* (MTP Press: Lancaster, 1980) 421–9.

63. Weinstein MR, Goldfield M, Cardiovascular malformations with lithium use during pregnancy, *Am J Psychiatry* 1975; **132**:529–31.

64. Zalzstein E, Koren G, Einarson T, Freedom RM, A case-control study on the association between first trimester exposure to lithium and Ebstein's anomaly, *Am J Cardiol* 1990; **65**:817–18.

65. Jacobson SJ, Jones K, Johnson K et al, Prospective multicentre study of pregnancy outcome after lithium exposure during first trimester, *Lancet* 1992; **339**:530–3.

66. Cohen LS, Friedman JM, Jefferson JW et al, A reevaluation of risk of in utero exposure to lithium, *JAMA* 1994; **271**:146–50.

67. Schou M, What happened later to the lithium babies? A follow-up study of children born without malformations, *Acta Psychiatr Scand* 1976; **54**:193–7.

68. Wisner KL, Perel JM, Psychopharmacological treatment during pregnancy. In: Jensvold MF, Halbreich U, Hamilton JA, eds, *Psychopharmacology and Women: Sex, Gender and Hormones* (American Psychiatric Press: Washington DC, 1996) 191–224.

69. Sitland-Marken PA, Rickman LA, Wells BG, Mabie WC, Pharmacologic management of acute mania in pregnancy, *J Clin Psychopharmacol* 1989; **9**:78–87.

70. Troyer WA, Pereira GR, Lannon RA et al, Association of maternal lithium exposure and premature delivery, *J Perinatol* 1993; **13**:123–7.

71. Battino D, Binelli S, Bossi L et al, Plasma concentrations of carbamazepine and carbamazepine 10,11-epoxide during pregnancy and after delivery, *Clin Pharmacokinet* 1985; **10**:279–84.

72. Dam M, Christiansen J, Munck O, Mygind KI, Anti-epileptic drugs: metabolism in pregnancy, *Clin Pharmacokinet* 1979; **4**:53–62.

73. Philbert A, Pedersen B, Dam M, Concentration of valproate during pregnancy, in the newborn and in breast milk, *Acta Neurol Scand* 1985; **72**:460–3.

74. Omtzigt JG, Nau H, Los FJ et al, The disposition of valproate and its metabolites in the late first trimester and early second trimester of pregnancy in maternal serum, urine, and amniotic fluid: effect of dose, co-medication, and the presence of spina bifida, *Eur J Clin Pharmacol* 1992; **43**:381–8.

75. Dickinson RG, Harland C, Lynn KR et al, Transmission of valproic acid (Depakene) across the placenta: half-life of the drug in mother and baby, *J Pediatr* 1979; **94**:832–5.

76. Delgado-Escueta AV, Janz D, Consensus guidelines: preconception counseling, management and care of the pregnant woman with epilepsy, *Neurology* 1992; **45** (suppl 5):149–60.

77. Rosa FW, Spina bifida in infants of women treated with carbamazepine during pregnancy, *N Engl J Med* 1991; **324**:674–7.

78. Lindhout D, Meinardi H, Meijer JW, Nau H, Antiepileptic drugs and teratogenesis in two consecutive cohorts: changes in prescription policy paralleled by changes in pattern of malformations, *Neurology* 1992; **42** (suppl 5): 94–110.

79. Nakane Y, Okuma T, Takahashi R et al, Multi-institutional study on teratogenicity and fetal toxicity of antiepileptic drugs: a report of a collaborative study group in Japan, *Epilepsia* 1980; **21**:663–80.

80. Shaw GM, Wasserman CR, O'Malley CD et al, Orofacial clefts and maternal anticonvulsant use, *Reprod Toxicol* 1995; **9**:97–8.

81. Scolnik D, Nulman I, Rovet J et al, Neurodevelopment of children exposed in utero to phenytoin and carbamazepine monotherapy, *JAMA* 1994; **271**:767–70.

82. Granstrom ML, Development of the children of epileptic mothers—preliminary results from the prospective Helsinki study. In: Janz D, Bossi L, Dam M et al, eds, *Epilepsy, Pregnancy, and the Child* (Raven Press: New York, 1982) 403–8.

83. Hiilesmaa VK, Teramo K, Granstrom ML, Bardy AH, Fetal head growth retardation associated with maternal anti-epileptic drugs, *Lancet* 1981; **2**:165–7.

84. Merlob P, Mor N, Litwin A, Transient hepatic dysfunction in an infant of an epileptic mother treated with carbamazepine during pregnancy and breastfeeding, *Ann Pharmacother* 1992; **26**:1563–5.

85. Legius E, Jaeken J, Eggermont E, Sodium valproate, pregnancy and infantile fatal liver failure, *Lancet* 1987; **2**:1518–19.

86. Borkenstein M, Haidvogl M, Treatment of ingestion of diphenhydramine, *J Pediatr* 1978; **92**:167–8.

87. Magee LA, Schick B, Donnenfeld AE et al, The safety of calcium channel blockers in human pregnancy: a prospective multicenter cohort study, *Am J Obstet Gynecol* 1996; **174**:823–8.

88. Kanto JH, Use of benzodiazepines during pregnancy, labour and lactation, with particular reference to pharmacokinetic considerations, *Drugs* 1982; **23**:354–80.

89. Safra MJ, Oakley GP Jr, Association between cleft lip with or without cleft palate and prenatal exposure to diazepam, *Lancet* 1975; **2**:478–80.

90. Milkovich L, van den Berg BJ, Effects of prenatal meprobamate and chlordiazepoxide hydrochloride on human embryonic and fetal development, *N Engl J Med* 1974; **291**: 1268–71.

91. Bracken MB, Holford TR, Exposure to prescribed drugs in pregnancy and association with congenital malformations, *Obstet Gynecol* 1981; **58**:336–44.

92. Hartz SC, Heinonen OP, Shapiro S et al, Antenatal exposure to meprobamate and chlordiazepoxide in relation to malformations, mental development, and childhood mortality, *N Engl J Med* 1975; **292**:726–8.

93. Laegreid L, Olegard R, Conradi N et al, Congenital malformations and maternal consumption of benzodiazepines: a case-control study, *Dev Med Child Neurol* 1990; **32**: 432–41.

94. St Clair SM, Schirmer RG, First-trimester exposure to alprazolam, *Obstet Gynecol* 1992; **80**:843–6.

95. Viggedal G, Hagberg BS, Laegreid L, Aronsson M, Mental development in late infancy after prenatal exposure to benzodiazepines—a prospective study, *J Child Psychol Psychiatry* 1993; **34**:295–505.

96. Fisher JB, Edgren BE, Mammel MC, Coleman JM, Neonatal apnea associated with maternal clonazepam therapy: a case report, *Obstet Gynecol* 1985; **66**:34S–5S.

97. Stahl MM, Saldeen P, Vinge E, Reversal of fetal benzodiazepine intoxication using flumazenil, *Br J Obstet Gynaecol* 1993; **100**:185–8.

98. Cowe L, Lloyd DJ, Dawling S, Neonatal convulsions caused by withdrawal from maternal clomipramine, *Br Med J* 1982; **284**:1837–8.

18

Postpartum psychiatric disorders
Deborah Sichel

Introduction

Postpartum psychiatric disorders comprise a number of different mood and anxiety disorders which are characterized by the onset of emotional symptoms in the weeks or months following birth. Each disorder is associated with a particular symptom constellation that suggests the clinical diagnosis. For reasons that are not entirely clear, these disorders have been globally under-recognized and undertreated. Fortunately, a flourishing interest in research and treatment in recent years is likely to change the past indifference to women who are at risk for postpartum psychiatric illness.

Although the traditional understanding of postpartum illnesses has focused on the mood disturbances,[1-4] more recent reports show that anxiety disorders also appear in the postpartum period and that they are often complicated by the comorbid onset of depressive disturbance.[5,6]

Most studies of postpartum illness have included those with symptom emergence until 6 months postpartum, although it is likely that only the early-onset disorders (i.e. onset within the first 2–6 weeks postpartum) may actually reflect a sensitivity to neuroendocrine factors specific to the postpartum period. Since depressive episodes are known to follow incidents of stressful life events,[7,8] the cumulative effects of this major life transition in the months after delivery possibly account for some of the later onset of the depressive and anxiety illnesses which emerge within the first postpartum year. Although it is reasonable to think that psychosocial factors are paramount in later-onset illness, they may also be important in early-onset disorders. Thus far, it has proved difficult to distinguish the factors that are operant in the onset of the illness. In time, differentiation between the early- and later-onset illnesses may be an important factor in determining the particular recurrent risks of a specific postpartum mood or anxiety disorder, as well as various effective methods of prophylaxis following subsequent deliveries.

Although there has been some debate about whether these disorders are distinct from depressive and anxiety disorders occurring at other times of the life cycle,[9,10] there is little argument about the fact that the postpartum period is a time of risk for the emergence of clinically serious episodes of mood and anxiety disorders. Certainly, the postpartum period is a time like no other in the female reproductive cycle, wherein a massive hormonal shift occurs simultaneously with newly emerging psychologically and developmentally challenging stressful tasks. Thus, inherent to this time are immense biological and psychosocial factors which impinge on the neuroendocrinology of the brain—all the events that we know to be associated with the emergence of a depressive or anxiety illness.

For many clinicians, the confusion about differentiating between normal postpartum emotional adjustment and postpartum psychiatric illness still lingers. This chapter reviews the current knowledge of postpartum psychiatric disorders and presents a new way for clinicians caring for pregnant women to better understand, diagnose, treat and prevent the various disorders that emerge peripartum.

Epidemiology

Epidemiological studies show that women experience double the rates of depression compared to men[11,12] (see Chapters 1 and 2). More recent studies not only confirm these previously determined rates, but also show that these elevated percentages are consistent within at least 13 countries,[13,14] suggesting that factors influencing depressive illness are common to all women and transcend culture. The rates of mood and anxiety disorders usually peak in women during the childbearing years, that is between the ages of 18 and 44.[15] Gater et al demonstrated that women who have borne children have higher rates of mood disorder than nulliparous women and that this elevation

never returns to the lower rates of non-childbearing status.[13] It is possible that one factor contributing to the rates of mood disorder in women may relate to the long-term effects of gonadal hormones in the brain, given recent evidence of the mood-stabilizing effects of oestrogen.[16]

O'Hara et al reported that postpartum women followed prospectively had a depression rate of between 8% and 12%.[17-19] Although he found that this paralleled the incidence of depression in the control group of non-childbearing women, it is important to note that these figures were derived from community samples. Other studies in England and Canada, with much larger samples of women, have suggested that the risk for the emergence of serious depressive illness in women after childbirth is substantially higher (between 12% and 15%) than in non-childbearing women.[20] Similarly, Wisner found that one out of seven depressive episodes for which women sought treatment was related to a childbearing event.[21]

The likelihood of a woman experiencing a depressive episode in the postpartum period is higher in women with a family history and/or personal history of depressive disturbance. The postpartum period is also a time when subsyndromal or partial affective symptoms increase substantially. Researchers and clinicians must address the possibility that childbearing may precipitate either the first significant episode of depression on a background of limited previous symptoms, or the re-emergence of a recurrent depressive episode.

Psychotic disorders are also more likely to be precipitated in association with childbearing. Kendell et al have demonstrated a dramatic increase in admissions to a psychiatric hospital of women experiencing psychosis within the first 3 months after delivery; beyond this critical period, the rates decline to those normally expected.[22] This finding, together with a high recurrence of postpartum mood disorders, suggests that there are subgroups of women with vulnerability specific to the early postpartum period.

The unique hormonal state during the peripartum period, which includes oestrogen, progesterone and cortisol withdrawal, may be an important factor in understanding the early onset of some postpartum mood disorders and the factors involved in recurrence. Increasing awareness about the temporal relationship between mood destabilization and a predictable reproductive event will permit identification of clinical groups at risk, as well as aid in the planning of prophylactic interventions. Identifying the impact of neurohormonal kindling mechanisms on limbic monoamine pathways and neuropeptide release will promote a more accurate understanding of how these subgroups of women become especially vulnerable to the onset of psychiatric illness in the postpartum period.

Despite the large number of women affected by mood disorders in the postpartum period, clinical recognition and diagnosis is often still poor. This is partly because of the lack of understanding by clinicians of postpartum disorders and partly because prenatal depression is often not recognized. Emotional wellbeing during pregnancy is a poor predictor of adverse postpartum outcome, since a woman may be at risk by virtue of a previous history of depression. Depressive symptoms during pregnancy are a robust indicator that postpartum illness will occur.[18,23,24]

Postpartum psychiatric disorders are not benign conditions. Emotional and cognitive disturbances in children of depressed mothers have been amply demonstrated and there is greater potential for impaired family development and psychopathology.[25,26] Lack of emotional wellbeing in the mother often impacts on her ability to adequately care for her baby. One particular problem, frequently unrecognized in paediatric clinical practice, is the association of maternal depression with the infant's failure to thrive. Yet, while the infant undergoes extensive medical work-up, this aspect of the dyad is rarely investigated.

Suicide or infanticide or both within the throes of a severe, undiagnosed postpartum illness is by far the biggest concern with this population. Recent data suggest that the early postpartum period is a time for increased risk of suicide, despite previous indications that the rates of suicide were low in the first postpartum year.[27,28] Thus, early diagnosis and treatment of a mother has enormous implications for her wellbeing, the development of the infant, and other children who are dependent on her.

Antepartum evaluation

From the obstetrician's clinical standpoint, evaluation of risk factors for postpartum psychiatric illnesses should begin with the first prenatal visit. The majority of women who experience postpartum illness have family histories of depression or anxiety disorder.[29,30] Many others have personally experienced some form of mood or anxiety problem, albeit mild or moderate in symptomatology, which often was never previously diagnosed. Together, these features confer the most significant determinants for the onset of a postpartum episode, which is usually the most severe episode of anxiety or depression for a woman.[31] Both family and personal history incorporate determinants of genetic vulnerability and whether or not symptomatic expression has already occurred in a particular woman. This could be understood as baseline risk, which the woman brings with her into every pregnancy.

Table 18.1 Questions to detect women at risk for postpartum depression.

Is there a family member who has or has had mood or emotional problems, problems with anxiety, or abuses alcohol (note, these conditions are often untreated)?

Have you ever experienced periods of sad or low mood, or lost interest in your usual activities?

If yes, were there changes in your sleep, appetite or concentration?

Have you ever thought about harming yourself, or have you attempted to harm yourself?

Have you at any time of your life believed that you have experienced depression, even though it has resolved on its own, or while you have received counselling?

Did you have difficulties coping and feeling like your usual self for any length of time following a previous birth of one of your children?

Is there evidence for a previous postpartum depression?

Have you ever had medications prescribed for anxiety or depression?

Asking a woman about 'psychiatric history' often elicits a negative answer. What clinicians understand as depression is often not the way in which a lay person identifies 'history'; therefore, a brief set of questions at the first visit might help to detect the baseline genetic and personal clinical risks (Table 18.1).

An affirmative answer to any of these questions places a woman in a potential risk category. A discussion about risk factors for a postpartum depression is important at this point, and a referral to psychiatry for postpartum prophylaxis should be considered.

Another set of questions will elucidate whether a woman has past experience of mood changes associated with fluctuating hormonal environments. The presence of moderate to severe premenstrual mood changes suggests the presence of a sensitive biological diathesis which may react adversely to the postpartum physiological process.

As the pregnancy progresses, the clinician should inquire about mood swings, tearfulness, anxiety, irritability, or appetite or sleep problems which seem to be unrelated to any physical discomfort or nocturia. Onset of these symptoms may indicate that there is emergence of depression during the pregnancy, which often implies a significant risk for postpartum depression. Irritability and agitation frequently predominate over sadness or low mood in pregnancy.

In the course of the pregnancy, a number of psychosocial events may impinge on baseline risk.[32] This is 'evolving risk'. Stressors may include a lack of social support, isolated living circumstances, financial concerns, marital conflict, domestic abuse and unexpected medical or obstetric complications. Thus by the end of the pregnancy, there may be an accumulation of significant life stressors affecting the pregnant woman. Following delivery, the rapidly changing neurohormonal milieu may finally tip an already 'loaded' situation, and a postpartum depression will emerge. The clinician should remember, however, that even in the absence of baseline risk factors, psychosocial factors can be severe enough to precipitate depressive illness peripartum, and the presence of depression in a pregnant woman is still the strongest predictor of postpartum illness.

Attention to these issues antepartum can go a long way in identifying women at risk, so that early treatment may be offered.

Pathophysiology

Biological studies

Although numerous investigations have attempted to implicate gonadal and thyroid hormones, prolactin, cortisol, endorphins, tryptophan and other peptides in the aetiology of postpartum depressive disorders, very few conclusive data have emerged.[33] This has to do in part with a snapshot approach within a complex, rapidly changing neuroendocrine milieu and the difficulties in correlating the serum levels of gonadal hormones with their impact on central monoamine and peptide pathways. Since gonadal hormones have been found to modulate monamine systems,[34,35] it is very likely that some precipitating factors are associated with the rates of change of gonadal hormones and not necessarily with the actual serum levels. Thus, abrupt withdrawal of oestrogen, progesterone, cortisol and peptides may well operate and impact negatively on pathways involved in mood stability (see Chapter 12). Genetic vulnerability is likely to be an important influential factor in how monoamine and peptide pathways react to different hormonal environments.

Hypothalamic–pituitary–thyroid axis function may be impaired in some postpartum patients. A prevalence rate of 6% for thyroid dysfunction of the autoimmune type has been noted in postpartum women.[36] Although some women may have positive thyroid antibodies or thyroid dysfunction concurrent with depression postpartum, there is no consistent evidence linking these phenomena. In most instances, both the depression and the thyroid problem require treatment.

Depression outside of the postpartum period is often associated with a dysregulated hypothalamic–pituitary–adrenal pathway, elevated cortisol levels and an inability of the pituitary to suppress cortisol levels. Postpartum increases in cortisol levels, however, are more difficult to interpret because cortisol levels are elevated in pregnancy, and increase with breast-feeding; increased suckling may also exaggerate cortisol levels.[37]

Wieck et al found an elevated growth hormone response to apomorphine challenge in women who were at risk for developing a postpartum psychosis.[38] This suggested that there may be a supersensitivity of dopamine receptors in the limbic system in these women; however, this finding was not replicated by others.[39]

A reduction of serum tryptophan on days 2–6 postpartum (which is associated with maternity blues), as well as at the 6-month follow-up, has been suggested; treatment with tryptophan, though, was not helpful.[40–42]

There are no biochemical studies pertinent to the emergence of anxiety disorders postpartum, although oestrogen and progesterone withdrawal may contribute to the worsening or new emergence of anxiety symptoms. In particular, withdrawal of progesterone, which binds to GABA receptors, may precipitate an increase in anxiety symptoms after delivery.[43] Klein has postulated that carbon dioxide levels during pregnancy are low, because of the increased respiratory effects of large amounts of circulating progesterone, effectively diminishing panic symptoms during pregnancy.[44] After delivery, carbon dioxide levels rapidly increase and return to normal, coincident with worsening or emergent panic symptoms. This may lead to a sense of suffocation. It is interesting to note that the intravenous fluid of choice given to women in labour is Ringer's lactate. Lactate induces panic attacks in individuals who demonstrate vulnerability to panic, so, in some women at risk for panic worsening, physicians may unwittingly be precipitating postpartum panic attacks.

There are no biological studies regarding the onset of obsessive-compulsive symptoms in the postpartum period, but recent explorations of the actions of oxytocin in the paralimbic cortical area offer some possible mechanisms for the onset of these symptoms. Normal maternal hypervigilance and nurturing behaviour is instinctively obsessive in nature, as survival of the young depends on constant maternal care and attention. The intactness of this process, contingent on adequate maternal bonding, appears to be mediated by oxytocin within the cingulate gyrus in rats and monkeys.[45] Overzealous vigilant behaviours leading to the emergence of obsessive-compulsive symptoms sufficient to induce distress, dysfunction and anxiety in the mother may represent a form of overshoot bonding response in genetically vulnerable women. This is, in a way, the opposite of what we see in women who demonstrate little capacity to attach to their infants.

Postpartum risk factors

Consistent risk factors for depressive disorders with postpartum onset are family and personal history of depression.[30] Prospective studies have demonstrated that lack of social support, marital conflict, medical and obstetric complications and temperamentally difficult infants are also correlated with the onset of postpartum depression.[19,46,47] Increased maternal age, breast-feeding, lower socio-economic class and education level have not been consistently correlated with depression.[48] Adolescents appear to have a significant rate of depression after delivery, assessed as 30% in one study.[49] This should not be surprising, since most adolescents are less able to cope with the burden of pregnancy and parenting, and often present with numerous psychosocial problems.

We recently conducted a chart review of the characteristics of 31 women consecutively admitted to a mother–baby unit in Boston.[50] Twenty-four of them had a history of psychiatric illness at the time of admission, as determined by a retrospective structured clinical interview using the *Diagnostic and Statistical Manual of Mental Disorders*, 4th edition criteria (DSM-IV).[51] Twelve women developed psychiatric illness during their pregnancies, but were not identified by their obstetric caregivers. Eighteen of the 31 women had bipolar illness, five postpartum major depression, and the others anxiety disorders complicated by depression. Of the 31 cases, 24 could have been predicted by history alone, and admission probably prevented with prophylactic medication measures instituted immediately after delivery. Aside from the cost of hospitalization at $1500 US a day, the enormous toll on the families would also have been averted. Thus, attention to psychiatric risk factors during the pregnancy makes good clinical practice as well as economic sense.

Postpartum mood and anxiety disorders—a new clinical classification

The majority of women seen in family practice, obstetric and psychiatric offices falls into one of the following groups when they present with emotional illness in the postpartum period.

Group 1: Maternity blues

Maternity blues is a self-limiting syndrome that affects 50–80% of women after delivery. Symptoms usually begin on the second or third day postpartum, peak on the fifth to seventh day, and should start to remit by the second week;[52] symptoms include labile mood with feelings of both joy and tearfulness, anxiety, sleep difficulties and irritability. Treatment includes reassurance, support, and enlisting family members to care for the infant to ensure some periods of catch-up sleep, even if the mother is breast-feeding. It is not detrimental to the breast-feeding relationship to introduce an occasional bottle of formula, allowing a mother some badly needed rest.

Occasionally, an extended period of the blues will continue into the fourth and fifth week postpartum. Strictly speaking, this longer-lasting period of mood disturbance is no longer blues, and qualifies for the diagnosis of minor depression, though some clinicians term this complicated blues.[53] It usually resolves by the fourth to eighth postpartum week. The clinical significance of the blues and the complicated type is that 25% of women will go on to have depression; thus, the blues may be a marker for later-onset postpartum depression.[17] Sometimes, depression will follow a subsequent pregnancy, with onset in the time frame of a previous episode of complicated blues.

Group 2: The 'pure' postpartum depression group

The first episode of depression in this group of women occurs in the early postpartum period, often within the first 4 weeks after delivery. There is usually a family history of depression or anxiety, but the woman herself appears not to have experienced any prior problems with depression. This group of women can be conceptualized as presenting with a 'pure' depression, because depression occurs only in the context of a postpartum period and appears to be more strongly associated with a biological vulnerability.[54] Although the risk for recurrence of depression (even outside the postpartum period) will be increased after this episode, depressive illness is likely to emerge again following a subsequent delivery. Depression onset is early, rapid and often severe.

These women tend to respond well to antidepressant therapy combined with supportive and interpersonal psychotherapy as well as health teaching.

Group 3: Women with a previous history of major or minor depression

This group includes women who demonstrate evidence of previous episodes of major or minor depression and/or a history of dysthymia, although it may not have been diagnosed. There is often a family history of depression or anxiety disorders. Although the postpartum episode is often the most severe episode yet experienced, a careful history will elicit previous evidence of mood disturbance, including premenstrual dysphoria. Onset may be within weeks of delivery, or later, after several months (Table 18.2).

In both groups 2 and 3, the diagnosis is major non-psychotic postpartum depression, but the distinction between groups 2 and 3 is a previous personal history of mood disturbance. Both carry a family history of depression.

An important and frequently misdiagnosed presentation in the postpartum period is the depressed phase of a bipolar diathesis which may be confused with postpartum depression.

Table 18.2 Symptoms of postpartum major depression.	
Feeling overwhelmed	Agitated
Irritable	Difficulty concentrating
Unhappy, sad, crying, hopeless	Poor sleep
Anxious, tense, worried	Poor appetite

As a result of the above symptoms, the patient blames herself and feels unnecessarily guilty, is unable to care for herself and/or the baby, shows a lack of interest in the baby or else is preoccupied with and constantly worried about the baby's health (and cannot be reassured), and in the extreme develops suicidal and/or infanticidal thoughts and plans.

Management

Initial assessment entails evaluation of symptom severity and safety of the mother. The Edinburgh Postnatal Depression Scale, a 10-item scale designed to specifically detect postpartum illness, can now be self-administered.[55] The Beck Depression scale, also self-administered, is useful in detecting severity and presence of depression.[56] It is at times misleading to believe that the mother will not harm herself due to the presence of the baby. New mothers can feel quite fragile and may interpret depression as meaning that they have failed in this fundamental task, the 'maternal role'. Women from dysfunctional families are especially vulnerable to these emotions, since their fantasy is to be the mother they did not have, in an attempt to 'redo' their own difficult childhoods. Hospitalization is warranted if the mother is assessed to be a danger to herself and/or to her baby and there is an inadequate family support structure.

Diagnostic testing

Thyroid function levels should always be measured, including antimicrosomal antibodies to rule out Hashimoto's thyroiditis. In most cases of Hashimoto's, depression and thyroid dysfunction co-occur, with each condition requiring treatment. The symptoms of both thyroid disease and anaemia can mirror those of major depression, and laboratory investigations should be used to eliminate an underlying medical cause.

Pharmacotherapy
Anti-anxiety medications
Relief of the intense discomfort of anxiety and agitation is important in the early treatment. The benzodiazepines are effective anti-anxiety agents, in adequate dosages. Long-acting agents, such as clonazepam, may be preferable to the shorter-acting agents, such as alprazolam, lorazepam and oxazepam, due to their greater potency. Sedation sometimes occurs, so doses should be titrated to each woman's needs. Typically, an average clonazepam dose ranges between 0.5 mg and 3 mg a day (see Chapter 17).

Antidepressant medications
These drugs should be started immediately,

concurrent with the anti-anxiety medications. The older tricyclic medications are still useful, in particular nortryptiline and desipramine, because they aid sleep in the agitated insomniac state. However, there is no evidence that one drug is superior to another in the treatment of postpartum depression. The newer agents, described below, are generally better tolerated than the older drugs.

The selective serotonin reuptake inhibiting antidepressants (SSRIs), including paroxetine, fluoxetine, fluvoxamine, sertraline and citalopram, are all effective treatments for depression.[57] Augmentation techniques to boost antidepressant response with lithium and tricyclics often convert an absent or a partial response to a full remission.

Venlafaxine and nefazodone target both serotonin and noradrenaline receptors and provide alternatives to the SSRIs, should the latter induce problematic side-effects.

Electroconvulsive therapy should be readily considered in a situation of persistent non-response to pharmacotherapy in both depression and psychotic depression, especially when the risks of suicide and/or infanticide are high.[58]

A recent, very preliminary report has suggested that transdermal oestrogen therapy (the patch) was effective in treating postpartum depression.[59] Half the women in that study were on antidepressant treatment, to which the oestrogen patch was added. Since they may have exhibited both an antidepressant and a placebo response, these results should be interpreted with caution. Although the addition of oestrogen to antidepressant therapy has been reported to effect a mild response in chronically, severely depressed women,[60,61] the doses administered in that study were high as compared with the oestrogen patch dose. It is possible that, in some cases, addition of oestrogen via patch or orally may augment the action of the antidepressant, either prior to the onset of

the first menstrual cycle after delivery or in anovulatory cycles when levels may be low. However, there is no information about oestrogen levels and their relationship to depression, and oestrogen administered alone has not been shown to exhibit an effective antidepressant response. More studies are needed to ascertain that oestrogen is indeed an effective augmentation technique in treatment-resistant postpartum depression.

Progesterone
The use of large doses of progesterone in suppository and oral micronized forms has long been touted as an effective treatment for premenstrual dysphoric disorder and postpartum depression.[62] Despite a worldwide following, accurate data collection on progesterone treatment has been poor, and double-blind studies using large doses have revealed no evidence of its efficacy.[63] In some situations, progesterone may actually worsen depression. Progesterone appears to be at best equal to placebo, and its use in the treatment of postpartum depression or premenstrual dysphoric disorder cannot be recommended at this time.

Breast-feeding
A number of case reports and case series at this time suggest that the use of antidepressant medication in breast-feeding mothers results in no or little accumulation of the parent drug or active metabolites in the baby's serum, when the mothers are taking therapeutic doses.[64–67] (For a comprehensive review of antidepressants and other medications during breast-feeding, see Chapter 19). Although these drugs were found in substantial quantities in the breast milk, accumulation in even young babies was quite limited. The majority of these reports indicate no adverse effects on infants' development, although there are few data on children's development after 36 months of age.[67] The

authors suggest that paediatricians should be made aware of the medications that women use while breast-feeding and that at least one infant serum level be measured.

In cases where a nursing mother requires antidepressant medication, optimal clinical care reflecting current evidence would include careful risk–benefit evaluation of the mother–infant pair and monitoring of the infant serum level at least once (see also Chapter 19).

Psychotherapy

Supportive psychotherapy is an important aspect of the treatment modality for a woman and her partner. These illnesses provoke tense, strained communication and misunderstanding in families. Women may elect to continue the psychotherapeutic process after recovery to resolve other issues in their lives. The best outcomes usually result from the use of pharmacotherapy provided within a caring, supportive relationship between clinician and patient.

Interpersonal psychotherapy (IPT)

O'Hara, studying this particular technique, suggests that IPT can be an effective treatment for postpartum depression.[68] Twelve sessions with a focus on relationships, support and problem-solving are provided. Further research is needed to establish the long-term treatment effects of IPT and to pinpoint which women are most likely to benefit. For example, most women with postpartum depression and a prior history of depression are at risk for future depressive episodes. IPT maintenance therapy or repeated IPT sessions in the event of another depressive episode may be necessary to prevent or limit recurrent depression (see Chapter 30).

Recurrence

Postpartum depressive disorders are frequently recurrent. A follow-up suggested that recurrence rates were between 1 in 3 and 1 in 4, but it is likely that the rates are even higher.[65] Women with the 'pure' onset may be particularly vulnerable to postpartum onset, whereas women who demonstrate a more recurrent pattern of depression outside of childbearing may show a more variable vulnerability. Wisner and Wheeler have suggested postpartum prophylaxis using antidepressants immediately after delivery in women who are deemed at high risk for recurrent postpartum depression.[69] Hopefully, prophylactic interventions will become the routine standard of care for obstetric patients at risk for the recurrence of postpartum depression.

Group 4: Postpartum psychosis

The onset of postpartum psychosis occurs at a rate of approximately 1 in 1000 births.[70] It usually presents acutely within the first 2–4 weeks postpartum. Although postpartum psychosis can appear in a context of no previous mood symptoms, the more common situation is a history of various patterns of mood swings. Mood swing disorders encompass bipolar 1 disorder, the most well-recognized form of manic depressive illness, bipolar 2 disorder, a less severe form of bipolar 1 disorder, and cyclothymic and hyperthymic mood states. Many women with bipolar 1 disorder will have been identified and treated with mood stabilizers, but occasionally this will be the index episode. Many women with these mood swing diatheses have histories of premenstrual irritability or significant mood instability during infertility treatments.

Symptom presentation (Table 18.3)

A careful history usually reveals onset within the first days after delivery. Prominent symptoms at that time are restlessness, exhilaration, and sleeplessness, which represent the hypomanic swing after delivery. Postpartum ward

Table 18.3 Symptoms of postpartum psychosis.	
Agitation, pressured speech	Delusions, either grandiose or paranoid
Hallucinations: auditory, command, visual, tactile, olfactory	Inability to sleep, confusion
	Poor appetite

staff usually attribute this behaviour to the excitement about the new baby. The full-blown illness appears within the next 2 weeks. Diagnostically, postpartum psychosis shares features of a manic psychosis, or if the illness has swung into the depressed phase, it appears as a psychotic depression. Glover et al suggest that the condition of the 'highs' predicts a post-partum depression,[71] but it is likely that these women actually have a bipolar 2 disorder, and the 'highs' represent the frequent hypomanic swing after delivery prior to the switch into the depressed phase.

Some investigators have described a waxing and waning course with lucid periods, which probably indicates a rapid-cycling diathesis in periods of normal mood.

Management

Postpartum psychosis is a dangerous illness that carries a risk of infanticide and suicide. It must be aggressively treated within a hospital setting. Mood-stabilizing medications (lithium, valproic acid or carbamazepine) should be started imme-diately along with antipsychotic drugs to stop the psychotic symptoms. The more potent, less sedating antipsychotic agents are preferable, such as perphenazine, haloperidol or fluphenazine. The newer, atypical antipsychotic olanzepine holds promise as a fast and effective antipsychotic agent in stemming the symptoms of postpartum psychosis;[48a] this may be due to its more selective effect on mesolimbic dopamine receptors. Once a treatment response with these agents is achieved, a depressive phase may emerge. Caution in adding antidepressant agents may be needed in order not to precipitate a hypomanic or rapid-cycling situation.

Postpartum psychosis carries a high rate (more than 90%) of recurrence after future pregnancies.[72] A number of studies have sug-gested that prophylaxis with lithium adminis-tered immediately after delivery prevents recurrence in 90% of the women at risk.[73,74] Although there are no formal studies, there is no reason why depakote would not be equally effective as a prophylactic agent, given its proven efficacy as a first-line antimanic agent.

The use of high-dose oestrogen in women at risk for early-onset puerperal depression and postpartum psychosis may also reduce the rate of recurrence,[16] but high-dose oestrogen may add to the risk of thromboembolism at a time when the chances of this complication are at their highest. Given that antidepressants and mood stabilizers are effective in substantially reducing the risks of recurrence, these represent much safer and universally available prophy-laxes compared with oestrogen.

Group 5: Comorbid emergence of postpartum depression

In this group of women, an anxiety disorder which may have been present for a long time (often mild and not diagnosed) is primary. Panic attacks, generalized anxiety or obsessive-compulsive disorder are evident from a history in the pregravid state. In the postpartum period, the anxiety disorder worsens and is followed by the emergence of depression. Occasionally, an anxiety or obsessive-compulsive disorder (OCD) will emerge for the first time in the postpartum period, also followed by depression.

Panic disorder

Until recently, the course, impact and prevalence of anxiety disorders related to pregnancy and the postpartum period have received little attention. Although some authors have noted improvement in panic symptomatology during pregnancy, others have described worsening.[75] Klein has noted that if women have no active panic symptoms prior to conception, they tend to remain well throughout the pregnancy.[44]

In contrast, the postpartum period appears to be consistently associated with worsening of panic symptoms.[75] Women with a history of mild pregravid panic symptoms have experienced their worst episodes of panic symptoms postpartum. Worsening of panic symptoms characteristically occurred within the first 2–3 postpartum weeks along with significant symptoms of depression.

Management

The treatment of panic attacks commonly includes pharmacotherapy with benzodiazepines, either alone or with antidepressant medications. The new SSRI medications are particularly effective for panic symptoms, even in the absence of depression. Frequently, pharmacotherapy is augmented with cognitive-behavioural therapy. Maintenance pharmacotherapy or cognitive-behavioural therapy may be needed to contain panic symptoms, since the primary disorder will always be present in varying degrees of severity.

Given consistent reports that panic symptoms are likely to worsen after delivery, women with a history of pregravid panic symptoms should be advised to consider preventive interventions with pharmacotherapy and/or cognitive-behavioural therapy after delivery.

Postpartum obsessive-compulsive disorder

A subgroup of women experience the onset of recurrent intrusive thoughts about harming their babies in gruesome ways, for example stabbing the baby, drowning, or throwing the child out of a window. Onset is usually within the first 6 weeks postpartum. Mothers typically become avoidant of their babies, and develop panic attacks and depression.[76] This syndrome must be differentiated from postpartum psychosis. Women with postpartum psychosis are unable to appreciate that their thoughts make no sense and demonstrate confusion, whereas women with OCD appreciate that their thoughts make no sense, and are not confused.

Women who develop this particular form of OCD usually become depressed after the onset of the thoughts. It appears to carry a high rate of relapse following subsequent deliveries. It is strongly recommended to begin prophylaxis with SSRI medications immediately after (the next) birth. The presentation of puerperal OCD should also be distinguished from a pregravid OCD which has worsened substantially after delivery.

Biological studies have yet to be done, but it is possible that there may be acute serotonin dysregulation triggered by falling levels of gonadal hormones. Dysregulation of serotonin pathways is now considered to be a significant aspect of OCD symptoms.[77]

Another possibility is that oxytocin, now implicated in bonding and nurturing behaviours, 'overshoots' and women develop an over-vigilant maternal response which becomes a pathological hypervigilance concerning potential harm to their infants. Elevated oxytocin levels have been noted in the cerebrospinal fluid of patients with OCD.[78]

Management

Treatment with the SSRI group of antidepressants is very effective in most situations. The dosages needed to stop the thoughts are often higher than required for treatment of depression. Fluoxetine may need to be used in doses of 40–80 mg, sertraline 200–300 mg, paroxetine 40–60 mg, clomipramine 150–250 mg, and fluvoxamine 100–300 mg. The use of long-acting benzodiazepines, particularly clonazepam, in the first stabilizing weeks is helpful in containing the severe concurrent anxiety until the SSRI medications are effective. Premenstrual recurrence is common in the months following stabilization. The author has found that the use of oral contraception worsens the OCD symptoms, so barrier or intrauterine device methods of contraception are generally recommended. Attempts to taper the medications should be attempted after 1 year. If the tapering is successful, clinicians should expect a high percentage of recurrence following future deliveries. The SSRI-type medications implemented immediately after delivery are very effective in preventing another episode.

Conclusion

Excellent prenatal care incorporates attention to the emotional health of the mother. It is not sufficient to pay attention only to her physical wellbeing during the pregnancy, since poor emotional health can adversely impact on the health of the baby, both antepartum and postpartum. As our knowledge about perinatal psychiatric illness has dramatically increased, we now know how to identify a significant number of the high-risk groups and are aware of effective prophylaxes for the different types of postpartum psychiatric illnesses.

The inclusion of a psychiatric history in prenatal care melds the two fields so that the best outcome for women and their babies can occur. Similarly, even when the pregnancy has gone well, a woman may be heading into the most significant illness of her life after delivery. Ironically, at a time when a mother may be most at risk, her needs too often take a back seat to those of her infant. As we progress into the next millennium, along with the wave of enthusiasm about women's health care we must understand that developing babies need emotionally intact mothers and that the infant's progress must be assessed within the dyad. Women's mental health care is integral to both women's health and the health of their families. A humane and compassionate society tends to the needs of both its children and their mothers. Achieving this end entails conviction, perseverance and collaboration among health-care specialties. It is not our choice but our obligation.

References

1. Pitt B, Maternity blues, *Br J Psychiatry* 1973; **122**:431–3.
2. Pitt B, Atypical depression following childbirth, *Br J Psychiatry* 1968; **114**:1325–35.
3. O'Hara MW, Postpartum mental disorders. In: Sciarra JJ, ed., *Gynecology and Obstetrics*, Vol. 6 (Harper Row: Philadelphia, 1991) 1–17.
4. O'Hara MW, Social support, life events, and depression during pregnancy and the puerperium, *Arch Gen Psychiatry* 1986; **43**:569–73.
5. Cohen LS, Sichel DA, Dimmock JA, Rosenbaum JF, Postpartum course in women with pre-existing panic disorder, *J Clin Psychiatry* 1994; **55**:289–92.
6. Villeponteaux VA, Lydiard RB, Laraia MT et al, The effects of pregnancy on preexisting panic disorder, *J Clin Psychiatry* 1992; **53**:201–3.
7. Dolan RJ, Calloway SP, Fonagy P et al, Life events, depression and hypothalamic pituitary adrenal axis function, *Br J Psychiatry* 1985; **147**:429–33.
8. Ezquiaqa E, Gutierrez JL, Lopez A, Psychosocial factors and the recurrence of depression, *J Affect Disord* 1987; **12**:135–8.
9. Whiffen VE, Is postpartum depression a distinct diagnosis? *Clin Psychol Rev* 1992; **12**:485–508.
10. Purdy D, Frank E, Should postpartum depression be given a more prominent place in the DSM IV? *Depression* 1993; **1**:59–70.
11. Kessler RC, McGonagle KA, Zhao S et al, Lifetime and 12 month prevalence of DSM-III-R psychiatric disorders in the United States. Results from the National Comorbidity Survey, *Arch Gen Psychiatry* 1994; **51**:8–19.
12. Weissman MM, Bland RC, Canino GJ et al, Cross national epidemiology of major depression and bipolar disorder, *JAMA* 1996; **276**:293–9.
13. Gater R, Tansella M, Korten A et al, Sex differences in the prevalence and detection of depressive and anxiety disorders in general health care settings, *Arch Gen Psychiatry* 1998; **55**:405–13.
14. Weissman MM, Bland R, Joyce PR et al, Sex differences in rates of depression: cross national perspectives, *J Affect Disord* 1993; **29**:77–84.
15. Weissman MM, Livingston Bruce M, Leaf PJ et al, Affective disorders. In: Robins LN, Rigeir DA, eds, *Psychiatric Disorders in America: The Epidemiological Catchment Area Study* (Free Press: NY, 1991) 53–80.
16. Sichel DA, Cohen LS, Robertson LM et al, Prophylactic estrogen in recurrent postpartum affective disorder, *Biol Psychiatry* 1995; **38**:814–18.
17. O'Hara MW, Neunaber DJ, Zekoski EM, Prospective study of postpartum depression: prevalence, course and predictive factors, *J Abnorm Psychol* 1984; **93**:158–71.
18. O'Hara MW, Schlechte JA, Lewis DA, Varner MW, Controlled prospective study of postpartum mood disorders: psychological, environmental and hormonal variables, *J Abnorm Psychol* 1991; **100**:63–73.
19. O'Hara MW, Swain AM, Rates and risk of postpartum depression – a meta-analysis, *Int Rev Psychiatry* 1996; **8**:37–54.
20. Whiffen VE, Gotlib IH, Comparison of postpartum and nonpostpartum depression: clinical presentation, psychiatric history and psychosocial functioning, *J Consult Clin Psychol* 1993; **61**:485–94.
21. Wisner KL, Peindl K, Hanusa BH, Relationship of psychiatric illness to childbearing status. A hospital based epidemiological study, *J Affect Disord* 1993; **28**:39–50.
22. Kendell RE, Chalmers JC, Platz C, Epidemiology of puerperal psychoses, *Br J Psychiatry* 1987; **150**:662–73.
23. Gotlib IH, Whiffen VE, Mount JH et al, Prevalence rates and demographic characteristics associated with depression in pregnancy and the postpartum, *J Consult Clin Psychol* 1989; **57**:269–74.
24. Kitamura T, Shima S, Sugawara M, Toda MA, Psychological and social correlates of the onset of affective disorders among pregnant women, *Psychol Med* 1993; **23**:967–75.
25. Cogill SR, Caplan HL, Alexandra H et al, Impact of maternal postnatal depression on cognitive development of young children, *Br J Psychiatry* 1986; **292**:1165–7.
26. Zuckerman B, Bauchner H, Parker S, Cabral H, Maternal depressive symptoms during pregnancy, and newborn irritability, *J Dev Behav Pediatr* 1990; **11**:190–4.
27. Appleby L, Suicide during pregnancy and in the

first postnatal year, *Br Med J* 1991; **302**:137–40.

28. Appleby L, Turnbull G, Parasuicide in the first postnatal year, *Psychol Med* 1995; **25**:1087–90.

29. Cutrona CE, Causal attributions and perinatal depression, *J Abnorm Psychol* 1983; **92**: 161–72.

30. Steiner M, Tam WYK. Postpartum depression in relation to other psychiatric disorders. In: Miller LJ, ed., *Postpartum Mood Disorders* (American Psychiatric Press: Washington, DC, 1999) 47–63.

31. Graff LA, Dyck DG, Schallow JR, Predicting postpartum depressive symptoms: a structural modelling analysis, *Percept Mot Skills* 1991; **73**:1137–8.

32. Kumar R, Robson KM, A prospective study of emotional disorders in childbearing women, *Br J Psychiatry* 1984; **144**:35–47.

33. Steiner M. Perinatal mood disorders: Position Paper, *Psychopharmacol Bull* 1998; **34**:301–6.

34. Biegon A, Reches A, Snyder L, McEwen BS, Serotonergic and noradrenergic receptors in the rat brain: modulation by chronic exposure to ovarian hormones, *Life Sci* 1983; **32**:2015–21.

35. Backstrom T, Bixo M, Hammarback S, Ovarian steroid hormones: effects on mood, behavior and brain excitability, *Acta Obstet Gynecol Scand Suppl* 1985; **130**:19–24.

36. Hall R, Pregnancy and autoimmune endocrine disease, *Baillieres Clin Endocrinol Metab* 1995; **9**:137–55.

37. Fleming AS, Carter C, Steiner M, Sensory and hormonal control of maternal behaviour in rat and human mothers. In: Pryce CR, Martin RD, Skuse D, eds, *Motherhood in Human and Nonhuman Primates* (Karger: Basel, 1994) 106–14.

38. Wieck A, Kumar R, Hirst AD et al, Increased sensitivity of dopamine receptors and recurrence of affective psychosis after childbirth, *Br Med J* 1991; **303**:613–16.

39. Meakin CJ, Brockington IF, Lynch S, Jones SR, Dopamine supersensitivity and hormonal status in puerperal psychosis, *Br J Psychiatry* 1995; **166**:73–9.

40. Handley SL, Dunn TL, Baker JM et al, Mood changes in puerperium and plasma tryptophan and cortisol concentrations, *Br Med J* 1977; **2**:18–20.

41. Handley SL, Dunn TL, Waldron G, Baker JM, Tryptophan, cortisol and puerperal mood, *Br J Psychiatry* 1980; **136**:498–508.

42. Baker JM, Handley SL, Waldron G, Dunn TL, Seasonal variation in plasma tryptophan in parturient women, *Prog Neuropsychopharmacol* 1981; **5**:515–18.

43. Freeman EW, Purdy RH, Coutifaris C et al, Anxiolytic metabolites of progesterone: correlation with mood and performance measures following oral progesterone administration to healthy female volunteers, *Neuroendocrinol* 1993; **58**:478–84.

44. Klein DF, Pregnancy and panic disorder, *J Clin Psychiatry* 1994; **55**:293–4.

45. Insel TR, Shapiro LE, Oxytocin receptor distribution reflects social organization in monogamous and polygamous voles, *Proc Natl Acad Sci* 1992; **89**:5981–5.

46. Cutrona CE, Troutman BR, Social support, infant temperament, and parenting self efficacy: a mediational model of postpartum depression, *Child Dev* 1986; **57**:1507–18.

47. Cox J, Rooney A, Thomas PF, Wrate RW, How accurately do mothers recall postnatal depression? Further data from a 3 year follow-up study, *J Psychosomatic Obstet Gynecol* 1984; **3**:185–7.

48. Davidson J, Robertson E, A follow-up study of postpartum illness, 1946–1978, *Acta Psychiatr Scand* 1985; **71**:451–7.

49. Troutman BR, Cutrona CE. Nonpsychotic postpartum depression among adolescent mothers, *J Abnorm Psychol* 1990; **99**:69–78.

50. Sichel DA, Driscoll JW, *Women's Moods – What every Woman should Know about Hormones, the Brain and Emotional Health* (William Morrow: New York, 1999).

51. American Psychiatric Association, *Diagnostic and Statistical Manual of Mental Disorder*, 4th edn (American Psychiatric Press: Washington, DC, 1994).

52. Kendell RE, McGuire RJ, Connor Y, Cox JL, Mood changes in the first three weeks after childbirth, *J Affect Disord* 1981; **3**:317–26.

53. Sichel DA, Postpartum psychiatric disorders. In: Carlson K, Eisenstat SA, Frigoletto FD Jr, Schiff I, eds, *Primary Care of Women* (Mosby: St Louis, MO, 1995) 394–9.

54. O'Hara MW, The nature of postpartum depres-

sive disorders. In: Murray L, Cooper PJ, eds, *Postpartum Depression and Child Development* (Guilford: New York, 1997) 3–31.

55. Cox JL, Holden JM, Sagovsky R, Detection of postnatal depression: development of the 10-item Edinburgh Postnatal Depression Scale, *Br J Psychiatry* 1987; **150**:782–6.

56. Beck AT, Steer, RA, *Manual for the Revised Beck Depression Inventory* (Psychological Corporation: San Antonio, TX, 1987).

57. Stowe ZN, Casaulla J, Landry J et al, Sertraline in the treatment of women with postpartum major depression, *Depression* 1995; **3**:49–55.

58. Nonacs R, Cohen LS, Postpartum mood disorders: diagnosis and treatment guidelines, *J Clin Psychiatry* 1998; **59** (suppl 2):34–40.

59. Gregoire AJ, Kumar R, Everitt B et al, Transdermal oestrogen for treatment of severe postnatal depression, *Lancet* 1996; **347**:930–3.

60. Klaiber EL, Broverman DM, Vogel W, Kobayashi Y, Estrogen therapy for severe persistent depression in women, *Arch Gen Psychiatry* 1979; **36**:550–4.

61. Oppenheim G, Estrogen in the treatment of depression: neuropharmacological mechanisms, *Biol Psychiatry* 1983; **18**:721–5.

62. Dalton K, *The Premenstrual Syndrome and Progesterone Therapy*, 2nd edn (William Heinemann: London, 1984).

63. Freeman E, Rickels K, Sondheimer SR, Polansky M, Ineffectiveness of progesterone suppository treatment for premenstrual syndrome, *JAMA* 1990; **264**:349–53.

64. Wisner KL, Perel JM, Serum nortryptiline levels in nursing mothers and their infants, *Am J Psychiatry* 1991; **148**:1234–6.

65. Wisner KL, Perel JM, Blumer J, Serum sertraline and n-desmethylsertraline levels in breast-feeding mother–infant pairs, *Am J Psychiatry* 1998; **155**:690–2.

66. Stowe ZN, Owens MJ, Landry JC et al, Sertraline and desmethylsertraline in human breastmilk and nursing infants, *Am J Psychiatry* 1997; **154**:1255–60.

67. Wisner KL, Perel JM, Findling RL, Antidepressant treatment during breastfeeding, *Am J Psychiatry* 1996; **153**:1132–7.

68. Stuart S, O'Hara MW, Interpersonal psychotherapy for postpartum depression: a treatment program, *J Psychother Prac Res* 1995; **4**:18–29.

69. Wisner KL, Wheeler SB, Prevention of recurrent postpartum major depression, *Hosp Community Psychiatry* 1994; **45**:1191–6.

70. Brockington I, *Motherhood and Mental Health* (Oxford University Press: Oxford, 1996) 241.

71. Glover V, Liddle P, Taylor A et al, Mild hypomania (the highs) can be a feature of the first postpartum week. Association with later depression, *Br J Psychiatry* 1994; **164**:517–21.

72. Kendall RE, Chalmers JC, Platz C, Epidemiology of puerperal psychoses, *Br J Psychiatry* 1987; **150**:662–73.

73. Stewart DE, Klompenhouwer JL, Kendell RE, van Hulst AM. Prophylactic lithium in puerperal psychosis—the experience of three centres, *Br J Psychiatry* 1991; **158**:393–7.

74. Cohen LS, Sichel DA, Robertson LM et al, Postpartum prophylaxis for women with bipolar disorder, *Am J Psychiatry* 1995; **152**:1641–5.

75. Cohen LS, Sichel DA, Faraone SV et al, Course of panic disorder during pregnancy and the puerperium: a preliminary study, *Biol Psychiatry* 1996; **39**:950–4.

76. Sichel DA, Cohen LS, Dimmock JA, Rosenbaum JF, Postpartum obsessive compulsive disorder, a case series, *J Clin Psychiatry* 1993; **54**:156–9.

77. Fineberg NA, Roberts A, Montgomery SA, Cowen PJ, Brain 5-HT function in obsessive-compulsive disorder. Prolactin responses to d-fenfluramine, *Br J Psychiatry* 1997; **171**:280–2.

78. Leckman JF, Goodman WK, North WG et al, Elevated cerebrospinal fluid levels of oxytocin in obsessive compulsive disorder. Comparison with Tourette's syndrome and healthy controls, *Arch Gen Psychiatry* 1994; **51**:782–92.

19

The use of psychiatric medications during breast-feeding

Zachary N Stowe, Alexis Llewellyn, Amy Hostetter and
Charles B Nemeroff

Introduction

In the USA, more than 60% of women plan to breast-feed when they leave the hospital after childbirth.[1] Many women plan to nurse for one of the following reasons: (1) reported benefits of breast-feeding; (2) perception of enhanced bonding with infants; (3) economics; and/or (4) social pressure. The American Academy of Pediatrics supports breast-feeding as the best and only source of nutrition necessary for the first 6 months of life.[1] More than 10% of women will experience psychiatric symptoms following their pregnancy. Despite this high prevalence rate, few studies have systemically measured psychiatric medication excretion into breast milk. The case reports and small case series that compose the majority of the literature to date render comparison of the data on various medications and the establishment of definitive treatment guidelines difficult. The use of psychiatric medications during lactation requires a careful and comprehensive risk/benefit assessment, taking into consideration all available treatment options, known data on the medication, the benefits of breast-feeding, the risk of untreated mental illness to the mother and child, and the value that the women and family place on breast-feeding. Pharmacological treatment during lactation remains controversial. Several reviews have compiled the available cases of psychotropic medication use in pregnancy and lactation;[2–22] however, reviews that focus solely on psychotropic medications during lactation are considerably more limited.[23–27] The lactation-specific studies, with limited exceptions, seldom address several potential confounding factors: (1) pregnancy and lactation are distinct metabolic and developmental periods, and the claim that data derived from one period are relevant to the other and vice versa is not supported by any available data; (2) assay methodology varies, and data from one assay may not be directly comparable to other documented cases; (3) the sensitivity of many commercially available assays may not reach the sensitivity and limits of detection of research-quality assays; (4) maternal factors, including the use of other prescribed or non-prescribed medications or smoking during both pregnancy and breast-feeding, are not documented; (5) most studies or case reports fail to document the portion of breast milk assayed (foremilk versus hindmilk) or the time at which the breast-milk sample is obtained in relation to the time post-dose of maternal medication ingestion, rendering direct comparison of studies difficult—there has been sparse appreciation of the pharmacokinetic complexity of medication excretion into breast milk. Despite these confounding factors, there have been few reports on adverse impacts of psychiatric medications on infants who were exposed via breast milk.

Nevertheless, it is premature to recommend specific medications for lactating women, due to the limited data available. In this chapter, we review the extant literature on the use of psychotropic medications during lactation and include articles focusing on infant serum measures or reports of infant outcome. We have also outlined the key elements of making comprehensive risk/benefit decisions in regard to making treatment decisions for lactating women. Preliminary guidelines are provided for choosing a medication which maximizes maternal mental health and minimizes infant exposure.

Breast-feeding and its benefits

Breast-feeding and the mother

Mothers are believed to benefit both psychologically and physiologically by nursing their infants. Breast milk is portable, economical, and resistant to spoilage while in the breast, so breast-feeding is an extremely efficient way to nourish infants. Moreover, nursing stimulates uterine contractions, due to suckling-induced oxytocin release which promotes the involution of the uterus after pregnancy. Nursing-induced

prolactin secretion delays the return of ovulation by blunting the ovarian response to follicle-stimulating hormone (FSH), and thereby delays the return of the menstrual cycle. The value that a mother places on nursing her infant should also be considered in her treatment planning. Although systematic studies have not been conducted on whether nursing enhances bonding between mother and infant, the possibility exists. In many women experiencing severe mood lability, nursing may be the sole activity which makes them feel good about themselves, reinforcing their ability to 'mother'. One group has reported that the incidence of breast cancer in premenopausal women was lowest in women who had breastfed the longest.[28] The potential maternal benefits of breast-feeding warrant further controlled investigation. A burgeoning literature has documented the short-term and long-term benefits of breast milk for the neonate.

Breast-feeding and the infant

There have been numerous studies documenting immunological benefits of breast milk for the infant. A retrospective cohort study of 776 mothers, at 6 months postpartum, matched for infant age, socio-economic status, maternal age, and cigarette consumption, found that breast-feeding had a protective effect against infant gastrointestinal, respiratory and all other illnesses except for trauma.[29] A decrease in the number of cases of otitis media (OM) associated with breast-feeding has been reported by several groups.[29–31] One review of 1220 infants' paediatric records shows that breast-feeding for at least 4 months protected infants from both single and recurrent cases of OM.[30] The dramatic correlation between breast-feeding and decreased incidence of OM in infants may be related to: (1) lower exposure to microorganisms; (2) improved nutrition; (3) feeding position; and/or (4) antibacterial qualities of breast milk possibly interfering with the attachment of *Haemophilus influenzae* and *Streptococcus pneumoniae* to nasopharyngeal epithelial cells.[31] Anti-adhesive properties of breast milk are thought to protect against infections elsewhere in the body as well. The rate of urinary tract infections in the first year of life is significantly reduced in breastfed infants.[32] An oligosaccharide in the urine of breastfed infants that causes inhibition of *Escherichia coli* adhesion to uroepithelial cells is the proposed mechanism of this reduction in urinary tract infections.[32,33] IQ testing of seven 2–8-year-old children born prematurely showed that preterm infants who breastfed had an 8.3 (over half of a standard deviation) point advantage over non-breastfed infants.[34] Thus, the data on benefits of breast-feeding to infants show both neurodevelopmental and immunological benefits.

Pharmacokinetics

The pharmacokinetics of medication excretion into breast milk and the infant can be conceptualized as three separate compartments. These are the maternal, breast-milk and infant compartments, all of which change and mature independently of one another.

Maternal compartment

Medication excretion into breast milk varies depending on the following maternal factors: (1) maternal volume of distribution; (2) medication dosing regimen; (3) maternal rate of medication metabolism; (4) the bioavailability of the medication in the circulation; and (5) the breast-feeding schedule. The rate at which pre-pregnancy physiological states return after pregnancy is highly variable. Medication ingested by the mother enters the bloodstream, where the 'free' non-protein-bound portion of the medication readily diffuses into breast milk. Dosage and frequency of medication administration, rate of maternal medication absorption and bloodflow to the breast will all affect the concentration of medication in breast milk. Following oral ingestion, the maternal serum concentration will vary, and it is the maternal serum concentration, not the dose, that determines breast-milk concentration. After entering the mother's circulatory system, medication enters the breast-milk compartment.

Breast-milk compartment

The individual physiochemical properties of a particular medication seem to be the best predictor of its availability in breast milk.[12] Lipid solubility typically determines the rate of diffusion of molecules into the breast milk, with more lipophilic medications diffusing more readily.[23] The molecular weight (MW) of the medication may limit its passage into the alveolar ducts, though such passive diffusion is not a significant factor for most psychotropic medications (MW < 500).

Breast milk is a unique fluid that undergoes marked alteration in composition over time. Milk pH is lower than plasma pH, which causes weak acids to diffuse slowly and weak bases to diffuse more readily into breast milk. Compounds diffuse down the concentration gradient between plasma and breast milk. Many central nervous system agents are organic bases, and become ionized under acidic conditions; the lower breast milk pH may cause these agents to concentrate in the milk, compared to maternal serum. Breast milk contains protein and lipids that demonstrate a concentration gradient, with the higher concentrations of lipids being in the later portion of the milk (hindmilk). The major determinant of the breast-milk concentration of medication involves the milk composition, which changes over time with maturity and also demonstrates a gradient in lipid content (foremilk to hindmilk). Our group and Yoshida et al have demonstrated the potential impact of such a gradient on the concentration of antidepressants in breast milk, with the higher concentrations found in hindmilk.[35,36] This gradient will be discussed further in regard to specific medications.

The milk/plasma (M/P) ratio provides a relative assessment of breast-milk concentration of medications. Providing an accurate comparison of medication, however, requires controlling for both the aliquot (fore–hind) and the time after maternal dose to determine the utility of the breast milk concentration.[16,35] The M/P ratio, therefore, may not be clinically useful in estimating infant exposure if aliquot and time since the last dose of the medication are unknown. Collection technique and methodology is vitally important in determining infant exposure and for developing techniques and feeding schedules for minimizing infant exposure to medications.

Infant compartment

The neonate possesses a physiological system that is metabolically immature and continually changing. Newborns are less able to metabolize and excrete medications compared to adults. Several factors may contribute to high serum concentrations in a nursing infant; these are discussed below. (1) Metabolites compete for the available enzymes, as neonates do not possess all metabolic enzymes at birth and may not possess the needed chemicals either to break down certain compounds expediently or to break them down at all.[23] Oxidation reactions and glucuronidation processes are immature

and develop at variable rates.[8,23,37] (2) A neonate's glomerular filtration rate and tubular secretion are less than those of an adult, and possibly lead to higher serum steady-state concentrations or accumulation of medications in the infant over time.[8,38] (3) The infant gastrointestinal tract has a higher gastric pH, a changing microbial environment, and slowed bowel motility and elimination rate, which produce irregular and unpredictable absorption.[37] (4) The bioavailability of medications is also altered in the infant secondary to the different pathophysiological composition in the bloodstream and altered plasma protein binding compared to adults.[37] Decreased protein binding increases the serum concentration of free drug in the infant.[37] (5) The infant has a different volume of distribution and a higher permeability of tissues and organs that may contribute to higher tissue concentrations of a medication. The infant may metabolize medications differently, as in the case of chlorpromazine, which may be a cause of concern.[39] In summary, the determinants of the actual infant daily exposure, to a given medication, are highly variable and may contribute to higher infant serum concentrations at steady state.

Earlier reviews utilized terms such as 'accumulation' and 'toxicity', but upon review of the literature, these terms cannot be truly substantiated. To demonstrate accumulation, repeated infant serum sampling would be required to confirm increasing serum concentrations. The limited cases of adverse effects of psychiatric medications on nursing infants reported are more representative of the medications' side-effect profiles and of acute toxicity. The infant data on vitamins, anticonvulsants and psychotropic medications suggest that infants achieve serum concentrations that are considerably higher than would be predicted from daily dose estimations and may even exceed maternal serum concentrations.[40] The potential for elevated steady-state concentrations in infants compared to adults underscores the need for infant serum monitoring and parent education about potential side-effects.

Limitations of current literature

Treatment decisions about pharmacology during lactation, by necessity, must be based mostly on case reports. Prior to interpretation of any of the current literature, the clinician should be familiar with the limitations of existing study methodology. These potential confounding factors include: (1) variations in assay sensitivity; (2) estimation of the infant dose based on breast-milk sampling with unknown or unreported aliquot (was it the foremilk or hindmilk portion of the breast-milk sample?); (3) no control for the maturity of the breast milk (was it taken in the first or sixteenth week postpartum?); (4) limited or no analysis of the medication's active metabolites; (5) no standardized methods for assessing an adverse effect in the infant; (6) documentation of nursing frequency and/or any supplemental infant nourishment. Many studies have not accounted for the use of medications in pregnancy, concomitant medications during breast-feeding or cigarette smoking. The vast majority, 95%, of breast-feeding mothers have been reported to take at least one medication during the first postpartum week, 17–25% of mothers take medications in the 2 weeks surrounding their fourth postpartum month, and up to 5% of mothers are on at least one medication for the entire time that they are breast-feeding their infant.[38,41] An increased incidence of attention deficit hyperactive disorder (ADHD) is reported in children with a cigarette-smoking parent.[42] Remarkably, up to 20–35% of breast-feeding mothers smoke cigarettes.[43] These data highlight the need to document the use of other drugs, both licit and illicit, when prescribing

medication to a lactating mother, and the need to consider possible drug–drug interactions. The clinician should keep two other points in mind when interpreting the extant literature: (1) case reports are biased towards any adverse effect that is not representative of larger clinical experience; and (2) the term 'undetectable' is solely a function of the limits of assay sensitivity, and does not necessarily indicate that the medication is absent.

Review of the literature on psychiatric medications in lactation

Antidepressants

A comprehensive review summarizing the reports on nursing infant serum concentrations during maternal treatment with antidepressants appeared in 1996.[26] Prior to that time, the majority of the literature on breast-feeding and infant serum concentrations involved cases with antidepressants, particularly the tricyclics.

Tricyclic antidepressants
The tricyclic antidepressants (TCAs) have been available for over four decades, and clinical studies have demonstrated their efficacy in a variety of psychiatric disorders, including major depression, obsessive-compulsive disorder and panic disorder. A detailed pharmacokinetic study of TCAs with infant serum and urine measures should serve as a template for interpreting the following literature.[36]

There are several case reports on the use of amitriptyline in breast-feeding women.[44–48] They note detectable concentrations of amitriptyline and its metabolite, nortriptyline, in the breast milk of women taking

75–175 mg/day of the parent compound. Detectable concentrations of either amitriptyline or nortriptyline could not be found in infant serum samples assayed with a sensitivity of 5–14 ng/ml. No adverse effects in the nursing infants were reported. One group reported an M/P ratio for nortriptyline of 0.74 and for E-10-hydroxynortriptyline of 0.70, and concluded that the metabolites of amitriptyline bound less to both plasma and milk proteins.[45] Similarly, Pittard found a lower M/P ratio for nortriptyline compared to amitriptyline, and suggested that hepatic reduction to more water-soluble substances might account for this difference.[48]

A case report on doxepin exposure during breast-feeding describes depression of respiratory function in an 8-week-old infant, associated with an increase in maternal TCA dose.[49] Breast-feeding was discontinued and the infant's respiratory function normalized within 24 h. Peak breast-milk concentrations of doxepin and N-desmethyldoxepin were observed 4–5 h after maternal dosing, and minimum concentrations were observed at 23–24 h after dosing. The total infant daily dose, based on 150 ml of breast milk per kilogram of infant weight, was 0.3% of the maternal dose.[39] However, infant serum concentrations of N-desmethyldoxepin, in this case, were comparable to maternal doxepin concentrations (3 μg/l). A second report included maternal plasma, infant plasma and breast-milk samples containing doxepin and N-desmethyldoxepin during an 8-week period.[50] Plasma taken from the infant, after 43 days of exposure to the medication, did not reveal detectable concentrations of doxepin (<5 μg/l) or N-desmethyldoxepin (15 μg/l). The authors calculated that the infant would have received 2.2% of the maternal doxepin dose. These estimated infant doses highlight the limited utility of M/P ratio reports.

A woman treated with clomipramine (125 mg/day during pregnancy) delivered an infant described as having had mild hypotonia, tremor, respiratory acidosis and air-trapping, all of which resolved at 6 days of age.[51] The same infant was breastfed and remained asymptomatic. Maternal and infant serum and breast-milk samples were obtained at delivery, and at 4, 6, 10, 14 and 35 days postpartum. Detectable concentrations of clomipramine were found in the infant at delivery, and declined post-delivery to achieve a 6% concentration of the maternal serum over the course of breast-feeding. These data suggest that medication accumulation did not occur and that pregnancy exposure could alter initial infant serum concentrations. The estimated infant dose, based on 1000 ml of breast milk ingested in a day and a mother's dose of 150 mg/day of clomipramine, was 0.4% of the maternal dose. In the cases of four women treated with clomipramine 75–125 mg/day, infant serum concentrations, collected after 3 weeks of stable maternal dosing, were below the assay sensitivity of 10 ng/ml for clomipramine and its three metabolites: N-desmethylclomipramine, 8-hydroxyclomipramine, and 8-hydroxyclomipramine.[52] All four infants were described as developing normally.

The largest collection of infant serum TCA measurements, conducted by a single group, is 12.[53,54] The women were treated with nortriptyline (50–110 mg/day), and infant sera were analysed for nortriptyline and its metabolites: E-10-hydroxynortriptyline and Z-10-hydroxynortriptyline. Nortriptyline was undetectable in all of the infant samples, and 10-hydroxynortriptyline was detected in only two infant sera. Both the parents and paediatricians described these infants as developing normally. The maternal serum concentrations of nortriptyline were as high as 201 ng/ml, and after 50 days of exposure there was no evidence of rising serum concentrations in the breastfed infants. The same group extended the data on nortriptyline with an additional group of six infants.[55] Similarly, Altshuler et al reported on a woman treated with nortriptyline and sertraline; neither compound was detectable in the infant serum.[56]

Amoxapine, a TCA metabolite of loxapine, is primarily used to treat depression but also demonstrates some antipsychotic properties. Gelenberg studied a female patient taking 250 mg/day at the time of breast-milk and serum sampling for the concentrations of amoxapine and 8-OH-amoxapine.[57] Forty-five minutes after maternal dosing at steady state (after 10 months of medication treatment), serum concentrations of 97 ng/ml of amoxapine and 375 ng/ml of the metabolite were observed; milk levels were below 20 ng/ml and 113 ng/ml, respectively. The second sampling, 1 month later, 11.5 h post maternal dose, revealed milk concentrations again below 20 ng/ml for amoxapine and at 168 ng/ml for the metabolite. There is little we can conclude from these data, because time-course data, gradient data and infant serum measures were not obtained.

Stancer and Reed measured desipramine and its metabolite, 2-hydroxydesipramine, in breast milk and infant plasma. This woman was treated with desipramine (300 mg/day) at this dose for 1 week at the commencement of sampling.[58] Concentrations in the maternal plasma and breast milk were similar, with serum ratios between the TCA and its metabolite of 0.91 and 0.93 and for milk of 1.2 and 1.0. Neither compound was detected in the serum of the 10-week-old infant. The authors suggested that a 4-kg infant would ingest about 1/100th of the maternal dose in a 24 h time period. No adverse effects were noted in the infant after 3 weeks of exposure. Sovner and Orsulak measured imipramine and desipramine concentra-

tions in a depressed woman also diagnosed and treated for hypothyroidism.[59] The woman did not report any adverse events affecting her child related to breast-feeding while on the TCA for 45 days. Six breast-milk samples and some maternal plasma samples were collected; the TCA and its metabolite were found in breast milk at levels similar to those in the plasma, despite different sampling times. Both of these TCAs are very lipophilic and are probably easily transferred into the breast milk. Thus, if therapeutic maternal serum concentrations of 200 ng/ml of both desipramine and imipramine were achieved, a 5-kg infant, who drinks 1000 ml of breast milk a day, would receive approximately 0.2 mg of desipramine plus imipramine per day.[47]

Misri and Sivertz reported on 19 nursing mothers treated with TCAs: imipramine ($n = 14$), nortriptyline ($n = 2$), amitriptyline ($n = 1$), desipramine ($n = 1$), and clomipramine ($n = 1$).[18] All of the women experienced symptom remission; remarkably, no note was made on any adverse outcomes for any infant as a result of medication exposure. However, the author noted that the need for hospitalization of some of these women may have had negative effects on maternal infant bonding and the family.

Selective serotonin reuptake inhibitors

The selective serotonin reuptake inhibitors (SSRIs), like the TCAs, have been shown to be effective in the treatment of a wide variety of psychiatric illnesses, and they are all excreted into breast milk. The SSRIs may be clinically preferable to the TCAs in breast-feeding women for many obvious reasons, including the TCAs' autonomic side-effects, which may decrease milk supply and lactational reflexes.[9] As a class, the SSRIs have the largest breast-feeding database relative to any other class of medication.

Fluoxetine demonstrates a time course of excretion into breast milk that parallels its absorptive phase from the gut.[60] In the case of a lactating woman treated with fluoxetine (20 mg/day) for postpartum depression, no adverse effects were noted in her infant's behaviour or nursing patterns, and after 2 months of exposure, the infant was described as having normal development.[61] No infant serum samples were obtained. In contrast, a father who was a paediatrician described increased irritability for the initial 2 weeks of nursing exposure in his son, yet the infant continued with normal weight gain and achieved all developmental milestones for his age.[62] Lester et al reported a case of infant colic in a 6-week-old whose mother continued to breast-feed while taking fluoxetine 20 mg/day. The mother kept a diary of the infant's behaviour that documented increased crying, decreased sleep, increased vomiting and watery stools when exposed to fluoxetine in breast milk.[63] The breast-milk concentrations of fluoxetine and norfluoxetine were 69 ng/ml and 90 ng/ml, respectively. The infant's serum contained 340 ng/ml of fluoxetine and 208 ng/ml of norfluoxetine. The author suggests that this case may represent adverse side-effects of fluoxetine in breast milk; however, infant colic is not unusual. In contrast, more recent studies with much larger samples have failed to find any adverse effects of fluoxetine exposure via breast milk and have found only low or undetectable infant serum fluoxetine concentrations.[60,64–66] One-year follow-up of four infants exposed to fluoxetine via breast milk demonstrated normal infant development using the Bayley and McCarthy scale.[65]

Our group conducted the largest study on SSRIs, in which both time-course and gradient data of sertraline and desmethylsertraline in breast milk were reported. The study demonstrates the ability to estimate sertraline and desmethylsertraline excretion in breast milk at any time after maternal dosing. This information allows a patient to reduce the infant's exposure to the SSRI by discarding the breast milk with peak concentration based on the time course of excretion. Twelve women's breast-milk samples were assayed in this study, with 11 maternal–infant serum pair concentrations measured. Detectable concentrations of sertraline were found in only four of the samples (the highest was 3 ng/ml) with assay sensitivity of 1 ng/ml. Desmethylsertraline was found in nine infant serum samples (the highest was 10 ng/ml), with assay sensitivity of 1 ng/ml. No adverse effects were reported in these infants.[35] Additional studies of sertraline in breast-feeding have failed to demonstrate any alteration in infant serum platelet serotonin,[67] but one group did report an elevated infant serum concentration,[68] similar to the results noted above with fluoxetine. The latter group concluded that this was an erroneous infant serum value, despite limited evidence supporting their assertion.

Additional reports for the remaining SSRIs have not included infant serum measures, but estimate infant dose, using maternal serum to breast milk ratios, to be 0.5% of maternal dose for fluvoxamine, based on milk and maternal plasma samples in one case, and 0.34% for paroxetine, also based on one case.[62,69,70] In collaboration with Cohen et al our group completed a study of paroxetine in breast-feeding that demonstrated the gradient from foremilk to hindmilk and no detectable paroxetine in the sera of 16 infants (Stowe et al, unpublished). No adverse effects were noted in the infants exposed. Similarly, a recent study failed to find venlafaxine in the serum of breastfed exposed infants[71] and demonstrated the complex pattern of breast-milk excretion, with both time-course and gradient effects. One study of citalopram in the sera of mother and breastfed infant and in breast milk found a milk-to-serum concentration ratio of −3 for both citalopram and its main metabolite desmethyl-citalopram.[72] However, the package labelling for citalopram cautions against breast-feeding, despite the sparse information supporting this warning.

The increasing database on SSRIs would suggest relative safety compared to other antidepressants. The limited number of adverse effects reported, with even fewer being confirmed as secondary to the medication, awaits confirmation with long-term follow up studies.

Monoamine oxidase inhibitors

The monoamine oxidase inhibitors (MAOIs) are seldom used as first-line treatment in lactating mothers, at least in part because of the dietary constraints and potential for hypertensive crisis.[7] Pons examined the use of moclobemide, a reversible monoamine oxidase-A inhibitor, in breast-feeding women, to determine the time course of the medication and its metabolites in breast milk. The highest concentrations of moclobemide and its metabolite in breast milk were found 3 h after maternal dose; milk concentrations were undetectable 12 h post-dose. The active metabolite was not detected in breast milk. The participants were six lactating women who received a single 300-mg dose within 3–5 days post-delivery. The researchers concluded that a 3.5-kg, breastfed infant would receive 1% of the maternal dose. A second group extended these results with nine nursing mothers, though infant sera were not obtained.[73] Both groups concluded that the low levels excreted into the breast milk were unlikely to be hazardous to the infant; however, long-term follow-up data are lacking.

Other antidepressants

Bupropion is a member of the aminoketone class of antidepressants. Milk and plasma samples from a woman treated with bupropion (100 mg, three times a day), who was breast-feeding her 14-month-old infant twice a day, revealed that this medication was quickly absorbed after ingestion, peak plasma concentrations being attained 2 h post maternal dose.[40] After 2 weeks of treatment, maternal serum and breast-milk samples obtained 30 min before the first morning dose, and at 1, 2, 4 and 6 h after maternal dose, revealed that bupropion concentrations in breast milk were much higher than in maternal plasma. The major metabolite, hydroxybupropion, was present in breast milk at 10% of its plasma concentration. The M/P ratio of bupropion ranged from 2.51 to 8.58, the hydroxybupropion M/P ratio ranged from 0.09 to 0.11, and the threohydroxybupropion M/P ratio ranged from 1.23 to 1.57. One infant serum sample collected 3.67 h after his last breast-feeding, and 9.5 h after the mother's last dose, revealed no measurable bupropion or its metabolites at an assay sensitivity of 0.05 µg/ml. No adverse effects or changes were noted in the infant, but it should be noted that bupropion treatment was only continued for 1 week after the sampling.

Trazodone is a triazolopyridine antidepressant. Six lactating women, between 3 and 8 months postpartum, were treated with a single dose of trazodone (50 mg). Blood and milk samples were obtained at 0.5, 1, 2, 3, 4, 5, 6, 9, 12, 24 and 30 h post maternal dose. The M/P ratio of trazodone was low, at 0.142 ± 0.045. The assay used did not measure the active metabolite 1-*m*-chlorophenyl-piperazine. The author calculated that, based on infant ingestion of 500 ml of breast milk in the 12 h after a dose, the baby would have been exposed to 0.03 mg of trazodone. The baby's dose would have been >1/150th the maternal dose.

There is an absence of data on mirtazapine, nefazadone and other TCAs and MAOIs.

Anxiolytics

When compared to affective disorders, anxiety disorders, such as panic disorder and generalized anxiety disorder, in the postpartum period, are understudied. Empirically, it is often said that the additional stress of caring for a newborn and disrupted sleep may increase anxiety. Treatment for anxiety disorders includes both cognitive-behavioural therapy and pharmacological approaches. Considerable literature exists on the use of many of the benzodiazepines in lactating women.

Fisher et al report on a case of a mother treated with clonazepam during pregnancy and lactation.[74] The infant was born at 36 weeks of gestation with apnoea, cyanosis, and hypotonia, which resolved by 10 days postpartum. The mother continued her clonazepam treatment and nursed from day 3 postpartum until day 14 postpartum. Multiple samples of breast milk were obtained to measure clonazepam concentrations; all contained 11–13 ng/ml of the medication. Infant serum obtained 120 h postpartum contained 2.9 ng/ml of clonazepam, and on day 14 postpartum the infant serum contained 1 ng/ml. No evidence of accumulation was found in either breast milk or the infant. The authors calculated that the ingestion of 770–1540 ml of breast milk daily would result in therapeutic levels of clonazepam in the child. The infant was neurodevelopmentally normal at 5 months postpartum but did have apnoea until 10 weeks postpartum; whether the apnoea was secondary to the clonazepam remains unclear. The authors recommend that all infants exposed to clonazepam during pregnancy or breast-feeding be monitored for apnoea or central nervous system depression, because clonazepam crosses the placenta. Soderman and Matheson reported a case of a mother treated with clonazepam

(2 mg) and phenytoin (200 mg, twice daily) during pregnancy and lactation.[75] Measurement of clonazepam was conducted using 10 ml of foremilk, 10 ml of hindmilk, maternal bloods, and the infant's blood, on postpartum days 2, 3 and 4. They used an assay with sensitivity of 3.2 µg/l, and the highest clonazepam concentration in breast milk was 10.7 µg/l, observed 4 h post maternal dose. The authors suggested that, based on an infant ingesting 0.15 mg/kg body weight, a maximum of 2.5% of the maternal weight-adjusted dose of clonazepam would be ingested. The infant's sera obtained on days 2–4 were mixed together, and a concentration of 4.7 µg/l of clonazepam was found. These levels are similar to the levels observed in the first study cited above. The authors of this latter study suggested that the concurrent use of phenytoin may have served to lower clonazepam concentrations by induction of liver enzymes that metabolize the benzodiazepines. Induction of hepatic enzymes in infants causes the half-life elimination rate of clonazepam to be similar to that of adults.[76]

Patrick et al reported a case of diazepam use in a breast-feeding mother who was treated with diazepam (10 mg, three times a day), starting on postpartum day 5.[77] On days 6–7 postpartum she discontinued breast-feeding; the baby lost 170 g in body weight and was lethargic in the 24 h period following discontinuation. The infant resumed normal activity and was regaining weight on the ninth day postpartum. Qualitative tests of infant urine obtained on the eighth day postpartum were positive for oxazepam, the metabolite of diazepam, and an electroencephalogram of the child that day showed evidence of sedative use. However, diazepam or oxazepam was detected in the breast milk, though this was most likely due to limited assay sensitivity. Erkkola and Kanto measured diazepam and its active, major metabolite, 10-desmethyldiazepam, in mother and infant sera and breast milk.[78] Three patients treated with diazepam (10 mg, three times a day) provided serum samples on their fourth and sixth postpartum days. The concentrations of diazepam and 10-desmethyldiazepam, in maternal serum, increased from day 4 to day 6. There were significantly higher concentrations of diazepam and N-desmethyldiazepam in maternal serum when compared to both breast milk and infant serum. No free oxazepam was detected in any of the biological samples. Both diazepam and 10-desmethyldiazepam concentrations in infant sera significantly decreased from day 4 to day 6. No lethargy or hypoventilation was observed in these three infants. The authors noted that interactions between bilirubin and diazepam might cause neurological damage or possibly kernicterus, and hyperbilirubinaemia has been observed in infants exposed to diazepam prenatally. Morselli et al studied the effect of diazepam (0.3 mg/kg) on premature infants, full-term infants, and children.[79] In premature and full-term infants, there was a decreased ability to both hydroxylate diazepam and excrete other metabolites of diazepam compared to adults. Diazepam serum levels were higher and persisted longer in premature infants when compared to children. Eliot et al reported that after a single dose of diazepam to a mother in labour, both diazepam and desmethyldiazepam could be detected in infant serum 10 days postpartum.[80] Cole and Hailey gave diazepam to nine breast-feeding mothers and collected breast milk, maternal serum, and infant's serum.[81] Three cases of mild jaundice were noted in the infants. Maternal milk and plasma levels of diazepam and desmethyldiazepam revealed a 2 : 1 ratio. Both compounds were detected in all of the biological fluids available in all subjects. The authors concluded that diazepam was metabolized more slowly in infants than in adults and, thus, accu-

mulation could occur. Brandt demonstrated in four mothers that both diazepam and its metabolite, desmethyldiazepam, passed into breast milk, yet oxazepam was not detectable by their assay.[82] The metabolite levels were consistently higher (by 10–47%) than the parent compound, perhaps due to the infant plasma protein-binding properties. Breast-milk concentrations of both diazepam and desmethyldiazepam were markedly lower than maternal plasma levels. The authors stated that the levels of both compounds were higher in evening milk than in morning milk, though plasma levels were lower in the evening. The authors hypothesized that this time course might occur because the evening milk had more fat and both compounds were more soluble in the higher-fat solutions. The authors calculated that if the maternal dose was 10 mg/day and the infant ingested 500 ml of milk a day, the maximum dose to the infant of diazepam plus desmethyldiazepam would have been 45 μg/day. The authors suggested that the quantity of diazepam and desmethyldiazepam ingested by an infant whose mother was prescribed diazepam (10 mg/day) was too small to result in any untoward effects in the infant; moreover, infants prescribed diazepam are prescribed doses 10–30 times higher than the estimated dose from this study. This group cautions that mothers receiving high doses of diazepam should discontinue breast-feeding, because the infant does metabolize the medication more slowly than an adult. Dusci et al studied a case of a woman taking high doses of both diazepam and oxazepam.[83] Maternal breast-milk and plasma levels, and her 1-year-old nursing infant's plasma levels of diazepam, N-desmethyldiazepam, temazepam and oxazepam, were measured. Ratios of the following maternal plasma-to-milk levels were found: diazepam 0.2, N-desmethyldiazepam 0.13, temazepam 0.14, and oxazepam 0.10.

The authors calculate, on a mg/kg basis, that the infant received 4.7% of the maternal dose. N-desmethyldiazepam 20 and 21 µg/l, temazepam 7 µg/l and oxazepam 7.5 and 9.6 µg/l were found in the infant's serum. The infant did not show any adverse physical or mental sequelae of benzodiazepine exposure. The results on diazepam are mixed, and prescribers are cautioned to monitor infants' exposure, due to the likely easy passage of the medication into breast-milk and the extended half-life of elimination in infants.

Wretlind studied oxazepam excretion in breast milk by obtaining samples of maternal plasma and breast milk at 10 and 34 h postdose, in a woman taking oxazepam (10 mg, three times a day).[84] The concentrations of oxazepam were 24 and 30 µg/l in the two samples, respectively. The infant's dose was estimated to be 1/1000th of the maternal dose. A study on breast-milk levels of oxazepam performed by Rane et al revealed similar concentrations of oxazepam in a mother prescribed the identical dose of oxazepam, with concentrations between 11 and 26 µg/l being found in the breast milk.[85] Because of the pharmacokinetic profile of oxazepam, with its low lipid solubility and short half-life in comparison to other benzodiazepines, the author concluded that infants received relatively low exposure to oxazepam.

Summerfield and Nielsen measured lorazepam concentrations in maternal plasma and in breast milk.[86] Four women were prescribed a single dose of lorazepam (3.5 mg) as premedication prior to sterilization surgery, and plasma and breast-milk samples were obtained 4 h later. The concentration of free drug in breast milk was between 8 and 9 ng/ml; this was between 14.8% and 25.7% of the lorazepam concentration found in maternal serum samples. The authors suggested that this one-time dose was 'safe', though the authors of

this monograph caution against the use of terms such as 'safe' in regard to medication in lactation.

Sedative hypnotics

Lebedevs et al measured temazepam concentrations in breast milk and maternal and infant serum levels in 10 mother–infant pairs treated with 10–20 mg at bedtime for at least 2 days.[87] The maternal serum concentrations were steady state. Several of the women were also taking concurrent medications. The time of sampling was within 2 weeks postpartum: a time of breast-milk composition variability. The M/P ratio for the samples was 0.12 in one of the 10 patients, and ranged between <0.09 and <0.63 in the other patients. The milk concentration of temazepam was below the level of detection, 5 µg/l, in several samples. Infants are less able to glucuronidate temazepam when compared to adults. Thus even if the medication was ingested, at the ratios seen, it is likely that the infant would receive negligible quantities of temazepam.

Hilbert et al measured the excretion of quazepam into the breast milk of four lactating mothers.[88] Mothers fasted overnight and then received quazepam (15 mg), and nursing was discontinued. Breast-milk and maternal plasma samples were obtained, and the mean M/P ratios of quazepam, and its metabolites 2-oxoquazepam and N-desalkyl-2-oxoquazepam, were 4.19, 2.02 and 0.09 respectively. The breast milk contained only 0.11% of quazepam plus metabolites of the actual administered quazepam dose. The authors calculated that the infant would have received 2.3% of the maternal dose.

Breast-milk levels of flunitrazepam for five women were found to be lower than maternal plasma levels at 11, 15 and 27 h after a single 2-mg maternal dose.[89] Accumulation might occur with repeated dosing, because of the medication's 20-h half-life. The authors did not observe any untoward effect on the newborn from this single dose.

Zolpidem, a novel sedative-hypnotic, acts on omega-1 receptor sites. The excretion of this medication into breast milk was examined by Pons et al.[90] Five women received a single 20-mg dose 30 min after dinner, and then milk and maternal plasma samples were obtained at various intervals. The half-life elimination was calculated to be 2.6 h. The amount of medication found in breast milk ranged from 0.004% to 0.019% of the maternally ingested dose. No accumulation in breast milk was found, but no actual study is available on infant serum levels or adverse effects in the infant.

The extant data on anti-anxiety medications are highly variable, but support the use of short-acting benzodiazepines without metabolites if such medications are required during lactation.

Mood stabilizers

Mood stabilizers are primarily used to control mania in bipolar patients. Breast-milk data exist for the three most commonly used anti-manic medications: valproate, carbamazepine, and lithium carbonate. Manic-depressive illness is equally common in women and men, but in women it first presents during the childbearing years.[91]

Lithium

The use of lithium during lactation has been categorically discouraged in several previous reports, and is considered to be contraindicated by the American Academy of Pediatrics (1994).[1] Lithium, like all psychotropic medications, readily passes into breast milk. The nurs-

ing infant is therefore exposed to this ion, yet there are remarkably few total cases reported of lithium use during breast-feeding.[92–96] Nursing infant serum lithium concentrations have been reported to be 10–50% of the mother's serum level.[95,96] Goldfield and Weinstein suggest that lithium is contraindicated in breast-feeding women because lithium concentrations in breast milk approach those found in maternal serum.[91] Schou and Amdisen measured lithium in the serum of infants who were exposed to lithium via breast milk.[94] The lithium concentration in breast milk was approximately half that in maternal serum. During the first postpartum week, the infant serum lithium concentration was approximately 50% of the mother's serum concentration, and thereafter declined to about 33% of the maternal serum concentrations. Sykes et al reported on a case of a woman treated with 800 mg/day of lithium carbonate at conception.[92] The woman's dose was reduced twice during pregnancy, and the infant was mildly hypotonic for 2 days after birth. Nevertheless, the mother chose to breast-feed. At birth, the infant serum lithium level was similar to the mother's but fell to 0.03 mmol/l by the sixth postpartum day and increased only slightly once breast-feeding was established. Although the mother's serum and breast-milk concentrations rose, there was not an appreciable rise in the infant serum concentration. The infant was assessed as having normal development after breast-feeding for 10 weeks. Linden and Rich suggested that infants receiving lithium through breast milk should be monitored for hypotonia, lethargy and cyanosis.[97] While the data are limited, there is evidence that management of women taking lithium while breast-feeding also warrants careful monitoring of the infant, especially the infant's hydration status.

Anticonvulsants

Both valproic acid and carbamazepine are considered to be compatible with breast-feeding by the American Academy of Pediatrics report[90] and are listed as compatible in reference books.[98] Alexander reported on a case of a woman treated with sodium valproate in pregnancy and who continued this treatment while breast-feeding.[99] The valproic acid infant serum concentration was approximately the same as the mother's at delivery, but fell to purportedly insignificant levels by the fifth postpartum day and was below the limits of detection by 29 days postpartum. Valproic acid was present in the breast milk on the fifth day postpartum at 50 mmol/l and fell to 21 mmol/l by day 29 postpartum. The authors suggest that valproic acid would be found in breast milk at between 5% and 10% of the maternal serum concentration. No adverse sequelae were noted in the infant as a result of breast-milk exposure to valproic acid.

Transient cholestatic hepatitis in an infant, associated with carbamazepine use in pregnancy and lactation, was reported by Frey et al.[100] The infant's mother was prescribed carbamazepine (600 mg/day) throughout her pregnancy and during the postpartum period. The child was admitted to hospital at 3 weeks postpartum, due to persistent jaundice which resolved after nursing was discontinued. Carbamazepine-induced hepatitis has been noted previously in both adults and children treated with that medication. In lactating women, M/P ratios of 0.24–0.69 have been reported with infant serum concentrations of 1.7 μmol/l.[101] Merlob et al described a case of an infant exposed to carbamazepine in utero and in breast milk. The mother received carbamazepine (400 mg/day) throughout pregnancy and during the postpartum period. Jaundice was noted in the infant on the first day of life.[102] Liver function tests were normal, with the exception of a very high level of liver enzyme GGT, which decreased slowly postpartum. The infant was fed breast milk for 9 days, at which time supplemental feeding was added. On postpartum day 2, carbamazepine concentrations were 5.5 μg/ml in the maternal serum, 2.8 μg/ml in the breast milk, and 1.8 μg/ml in infant serum. On postpartum day 63, medication concentrations were 6.5 μg/ml in the maternal serum, 2.2 μg/ml in the breast milk, and 1.1 μg/ml in the infant serum. The infant appeared to be developing normally at 2-, 4- and 6-month follow-up visits.

Mood stabilizers in lactation summary

The American Academy of Pediatrics Report (1994) is of concern with respect to the available data on mood stabilizers during lactation.[1] The sparse reports of lithium use, particularly when used not only during pregnancy, limit any definitive conclusions. The ratios of breast-milk concentration to maternal serum concentration observed for carbamazepine are similar to the ratios observed for lithium. The data on valproic acid suggest a progressive decrease in excretion into breast milk and lower infant serum concentrations compared to maternal serum measures. For all mood stabilizers, long-term follow-up data on the consequences of breast-feeding exposure are limited.

The issue of infant hydration is important in regard to lithium use during lactation; neither this issue nor any other constitutes an absolute contraindication to lithium. Advantages of lithium are that, with hydration, the serum concentration can be decreased rapidly, and the side-effects of lithium are more clinically discernible. While they are admittedly rare, both carbamazepine and valproic acid have the potential for serious or possibly lethal side-effects such as leukopenia and hepatitis that are difficult to detect prior to clinical symptomology. The authors typically do not encourage breast-feeding during treatment with mood stabilizers, partly because of the need for invasive infant monitoring. The need to gather data on lithium excretion into breast milk, including time course of excretion, infant serum concentration and incidence, if any, of adverse effects, in the absence of in utero exposure, is underscored by the clinical data. In general, valproic acid during lactation is preferable to both carbamazepine and lithium. The use of novel agents or switching to a second agent with purportedly greater relative safety during lactation is not without risk. First, such changes may result in exposing the developing infant to a second medication (e.g. lithium in pregnancy and valproic acid for lactation), and there are no data on the safety of such multiple exposures. Changing to a novel medication during the high-risk period may enhance the possibility of syndromal recurrence, thus increasing the risk by having both medication and illness exposure.

If mood-stabilizing medications are used in breast-feeding women, the infant is exposed and should have routine monitoring. The frequency of infant monitoring remains unclear; perhaps a reasonable approach would be monthly for 2–3 months, or following any increase in maternal daily dose, or if any side-effects are observed in the infant. Despite the benefits of breast-feeding, a low threshold for suspending breast-feeding or complete weaning is recommended. The reports of recurrent psychotic symptoms in women with postpartum-onset psychosis, particularly those with bipolar disorders, upon return of the menstrual cycle underscore the need to monitor women closely throughout the first postpartum year.[103–105]

Antipsychotic medications

Butyrophenones

Few studies exist on haloperidol excretion in breast milk. The first study was reported by Stewart et al, in which breast-milk concentrations of haloperidol in one woman were 5 ng/ml, 11 h after a 6-day average dose of 29.2 mg/day. Breast-milk concentrations on the twelfth day were 2 ng/ml, 9 h after a 12-mg dose.[106] The woman received 7 mg/day of haloperidol from day 13 to day 19 and then discontinued the medication. Three days after discontinuation, their assay did not detect haloperidol in her breast milk. The authors calculated that, based on the levels above, an infant ingesting 1–2 l of milk per day would receive a maximum dose of 0.0075 ng/day of haloperidol. Whalley et al also studied haloperidol excretion into breast milk in a woman receiving 10 mg/day in divided doses, while nursing an infant.[107] On the sixteenth postpartum day, chlorpromazine, 100 mg/day, was added to her haloperidol treatment regimen. Maternal plasma and breast-milk samples were obtained on the first, sixth, seventh and twenty-first days after initiation of treatment. The haloperidol concentrations in milk ranged from 0 to 23.5 µg/l. The author concluded that, based on the levels found in milk, the infant was possibly exposed to rather sizeable amounts of haloperidol. However, the child did not appear to suffer any adverse effects from the exposure and was reported to be developing normally at his 6-month and 1-year physician check-ups. The mother remained on the medication only until the sixth postpartum week but continued to nurse for 5 months.

Dibenzazepines

Barnas et al reported a case of a woman taking clozapine (100 mg/day) throughout most of her pregnancy and a lower dose (50 mg/day) in the last 9 weeks of her pregnancy.[108] She did not breast-feed, but breast-milk and maternal plasma samples were collected. One day post-delivery, the maternal plasma clozapine concentration was 14.7 ng/ml and the foremilk concentration was 63.5 ng/ml. Three days post-delivery, her dose was increased to 100 mg/day. On postpartum day 7, clozapine concentrations were 41.4 ng/ml in maternal plasma and 115.6 ng/ml in breast milk. Accumulation of clozapine was clearly noted in the 1-week samples. The authors attribute this to clozapine's high lipid solubility and lipophilic properties. Infants exposed to clozapine may be at risk for accumulation or 'floppy infant syndrome'.

Phenothiazine derivatives—aliphatic
Blacker et al measured breast-milk and maternal plasma levels in a woman treated, initially, with a single dose of 1200 mg of chlorpromazine.[109] A blood sample was obtained before the initial dose and 30, 60, 90 and 180 min post-dose. Breast-milk samples were obtained at 60, 120 and 180 min post-dose. The peak plasma concentration, found at 90 min post maternal dose, was 0.75 μg/ml. The peak breast-milk concentration, found at the 120 min post maternal dose collection, was 0.29 μg/ml. From these data, the group calculated that a 7-pound baby would receive 3 μg/kg daily. The paediatric dosage of chlorpromazine for children is 250 μg/kg every 4–6 h. The woman was continued on chlorpromazine, but her dose regimen was changed to 600 mg, twice a day, resulting in plasma and milk sample concentrations that were reduced to below their group's assay sensitivity. They suggested that divided dosing may result in lower concentrations of chlorpromazine in breast milk and perhaps enhanced safety to nursing infants. Wiles et al also measured

plasma and breast-milk concentrations of chlorpromazine in four lactating mothers.[110] Chlorpromazine was detected in all samples with a range of 7–98 ng/ml, and metabolites were also found in the samples; 7-hydroxy-chlorpromazine was found in two subjects, monodesmethylated chlorpromazine was found in one sample, and chlorpromazine sulphoxide was found in all four samples. Plasma levels were lower than breast-milk levels in two patients. Only two mothers were actually breast-feeding. One of these mothers reported no adverse effects on the infant (milk level of 7 ng/ml), but the second mother reported drowsiness and lethargy in her infant (milk level of 92 ng/ml). Mothers who nurse while receiving chlorpromazine should carefully monitor their infants for side-effects.

Kirk and Jorgensen reported three cases in which breast-milk and plasma levels of *cis-(Z)*-flupenthixol were measured.[111] Maternal doses were 2 mg/day, 40 mg/day, and 60 mg/day; two mothers provided one set of serum and milk samples, and a third provided two sets of serum and milk samples. The milk concentrations of the medication were approximately 30% higher than the serum concentration. The authors calculate that an infant who ingests 1 l of breast milk a day receives a dosage of 2 μg/day.

Phenothiazine derivatives—piperazine
Olesen et al reported on a case of perphenazine and lactation.[112] A mother was treated with perphenazine (12 mg, twice a day) for postpartum psychosis. The dose was reduced to 8 mg (twice a day, due to side-effects and high serum concentrations). The group measured breast-milk and maternal serum concentrations at both doses of medication at different time intervals. Maternal serum and milk levels increased and decreased congruently, and levels

were similar at all intervals. The mean milk/serum ratios were 0.7 and 1.1. Based on the results of their comparison between milk and serum concentrations, they calculated that an infant would receive approximately 0.1% of the maternal dose of perphenazine. The child in this case continued to breast-feed during the mother's entire 3-month course of perphenazine treatment, exhibited normal development and had no signs of adverse medication effects. The paucity of information on antipsychotic medications limits any definitive conclusions in regard to their use in lactation

The data on antipsychotic medication are remarkably limited, considering the duration of their availability. The introduction of newer agents devoid of significant effects on serum prolactin and their increasing use in affective disorders may increase the number of patients on these medications conceiving—hence there will be a need to obtain further data with respect to breast-feeding.

Discussion

The myriad of case reports, case series and variability in methodology render definitive guidelines for medication use during lactation premature. Although the overall sample sizes are limited, they are quite comparable to the available data on most other, non-psychiatric, medications. There are several key points that warrant comment. (1) The terminology in previous reports (e.g. toxicity, accumulation, negligible exposure) has not been validated and is therefore highly suspect. (2) The majority of reports do not report any adverse effects on the nursing infant. (3) The details and scientific methodology of obtaining and analysing breast-milk and infant serum concentrations of medications are rapidly advancing. (4) With all

psychotropic medication use during lactation, the infant should be monitored on a routine basis, at a minimum frequency as often as an adult would be monitored, during and after medication exposure. However, the clinician should not assume that undetectable is synonymous with infant non-exposure, and nor should elevated infant serum concentrations result in reflexive discontinuation of medication without review of the risk/benefit assessment. (5) Postpartum women should be cautioned about subsequent conception while breast-feeding and while being treated with psychiatric medications. (6) It is unlikely that any data would preclude a comprehensive risk/benefit assessment (Table 19.1).

Based on the available literature, we recommend the following guidelines when deciding on the use of psychiatric medications during breast-feeding: (1) Document all other medications, alcohol, drugs and potentially hazardous environmental exposures that occur during this time period, because they may influence infant development alone or in combination with the medication under study. (2) Use one medicine if at all possible. Data on combination therapy are virtually non-existent. Choose monotherapy of a medicine with few side-effects, if at all possible, to avoid the need for a second medicine. (3) Use a medication of prior positive response in the patient whenever possible. The issue of lactation and the documented worsening of illness in the postpartum period make this a poor time for experimenting with new medications or new treatment plans. The clinician should try to avoid exposing the infant to a second medication, as mentioned above, and should try to avoid a partial response in the patient. The exceptions to this prior response rule would be with the MAOIs, clozapine, and possibly lithium (see mood stabilizer summary), because they are likely to cause side-effects, and more extensive monitoring in the

Table 19.1 Risk/benefit assessment—Lactation: summary.

Known data

- >60% of women plan to breast-feed in the postpartum period
- 5% of women will take at least one prescription medication for the duration of breast-feeding
- 20% of women smoke cigarettes for the duration of breast-feeding
- There are immunological benefits of breast-feeding for the infant
- Breast-feeding is purportedly the ideal and only source of nutrition necessary for infants
- There is a high rate of new-onset and relapse psychiatric illness in the postpartum period
- Untreated maternal mental illness, particularly major depression, can negatively affect infant attachment and development
- All psychiatric medications are excreted through breast milk, and the infant will be exposed
- Breast-feeding is not a 100% effective method of contraception, women should be reminded that conception is possible

Increasing data

- The pharmacokinetics of psychotropic medication excretion into breast milk are complex
- Nursing infants are exposed to less medication than the maternal daily dose
- Infant monitoring may require infant serum sampling, among other tests (e.g. EKG, hydration status)
- Reports of adverse effects on infants from exposure are limited to a few case reports
- Commercial laboratory assay sensitivity is typically less than that of research-quality assays

Unknown data

- The clinical significance of detectable medications in the infant; such values may reflect metabolic issues in the infant
- The long-term neurobehavioural outcome of children exposed to psychiatric medications via breast milk
- The long-term impact on infant development of untreated maternal mental illness

infant would be necessary. (4) We recommend the use of a medication with some published data, whenever possible, in the absence of a medication with prior positive response in the patient. As new medications of a class are developed, the relative safety of previous members of that class cannot be assumed to predict safety of the new medication class. (5) It may be preferable to choose a medication without documented metabolites. (6) Medications which allow for dosing flexibility and careful dose titration are preferable. Medications with multiple dosages available may help to minimize the infant dose while using the lowest effective dose to treat the mother. (7) Limit the need for frequent invasive infant monitoring. We support monitoring of the infant serum concentrations of medications. Medications such as lithium and clozapine that warrant more frequent venous sampling or extensive tests (e.g. ECG or hydration status) may pose additional risks to the infant. (8) Use a familiar medication after following rules 1–7. A physician should choose a medication with an efficacy and side-effect profile that he or she is familiar with. The clinician will be better able to identify side-effects in the mother or infant and provide reassurance to the mother.

These guidelines and the risk/benefit assessment may be of use to a clinician discussing medication exposure in lactation with parents. It is our hope that improving methodology and analysis techniques will eventually produce more definitive data for use in determining infant exposure and outcome. Long-term studies on the consequences of infant exposure to psychotropic medications are needed.

Acknowledgments

This paper was supported by NIMH grant MH-51761, an Unrestricted Educational Grant from Pfizer Pharmaceuticals and the American Psychiatric Association SmithKline Beecham Young Faculty Award (ZNS).

References

1. American Academy of Pediatrics Committee On Drugs, The transfer of drugs and other chemicals into human milk, *Pediatrics* 1994; 93:137–50.
2. Cohen LS, Heller VL, Rosenbaum JF, Treatment guidelines for psychotropic drug use in pregnancy, *Psychosomatics* 1989; 30:25–33.
3. Cohen LS, Psychotropic drug use in pregnancy, *Hosp Community Psychiatry* 1989; 40:566–7.
4. Kerns LL, Treatment of mental disorders in pregnancy: a review of psychotropic drug risks and benefits, *J Nerv Ment Dis* 1986; 174:652–9.
5. Miller LJ, Clinical strategies for the use of psychotropic drugs during pregnancy, *Psychiatr Med* 1991; 9:275–98.
6. Miller LJ, Psychiatric medication during pregnancy: understanding and minimizing the risks, *Psychiatr Ann* 1994; 24:69–75.
7. Wisner KL, Perel JM, Psychopharmacologic agents and electroconvulsive therapy during pregnancy and the puerperium. In: Cohen RL, ed., *Psychiatric Consultation in Childbirth Settings: Parent- and Child-oriented Approaches* (Plenum Medical Book Company: New York, 1988) 165–206.
8. Morselli PL, Franco-Morselli R, Bossi L, Clinical pharmacokinetics in newborns and infants: age related differences and therapeutic implications, *Clin Pharmacokinet* 1980; 5: 485–527.
9. Mortola JF, The use of psychotropic agents in pregnancy and lactation, *Psychiatr Clin North Am* 1989; 12:69–87.
10. Robinson GE, Stewart DE, Flak E, The rational use of psychotropic drugs in pregnancy and postpartum, *Can J Psychiatry* 1986; 31:183–90.
11. Stowe ZN, Nemeroff CB, Psychopharmacology during pregnancy and lactation. In: Schatzberg AF, Nemeroff CB, eds, *Textbook of Psychopharmacology* (American Psychiatric Press Inc.: Washington, DC, 1995) 823–37.
12. Kacew S, Adverse effects of drugs and chemicals in breast milk on the nursing infant, *J Clin Pharmacol* 1993; 33:213–21.
13. Knowles JA, Excretion of drugs in milk—a review, *Pediatr Pharmacol Ther* 1965; 66: 1068–82.
14. Vorherr H, Drug excretion in breast milk, *Postgrad Med* 1974; 56:97–104.
15. O'Brien TE, Excretion of drugs in human milk, *Am J Hosp Pharm* 1974; 31:844–54.

16. Anderson PO, Drug use during breast-feeding, *Clin Pharm* 1991; **10**:594–624.

17. Ito S, Blajchman A, Stephenson M et al, Prospective follow-up of adverse reactions in breast-fed infants exposed to maternal medication, *Am J Obstet Gynecol* 1993; **168**:1393–9.

18. Misri S, Sivertz K, Tricyclic drugs in pregnancy and lactation: a preliminary report. *Int J Psychiatry Med* 1991; **21**:157–71.

19. Wilson JT, Determinants and consequences of drug excretion in breast milk, *Drug Metab Rev* 1983; **14**:619–52.

20. Wilson JT, Brown RD, Cherek DR et al, Drug excretion in human breast milk: Principles, pharmacokinetics and projected consequences, *Clin Pharmacokinet* 1980; **5**: 1–66.

21. VanBlerk GA, Majerus TC, Myers RA, Teratogenic potential of some psychopharmacologic drugs: a brief review, *Int J Gynaecol Obstet* 1980; **17**:399–402.

22. Murray L, Seger D, Drug therapy during pregnancy and lactation, *Emerg Med Clin North Am* 1994; **12**:129–49.

23. Buist A, Norman TR, Dennerstein L, Breast-feeding and the use of psychotropic medication: a review, *J Affect Disord* 1990; **19**: 197–206.

24. Baum AL, Misri S, Selective serotonin-reuptake inhibitors in pregnancy and lactation *Harv Rev Psychiatry* 1996; **4**:117–25.

25. Pons G, Rey W, Matheson I, Excretion of psychoactive drugs into breast milk: Pharmacokinetic principles and recommendations, *Clin Pharmacokinet Special Populations* 1994; **27**:270–89.

26. Wisner KL, Perel JM, Findling RL, Antidepressant treatment during breast-feeding, *Am J Psychiatry* 1996; **153**:1132–7.

27. Ananth J, Side effects in the neonate from psychotropic agents excreted through breast-feeding, *Am J Psychiatry* 1978; **135**:801–5.

28. Byers T, Graham S, Rzepka T, Marshall J, Lactation and breast cancer. Evidence for a negative association in premenopausal women, *Am J Epidemiol* 1985; **121**:664–74.

29. Beaudry M, Dufour R, Marcoux S, Relation between infant feeding and infections during the first six months of life, *J Pediatr* 1995; **126**:191–7.

30. Duncan B, Ey J, Holberg CJ et al, Exclusive breast-feeding for at least 4 months protects against otitis media, *Pediatrics* 1993; **91**:867–7.

31. Sassen ML, Brand R, Grote JJ, Breast-feeding and acute otitis media, *Am J Otolaryngol* 1994; **15**:351–7.

32. Pisacane A, Graziano L, Mazzarella G et al, Breastfeeding and urinary tract infection, *J Pediatr* 1992; **120**:87–9.

33. Coppa GV, Gabrielli O, Giorgi P et al, Preliminary study of breast-feeding and bacterial adhesion to uroepithelial cells, *Lancet* 1990; **335**:569–71.

34. Lucas A, Morley R, Cole TJ et al, Breast milk and subsequent intelligence quotient in children born preterm, *Lancet* 1992; **339**:261–4.

35. Stowe ZN, Owens MJ, Landry JC et al, Sertraline and desmethylsertraline in human breast milk and nursing infants, *Am J Psychiatry* 1997; **154**:1255–60.

36. Yoshida K, Smith B, Craggs M, Kumar RC, Investigation of pharmacokinetics of possible adverse effects in infants exposed to tricyclic antidepressants in breast milk, *J Affect Disord* 1997; **43**:225–37.

37. Morselli PL, Clinical pharmacokinetics in neonates, *Clin Pharmacokinet* 1976; **1**:81–98.

38. O'Dea RF, Medication use in the breast-feeding mother, *NAACOGS Clin Issues Perinat Women's Health Nurs* 1992; **3**:598–604.

39. Atkinson AJ, Stec GP, Lertora JJ et al, Impact of active metabolites on monitoring plasma concentrations of therapeutic drugs, *Ther Drug Monitoring* 1980; **2**:19–27.

40. Briggs GG, Samson JH, Ambrose PJ, Schroeder DH, Excretion of bupropion in breast milk, *Ann Pharmacother* 1993; **27**: 431–3.

41. Cunningham AS, Jelliffe DB, Jelliffe EF, Breast-feeding and health in the 1980's: a global epidemiologic review, *J Pediatr* 1991; **118**: 659–66.

42. Milberger S, Biederman J, Faraone SV et al, Is maternal smoking during pregnancy a risk factor for attention deficit hyperactivity disorder in children? *Am J Psychiatry* 1996; **153**:1138–42.

43. Pichini S, Altieri I, Zuccaro P, Pacifici R, Drug monitoring in non-conventional biological

fluids and matrices, *Clin Pharmacokinet* 1996; 30:211–28.

44. Bader TF, Newman K, Amitriptyline in human breast milk and the nursing infant's serum, *Am J Psychiatry* 1980; **137**:855–6.

45. Breyer-Pfaff U, Nill K, Entenmann KN, Gaertner HJ, Secretion of amitriptyline and metabolites into breast milk, *Am J Psychiatry* 1995; **152**:812–13.

46. Brixen-Rasmussen L, Halgrener J, Jorgensen A, Amitriptyline and nortriptyline excretion in human breast milk, *Psychopharmacology* 1982; **76**:94–5.

47. Erickson SH, Smith GH, Heidrich F, Tricyclics and breast feeding, *Am J Psychiatry* 1979; **136**:1483–4.

48. Pittard WB, O'Neal W, Amitriptyline excretion in human milk, *J Clin Psychopharmacol* 1986; **6**:383–4.

49. Matheson I, Pande H, Alertsen AR, Respiratory depression caused by N-desmethyldoxepin in breast milk, *Lancet* 1985; **2**:1124.

50. Kemp J, Ilett KF, Booth J, Hackett LP, Excretion of doxepin and N-desmethyldoxepin in human milk, *Br J Clin Pharmacol* 1985; **20**:497–9.

51. Schimmell MS, Katz EZ, Shaag Y et al, Toxic neonatal effects following maternal clomipramine therapy, *J Toxicol Clin Toxicol* 1991; **29**:479–84.

52. Wisner KL, Perel JM, Foglia JP, Serum clomipramine and metabolite levels in four nursing mother–infant pairs, *J Clin Psychiatry* 1995; **56**:17–20.

53. Wisner KL, Perel JM, Serum nortriptyline levels in nursing mothers and their infants, *Am J Psychiatry* 1991; **148**:1234–6.

54. Wisner KL, Perel JM, Nortriptyline treatment of breast-feeding women, *Am J Psychiatry* 1996; **153**:295.

55. Wisner KL, Perel JM, Findling RL, Hinnes RL, Nortriptyline and its hydroxymetabolites in breast-feeding mothers and newborns, *Psychopharmacol Bull* 1997; **33**:249–51.

56. Altshuler LL, Cohen L, Szuba MP et al, Pharmacologic management of psychiatric illness in pregnancy: dilemmas and guidelines, *Am J Psychiatry* 1996; **153**:592–606.

57. Gelenberg AJ, Amoxapine, a new antidepressant, appears in human milk, *J Nerv Ment Dis* 1979; **167**:635–6.

58. Stancer HC, Reed KL, Desipramine and 2-hydroxydesipramine in human breast milk and the nursing infant's serum, *Am J Psychiatry* 1986; **143**:1597–600.

59. Sovner R, Orsulak PJ, Excretion of imipramine and desipramine in human breast milk, *Am J Psychiatry* 1979; **136**:451–2.

60. Taddio A, Ito S, Koren G, Excretion of fluoxetine and its metabolite norfluoxetine, in human breast milk, *J Clin Pharmacol* 1996; **36**:42–7.

61. Burch KJ, Wells BG, Fluoxetine/norfluoxetine concentration in human milk, *Pediatrics* 1992; **89**:676–7.

62. Isenberg KE, Excretion of fluoxetine in human breast milk, *J Clin Psychiatry* 1990; **51**:169.

63. Lester BM, Cucca J, Andreozzi L et al, Possible association between fluoxetine hydrochloride and colic in an infant, *J Am Acad Child Adolesc Psychiatry* 1993; **32**: 1253–5.

64. Kim J, Misri S, Riggs KW et al, Steroselective excretion of fluoxetine and norfluoxetine in breast milk and neonatal exposure, presented at American Psychiatric Association Annual Meeting, San Diego, 1997.

65. Yoshida K, Smith B, Craggs M, Kumar RC, Fluoxetine in breast-milk and developmental outcome of breast-fed infants, *Br J Psychiatry* 1998; **172**:175–8.

66. Birnbaum CS, Cohen LS, Grush LR et al, Serum concentrations of antidepressants and benzodiazepines in nursing infants: A case series, *Pediatrics* 1999; **104**:1–6.

67. Eppersen CN, Anderson GM, McDougle CJ, Sertraline and breast-feeding, *N Engl J Med* 1997; **336**:1189–90.

68. Wisner KL, Perel JM, Blumer J, Serum sertraline and N-desmethylsertraline levels in breast-feeding mother–infant pairs, *Am J Psychiatry* 1998; **155**:690–2.

69. Wright S, Dawling S, Ashford JJ, Excretion of fluvoxamine in breast milk, *Br J Clin Pharmacol* 1991; **31**:209.

70. Spigset O, Carleborg L, Norstrom A, Sandlund M, Paroxetine level in breast milk, *J Clin Psychiatry* 1996; **57**:39.

71. Ilett KF, Hackett LP, Roberts MJ et al, Distribution and excretion of venlafaxine and

O-desmethylvenlafaxine in human milk, *Br J Clin Pharmacol* 1998; **45**:459–62.

72. Jensen PN, Olesen OV, Bertelsen A, Linnet K, Citalopram and desmethylcitalopram concentrations in breast milk and in serum of mother and infant, *Ther Drug Monit* 1997; **19**:236–9.

73. Buist A, Dennerstein L, MacGuire KP, Norman TR, Plasma and human milk concentrations of moclobemide in nursing mothers, *Human Psychopharmacol Clin Exp* 1998; **13**: 570–82.

74. Fisher JB, Edgren BE, Mammel MC, Coleman JM, Neonatal apnea associated with maternal clonazepam therapy: a case report, *Obstet Gynecol* 1985; **66**:34S–5S.

75. Soderman P, Matheson I, Clonazepam in breast milk, *Eur J Pediatr* 1988; **147**:212–13.

76. Andre M, Boutroy MJ, Dubruc C et al, Clonazepam pharmacokinetics and therapeutic efficacy in neonatal seizures, *Eur J Clin Pharmacol* 1986; **30**:585–9.

77. Patrick MJ, Tilstone WJ, Reavey P, Diazepam and breast-feeding, *Lancet* 1972; **1**:542–3.

78. Erkkola R, Kanto J, Diazepam and breast-feeding, *Lancet* 1972; **1**:1235–6.

79. Morselli PL, Principi N, Tognoni G et al, Diazepam elimination in premature and full term infants and children, *J Perinat Med* 1973; **1**:133–41.

80. Eliot BW, Hill JG, Cole AP, Hailey DM, Continuous pethidine/diazepam infusion during labour and its effects on the newborn, *Br J Obstet Gynaecol* 1975; **82**:126–31.

81. Cole AP, Hailey DM, Diazepam and active metabolite in breast milk and their transfer to the neonate, *Arch Dis Child* 1975; **50**:741–2.

82. Brandt R, Passage of diazepam and desmethyl-diazepam into breast milk, *Arzneimittelforschung* 1976; **26**:454–7.

83. Dusci LJ, Good SM, Hall RW, Ilett KF, Excretion of diazepam and its metabolites in human milk during withdrawal from combination high dose diazepam and oxazepam, *Br J Clin Pharmacol* 1990; **29**:123–6.

84. Wretlind M, Excretion of oxazepam in breast milk, *Eur J Clin Pharmacol* 1987; **33**:209–10.

85. Rane A, Sundwall A, Tomson G, Withdrawal symptoms in a neonate after intrauterine exposure to oxazepam, *Lakartidningen* 1979; **76**:4416–7.

86. Summerfield RJ, Nielsen MS, Excretion of lorazepam into breast milk, *Br J Anaesth* 1985; **57**:1042–3.

87. Lebedevs TH, Wojnar-Horton RE, Yapp P et al, Excretion of temazepam in breast milk, *Br J Clin Pharmacol* 1992; **33**:204–6.

88. Hilbert JM, Gural RP, Symchowicz S, Zampaglione N, Excretion of quazepam into human breast milk, *J Clin Pharmacol* 1984; **24**:457–62.

89. Kanto J, Aaltonen L, Kangas L et al, Placental transfer and breast milk levels of flunitrazepam, *Curr Ther Res* 1979; **26**:539–46.

90. Pons G, Francoual C, Guillet P et al, Zolpidem excretion in breast milk, *Eur J Clin Pharmacol* 1989; **37**:245–8.

91. Goldfield MD, Weinstein MR, Lithium carbonate in obstetrics: guidelines for clinical use, *Am J Obstet Gynecol* 1973; **116**:15–22.

92. Sykes PA, Quarrie J, Alexander FW, Lithium carbonate and breast-feeding, *Br Med J* 1976; **2**:1299.

93. Woody JN, London WL, Wilbanks GD, Lithium toxicity in a newborn, *Pediatrics* 1971; **47**:94–6.

94. Schou M, Amdisen A, Lithium and pregnancy—III. Lithium ingestion by children breast-fed by women on lithium treatment, *Br Med J* 1973; **2**:138.

95. Weinstein MR, Goldfield M, Lithium carbonate treatment during pregnancy, *Dis Nerv Syst* 1969; **30**:828–32.

96. Weinstein MR, Goldfield MD, Cardiovascular malformations with lithium use during pregnancy, *Am J Psychiatry* 1975; **132**:529–31.

97. Linden S, Rich CL, The use of lithium during pregnancy and lactation, *J Clin Psychiatry* 1983; **44**:358–61.

98. Briggs GG, Freeman RK, Yaffe SJ, eds, *Drugs in Pregnancy and Lactation* (Williams & Wilkins: Baltimore, 1994).

99. Alexander FW, Sodium valproate and pregnancy, *Arch Dis Child* 1979; **54**:240.

100. Frey B, Schubiger G, Musy JP, Transient cholestatic hepatitis in a neonate associated with carbamazepine exposure during pregnancy and breast-feeding, *Eur J Pediatr* 1990; **150**:136–6.

101. Briggs GG, Pharm B, Freeman RK, Yaffe SJ, Update: drugs in pregnancy and lactation, *Drugs Pregnancy Lactation Update* 1996; **9**:9–18.

102. Merlob P, Mor N, Litwin A, Transient hepatic dysfunction in an infant of an epileptic mother treated with carbamazepine during pregnancy and breast-feeding, *Ann Pharmacother* 1992; **26**:1563–5.

103. Brockington IF, Meakin CJ, Clinical clues to the aetiology of puerperal psychosis, *Prog Neuropsychopharmacol Biol Psychiatry* 1994; **18**:417–29.

104. Brockington IF, Kelly A, Hall P, Deakin W, Premenstrual relapse of puerperal psychosis, *J Affect Disord* 1988; **14**:287–92.

105. Brockington IF, Oates M, Rose G, Prepartum psychosis, *J Affect Disord* 1990; **19**:31–5.

106. Stewart RB, Karas B, Springer PK, Haloperidol excretion in human milk, *Am J Psychiatry* 1980; **137**:849–50.

107. Whalley LJ, Blain PG, Prime JK, Haloperidol secreted in breast milk, *Br Med J* 1981; **282**:1746–7.

108. Barnas C, Bergant A, Hummer M et al, Clozapine concentrations in maternal and fetal plasma, amniotic fluid, and breast milk, *Am J Psychiatry* 1994; **151**:945.

109. Blacker KH, Weinstein BJ, Ellman GL, Mother's milk and chlorpromazine, *Am J Psychiatry* 1962; **119**:178–80.

110. Wiles DH, Orr MW, Kolakowska T, Chlorpromazine levels in plasma and milk of nursing mothers, *Br J Clin Pharmacol* 1978; **5**:272–3.

111. Kirk L, Jorgensen A, Concentrations of cis(Z)-flupenthixol in maternal serum, amniotic fluid, umbilical cord serum, and milk, *Psychopharmacology* 1980; **72**:107–8.

112. Olesen OV, Bartels U, Poulsen JH, Perphenazine in breast milk and serum, *Am J Psychiatry* 1990; **147**:1378–9.

20

Pregnancy loss

John T Condon

Introduction

Scope of this review

The term 'abortion' has become somewhat obsolete, because of both its ambiguity and the ethical and political connotations it has acquired. In this chapter, I will review the literature in three areas. First, the psychological sequelae of *spontaneous miscarriage* occurring under 20 weeks of gestation will be examined. Within this category, I will include the phenomenon of 'recurrent miscarriage', previously referred to as 'habitual abortion'. Second, the sequelae of *termination of pregnancy* (also known as 'abortion', 'induced abortion', 'therapeutic abortion' or 'medical abortion') will be addressed. Included within this category will be termination of pregnancy for genetic (or other 'medical' reasons) *vis-à-vis* psychosocial reasons, a distinction which may become increasingly blurred as intrauterine diagnostic technology advances. Also included is the very recent literature on multiple pregnancy reduction. The term 'elective termination' will be

avoided because of its ambiguity and its implication of 'choice', which is often unfounded. Third, the recent literature dealing with late pregnancy loss, including intrauterine death (beyond 20 weeks of gestation), stillbirth and neonatal death, will be summarized.

Excluded from this review is pregnancy loss occurring in the context of infertility management, which is best considered within the context of the psychological aspects of infertility.

Theoretical framework

A conceptual framework arising from the literature on grief and bereavement is the most appropriate starting point for understanding psychological reactions to pregnancy loss.[1] Such a model presupposes the existence of emotional attachment to the unborn baby, and postulates that the loss represents the breaking of this attachment bond. Elsewhere, I have reviewed the literature on antenatal attachment, traced its development as gestation progresses and developed a self-report questionnaire for its measurement.[2-4] Muller[5] has reviewed the contributions of others to the literature in this area.

My own work, and that of others, suggests that a substantial increase in antenatal emotional attachment occurs around 16–20 weeks of gestation. This coincides with the first experience of fetal movement, and also the routine ultrasound examination which is performed in many Western obstetric settings. Both of these events, reinforcing the reality of fetal existence, probably contribute to this steep rise in attachment.

The attachment construct is complex, as is its assessment. A clinically useful distinction is between 'quantity' and 'quality' of antenatal attachment.[3] The latter refers to the nature of the feelings towards the unborn baby, which may range from intense affection and closeness through ambivalence to intense dislike (some women report an absence of any feelings). 'Quantity' refers to the degree of preoccupation with the baby and the frequency with which feelings towards it are experienced. For example, a woman with two other children under the age of 3 may experience very positive feelings towards the fetus, but have little time to indulge in these. In contrast, we have identified a subgroup of women who have highly ambivalent or negative feelings, yet spend a great deal of time 'anxiously preoccupied' with their fetus.[3]

The bereavement framework facilitates understanding of the complex emotional reactions which may accompany pregnancy loss, typically sadness, anger and guilt. In addition, it facilitates recognition of the subgroup of women who may be at risk of having pathological grief reactions. Finally, it provides a psychotherapeutic framework for assisting the resolution of the loss.

Thus, the bereavement model is central to our understanding of pregnancy loss. However, as described by Leon,[6] it can be usefully complemented by other theoretical perspectives. Pregnancy loss potentially interferes with an important developmental milestone in a woman's life and impacts upon her sense of self as a woman. From an object-relations perspective, the maternal–fetal relationship has become more 'real' with the advent of ultrasonography, potentially intensifying the sense of loss. Such a perspective also fosters understanding of the ambivalence which may characterize this relationship, stemming in part from the sacrifices which many Western women must make if they embark upon the transition to motherhood. An ego-psychological perspective focuses attention upon the defence and coping mechanisms (adaptive and maladaptive) which women may utilize when confronted with pregnancy loss. Of particular interest is the withholding of attachment to the fetus during subsequent pregnancy.[7]

Methodological shortcomings of research into pregnancy loss

Over the last two decades there has been a vast increase in the literature dealing with the psychological sequelae of pregnancy loss. Although consensus is emerging in several important areas (e.g. elective termination of pregnancy), many areas remain both confused and confusing, and inconsistent findings are commonplace. There are many factors which might account for these inconsistencies. Samples are often small, biased and non-representative; for example, those who decline to participate (or drop out) may be more distressed or dysfunctional. Samples are often heterogeneous, combining women with early/late pregnancy loss, single/recurrent loss and planned/unplanned pregnancy, and primiparous/multiparous women. Subjects are rarely assessed prior to pregnancy loss, because such longitudinal studies require very large initial sample sizes and hence are difficult and expensive. Control groups are often absent or poorly matched to subjects. The reliability and validity of outcome measures are often suspect, especially in relation to distinguishing 'depression' from 'normal grief' and in the measurement of constructs such as 'guilt'.

Follow-up periods greater than 2–3 months are uncommon. There is frequently a failure to take account of confounding factors which might contribute to both pregnancy loss (or request for termination of pregnancy) and distress or psychological symptoms.

Finally, social support is often not assessed, and nor is account taken of the 'support' and debriefing which women may derive from involvement in the research per se (e.g. via interview assessments).

Spontaneous miscarriage

Spontaneous miscarriage is the most common complication of pregnancy, and approximately 15% of confirmed pregnancies miscarry, most in the first trimester, with an average gestation of approximately 11 weeks. Almost all such women subsequently undergo an operative procedure under general anaesthetic to remove any residual products of conception. For the vast majority of these women this represents their first hospitalization, general anaesthetic and operation, yet this aspect is rarely mentioned in the research literature. This omission highlights the importance of considering what Lee and Slade[8] have referred to as the 'totality' of the miscarriage experience in terms of the event itself, the circumstances in which it took place, the response of the male partner, family and health professionals and its meaning to the woman herself.

Psychological sequelae

There is a consensus in the more recent literature that 'distress' commonly follows spontaneous miscarriage.[9] However, there is considerable disagreement between studies regarding the intensity and nature of this distress (e.g. grief versus depression), its duration and what factors predict its intensity and duration. Many writers have argued that health professionals devalue the significance of miscarriage for the women involved, underestimate its emotional impact (both short and long term), and fail to provide the much-needed support.[9] In contrast, two of the pioneers in the area of perinatal bereavement warn of 'another iatrogenic danger with every miscarriage liable to be magnified into a catastrophe' and state that 'the overzealous may interfere with the healthy resilience that enables most people to get over an early miscarriage without becoming psychiatrically disturbed'.[10]

In one of the first studies to utilize well-validated measures, Friedman and Gath[11] found that almost 50% of their sample of 67 women satisfied diagnostic caseness for depression when interviewed 4 weeks after miscarriage using the Present State Examination. Previous miscarriage and nulliparity were identified as risk factors. The characteristics of this sample are well described, and there are no obvious reasons why it should be considered biased or atypical. Eighty women were approached and 67 (i.e. 84%) participated.

One study[12] assessed 65 women at 1, 6 and 12 weeks following early miscarriage using a well-validated self-report questionnaire for depression and anxiety. Only 2 of 67 consecutive women admitted to hospital refused to participate. The study found that 41% and 22% were experiencing clinically significant levels of anxiety and depression (respectively) at the first assessment, considerably in excess of the levels to be expected in the general population. At the 6-week assessment the prevalences had dropped to less than half those found initially. The prevalence of depression continued to fall at the 12-week assessment (6%) but that of anxiety had (paradoxically) increased (32%). The authors speculate that the latter may be due to couples addressing the issue of whether to reattempt pregnancy at around 3 months post-miscarriage.

A number of studies of miscarriage have utilized the Perinatal Grief Scale,[13] which attempts to assess grieving as distinct from depression. Beutel et al[14] attempted to follow a cohort of 125 women for 1 year after miscarriage. Ninety women completed the study. Two control groups of 80 pregnant and 125 community women were utilized. Assessments made shortly after miscarriage indicated that 20% exhibited a grief reaction, 12% suffered depression and 20% appeared to demonstrate both. At the 1-year follow-up, depression, but not grief, was predictive of psychosocial dysfunction. This study provides a useful discussion of the differentiation between grief and depression.

In one of the first controlled studies, approximately 380 women were assessed at 2 weeks, 6 weeks and 6 months after miscarriage.[15] The study utilized a matched group of community controls and also a matched group of pregnant women controls. Clinically significant levels of depressive symptomatology were three to four times more prevalent in the miscarriage group than in the control groups at 2 weeks. When the women were re-interviewed at 6 weeks or 6 months, these differences were no longer significant. However, in a subgroup of miscarriage women interviewed for the first time at 6 weeks or 6 months, elevated depressive symptom levels were found. The authors postulate that the interview itself may have been therapeutic and thus reduced depressive symptoms in the re-interviewed cohort.

A study of 144 French women found a prevalence of 51% of DSM-III major depressive episode 3 months after miscarriage as assessed by recorded interviews.[16] A study of Chinese women,[17] using DSM-III-R criteria, found a 12% prevalence of major depression 6 weeks after miscarriage. The DSM cautions against diagnosing major depression within 2 months of 'bereavement', the latter being defined as 'death of a loved one'. Some have questioned whether fetal loss can be legitimately construed as 'death of a loved one'.[18]

In a controlled study[19] of 69 consecutive women who had been admitted to hospital following miscarriage and 62 antenatal clinic attenders at the same hospital, women were assessed shortly after miscarriage and at 6 weeks thereafter using the General Health Questionnaire and the Hospital Anxiety and Depression Scale. Miscarriage women had higher levels of anxiety and somatic symptoms at both assessments; however, the findings for depression were somewhat equivocal. The authors argue that anxiety is an important sequel of miscarriage and has been overlooked in most previous studies, which have focused on depression. Risk factors identified were a previous miscarriage, childlessness and unplanned pregnancy.

There is only one prospective controlled investigation of the sequelae of spontaneous miscarriage. This is an important study, since some have argued that the depression found in women after miscarriage might be simply a continuation of preexisting depression, and that the latter might be a contributing factor to the miscarriage. Approximately 2000 Dutch women were assessed using the Symptom Check List 90 in early pregnancy. Approximately 200 miscarried and these were reassessed on four occasions during the 18 months following the loss and compared with a similarly sized group who had delivered a live baby. When pregnancy symptom levels were controlled for, miscarriage women still showed significantly higher levels of depression, anxiety and somatization during the 6 months following their loss compared to women having live births. However, at 1 year the symptom levels of the two groups were comparable.

A very recent and methodologically rigorous study[21] assessed the 6-month incidence of new or recurrent episodes of major depression (using the Diagnostic Interview Schedule) in 229 women following miscarriage and in a matched group of community women of similar size. Incidences of 10.9% and 4.3% were found in the miscarriage and community groups respectively, equating with a relative risk of 2.5 (95% confidence limits 1.2–5.1). The relative risk for childless women was twice this value.

Recurrent miscarriage ('habitual abortion') affects approximately 1% of couples and is usually defined as three or more consecutive miscarriages. Obviously, in this context, the couple must deal not only with fetal loss, but also with the possibility of fertility loss. Katz and Kuller[22] have recently reviewed the literature in this area. The complex psychosocial sequelae of recurrent miscarriage are best considered as a subset of emotional reactions to infertility.

Many authors have advocated that women should be routinely assessed after miscarriage and be offered counselling. Lee et al,[23] in the only randomized controlled trial of debriefing after miscarriage, were unable to demonstrate any positive effect of debriefing upon emotional adaptation at 4 months. These authors make two important points in discussion. First, debriefing may have a positive impact for some, and a negative impact for others (e.g. by interfering with adaptive suppression, distraction). Thus, these effects may cancel out. Second, an important component of the debrief may be detailed explanation, which can only be provided by the obstetric staff involved, and is unavailable from the counsellor, whose medical knowledge is limited.

Pregnancy following miscarriage

A useful summary of the previous literature in this controversial area has recently been provided by Cuisinier et al;[24] they also report results from their follow-up study of approximately 200 women who miscarried and conceived again within 18 months of the loss. The main instrument used was the Perinatal Grief Scale.[13] Two main findings emerged from this study. First, pregnancy resulted in significant reductions in grief, regardless of the time lapse between loss and subsequent conception. Second, very few women appeared to suffer reactivation of grief following the birth or to regard the new infant as a replacement. The authors, acknowledging some methodological limitations of the study, suggest that the traditional advice to parents to wait 3–6 months before conceiving may be ill-founded. This issue is further addressed below.

Conclusion

Clearly, there is wide disparity in these findings in terms of the nature, intensity and duration of the psychological implications of miscarriage. However, it does seem apparent that a substantial number of women do experience adverse reactions which commonly extend over several months. The extent to which these equate with grief, as opposed to other dysphoric states such as depression, is unclear. A minority of women, probably less than 10%, appear to suffer more enduring adverse reactions extending beyond 6 months. The literature also suggests that health professionals have an inadequate awareness of these sequelae.

Termination of pregnancy

In 1991, Blumenthal[25] found over 200 reports on the psychological sequelae of termination of pregnancy in the literature. Since that time, probably another 70 papers have been published. Much of this research suffers from the kind of methodological weaknesses outlined in the introduction. In addition, two further obstacles render the interpretation of these findings difficult. First, the intense controversy and debate surrounding legal, moral and ethical aspects of this issue have sometimes introduced bias and a lack of scientific objectivity. Given the large size of this body of literature, findings can easily be selectively quoted to support a particular viewpoint. Second, inadequate attention has been paid to the heterogeneous nature of the procedures considered under the general rubric 'termination of pregnancy'. Such differences can crucially influence psychological sequelae and include: first- versus second-trimester termination; legal versus illegal abortion; termination of an unwanted versus wanted pregnancy; termination of a wanted pregnancy because of fetal abnormality versus psychosocial pressures; termination which conflicts with strongly held religious or moral values versus one which does not; terminations requiring likely psychiatric disturbance as a prerequisite for obtaining the procedure versus 'abortion on demand'. Given this heterogeneity, it is not surprising that contradictory findings exist.

Clearly, many of these factors which define the context in which termination occurs will vary widely between cultures and also between subgroups within a culture. Hence, generalization of findings should be made cautiously.

The psychological sequelae of termination

Many studies prior to the early 1960s showed an adverse impact of termination of pregnancy upon mental health and wellbeing.[25] These studies tended to be methodologically flawed,

and in many cases were undertaken in a climate where termination was illegal, with the accompanying physical complications, humiliation and need for subterfuge. Demonstrable psychiatric disturbance was often a prerequisite for obtaining termination. Simon and Senturia[26] have critically reviewed this early literature, highlighting the methodological shortcomings. In Sweden, where abortion was legal, early studies tended to find fewer adverse sequelae. For example, a study[27] in 1955 of 479 women interviewed after the procedure and followed up for 2–4 years found that 75% did not report self-recrimination or guilt, 11% acknowledged significant regret and guilt, and long-term incapacitating psychological sequelae were rare (1%). This study also found that a previous history of psychiatric illness was a risk factor for adverse sequelae, a finding that has been replicated in many subsequent studies.

American studies from the late 1960s and early 1970s were also methodologically weak, but consistent findings began to emerge.[25] Obviously, these require cautious interpretation; however, serious adverse sequelae appeared to affect only a relatively small minority of women, transient distress seemed fairly common, and the notion emerged that termination may have a positive impact in alleviating the depression and anxiety associated with unwanted pregnancy. These studies paved the way for the legalization of abortion in the USA in 1973.

Comprehensive reviews of the literature on the sequelae of termination over the last 2 decades have been published,[25,28,29] the most thorough and least biased being that by Zolese and Blacker.[29] Findings remain, to some extent, conflicting; however, there is a reasonably strong consensus that serious adverse psychological sequelae affect 5–10% of women, but transient grief reactions (lasting up to several months) are common. The significance of this figure of 5–10% has been variously interpreted. Those supporting abortion tend to dismiss it (equating it with 'very rare' or 'small minority'), while those opposing abortion deem it catastrophic, given that approximately 60 million abortions are performed worldwide annually. For this author, it suggests a need for further research to better define the characteristics of this at-risk group and, clinically, a need for adequate pre- and post-abortion assessment and counselling.

Several more recent studies warrant specific mention. A very large recent study[30] carried out in the UK under the auspices of the Royal College of General Practitioners compared 6410 women who had a termination of pregnancy with 6151 women who did not. The rates of psychiatric disorder over several years were not significantly different between the two cohorts. In both groups, significantly elevated rates were found in women with a past history of psychiatric illness, replicating the conclusions of Zolese and Blacker.[29] However, in women with no previous history of psychiatric illness, deliberate self-harm was more common in the termination cohort. The authors attribute this to confounding factors (such as preexisting psychosocial dysfunction) associated with both the request for termination and self-harm.

In a study by Greer et al,[31] a cohort of 360 women were assessed at 3, 15 and 24 months post-termination. Only 60% of the subjects could be traced at 2 years. The cumulative incidence of new cases receiving psychiatric treatment was 6.5%; however, only 1 in 10 of these attributed their symptoms to the termination. 'Guilt' was identified in 13% at 3 months and 7% at 2 years. The obvious methodological shortcomings, including the lack of a control group, dictate cautious interpretation of these data.

Other recent, more methodologically sound, studies have also failed to find increased incidence of psychiatric disorder following termination of pregnancy.[25,28,29,32] There is some evidence that termination carries less risk of psychiatric disorder than childbirth.[33]

Risk factors for adverse sequelae which have been identified in more than one study include past psychiatric illness, termination of a wanted pregnancy for medical or psychosocial reasons (i.e. an absence of free choice) and a lack of social support.[25,28,29] Tietze[34] has made the important point that the presence of one or more risk factors should not constitute a contraindication to termination, but rather an indication for more thorough monitoring and supportive intervention both prior to and after termination.

The evidence that termination of pregnancy is psychologically 'therapeutic' requires more cautious interpretation for several reasons. First, the baseline assessment is invariably made during the crisis which usually accompanies the request for termination. Second, a decrease in negative mood states does not necessarily equate with an increase in positive mood states, and measures of the latter (e.g. 'relief') are far less well developed (in terms of reliability and validity) than the former. Nevertheless, studies which have attempted comparisons of women whose request for termination has been granted with those whose request has been denied tend to find higher rates of psychological disturbance in the latter group.

Such findings in women who have been refused termination (often on the grounds of their good psychological health) must be interpreted with considerable care. In particular, the representativeness of a sample of (presumably) alienated women who agree to participate in a research project must be questioned. Dagg[32] has reviewed this literature (as have others[25,28,29]). It seems clear that a large proportion (up to 40%) of these women succeed in eventually obtaining a termination. The findings suggest that substantial levels of both psychosocial dysfunction and impaired maternal–infant relationship may exist in this group; however, its aetiology must be considered uncertain.

Two studies have attempted to follow the progress of children born to women who were denied termination of pregnancy. A Swedish study compared 120 such children with 120 controls at 15, 21 and 35 years.[35,36] The control subjects showed significantly higher levels of achievement and lower levels of psychosocial dysfunction (including psychiatric illness). A Czechoslovakian study[37,38] compared 220 such children with 220 well-matched controls at 9 and 22 years. The adverse findings of the Swedish study were confirmed, and significantly higher rates of criminality were also evident in the index children compared to controls at age 22.

There is little literature comparing different methods of termination of pregnancy. In a recent prospective trial,[39] 363 women were (partially) randomized to either vacuum aspiration or pharmacologically induced 'labour'. The latter does not involve general anaesthesia, and the woman is aware of the procedure, may experience pain and may see the aborted fetus. No differences in psychological sequelae could be detected at follow-up after 16 days. The authors provide a useful review of this area.

Termination because of fetal abnormality

Fetal abnormality may be detected by ultrasound examination, amniocentesis or chorion villus sampling (CVS). The latter enables earlier termination, but carries a higher risk of precipitating miscarriage regardless of whether the fetus is abnormal. The author could not locate any study comparing the psychological seque-

lae of amniocentesis with those of CVS. One study[40] has suggested that there are *a priori* differences between women who choose one method rather than the other.

Several recent studies have compared the psychological sequelae of termination due to fetal abnormality with those following perinatal loss. Using a battery of well-validated measures, Salvesen et al[41] conducted such a comparison, following both groups for 1 year. They found no differences between the two groups in levels of anxiety, depression and other psychological measures.

A case-control design[42] was used to compare 23 women 2 months after termination for fetal abnormalities with a demographically similar group 2 months after perinatal bereavement. After correcting for age differences between the two groups, no significant differences in grief response or depression were detected. The authors suggest that, given that both groups experienced the same intensity of grief, greater attention should be devoted to the management of women who undergo termination of pregnancy because of fetal abnormality.

Termination during the second trimester of pregnancy (e.g. following amniocentesis) warrants special consideration. With technological advances in the diagnosis of fetal abnormalities, it is possible (but not inevitable) that this kind of termination may become more common. Such pregnancies are usually not terminated by free choice. Moreover, maternal–fetal attachment during the second trimester may be stronger and have been enhanced by the experience of fetal movement or ultrasound examination. There is also some evidence that awareness of fetal abnormality may increase the risk of adverse sequelae.[43] Finally, the various obstetric procedures utilized are more invasive and more likely to lead to physical and psychological complications. In particular, induction of labour, followed after several hours by the delivery of a recognizably human fetus, potentially equates with a level of stress not encountered in first-trimester termination. Misri and Anderson have provided a review of second-trimester termination.[44]

Implications of advances in antenatal diagnosis

Advances in reproductive technology frequently outstrip understanding of their ethical and psychological implications. Two examples in the area of termination which illustrate this are antenatal detection of cystic fibrosis (CF) and multifetal pregnancy reduction.

Children with CF are usually cognitively intact, have an average lifespan of 40 years, yet suffer distressing and debilitating symptoms throughout their lives. The dilemmas posed are obvious; however, it is of interest that a recent survey[45] in the UK found that 68% of CF sufferers and 84% of their parents supported the option of termination being offered if an affected pregnancy was detected at antenatal diagnosis.

Ovulation induction has assisted many infertile couples to conceive. However, it carries a substantial risk of multiple pregnancy with the accompanying risks of maternal complications, prematurity and increased perinatal mortality. Multiple pregnancy reduction usually involves injection of a lethal solution into the heart of one or more selected fetuses between 7 and 13 weeks. The dead fetus is then gradually resorbed within the uterus, leaving its siblings with an enhanced chance of survival. A small but growing literature[46–48] (including psychoanalytic contributions[49]) addresses the possible psychological sequelae in women undergoing this procedure. The current findings suggest that, provided the remaining fetuses survive, long-term adverse psychological sequelae are rare. However, the procedure is experienced as stressful and distressing, and a significant grief reaction, lasting up to 1 month, affects the majority of women. Having viewed the multifetal pregnancy on ultrasound has been postulated as one risk factor for more prolonged reactions.

Conclusions

There seems little doubt that only a small minority of women suffer any substantial long-term adverse sequelae following termination of pregnancy. However, given the very large number of terminations performed, this potentially represents a large number of women. High-quality, prospective studies are required to better define the size and characteristics of this at-risk group. There is a conspicuous lack of sound research into prevention in women who might be at risk of adverse psychological sequelae.[50]

Advances in antenatal diagnosis and obstetric technology, as exemplified by multifetal pregnancy reduction, will undoubtedly continue and possibly lead to a blurring of the boundary between 'genetic' and 'psychosocial' termination. Ethical implications will remain difficult and complex. However, ongoing research into the psychological sequelae, for the woman and others involved, can provide data relevant to consideration of the ethical dilemmas.

Intrauterine death, stillbirth and perinatal bereavement

The term stillbirth will be used to refer to the delivery of a dead baby who was living at the commencement of labour. Intrauterine death implies death prior to the commencement of labour and usually refers to a gestation longer than 20 weeks. Perinatal bereavement refers to the subsequent death of a live-born baby after a period which differs between authorities from 7 to 28 days. Some authors use 'perinatal bereavement' to cover all three types of late pregnancy loss.

Research addressing possible psychological sequelae suffers from many of the same methodological problems outlined in the introduction. Two further complications arise in this particular area. First, the management of late pregnancy loss has altered dramatically over the last 25 years in most Western hospitals. The former practice of staff deliberately preventing or discouraging parents from having visual and tactile contact with the dead baby has given way to protocols which encourage such contact, as well as offering parents photographs and other mementos of the baby. The older practice of 'hospital disposal' of the body has also been replaced by options involving funeral services, etc.[51,52] As pointed out by Zeanah[53] and others,[54] the impact of this more humanitarian approach has not been adequately researched and such investigation is probably no longer ethically feasible. Very few studies even define what kinds of psychological management occurred in the hospital. However, it is important to note that many of the earlier studies, which found very high rates of psychological morbidity in women suffering late pregnancy loss, were conducted prior to the inception of these major changes.

A second complication is the high levels of postnatal depression which have been found in women following the birth of a *surviving* infant (typically 10–15%).[55] Hence, it would seem that the only appropriate control group is a matched group of postnatal women.

A most comprehensive and detailed critical review of this literature to 1988 (including tabulations of all the major studies) has been provided by Zeanah.[53] His main conclusions will be summarized here and the remainder of the

chapter will focus on studies from the last decade.

Literature to 1988

There is general agreement that late pregnancy loss involves very considerable emotional pain and suffering for the majority of parents who experience it. There is also agreement that the intensity of grief appears to be greater in the mother than in the father; however, the possibility that grief may be expressed differently in males cannot be excluded. Methodological problems preclude any firm conclusions regarding differences between the responses to the different types of late pregnancy loss.

Zeanah found only four studies[56–59] which had assessed parents on more than one occasion following their loss. All of these studies suffer significant shortcomings, including substantial drop-out rates. However, all suggest a significant decline in both symptom levels and the number of women affected over the course of the first year. In addition, taken as a whole, they suggest that a substantial minority of bereaved women (20–30%) remain significantly symptomatic at the end of the first year.

Several studies have attempted to identify risk factors for disordered mourning. Lack of social support (both within and outside the partner relationship) has been identified in several studies,[58,60–62] as have adverse life events during pregnancy.[60]

Exploring the effect of intervention, Forrest et al[59] randomly allocated 50 perinatally bereaved women to either routine care or planned support. Assessments were made at 6 and 14 months. At the 6-month assessment, 10 of 19 women in routine care, but only 2 of 16 in supportive care, satisfied criteria for psychiatric disorder. At 14 months, 20% of the sample remained adversely affected, but there were no longer any significant differences between the two groups. This is arguably the most methodologically sound intervention study from this era.

As pointed out by Zeanah,[53] the literature from this era inadequately distinguishes grief and depression, and tends to focus on affective symptomatology at the expense of broader indicators of psychological distress or wellbeing.

Literature 1989–97

Most of the relatively small number of studies over this period took place in settings where parents were offered the opportunity to have contact with the dead baby and offered photographs and mementos. Instruments which attempt to distinguish grief and depression have been developed, such as the Perinatal Grief Scale[13] and the Perinatal Bereavement Scale,[63] and utilized in several studies.

A study by Theut et al[63] compared nine perinatally bereaved women with 16 women who had had a spontaneous miscarriage. Assessment was in the third trimester of a subsequent pregnancy using the Perinatal Bereavement Scale. The miscarriage group showed significantly lower levels of unresolved grief.

A series of papers[64–66] have described an Australian study following (over 8 months) a mixed cohort of approximately 250 women of whom 200 were bereaved by either stillbirth or perinatal death and 50 had lost a child by sudden infant death syndrome (SIDS). The study is important in that it is longitudinal, utilizes a matched control group of similar size, and uses standardized measures. The authors found the highest levels of anxiety and depression in the women bereaved by SIDS. At 2 months, high levels of anxiety and depression were four to seven times more likely in the perinatally bereaved women than in controls. By 8 months, these figures had decreased to two to

four, and the stillbirth group did not differ significantly from controls. The study is also of interest in that it consistently indicates higher levels of distress in women suffering perinatal bereavement (i.e. death within the first 28 days) as opposed to stillbirth. It confirms the finding of earlier studies of consistently higher levels of distress in mothers relative to fathers.

The same group has recently published a further follow-up of this cohort at 15 and 30 months post-bereavement.[67] Approximately 20–25% of the original cohort of perinatal bereaved and control women were lost to follow-up. However, there is no evidence that these differed on earlier measures of anxiety or depression. In women bereaved by late pregnancy loss, there was no difference from controls in rates of depression by 15 months. Anxiety remained significantly elevated at 15 months, but had also normalized by 30 months. The authors believe that anxiety is a more ubiquitous form of distress than depression following late pregnancy loss.

Another recent controlled study[68] compared 380 Swedish women 3 years after bereavement by stillbirth or intrauterine death with a similar number of controls. The results contradicted the findings of earlier studies, which suggested very high levels of long-term morbidity. The ratio of bereaved women with high anxiety to non-bereaved controls was 2.1 (95% confidence limits, 1.2–3.9). A delay of greater than 25 h between diagnosis of in utero death and subsequent delivery was identified as a significant risk factor for persistent anxiety at 3 years, as was the mother not being able to see the baby for as long as she wished. The authors found similar, but less pronounced, effects for depression.

In a study by Graham et al,[69] 28 women were interviewed during the first 4 weeks following late pregnancy loss. The authors found that higher levels of depression were associated with childlessness, self-blame for the death and not having seen the infant. They make the important point that the latter variable could not be randomized, and level of distress may have influenced the decision of whether or not to view the infant. The paper provides a useful discussion of self-blame and guilt in this setting.

A study by Murray and Callan[61] assessed 130 parents attending a perinatal bereavement support group an average of 2 years after bereavement. The findings highlight that more than 50% felt that they had been allowed insufficient time with their dead baby. A consistent predictor of better outcome was high level of perceived support from hospital staff. The sample is clearly non-representative and hence the findings must be interpreted cautiously. Other authors[51,52] have stressed the importance of support from the obstetric team *directly involved* rather than professional counsellors. Crowther (writing in 1995)[70] found that only 29% of their stillbirth and neonatal death sample were satisfied with the information they had been given.

Several authors[53,62] have addressed the impact of perinatal loss upon the partner relationship. Findings are variable, with both improvement and deterioration being found.[53] The most recent controlled study of this issue[65] involved 809 parents and found significantly increased relationship break-up following perinatal loss, as well as a deterioration in relationship functioning in those who remained together. Interestingly, the authors found a significant deterioration also in the control parents whose infant had survived, such that, by 6 months, there were no differences in relationship functioning between the two groups.

The vexed question of whether to postpone subsequent pregnancy after pregnancy loss has always been controversial, and remains so. Zeanah[53] has summarized the history of this

recommendation, including the writings of Lewis[71] on how early pregnancy may inhibit grieving and the notion of the 'replacement child syndrome'. The studies reviewed by Zeanah[53] provide conflicting findings and most are methodologically weak. Three tentative conclusions can be drawn from these studies together with more recent findings.[70,72] First, the usual recommendation to 'wait at least 6 months' is an over-generalization and bereft of empirical support. Second, individual differences are very real and very substantial. Thus, couples need to be helped to explore their options in terms of their own individual grief progression and circumstances. Third, dogmatic advice, if given, is rarely followed.

Management issues

An extremely comprehensive annotated bibliography of the literature between 1960 and 1990 has been published by Bourne and Lewis,[73] who have provided much of the impetus for the humanitarian reforms in management over several decades. This is a valuable resource for both clinicians and researchers who are involved with late pregnancy loss.

The framework of grief and mourning greatly facilitates our understanding of the psychological reactions of women suffering pregnancy loss, as well as providing a psychotherapeutic model for treatment. However, in my clinical experience, sole preoccupation with this model can sometimes lead to the coexistence of severe psychiatric illness being overlooked in bereaved women. Pregnancy loss does not render a woman immune from serious disorders such as major depression, psychosis or post-traumatic stress disorder which might warrant biological or other treatments. The first task of the clinician is to exclude such disorders before embarking solely upon grief therapy. Elsewhere, I have addressed the practicalities of distinguishing grief and depression.[51]

In this author's view, much of the psychological morbidity associated with late pregnancy loss is preventable. There are two distinct aspects of prevention. First, many young adults have totally unrealistic expectations about pregnancy and childbirth. They believe that stillbirth is an extremely rare event and that, if a baby is born alive, current neonatal technology will ensure its survival. The media parades the triumphs of the technology, while overlooking its failures. Better education in these areas would reduce psychological morbidity as well as litigation in obstetrics and neonatology.[74]

Second, as I have described elsewhere,[51] the events surrounding the death, including the behaviours and attitudes of obstetric and neonatal staff, are critically important in influencing the psychological outcome.[75]

In grief therapy, the pregnancy experience (including its 'wantedness') should be explored in some detail, as should any previous pregnancy losses and their meaning to the patient. The reactions of significant others to these issues also warrant careful exploration. Feelings towards the *unborn baby per se* (rather than towards 'the pregnancy') should also be gently probed.

In subsequent sessions, the events occurring at the time of loss (e.g. in the delivery room) are covered, including the perceived reactions of staff and family.

As I have described in detail elsewhere,[54] the whole issue of *what (or who) was lost* often needs to be a central focus in this kind of grief therapy. The parents often need to be helped to develop an internalized representation of the unborn baby. This aspect is often inadequately dealt with by therapists, since, in more conventional grief, the deceased is well known to the bereaved and there is much less need for this phase.

As in all mourning, that following pregnancy loss may become blocked at various phases. An absence of grieving may subsequently present as depression or other psychological symptoms. Alternatively, the grieving may appear to be proceeding normally but the women seem unable to achieve resolution. Such women, often years after the loss, feel like 'it only happened yesterday' and become overwhelmed and tearful at any reminder of the loss.

If grief has been minimally expressed, and the onset of other symptoms is closely linked to the loss, the therapist's task is often to assist the woman to initiate grieving. Sometimes only 'permission to grieve' is required, the woman having equated the expression of grief with 'weakness' or 'stupidity'. In other cases, encouraging a chronological account of events in an empathic environment will achieve the desired objective.

Prolonged grief is more difficult to treat. Clearly, the woman is very much in touch with her sadness. However, often such women have not adequately dealt with anger and/or guilt surrounding their loss. Experience and sensitivity are required to gently help the woman to focus on the specific aspects of the pregnancy (or death) which have engendered these emotions and enable her to express them in the setting of a 'safe' patient–therapist relationship.

Anger is very frequently a component of the reaction to pregnancy loss. It may be directed at staff, the male partner, other women who have not lost their pregnancies, god, fate, the baby or the therapist. This anger may or may not have some justification. However, regardless of whether it may be justified, the most important aspect of dealing with it is the therapist's acceptance of the anger in a non-defensive and empathic manner.

Guilt and shame are almost ubiquitous in

this group of women. At the most basic level, shame arises from the fundamental belief that 'good mothers don't let their babies die'. There may have been behaviours during pregnancy (or preceding the death) which now exacerbate guilt, and lead to the woman believing that she 'killed' the baby. In our society, from children's earliest stories and fables, good people 'live happily ever after' and bad people are meant to die or suffer. Hence, it is hardly surprising that, when tragedy strikes, the notion that 'bad things happen to bad people' rapidly enters conscious awareness. This can lead to the baby's death being experienced as a punishment for real or imagined past transgressions. Finally, for some women, guilt and self-blame can be a mechanism which, at an unconscious level, 'solves' the problem of possible recurrence. Thus, if the woman herself 'caused' the death, she does not have to confront the possibility that such events may occur in a random, unpredictable and inexplicable manner. Moreover, the power to prevent a recurrence rests with her.

Guilt is one of the most difficult emotions to work with in this type of therapy. Logic and reassurance are rarely helpful, and have usually been already repeatedly received by the woman.

Guilt may be dealt with in a number of maladaptive ways, including self-punishment and projection. The latter is unfortunately commonplace in obstetric tragedies, and contributes to the high rates of litigation against this medical specialty.[74] Reparation and altruism may, depending on their form and extent, be either adaptive or maladaptive. It is interesting to observe that from our very earliest preverbal years we express sadness by crying, and anger by screaming, hitting, biting, etc. With the acquisition of language, we are taught how to deal with guilt by saying 'I'm sorry'. In my own clinical work with perinatally bereaved, guilt-ridden women, I have been struck by how many of them, in therapy, seem to reach a point where they themselves experience a need to 'apologize' to their dead baby. A monologue with this theme at the graveside (or some other place associated with the death) is sometimes highly effective in relieving an intense sense of guilt. The origin of the guilt is (usually) irrational. So, it would seem, must sometimes be its cure.

Textbooks (and many respected authorities) in the field of bereavement and grief therapy instruct us to explain to our patients that the objective of the therapy is to 'say goodbye to' or 'let go of' the deceased. In my experience, perinatally bereaved women have great difficulty in relating to such objectives. As one patient stated: 'How can you say goodbye, when you've never said hello?'

George Vaillant has written a remarkable and very lucid paper[76] dealing with this precise issue. Vaillant's message, relevant for all of us who work with bereaved patients, is summarized by the following quotation: 'The psychological work of mourning is to remember more than it is to say goodbye.... Grief work is remembering, not forgetting; it is a process of internalising, not extruding.'

References

1. Raphael B, *The Anatomy of Bereavement* (Basic Books: New York, 1983).
2. Condon JT, The parental–foetal relationship—a comparison of male and female expectant parents, *J Psychosom Obstet Gynaecol* 1985; 4:271–84.
3. Condon JT, The assessment of antenatal emotional attachment: development of a questionnaire instrument, *Br J Med Psychol* 1993; 66:167–83.
4. Condon JT, Corkindale C, The correlates of antenatal attachment in pregnant women, *Br J Med Psychol* 1997; 70:359–72.
5. Muller ME, A critical review of prenatal attachment research, *Scholarly Inquiry Nurs Pract* 1997; 6:5–26.
6. Leon IG, The psychoanalytic conceptualization of perinatal loss: a multidimensional model, *Am J Psychiatry* 1992; 149:1464–72.
7. Phipps S, The subsequent pregnancy after stillbirth: anticipatory parenthood in the face of uncertainty, *Int J Psychiatry Med* 1985; 15:243–64.
8. Lee C, Slade P, Miscarriage as a traumatic event: a review of the literature and new implications for intervention, *J Psychosom Res* 1996; 40:235–44.
9. Frost M, Condon JT, The psychological sequelae of miscarriage: a critical review of the literature, *Aust NZ J Psychiatry* 1996; 30:54–62.
10. Bourne S, Lewis E, Perinatal bereavement, *Br Med J* 1991; 302:1167–8.
11. Friedman T, Gath D, The psychiatric consequences of spontaneous abortion, *Br J Psychiatry* 1989; 155:810–13.
12. Prettyman RJ, Cordle CJ, Cook GD, A three-month follow-up of psychological morbidity after early miscarriage, *Br J Med Psychol* 1993; 66:363–72.
13. Toedter LJ, Lasker JN, Alhadeff JM et al, The perinatal grief scale: development and initial validation, *Am J Orthopsychiatry* 1988; 58:435–49.
14. Beutel M, Deckardt R, von Rad M, Weiner H, Grief and depression after miscarriage: their separation, antecedents, and course, *Psychosom Med* 1995; 57:517–26.
15. Neugebauer R, Kline J, O'Connor P et al, Depressive symptoms in women in the six months after miscarriage, *Am J Obstet Gynecol* 1992; 166:104–9.
16. Garel M, Blondel B, Lelong N, Kaminski M, Depressive disorders after a spontaneous abortion, *Am J Obstet Gynecol* 1993; 168:1005–6.
17. Lee DT, Wong CK, Cheung LP et al, Psychiatric morbidity following miscarriage: a prevalence study of Chinese women in Hong Kong, *J Affect Disord* 1997; 43:63–8.
18. Lynch DJ, Johnson LW, Major depressive disorder following miscarriage, *JAMA* 1997; 277:1517.
19. Thapar AK, Thapar A, Psychological sequelae of miscarriage: a controlled study using the general health questionnaire and the hospital anxiety and depression scale, *Br J Gen Pract* 1992; 42:94–6.
20. Janssen HJ, Cuisinier MC, Hoogdium KA, de Graauw KP, Controlled prospective study on the mental health of women following pregnancy loss, *Am J Psychiatry* 1996; 153:226–30.
21. Neugebauer R, Kline J, Shrout P et al, Major depressive disorder in the 6 months after miscarriage, *JAMA* 1997; 277:383–8.
22. Katz VL, Kuller JA, Recurrent miscarriage, *Am J Perinatol* 1994; 11:386–97.
23. Lee C, Slade P, Lygo V, The influence of psychological debriefing on emotional adaptation in women following early miscarriage: a preliminary study, *Br J Med Psychol* 1996; 69:47–58.
24. Cuisinier M, Janssen H, de Graauw C et al, Pregnancy following miscarriage: course of grief and some determining factors, *J Psychosom Obstet Gynecol* 1996; 17:168–74.
25. Blumenthal SJ, Psychiatric consequences of abortion: overview of research findings. In: Stotland NL, ed., *Psychiatric Aspects of Abortion* (American Psychiatric Press: Washington, 1991) 17–38.
26. Simon NM, Senturia AG, Psychiatric sequelae of abortion, review of the literature 1935–64, *Arch Gen Psychiatry* 1966; 15:378–89.
27. Ekblad M, Induced abortion on psychiatric grounds: a follow-up study of 479 women, *Acta Psychiatr Neurol Scand Suppl* 1955; 99:1–238.

28. Romans-Clarkson SE, Psychological sequelae of induced abortion, *Aust NZ J Psychiatry* 1989; **23**:555–65.

29. Zolese G, Blacker CV, The psychological complications of therapeutic abortion, *Br J Psychiatry* 1992; **160**:742–9.

30. Gilchrist AC, Hannaford PC, Frank P, Kay CR, Termination of pregnancy and psychiatric morbidity, *Br J Psychiatry* 1995; **167**:243–8.

31. Greer HS, Lal S, Lewis SC et al, Psychosocial consequences of therapeutic abortion: Kings termination study III, *Br J Psychiatry* 1976; **128**:74–9.

32. Dagg PK, The psychological sequelae of therapeutic abortion—denied and completed, *Am J Psychiatry* 1991; **148**:578–85.

33. Stotland NL, Psychiatric issues in abortion, and the implications of recent legal changes for psychiatric practice. In: Stotland NL, ed., *Psychiatric Aspects of Abortion* (American Psychiatric Press: Washington, 1991) 1–16.

34. Tietze C, Contraceptive practice in the context of a non-restrictive abortion law: age-specific pregnancy rates in New York City, 1971–1973, *Fam Plann Perspect* 1975; **7**:197–202.

35. Forssman H, Thuwe I, One hundred and twenty children born after application for therapeutic abortion refused. Their mental health, social adjustment and educational level up to the age of 21, *Acta Psychiatr Scand* 1966; **42**:71–88.

36. Forssman H, Thuwe I, The Goteborg cohort, 1939–77. In: David HP, Dytrych Z, Matejcek Z et al, eds, *Born Unwanted: Developmental Effects of Denied Abortion* (Springer: New York, 1988).

37. Matejcek Z, Dytrych Z, Schuller V, Follow-up study of children born to women denied abortion, *Ciba Found Symp* 1985; **115**:136–49.

38. Dytrych Z, Matejcek Z, Schuller V, The Prague cohort: adolescence and early adulthood. In: David HP, Dytrych Z, Matejcek Z et al, eds, *Born Unwanted: Developmental Effects of Denied Abortion* (Springer: New York, 1988).

39. Henshaw R, Naji S, Russel I, Templeton A, Psychological responses following medical abortion (using mifepristone and gemeprost) and surgical vacuum aspiration. A patient-centered, partially randomised prospective study, *Acta Obstet Gynecol Scand* 1994; **73**:812–18.

40. Burke BM, Kolker A, Clients undergoing chronic villus sampling versus amniocentesis: contrasting attitudes towards pregnancy, *Health Care Women Int* 1993; **14**:193–200.

41. Salvesen KA, Oyen L, Schmidt N et al, Comparison of long-term psychological responses of women after pregnancy termination due to foetal anomalies and after perinatal loss, *Ultrasound Obstet Gynecol* 1997; **9**:80–5.

42. Zeanah CH, Dailey JV, Rosenblatt MJ, Saller DN Jr, Do women grieve after terminating pregnancies because of fetal anomalies? A controlled investigation, *Obstet Gynecol* 1993; **82**:270–5.

43. Donnai P, Charles N, Harris R, Attitudes of patients after 'genetic' termination of pregnancy, *Br Med J Clin Res Ed* 1981; **282**:621–2.

44. Misri S, Anderson E, Second trimester abortion. In: Stotland NL, ed., *Psychiatric Aspects of Abortion* (American Psychiatric Press: Washington, 1991) 159–70.

45. Conway SP, Allenby K, Pond MN, Patient and parental attitudes towards genetic screening and its implications at an adult cystic fibrosis centre, *Clin Genet* 1994; **45**:308–12.

46. Schreiner-Engel P, Walther VN, Mindes J et al, First-trimester multifetal pregnancy reduction: acute and persistent psychologic reactions, *Am J Obstet Gynecol* 1995; **172**:541–7.

47. McKinney M, Downey J, Timor-Tritsch I, The psychological effects of multifetal pregnancy reduction, *Fertil Steril* 1995; **64**:51–61.

48. Ormont MA, Shapiro PA, Multifetal pregnancy reduction: a review of an evolving technology and its psychosocial implications, *Psychosomatics* 1995; **36**:522–30.

49. McKinney MK, Tuber SB, Downey JI, Multifetal pregnancy reduction: psychodynamic implications, *Psychiatry* 1996; **59**:393–407.

50. Lilford RJ, Stratton P, Godsil S, Prasad A, A randomised trial of routine versus selective counselling in perinatal bereavement from congenital disease, *Br J Obstet Gynaecol* 1994; **101**:291–6.

51. Condon JT, Prevention of emotional disability following stillbirth—the role of the obstetric team, *Aust NZ J Obstet Gynaecol* 1987; **27**:323–9.

52. Weiss L, Frischer L, Richman J, Parental adjustment to intrapartum and delivery room loss. The role of a hospital-based support program, *Clin Perinatol* 1989; **16**:1009–19.

53. Zeanah CH, Adaptation following perinatal loss: a critical review, *J Am Acad Child Adolesc Psychiatry* 1989; **28**:467–80.

54. Condon JT, Management of established pathological grief reaction after stillbirth, *Am J Psychiatry* 1986; **143**:987–92.

55. O'Hara MW, Zekoski EM, Postpartum depression: a comprehensive review. In: Kumar R, Brockington IF, eds, *Motherhood and Mental Illness: 2, Causes and Consequences* (Wright: London, 1988) 17–63.

56. Jensen JS, Zahourek R, Depression in mothers who have lost a newborn, *Rocky Mountain Med J* 1972; **69**:61–3.

57. Harmon RJ, Glicken AD, Siegel RE, Neonatal loss in the intensive care nursery: effects of maternal grieving and a program for intervention, *J Am Acad Child Psychiatry* 1984; **23**:68–71.

58. LaRoche C, Lalinec-Michaud M, Engelsmann F et al, Grief reactions to perinatal death – a follow-up study, *Can J Psychiatry* 1984; **29**:14–19.

59. Forrest GC, Standish E, Baum JD, Support after perinatal death: a study of support and counselling after perinatal bereavement, *Br Med J Clin Res* 1982; **285**:1475–9.

60. Nicol MT, Tompkins JR, Campbell NA, Smye GJ, Maternal grieving response after perinatal death, *Med J Aust* 1986; **144**:287–9.

61. Murray J, Callan VJ, Predicting adjustment to perinatal death, *Br J Med Psychol* 1988; **61**:237–44.

62. LaRoche C, Lalinec-Michaud M, Engelsmann F et al, Grief reactions to perinatal death: an exploratory study, *Psychosomatics* 1982; **23**: 510–18.

63. Theut SK, Pedersen FA, Zaslow MJ et al, Perinatal loss and parental bereavement, *Am J Psychiatry* 1989; **146**:635–9.

64. Vance JC, Foster WJ, Najman JM et al, Early parental responses to sudden infant death, stillbirth or neonatal death, *Med J Aust* 1991; **155**:292–7.

65. Najman JM, Vance JC, Boyle F et al, The impact of a child death on marital adjustment, *Soc Sci Med* 1993; **37**:1005–10.

66. Vance JC, Najman JM, Thearle MJ et al, Psychological changes in parents eight months after the loss of an infant from stillbirth, neonatal death, or sudden infant death syndrome—a longitudinal study, *Pediatrics* 1995; **96**:933–8.

67. Boyle FM, Vance JC, Najman JM, Thearle MJ, The mental health impact of stillbirth, neonatal death or SIDS: prevalence and patterns of distress among mothers, *Soc Sci Med* 1996; **43**:1273–82.

68. Radestad I, Steineck G, Nordin C, Sjogren B, Psychological complications after stillbirth—influence of memories and immediate management: population based study, *Br Med J* 1996; **312**:1505–8.

69. Graham MA, Thompson SC, Estrada M, Yonekura ML, Factors affecting psychological adjustment to a fetal death, *Am J Obstet Gynecol* 1987; **157**:254–7.

70. Crowther ME, Communication following a stillbirth or neonatal death: room for improvement, *Br J Obstet Gynaecol* 1995; **102**:952–6.

71. Lewis E, Inhibition of mourning by pregnancy: psychopathology and management, *Br Med J Clin Res* 1979; **2**:27–8.

72. Davis DL, Stewart M, Harmon RJ, Postponing pregnancy after perinatal death: perspectives on doctor advice. *J Am Acad Child Adolesc Psychiatry* 1989; **28**:481–7.

73. Bourne S, Lewis E, *Psychological Aspects of Stillbirth and Neonatal Death: An Annotated Bibliography* (Tavistock: London, 1992).

74. Condon JT, Medical litigation. The aetiological role of psychological and interpersonal factors, *Med J Aust* 1992; **157**:768–70.

75. Condon JT, Predisposition to psychological complications after stillbirth: a case report, *Obstet Gynaecol* 1987; **70**:495–7.

76. Vaillant GE, Loss as a metaphor for attachment, *Am J Psychoanal* 1985; **45**:59–67.

21

Anxiety and depression in subfertility

Koen Demyttenaere

Introduction

Parenthood is believed to be one of the major role transitions in adult life for both men and women. The experience of subfertility can be viewed as a developmental transition or as a non-event transition.[1,2] A transition is defined as 'an event or non-event that alters the individual's perception of self and of the world, that demands a change in assumptions or behaviour, and that may lead either to growth or to deterioration'.[3]

Thus, fertility difficulties, along with their often invasive investigations and treatment, are widely believed to cause significant psychological stress. To date, research has been aimed at examining the role of psychological factors in the cause and consequences of subfertility. This chapter, after describing why subfertility and its treatment can be experienced as very distressing, will focus on the anxiety and depression levels in subfertile patients and their effect upon fertility and treatment outcome. The role and effects of counselling will also be discussed briefly.

The nature of the stress in subfertility and subfertility treatment

The nature of the stress experienced by couples facing infertility can be described on several levels: the stress of the non-event transition (the non-fulfilment of the wish for a child), the stress of the subfertility situation and the stress of the subfertility treatment.

The stress of the non-fulfilment of the wish for a child

There has been much investigation of the emotional sequelae of subfertility (depression, anger and anxiety; marital and psychosexual dysfunction; social isolation), but relatively little attention has been paid to the assessment of cognitive factors and their impact on adjustment to subfertility. Indeed, what has not yet been clearly determined is why some couples appear to respond to this life event with relative ease, whereas others experience intense intra- and interpersonal distress. Since there are few available research data, we can turn to theoretical concepts useful in clinical practice. The wish for parenthood is not one act and attitude, as the popular idea of 'fatherhood/motherhood' would persuade us to believe, but a sequence whose stages may differ vastly in the challenges they imply and the gratifications they provide. It is a multitude of motive combinations, some of which have little to do with bringing up and caring for a child.[4]

Psychodynamic considerations

An important aspect of the wish for a child is the notion of *imaginary child*. The wish for a child (the imaginary child), like all wishes, has an individual history. Earlier needs and fantasies prepared for it. In the process, it was transformed so that the manifest appearance of the present wish has little in common with the need-images from which it came. An interesting notion is *inner duality*.[5] Inner duality pertains to our capacity for splitting the self into two prototypical roles so that it can re-enact and revise certain elementary relationships. The pregnant woman (or the woman who desires to become pregnant) who speaks to her yet unborn child is both mother and child at the same time. She experiences herself from both sides: she can be alternately mother and child, thereby giving and receiving affection without reservation. She is not only mother and baby, but, by means of her identifications, also the image of her own mother and the image of herself as a child. This process has also been labelled the psychological mitosis of pregnancy (splitting in unity).[6] These mechanisms and their anticipation can partly explain the interindividual differences in handling the stress of subfertility, since they will influence the beliefs and representations that couples will have concerning this non-event transition.

Relational aspects

Both the transition and the non-transition to parenthood can potentially threaten or protect the marital equilibrium. Collusive partner relationships have been described as being when both partners choose each other on the basis of a common unconscious conflict, and where one partner always plays a progressive role and the other a regressive role; such couples often have difficulties with event (pregnancy, parenthood) and non-event (subfertility) transitions.[7]

In general, infertile women show higher distress than their infertile partners: for women, infertility results in a greater loss of identity,[8] in more pronounced feelings of defectiveness and reduced competence,[9,10] and in higher anxiety and depression levels.[11] Compared with infertile men, infertile women are more likely to avoid children, pregnant women, and other reminders of the fertile world.[12-14] From clinical experience with couples in crisis over their infertility, gender differences in psychosocial responses are often the final event triggering a crisis: she is surprised and disappointed that he is not more concerned, affected and touched by the problem. He is disappointed that she is so distressed, preoccupied or affected by the experience. In short, each wishes the other would adopt his/her coping strategies.[11] For women, there is a big difference between infertility and other problems, while men are affected by infertility in much the same way as by other problems.[15]

Others have investigated the response to the infertility situation as a stigma (a negative sense of social difference from others that is so outside the socially defined norm that it is both deeply discrediting and devalues the individual), a perception of loss (of the experience of pregnancy, procreation, childbearing, or ability to raise a biological child), and a loss of self-esteem (issues of mastery and competence in the performance of social roles).[16] Stigma, perception of loss and loss of self-esteem were experienced by women regardless of diagnosis, and similarly by men who had reproductive impairment. This means that men's response to infertility closely approximates women's if infertility has been attributed to a male factor, but differs considerably if a male factor is not found.

There is also an interesting gender difference in the need for counselling reported by men and women: 98% of women and 95% of men reported that counselling should be offered at an infertility clinic, but only 72% of the women and 53% of the men reported that counselling was needed for themselves.[17]

Transgenerational aspects

The wish for a child challenges personal, relational and family homeostasis. Key moments that challenge the adaptive evolution of a family system include birth, death, wedding and divorce, i.e. someone entering or desiring to enter the system, or likewise leaving or desiring to leave this system. The wish for a child is hence the mathematical result of all covert credits and debits to the two families of origin.

The notions of transgenerational guilt, debt, gratitude and loyalty are essential in the estimation of the advantages and disadvantages of having a child.[18] When a family is unclear about who is in and who is out, the family's boundaries are said to be ambiguous. Boundary ambiguity in subfertility occurs on different levels.[19] First, the imaginary child is experienced as a psychologically present but physically absent member of the subfertile couple. Second, the subfertile couple is often as frustrated in this non-event transition of not becoming parents as the couple's parents are in their developmental task of becoming mentors and grandparents. Changing loyalties form a part of adulthood that often becomes confused and muddled for the subfertile couple: a hus-

band or wife may remain torn in his/her loyalty between their families of origin and their spouse (and thus become a marginal person in the marriage). Theoretically, this can be viewed as the failure to differentiate from one's family of origin or as being part of an enmeshed family system. Some subfertile couples transfer this enmeshed pattern from their families of origin to the marital relationship, and the boundaries between the two partners become confused. Third, filiation boundary ambiguity can result from a confusion of genetic links within the family (donor insemination, adoption). It requires a recognition of the difference between biological and psychosocial parenthood, for the couple as well as the couple's family and social surroundings.

The stress of the subfertility situation

Subfertility can be regarded as an uncontrollable and unpredictable event. Years of monthly hope and disillusion, and years of monthly abortions of the imaginary child, usually lead to a deterioration of the feeling of control over bodily processes. Subfertility can also be regarded as a complex grief process.[20] Subfertility means the experience of a handicap—a loss—and is often associated with feelings of emptiness, inferiority, punishment, shame, and guilt. Time is needed before a couple can accept their subfertility and before they can make adequate decisions about possible alternatives. Memories of grieving—such as the death of a family member—are different from those for a non-event transition such as childlessness.[21] Gender role and sexual functioning are often (temporarily) impaired by subfertility treatment. Absence of sexual activity (e.g. due to vaginismus or erectile dysfunction) can be a cause of infertility (3–5% of couples presenting at an infertility clinic). Mid-cycle sexual dysfunction, i.e. the inability to have sexual intercourse in the periovulatory period, can be ascribed to several aetiological factors, e.g. 'this is the night syndrome', change in purpose of sexual interaction, stress of clinical testing by a third party, and self-doubt about adequate performance.[22]

The stress of the subfertility treatment

Couples (as well as subfertility specialists) have been observed to frequently overestimate the likelihood of treatment success, which often results in violated expectations. A recent 1-year comparative study of couples ($n = 281$) undergoing assisted reproductive treatment found that, in general, treatment-related distress and levels of depression were higher for women than for men.[23] Investigators found moderate to high levels of grief and depression before, during and after treatment in a study of 100 women undergoing in vitro fertilization (IVF) or ovulation-induction medication.[24] In general, the women in this latter study used isolation coping behaviours (e.g. self-talk, sleep).

It is remarkable that, in most papers, the psychological impact of ovarian (hyper)stimulation is often overlooked. This is especially true for IVF, where the ovarian (hyper)stimulation is preceded by a pituitary desensitization often resulting in climacteric symptoms. The intense emotions around the storage of oocytes outside the intimacy of the body or the storage of frozen embryos have also been poorly investigated.

Anxiety and depression levels in subfertile women

There is still controversy over whether subfertile individuals differ from fertile controls on measures of anxiety or depression. In a recent study with 98 women participating in an IVF programme, we found that depression levels in subfertile women as assessed by the Zung Self-Rating Depression Scale (Zung SDS) were very high: 54.1% of these women presented with mild depression and 19.4% showed moderate to severe depressive symptomatology.[25] This is in accord with other findings in the literature, in which the reported prevalence of depressed patients at a subfertility clinic was always high (usually twice the prevalence of depression in controls) (see Hunt and Monach 1997[20] for a review).

The prevalence of depression, however, depends on the psychometric test employed. In two studies that used the Centre for Epidemiological Studies Depression Scale, depression was found in 25% of women treated with IVF[26] and 25.8% (versus 13.2% of controls) of women attending an infertility clinic.[27] In the latter study, depressive symptomatology was also assessed using the Beck Depression Inventory (BDI), which demonstrated that 36.7% (versus 18.4% of controls) of the women attending the infertility clinic were depressed.[27] Yet, other studies that utilized the BDI,[28] the 'elated–depressed' subscale of the Profile of Mood States (POMS),[29] or the Institute for Personality and Ability Testing (IPAT) depression scale,[30] failed to demonstrate significant differences between subfertile and fertile women.

The same controversy exists for anxiety levels: some studies demonstrate higher anxiety levels in subfertile women compared with fertile women,[31,32] while others do not.[29,30]

The discrepancies in reported rates of psychopathology could be due to methodological issues. First, the population norms (so-called fertile controls) are usually not controlled for their fertility status and hence include at least 15% of subfertile women. Second, anxiety and depression levels could well vary with the different stages of work-up and treatment. One study demonstrated that fewer women (15%) are clinically depressed during a first IVF cycle (inductees) than during the following cycles (25%) (veterans), whereas the community norm for clinical depression was 12%.[26]

While there is some evidence that depression scores may decrease with longer duration of infertility treatment,[25] others have found that depression may increase over the longer (treatment) term.[33] Some have suggested that an association between decreased depression and longer course of reproductive treatment may be due to progressive adaptation to the idea of remaining childless.[25] Other factors that may influence anxiety or depression levels in women include age, number of IVF attempts, personality aspects, self-esteem, marital satisfaction, job position and satisfaction, and culture-specific phenomena.[25,34,35]

One of the few available follow-up studies on subfertile women demonstrated that 66% of the women and 40% of the men reported depression following IVF failure; one-third of the respondents were still depressed 18 months after their failed IVF attempt.[36] A history of (female) subfertility may influence spousal support during a subsequent pregnancy; further, a longer time to conception and (lack of) spousal support during pregnancy have been associated with increased risk for postnatal depression.[37] There is some evidence of risk for post-traumatic stress disorder in the postpartum period following infertility treatment.[38] Others, however, have found no significant differences in adaptation to pregnancy or motherhood in previously subfecund women compared with fecund controls.[39]

In general, subfertile women tend to present with suppressed stress levels, since they are more likely than other patients to give socially desirable answers (they are afraid of being kicked out of the programme).[40] In addition, retrospective—compared with prospective—assessment of anxiety levels during the luteal phase of an IVF cycle resulted in higher levels of reported anxiety.[41]

Since not all couples are distressed by infertility, it is important to look at research that examines particular characteristics of couples who are distressed by infertility and infertility treatment. One study demonstrated greater psychosocial stress (anxiety, hostility, and phobic anxiety) in women with non-anatomical infertility than in women with anatomical infertility.[42] The authors found this result to be consistent with the hypothesis that psychosocial stress contributes significantly to the aetiology of some forms of infertility. An alternative explanation could be that suffering from non-anatomical infertility (especially unexplained infertility) is more stressful than suffering from anatomical infertility: the grief process is usually easier in a clearcut situation than in more ambiguous situations of (anticipated) loss. Another study demonstrated that higher levels of anxiety are found in infertile women remaining in the introversive stage of the grief process (characterized by shock, denial, and loneliness) than in infertile women reaching the acceptance phase of the grief process.[43]

Gender differences in depression and anxiety levels have been reported: 40% of women and 16% of men attending an infertility clinic had scores indicative of clinically significant depression, suggesting that women react differently than men when faced with a subfertility problem.[44] In both men and women, personal control over the situation, the confidence that one will have a child, lower past treatment costs, and a lower number of tests and treatments received, were protective factors against higher anxiety levels. Higher levels of stress in women were correlated with the importance of children and dissatisfaction with social support network, whereas in men, higher stress levels were correlated with the anticipated future treatment costs, a lower income, and the attribution of responsibility to the self.[45] These data suggest that a high proportion of infertile women and men present with high depression and/or anxiety levels, but that some characteristics (such as the aetiology of infertility, the stage of the grief process, and gender) render some infertile individuals more vulnerable to mood disturbance than others.

The influence of anxiety, depression and coping style upon fertility

Whether psychological characteristics influence fertility or outcome of infertility treatment remains a matter of debate.[46] It was often suggested that unexplained infertility equals *psychogenic infertility*. This stems from an old-fashioned way of thinking, when psychogenic infertility or functional infertility was defined by exclusion, i.e. when no organic causes were found. Anecdotal data suggest that major stressors (e.g. war situation, incarceration in concentration camps, admittance to an intensive care unit) and minor stressors (e.g. starting college, the so-called first kiss amenorrhoea) can provoke amenorrhoea.

Several epidemiological studies suggest a link between anxiety or depression and subfertility. In a case-control study of risk factors for primary infertility, the relative risk of ovulatory infertility was more than two times greater in users of antidepressants for 1–2 years, and more than four times greater in users of antidepressants for more than 2 years.[47] However, several limitations of these data must be considered. Since information on exposure history was obtained by self-report, misclassification of

pharmaceutical use may have occurred (which could lead to an underestimation of the actual risks associated with drug use). Moreover, an additional confounding factor is possible, since depression itself has been associated with hormonal disturbances, although there is little evidence of a relationship between disturbance of reproductive hormones and depression.

Decreased libido may be another consequence of depression that could affect infertility. For example, women with a history of depressive symptoms were nearly twice as likely to report infertility relative to women without a history of depressive symptoms after controlling for potential confounders (age, sedentary lifestyle, and cigarette smoking).[48] Again, limitations of these data should be considered. Although the adjusted odds ratio for the history of depression is elevated, it is not an exceptionally high risk gradient. Of greater concern is the definition of 'depressive symptoms'; this was construed as an affirmative reply to the question: 'Have you ever felt so sad, discouraged, or hopeless, or had so many problems that you wondered if anything was worthwhile?' It is surprising that only 58 of the 339 women met this criterion, given that there was no minimum duration requirement or any age restriction.[49]

The few studies in the literature using standardized psychometric tests to assess the influence of stress, anxiety or depression levels upon fertility show contradictory results. For example, investigators prospectively monitored mood and anxiety in 13 women from the general community who were attempting pregnancy; during the month of conception, all subjects exhibited significantly improved mood states and significantly lower state anxiety levels compared with previous non-conception cycles.[50] A prospective study that examined the effect of chronic stress levels (trait anxiety) upon conception rates in ovulatory cycles of normally fertile women treated with donor insemination (AID) for male infertility demonstrated that higher trait anxiety levels significantly predict a lower pregnancy rate. Regression analysis revealed that 16% of the variability in the AID cycle leading to conception was determined by the trait anxiety level.[31]

In two studies of anxiety and IVF, state anxiety levels at the moments of oocyte retrieval and embryo transfer were significantly higher in non-conceiving than in conceiving women.[51,52] An association between higher trait anxiety, hostile mood and lower cumulative pregnancy rate was found in a recent study of 90 women undergoing IVF.[53] Following the initial assessment—and controlling for the number of treatment cycles—a significant difference in the rate of pregnancy was observed per year of IVF treatments between clinically depressed and non-depressed women (13% versus 29% respectively). Depressed women were also more frequently drop-outs from treatment programmes (21% versus 10% respectively). Taken together, these results suggest that a dual mechanism might be involved in the lower pregnancy rates in depressed women starting IVF.[25]

Several investigations into the effect of stress on fertility during IVF, on the other hand, have found that non-pregnant and pregnant women revealed similarities in (trait and state) anxiety levels and in hormonal markers of stress,[54,55] suggesting that high levels of anxiety during IVF treatment may not be associated with the chance of pregnancy.

We have already suggested that the problem of repressed anxiety or repressed depression could explain part of the discrepancies found in the relationship between affect and outcome in subfertility treatment. Another methodological problem is the diversity within patient samples (e.g. different aetiologies of infertility): a woman could react differently if she is the perceived cause of the infertility or if the perceived

cause is mainly her partner. In our recent study investigating the link between psychological variables and IVF outcome in 98 women, the depression scores in women with a female indication for IVF were comparable with those found in women with a male indication for IVF.[25] This is in accordance with previous literature.[27] Others, however, have found that women with male factor infertility tended to express anger towards their husbands, whereas those with female factor infertility presented with depressive symptoms.[56]

The analysis of coping style, depressive symptomatology and IVF outcome within the subgroups of women with a female or a male indication for IVF produced several unexpected results. We observed a complex relationship between depression scores and IVF outcome. While there was no significant difference in the total Zung SDS scores between the pregnant and the non-pregnant groups (total $n = 98$), higher depression scores were associated with (1) a lower pregnancy rate in couples where the indication for IVF was female subfertility, and (2) a higher pregnancy rate in couples where the indication for IVF was male subfertility,[25] suggesting that the individual items on the Zung SDS that resulted in a similar total score for both groups were different.

A more detailed post hoc analysis of the inter-correlations between coping styles and the Zung SDS score supports this postulate. Thus, if the woman attributes the cause of infertility to herself, general protective coping mechanisms (i.e. active coping and comforting ideas) seem to be helpful in preventing depressive symptomatology, whereas expression of negative emotions (i.e. directing anger at herself as the source of the problem) seems to worsen her psychological situation. On the other hand, if the woman attributes the cause of the infertility to her partner, general protective coping mechanisms are not helpful in preventing depressive symptomatology, but the expression of negative emotions serves to protect her, since anger is projected onto her partner.

The aforementioned is in concordance with clinical experience. One of the strongest taboos between subfertile couples is the cause of the subfertility problem (e.g. Who is responsible for the problem? Who is guilty? Why did I choose a subfertile partner?). It is remarkable that couples can seldom address these questions or express their negative feelings and emotions. It is our clinical experience that the decision-making (i.e. when to start IVF, when to stop it) is particularly difficult in couples with male subfertility. The cause of the subfertility may be male, but it is the woman who undergoes invasive therapy; if she gets pregnant, she can 'hide' the male's problem, but if she does not remain in IVF, the male problem becomes even more apparent. Moreover, the man often does not insist on another IVF trial, since his wife has to suffer, but he also does not insist on stopping treatment, since he then withholds a child from his wife.

The role of counselling

In general, there is accumulating evidence of the positive effect of counselling—supportive type or a more structured style, with individual, couple or group format—on the psychological adjustment to infertility and on the likelihood of conception. Investigators have identified some characteristics of the couples at risk for depression that may play a role in the therapeutic process, e.g. an unsuccessful treatment outcome, repeated treatment cycles, a low socio-economic status, and foreign nationality.[23] Yet, many questions regarding the role and effect of counselling in subfertility and subfertility treatment remain: What are the couple's needs? What constitutes success in terms

of counselling outcome? Should counselling be aimed at providing emotional support for the couple or should the emphasis be on helping them to accept their childlessness? The recently published Fertility Problem Inventory, a global measure of perceived infertility-related stress (the five domains include social concern, sexual concern, relationship concern, need for parenthood, and rejection of childfree lifestyle), may assist a variety of health clinicians in therapy planning and follow-up.[57]

There is rudimentary evidence of a positive effect of non-specific counselling on pregnancy rates in couples with unexplained subfertility: 6 couples out of 10 in the counselling group versus 1 out of 9 in the control group were pregnant after 18 months.[58] Another preliminary report also supported a clear connection between anxiety, treatment and subsequent conception.[59] In this two-part study, 42 women with unexplained subfertility were followed for 1 year, and biweekly assessments of situational anxiety were performed. During this time, 12 of the 42 women became pregnant. A time-series analysis of the anxiety scores revealed that spontaneous decreases in anxiety were significantly related to pregnancy, and increases in situational anxiety to non-pregnancy. In the second study phase, 14 women with unexplained infertility were randomized into either a non-treatment control group or an experimental group. The experimental group underwent a 16-session individual behavioural treatment programme that included relaxation–response training, cognitive restructuring, and self-instructional management. By the end of the 3-month project, four of the seven experimental patients had become pregnant, while none of the control patients conceived. There is, however, an important selection bias in this type of study: couples accepting counselling or accepting such a protocol are only a subgroup of the couples attending a subfertility clinic.

The effect of counselling for couples undergoing subfertility treatment has been examined rudimentarily. Three sessions of counselling (before, during and on conclusion of a first IVF treatment cycle) did not lead to any further reduction in levels of anxiety or depression compared with couples who received information about the treatment programme only.[60] Yet, the effectiveness of a brief, professionally led support group for subfertile patients (eight weekly sessions of 2 h, with closed groups of 6–12 people) has been shown clearly in a group of 64 patients: there were significant reductions in depression scores in the female participants.[61]

A novel mind–body programme for (female) infertility, which was based on an established 10-week programme at the New England Deaconess Hospital, also demonstrated that a behavioural treatment approach might be efficacious in the treatment of the emotional aspects of infertility: all dimensions of the POMS as well as the Spielberger State Trait Anxiety Inventory changed significantly from entry to exit. The initial treatment group showed statistically significant decreases in anxiety, depression, and fatigue, as well as an increase in vigour. Moreover, 34% of these women became pregnant within 6 months of completing the programme (the authors, however, did not mention details of the somatic treatment or pregnancy rates in a control group).[62]

In a controlled comparative study of emotion-focused versus problem-focused group therapy (six sessions) for infertile women ($n = 29$), researchers found that, compared with a no-treatment control condition, both therapies were efficacious in women's adjustment to infertility, with slight differences in the improvements derived from each.[63] There is also early evidence of the benefits of a group treatment programme (24 weeks), with a psycho-educational format, for women with obesity and infertility.[64] In addition to weight loss, there was significant improvement on measures of self-esteem, anxiety, depression, and general health. In the 21–36-month follow-up period, 29 out of 35 women—who desired to conceive and were previously unsuccessful—became pregnant.

Summary

Subfertility and its ramifications can cause significant intra- and interpersonal psychological stress. Higher levels of stress in women are associated with the importance of children, dissatisfaction with their social support network, and non-anatomical infertility. Yet, controversy remains whether women who are subfertile manifest higher levels of anxiety and/or depression compared with fertile women. There is also debate regarding the influence of anxiety and depression on fertility. Notwithstanding, there is accumulating evidence of an association between reduction of psychological distress with counselling and achieving pregnancy. Utilization of the Fertility Problem Inventory can assist clinicians in the assessment and treatment of fertility-related stress.

References

1. Matthews R, Matthews A, Infertility and involuntary childlessness: the transition to nonparenthood, *J Mar Fam* 1986; **48**:641–9.
2. Koropatnick S, Daniluk J, Pattinson HA, Infertility: a non-event transition, *Fertil Steril* 1993; **59**:163–71.
3. Schlossberg NK, A model analyzing human adaptation to transition, *Counsel Psychol* 1981; **9**:2–18.
4. Demyttenaere K, *Psychoendocrinological Aspects of Reproduction in Women* (Peeters Press: Leuvain, 1990).
5. Wyatt F, Clinical notes on the motives for reproduction, *J Social Issues* 1967; **23**:29–56.
6. Bibring GL, Some considerations on the psychological processes in pregnancy, *Psychoanal Studies Child* 1959; **14**:113–28.
7. Willi J, *Die Zweierbeziehung* (Rowohlt Verlag: Reinbek bei Hamburg, 1975).
8. Olshansky EF, Identity of self as infertile: an example of theory-generating research, *Adv Nurs Sci* 1987; **9**:54–63.
9. Valentine D, Psychological impact of infertility: identifying issues and needs, *Soc Work Health Care* 1987; **11**:61–9.
10. Mahlstedt P, Macduff S, Bernstein J, Emotional factors and the in-vitro-fertilization and embryo transfer process, *J In Vitro Fert Embryo Transf* 1987; **4**:232–6.
11. Wright J, Duchesne C, Sabourin S et al, Psychosocial distress and infertility: men and women respond differently, *Fertil Steril* 1991; **55**:100–8.
12. Greil AL, Leitko TA, Porter KL, Infertility: his and hers, *Gender Society* 1988; **2**:172–99.
13. Sabatelli RM, Meth RL, Gavazzi SM, Factors mediating the adjustment to involuntary childlessness, *Family Relations* 1988; **37**:338–43.
14. Berg BJ, Wilson JF, Weingartner PJ, Psychological sequelae of infertility treatment: the role of gender and sex-role identification, *Soc Sci Med* 1991; **33**:1071–80.
15. Andrews FM, Abbey A, Halman LJ, Is fertility-problem stress different: the dynamics of stress in fertile and infertile couples, *Fertil Steril* 1992; **57**:1247–53.
16. Nachtigall RD, Becker G, Wozny M, The effects of gender-specific diagnosis on men's and women's response to infertility, *Fertil Steril* 1992; **57**:113–21.
17. Boivin J, Is there too much emphasis on psychosocial counseling for infertile patients? *J Assist Reprod Genet* 1997; **14**:184–6.
18. Boszormenyi-Nagy I, Spark GM, *Invisible Loyalties* (Harper and Row: New York, 1973).
19. Hammer Burns L, Infertility as a boundary ambiguity, *Family Process* 1987; **26**:359–65.
20. Hunt J, Monach JH, Beyond the bereavement model: the significance of depression for infertility counselling, *Hum Reprod* 1997; **2**:188–94.
21. Patterson JE, But not alone: the grief of infertility, *JAMA* 1986; **255**:2293–4.
22. Drake TS, Grunert GM, A cyclic pattern of sexual dysfunction in the infertility investigation, *Fertil Steril* 1979; **32**:542–5.
23. Beutel M, Kupfer J, Kirchmeyer P et al, Treatment-related stresses and depression in couples undergoing assisted reproductive treatment by IVF or ICSI, *Andrologia* 1999; **31**:27–35.
24. Lukse MP, Vacc NA, Grief, depression, and coping in women undergoing infertility treatment, *Obstet Gynecol* 1999; **93**:245–51.
25. Demyttenaere K, Bonte L, Gheldof M et al, Coping style and depression levels influence outcome in IVF, *Fertil Steril* 1998; **69**:1026–33.
26. Thiering P, Beaurepaire J, Jones M et al, Mood state as a predictor of treatment outcome after in vitro fertilization/embryo transfer technology, *J Psychosom Res* 1993; **37**:481–91.
27. Domar AD, Broome A, Zuttermeister PC et al, The prevalence and predictability of depression in infertile women, *Fertil Steril* 1992; **58**:1158–63.
28. Cook R, Parsons J, Mason B, Golombok S, Emotional, marital and sexual problems in couples embarking upon AID and IVF treatment for infertility, *J Reprod Infant Psychol* 1989; **7**:87–93.
29. Edelmann RJ, Connolly KJ, Bartlett H, Coping strategies and psychological adjustment of couples presenting for IVF, *J Psychosom Res* 1994; **38**:355–64.
30. Paulson JD, Haarmann BS, Salerno RL, Asmar P, An investigation of the relationship between emotional maladjustment and infertility, *Fertil Steril* 1988; **49**:258–62.

31. Demyttenaere K, Nijs P, Steeno O et al, Anxiety and conception rates in donor insemination, *J Psychosom Obstet Gynecol* 1988; **8**:175–81.

32. Demyttenaere K, Nijs P, Evers-Kiebooms G, Koninckx PR, Coping, ineffectiveness of coping and the psychoendocrinological stress responses during in-vitro-fertilization, *J Psychosom Res* 1991; **35**:231–43.

33. Chiba H, Mori E, Morioka Y et al, Stress of female infertility: relations to length of treatment, *Gynecol Obstet Invest* 1997; **43**:171–7.

34. Bringhenti F, Martinelli F, Ardenti R, La Sala GB, Psychological adjustment of infertile women entering IVF treatment: differentiating aspects and influencing factors, *Acta Obstet Gynaecol Scand* 1997; **76**:431–7.

35. Aghanwa HS, Dare FO, Ogunniyi SO, Sociodemographic factors in mental disorders associated with infertility in Nigeria, *J Psychosom Res* 1999; **46**:117–23.

36. Baram D, Tourtelot E, Muechler E, Huang K, Psychological adjustment following unsuccessful IVF, *J Psychosom Obstet Gynecol* 1988; **9**:181–90.

37. Demyttenaere K, Lenaerts H, Nijs P, Van Assche FA, Individual coping style and psychological attitudes during pregnancy predict depression levels during pregnancy and during postpartum, *Acta Psychiatr Scand* 1995; **91**:95–102.

38. Bartlik B, Greene K, Graf M et al, Examining PTSD as a complication of infertility, *Medscape Womens Health* 1997; **2**:1.

39. Halman LJ, Oakley D, Lederman R, Adaptation to pregnancy and motherhood among sub-fecund and fecund primiparous women, *Matern–Child Nurs J* 1995; **23**:90–100.

40. Haseltine FP, Mazure C, De L'Aune W et al, Psychological interviews in screening couples undergoing in vitro fertilization, *Ann NY Acad Sci* 1985; **442**:504–22.

41. Boivin J, Takefman JE, Stress level across stages of in vitro fertilization in subsequently pregnant and nonpregnant women, *Fertil Steril* 1995; **64**:802–10.

42. Wasser SK, Sewall G, Soules MR, Psychosocial stress as a cause of infertility, *Fertil Steril* 1993; **59**:685–9.

43. Mori E, Nadaoka T, Morioka Y, Saito H, Anxiety of infertile women undergoing IVF-ET: relation to the grief process, *Gynecol Obstet Invest* 1997; **44**:157–62.

44. Link PW, Darling CA, Couples undergoing treatment for infertility: dimensions of life satisfaction, *J Sex Marital Ther* 1986; **12**:46–59.

45. Abbey A, Halman LJ, Andrews FM, Psychosocial, treatment and demographic predictors of the stress associated with infertility, *Fertil Steril* 1992; **57**:122–8.

46. Brkovich AM, Fisher WA, Psychological distress and infertility: forty years of research, *J Psychosom Obstet Gynaecol* 1998; **19**:218–28.

47. Grodstein F, Goldman MB, Ryan L, Cramer DW, Self-reported use of pharmaceuticals and primary ovulatory infertility, *Epidemiology* 1993; **4**:151–6.

48. Lapane KL, Zierler S, Lasater TM et al, Is a history of depressive symptoms associated with an increased risk of infertility in women? *Psychosom Med* 1995; **57**:509–13.

49. Rubinow DR, Roca CA, Infertility and depression, *Psychosom Med* 1995; **57**:514–16.

50. Sanders KA, Bruce NW, A prospective study of psychosocial stress and fertility in women, *Hum Reprod* 1997; **12**:2324–9.

51. Demyttenaere K, Nijs P, Evers-Kiebooms G, Koninckx PR, Coping and the ineffectiveness of coping influence the outcome of in vitro fertilization through stress responses, *Psychoneuroendocrinology* 1992; **17**:655–65.

52. Merari D, Feldberg D, Elizur A et al, Psychological and hormonal changes in the course of in vitro fertilization, *J Assist Reprod Genet* 1992; **9**:161–9.

53. Sanders KA, Bruce NW, Psychosocial stress and treatment outcome following assisted reproductive technology, *Hum Reprod* 1999; **14**:1656–62.

54. Harlow CR, Fahy UM, Talbot WM et al, Stress and stress-related hormones during in-vitro fertilization treatment, *Hum Reprod* 1996; **11**:274–9.

55. Milad MP, Klock SC, Moses S, Chatterton R, Stress and anxiety do not result in pregnancy wastage, *Hum Reprod* 1998; **13**:2296–300.

56. Edelmann RJ, Connolly KJ, Psychological aspects of infertility, *Br J Med Psychol* 1986; **59**: 209–19.

57. Newton CR, Sherrard W, Glavac I, The Fertility Problem Inventory: measuring perceived infertility-related stress, *Fertil Steril* 1999; **72**:54–62.

58. Sarrel PM, De Cherney AH, Psychotherapeutic intervention for treatment of couples with secondary infertility, *Fertil Steril* 1985; **43**:897–900.

59. Rodriguez B, Bermudez L, Ponce de Leon E, Castro L, The relationship between infertility and anxiety: some preliminary findings. Presented at the II World Congress of Behavior Therapy, Washington DC, 1983.

60. Connolly KJ, Edelmann RJ, Bartlett H et al, An evaluation of counselling for couples undergoing treatment for in-vitro-fertilization, *Hum Reprod* 1993; **8**:1332–8.

61. Stewart DE, Boydell KM, McCarthy K et al, A prospective study of the effectiveness of brief professionally-led support groups for infertility patients, *Int J Psychiatry Med* 1992; **22**:173–82.

62. Domar AD, Seibel MM, Benson H, The mind/body program for infertility: a new behavioral treatment approach for women with infertility, *Fertil Steril* 1990; **53**:246–9.

63. McQueeney DA, Stanton AL, Sigmon S, Efficacy of emotion-focused and problem-focused group therapies for women with fertility problems, *J Behav Med* 1997; **20**:313–31.

64. Galletly C, Clark A, Tomlinson L, Blaney F, Improved pregnancy rates for obese, infertile women following a group treatment program. An open pilot study, *Gen Hosp Psychiatry* 1996; **18**:192–5.

22

The perimenopause
Beth Alder

Introduction

There is some controversy about the psychological importance of the perimenopause. The perimenopause is both a psychosocial transition and an endocrinological event. Changes in mood in the perimenopause in middle-aged women may be related to endocrine change, social context or the ageing process, or all three. Most women go through the menopause without complaints, but the perimenopause is still associated with ill-health in spite of the lack of epidemiological evidence.

During the 10 years or so of the perimenopause, there are changes in hormones, changes in psychological disorders (especially depression), changes in sexual interest and activity, and changes in psychiatric illness. Are these related to the time of the menopause and, if so, how should they be managed? Are these relationships different during the climacteric from those at other times of hormonal change, such as at menarche or in the puerperium? Does hormone replacement therapy (HRT) affect mood? The clinical question may be what is the

extent to which symptoms can be attributed to the menopause (as an endocrinological event), and which symptoms can be attributed to underlying psychological processes or the ageing process itself? Social context and life events may also be highly relevant. The menopause is just one aspect of change in women's lives as they go through middle-age.

There has recently been an increase in research into the menopause and post-menopause. This may have been fuelled by the interest of baby boomers and by demographic changes. More women are living for longer, so that the number of women with post-menopausal status is increasing. There have also been major developments in treatment of oestrogen deficiency symptoms by HRT. New compounds and methods of delivery have been developed and there has been huge investment by the pharmaceutical industry. The results of clinical trials of oestrogen therapy give us evidence about group effects, which are generally positive. Clinical experience finds that some women, but not others, respond dramatically with an improvement in mood after oestrogen therapy. Finally, expectations of health have changed and women may no longer be content to tolerate symptoms in the 'change of life' that are incompatible with expectations of an equal role in society.

The association of psychological and physical complaints with the time of the menopause has led to the construction of a menopausal syndrome, which implies causality. It is then but a small step to associate this with oestrogen deficiency or endocrinopathology.[1] Individual differences in response to hormone changes have been noted at other times of endocrinological change. Some women may be particularly susceptible to change in hormone status and they may be more liable to premenstrual syndrome, postnatal depression and mood changes in the menopause.[2]

Ussher, in a seminal text,[3] argues strongly that biological reductive explanations are insufficient and that the understanding of women's mental health has been dominated by the biological model of reproduction. Feminist literature has challenged the medical model of the menopause.[4] This chapter will explore the phenomenon of the perimenopause and associated mood changes, and place them in a biopsychosocial context. This approach, which integrates rather than separates, has been used extensively in health psychology and behavioural medicine, for example in textbooks.[5,6]

Definitions

The menopause is defined as occurring at the time of a woman's last menstrual period. The WHO defines it as 'the permanent cessation of menstruation resulting from loss of ovarian follicular activity'. The average age in Western women is 51 years, range 48–58. The perimenopause is defined as the period of time immediately before menopause when

endocrinological, biological and clinical features of approaching menopause commence, and lasts until the first year after the menopause. The postmenopause is defined as dating from the time of menopause, although the menopause cannot be determined until after a period of 12 months of spontaneous amenorrhea has been observed.[7]

All women will go through a natural menopause if they have not previously had their ovaries removed. It has been estimated that in the 1990s there will be 40 million women over the age of 50 years. Ninety per cent of women will enter the perimenopause at a median age of 47.5 years, with a mean duration of 3.8 years. The Massachusetts Women's Health Study found the median age of natural menopause to be 51.3 years.[9,10] Irregular menstruation can occur for many years preceding the last period and is described as the premenopause. As ovulation becomes intermittent, there is a loss of production of oestrogen from the ovaries. More cycles become anovulatory and the length of the follicular phase increases. Levels of FSH (follicle-stimulating hormone) rise during the follicular phase to over 10 times the premenopausal level. This rise in FSH may be used as a marker of the menopause but the levels can be variable and two or three measurements may be needed. The raised FSH levels may stimulate the stroma cells of the ovaries to produce more testosterone, giving an androgenic surge. Many women experience some androgenic effects such as hirsutism, thinning hair, deeper voice, skin changes, decreased breast size and weight gain.[8] High levels of FSH do not necessarily predict absolute sterility, because there may be a later ovulation. Women may not know that they are not ovulating, as they may menstruate, and they do not know that they have passed the menopause until 1 year after the last period.

Surgical menopause

Surgical menopause occurs as a result of bilateral oophorectomy at the time of hysterectomy. The rates of hysterectomy in the USA are high although they are lower in Europe. In 1988 it was estimated that 37% of women in the USA had had a hysterectomy by age 60.[11] Ovaries may be removed at the same time to prevent ovarian cancer. Premenopausal women are more likely to have their ovaries conserved but there are variations in medical practice. Surgical menopause may have different physical and psychological health outcomes from natural menopause. Premature menopause is defined as being before the age of 40 and may be associated with psychological problems of the consequent infertility. The changes in the perimenopause are described in Table 22.1.[8]

The social context of the perimenopause

The historical context

Historically, the image of the menopause has been negative. During the eighteenth century in Europe, life-expectancy increased and women began to live beyond the menopause. In France, doctors became interested in the perimenopause and the term 'menespausie' was coined by Gardanne in 1812; he later changed this to menopause. Soon and Teoh[12] give an interesting account of the history of the menopause. In 1857, Tilt suggested that nervous disorders, cancers and structural diseases were prevalent during or after the 'change of life'. He described the suffering as 'generally tedious, recurrent, and destructive of peace and happiness'. His remedy for nervous disorders was sedatives and tonics for 'sinking in the pit of the stomach'.

Table 22.1 Changes in the perimenopause with increasing age.[8]

Biological
  Depletion of follicles
  Irregular ovulatory cycles
  Increase in percentage of anovulatory cycles
  Increase in chromosomal abnormalities
  Increase in spontaneous abortions

Endocrinological
  Decreased cyclical production of oestradiol, progesterone and inhibin
  Increased levels of FSH and luteinizing hormone
  Change in oestradiol/oestrone ratio, and oestrogen/androgen ratio

Clinical
  Alterations in menstrual cycle intervals
  Increase in vasomotor symptoms and vaginal dryness
  Changes in menstrual flow

Psychological
  Increase in somatic symptoms
  Awareness of ageing process
  Psychosocial changes and life events

The endocrine context

The understanding of the endocrine basis of the menopause came in the 1920s and the influential book *Feminine Forever* was published in 1966.[13] This was a polemical book and persuaded many women in the USA to seek HRT. Wilson made a number of claims that have not been substantiated. He described the menopause as chemical castration, and said that oestrogen therapy was essential to remain feminine forever. Production of oestrogen secreted from the ovaries and adrenals continues after the menopause. Sexual attractiveness and interest, especially in a stable relationship, are not entirely based on physical attributes. Wilson suggested that the menopause caused 'emotional upheavals'. Emotional upheavals (as we shall see later in this chapter) may result from external factors and are not typical of most middle-aged women. The use of unopposed oestrogen replacement therapy continued in the 1970s until it was found that it increased the risk of endometrial cancer. The uptake of HRT fell dramatically but has risen again since the addition of progesterone to oestrogen, which protects the endometrium.

The cultural context

The change of life may still be associated with negative meaning. It may be associated with awareness of the ageing process, and changes in hair and skin and physical stamina. The empty nest, feelings of loss of femininity and a partner who may seek a younger woman to revive his sexual interests may all contribute to a negative experience. On the other hand, in some cultures the menopause can mean a rise in social status. Women in Asia tend to report fewer symptoms than women in Western societies.[14] Rural Mayan Indians do not report menopausal symptoms in spite of similar endocrine changes to those in American women.[15] A disease construction of menopause may allow women to get help from doctors if they experience stress in mid-life, but the majority of women who are well in mid-life may not benefit from being classified as suffering from a hormone deficiency.

The family context

Around the time of menopause, women may be free from early adult worries about adult identity, the duties of child-rearing and the risks of pregnancy, but they may have other problems. Women may worry about domestic responsibilities, which continue to fall on women's shoulders in spite of changes in gender behaviour.[16] Responsibilities at home include caring for ageing parents and for teenage or grown-up children. Although the empty nest syndrome describes the feelings when children leave home,[17] economic necessity may mean that children stay on in the parental home. If their marriages break down, they may return to the parental home, and this has been described as the 'crowded nest'.[18] The review by Greene found that pre-existing marital dissatisfaction and financial problems were associated with menopausal symptoms, but not children leaving home.[19]

If a women presents with menopausal complaints, it is important to ask about her family circumstances. Caring for elderly parents rests mainly with women. In the UK, more caregivers (non-disease and non-age specific) are female and the average caregiver is middle-aged.

In the middle years, women are likely to suffer the loss of their parents, and may suffer successive bereavements. McKinlay et al[9] found that life events in mid-life that were unrelated to the menopause had strong associations with depressed mood, but not the timing of the menopause.

Symptoms of the perimenopause

The menopause syndrome

Hot flushes, night sweats and vaginal dryness are the only symptoms that have been clearly shown to be related to the endocrinological event of the menopause. However, many symptoms have been associated with the perimenopause and attributed to hormonal changes. These include irritability, headaches, depression, anxiety, problems of memory and concentration, and loss of libido. Sometimes these are described as 'the menopause syndrome'.

Vasomotor symptoms

For most women, the first sign of the perimenopause will be irregular menstruation, possibly accompanied by hot flushes or flashes. These are felt as a rising sensation of heat in the chest, neck and face. There is a rise in peripheral bloodflow and heart rate.[20] Skin conductance in the chest increases, but subjective hot flushes do not necessarily accompany physiological flushes. In laboratory experiments, physiological and subjective measurements were taken in menopausal women with frequent hot flushes.[21] Not all physiological hot flushes were reported subjectively and not all subjective hot flushes were accompanied by physiological markers. This may have been because they were in a laboratory situation. Negative attitudes may mean that women focus on perception of temperature. Symptom reporting may increase with negative affect because of high introspection, and mild symptoms may be interpreted as being severe. In experimental studies, Pennebaker[22] has shown that if attention is directed onto bodily sensations, symptom reporting is increased.

Hot flushes may be accompanied by sweating, and the woman may feel that her clothes are restrictive. Sweaters are put on and off and women are advised to wear loose clothing made of natural fibres. A menopausal woman may be more aware of the flush than others surrounding her, and other people may not detect a change in her appearance.

The aetiology of hot flushes is unknown. Genazzani et al[23] suggest that there is an increased activity of the noradrenergic system and reduction of dopamine activity, which modulate both gonadotrophin-releasing hormone (GnRH) and luteinizing hormone (LH) pulsatile release and the vasomotor/thermoregulatory system. The agonists naxolone and clonidine reduce the frequency of postmenopausal symptoms. Opioid peptides also play a part in the regulation of GnRH synthesis and pulsatile release. Hot flushes are likely to be affected by psychological and social factors. In a small study of 10 women, it was found that the reporting of hot flushes was influenced by daily stress levels; external temperature was associated with hot flushes in only one woman.[24] In a study of the reporting of hot flushes,[25] 17 women kept daily records for a week and carried a thermometer on their external clothing. About half of the flushes were preceded by feelings of anxiety, and one-fifth occurred after moving to a warmer environment. Hot flushes lasted no longer than the anxious state when in the warm room. There were no significant correlations between the frequency of flushes and the duration of flush. Anxious flushes may be more apparent to women, thus influencing self-reporting rates.

Hot flushes are not necessarily troublesome.[26,27] Only 10–15% of a sample of 101 women in general practice who reported hot flushes described them as problematic. Physical discomforts, disruption of sleep and social embarrassment are the main problems. Women who reported hot flushes tended to report higher levels of anxiety and depression than women who did not rate them as problematic. Levels of self-esteem were lower in these women but it is not clear whether the reporting of symptoms is the cause or the effect of these individual differences. Night sweats are probably similar to hot flushes but occur at night and are associated with waking. Women may report being drenched in sweat, disturbing their partners and having to change their night-clothes. They also report fatigue and irritability during the day. If women are physically and socially disturbed by hot flushes during the day and night sweats disrupt their sleep at night, it should not be surprising that mood disturbances occur.

Measurement of menopausal symptoms

Early studies

Many of the early studies on psychological changes in the perimenopause used inadequate psychometric assessments. In the last 40 years a number of research studies used an index of climacteric symptoms known as the Kupperman index or the Blatt–Kupperman index. In 1953 Kupperman and his co-workers described a numerical summation of 11 menopausal complaints and termed it the Menopausal Index.[28] This was based on their experience in treating women with menopausal complaints. A modification to the Menopausal Index, which allowed for some symptoms to be weighted more than others, was used in subsequent papers on menopausal symptoms.[29] It includes the following symptoms: vasomotor, paraesthesia, insomnia, nervousness, melancholia, vertigo, weakness (fatigue), arthralgia and myalgia, headaches, palpitation, and formication.

Ballinger published a major review on the psychiatric aspects of the menopause and pointed out that most of the general population surveys of the 1960s and 1970s used symptom checklists based on the Blatt–Kupperman index, although she failed to comment on its limitations.[30] In a review of the evidence for the psychological effects of tibolone on menopausal symptoms, many studies used the index.[31] The Kupperman index continues to be used today, but has severe limitations and a number of methodological problems. The index was a combination of self-report and physician ratings; it omitted measures of vaginal dryness and loss of libido; no demographic data of the sample were given; weighting was used without statistical justification; terms were ill-defined; categories included overlapping scores; and, most importantly, scores were summed without being based on independent factors.[32] Neugarten and Kraines[33] classified 28 symptoms of the menopause derived from clinicians' reports into three groupings: somatic, psychological and psychosomatic. A consensus classification by the International Menopause congress in 1976[34] classified symptoms by their supposed aetiology. They were those related to oestrogen deficiency, socio-cultural factors or psychological factors.

Factor analytic studies

Factor analysis has been used to analyse menopausal symptoms as a basis for the derivation of a scale. Greene factor analysed the responses of women attending a menopause clinic to a list of 30 menopausal symptoms. Three factors, labelled psychological, general somatic and vasomotor symptoms, were identified, and the Greene Climacteric Scale (GCS) of 21 items was derived. This was later published with six subscales.[35] Three other analyses were published in the 1980s, and all identify one or more factors comprising psychological complaints. These include psychological disorders, somatic/anxiety,[36] mood lability, nervousness,[37] depressed mood, cognitive difficulties, anxiety/fears, sexual functioning and sleep problems.[38] However, these studies tended to rely on clinical samples and the items were drawn from pre-existing reports. Holte and Mikkelsen[39] sent a symptom checklist to over 2000 women aged 44–55 in Norway. Factor analysis identified five factors: somatic complaints, nervousness, mood lability, vasomotor symptoms, and urogenital complaints. Vasomotor symptoms (sweating, hot flushes) and vaginal dryness were the only variables significantly associated with the stage of the menopause.

Rating can be difficult. Perz[40] points out that the CRS confounds symptom severity per se by the perception of distress. The women were asked to rate the extent to which they were bothered by the symptoms. The women's assessment of bother may not be the same as the intensity of the symptom. Three-point scales may inflate the level of intercorrelations.

Perz improved on the methodology and devised a menopausal checklist. She recruited a sample of 40 women from a newspaper advertisement, and identified a list of 120 items from the literature. These were reduced to a 56-item checklist. The symptoms were given operational definitions, and some examples are shown in Table 22.2. They were assessed on the frequency of occurrence and severity of symptoms. Three factors were found, described as psychological, general somatic and vasomotor. Thus all the factor analytic studies produced psychological symptoms as an important factor in the menopause syndrome, although Perz points out that symptomatology alone does not equate with a disorder.

Menopausal scales may not detect clinical depression, and few studies have used standardized psychiatric diagnostic tests. However, psychiatric assessments may not be able to distinguish somatic symptoms from psychological symptoms. Sleep disturbance may reflect night sweats rather than psychological distress. Menopausal scales that give a profile of the woman may help to identify the problems.

Table 22.2 Examples of items from the symptom checklist.[40]

Symptom	Operational definition
Tiredness or fatigue	Feeling tired or lacking in energy
Nervousness	Feeling jumpy or agitated
Irritable	Easily upset or annoyed
Crying spells	Crying or wanting to cry without reason
Loss of interest	Lost interest in most things and activities
Worry about nervous breakdown	Preoccupation with thoughts that you are having severe emotional problems

However, trying to identify mood disorders that are specifically related to the perimenopause raises a problem known as the 'domino effect'.

The domino effect

The psychological benefits of HRT may occur because they are secondary to the relief of vasomotor symptoms and a reduction in vaginal dryness. In an American study of 426 pre- and perimenopausal American women, depression (measured by the CES-D scale) was significantly associated with hot flushes (measured by self-report) but not hormone levels.[41] These findings support the domino effect. However, a Swedish study found no relationship between vasomotor symptoms and mental distress.[42] Most studies which investigate the psychological benefits of HRT are carried out on women who report vasomotor symptoms at baseline. Any improvement in mood could be due to domino effects.

In the absence of vasomotor symptoms, it would be possible to investigate whether mood enhancement is due to a direct psychotropic and/or placebo effect. If mood enhancement occurs as a result of a domino effect resulting from improvement in vasomotor symptoms, there should be no change in mood. Thirteen asymptomatic climacteric women who were taking HRT for the prevention of osteoporosis or cardiovascular disease were assessed in a pilot study to investigate the effects of HRT on mood in the absence of changes in climacteric symptoms. The results showed that mood, sexuality and self-esteem did not significantly change in the absence of any improvement in climacteric symptoms, suggesting that HRT did not exert psychotropic or placebo effects. Mood enhancement in symptomatic women treated with HRT is more likely to be due to a domino effect. In a study of hormones, sexuality and wellbeing in 140 women aged 40–60, it was found that tiredness was the only significant predictor of depression (measured by the Multiple Affect Adjective Check List (MAACL)).[43] Vasomotor symptoms were positively correlated with tiredness, and this suggests that the adverse effects that vasomotor symptoms have on wellbeing are mainly mediated by tiredness.[44]

Studies of general symptoms in the perimenopause

The very early cross-sectional studies found a high incidence of symptomatology, and this may have exaggerated the size of the problem.[45,46] Lower rates have been reported in more recent cross-sectional studies. Variations in figures may depend on the definitions used, and the sampling technique. Greene[19] reviewed 14 cross-sectional studies and found that vasomotor symptoms, but not psychological symptoms, were associated with the time of the menopause. Hagstad and Jansen surveyed a random sample of the female population aged 40–64 in Goteborg in Sweden.[47] Eighty-one per cent (1413/1746) responded to a questionnaire and attended for interview. Women who had had a surgical menopause had more vasomotor symptoms than those with a natural menopause. Less than half (47%) of those postmenopausal women who had ever had flushes reported them as moderate or severe. Perimenopausal women (bleeding 2–5 months previously) had a significantly higher frequency of hot flushes and sweating than menstruating women (bleeding in the last 2 months). Kaufert et al[48] described the methodological problems in establishing the prevalence of menopausal symptoms. Definitions of menopausal status vary, scales are unstandardized, and populations are often recruited from clinics, volunteers, or general practice surgeries. In Australia, a cross-sectional interview study of women selected from the electoral roll (64% response) found relatively low reporting of hot flushes (25%), but 37% reported irritability, 36% mood swings and 28% depression over the last 2 weeks. However, the sample included 31% HRT users and they did not appear to have lower rates of symptoms, although the analysis is unclear.[49]

In a careful cross-sectional study, Hunter et al surveyed 850 pre-, peri- and postmenopausal women.[30] The questionnaire established independent symptom clusters of depressed mood, somatic symptoms, cognitive difficulties, vasomotor symptoms, anxiety/fears, sexual problems and sleep problems. Multiple regression analysis showed that vasomotor symptoms and sexual problems were best predicted by menopausal status alone, but that social class was a strong predictor of the other symptoms. Absence of employment also strongly predicted somatic symptoms and anxiety symptoms. They note that the increased prevalence of symptoms in peri- and postmenopausal women was small. The association between menopausal status and symptoms may be related to declining levels of oestrogen, but the psychological and somatic symptoms could be secondary reactions to vasomotor symptoms.

Cross-sectional studies, although criticized as being a weak design,[50] have confirmed that vasomotor symptoms and sometimes insomnia increase across the menopause transition and general symptoms reporting increases in the perimenopause.[9,51] However, in general there is little change for most women apart from vasomotor symptoms and vaginal dryness.[48,52,53]

The perimenopause and depression

Investigation of the relationship between the timing of the menopause and depressed mood has been beset by methodological problems. Problems in measurement of symptoms in the perimenopause have been described above, and few studies have used standardized criteria and objective assessments. Women attending menopause clinics may not be typical. High levels of depressive disorder have been reported in women attending gynaecology clinics.[54,55] In a review, Pearce et al point out the importance of assessing and controlling for environmental factors and social stresses.[56] In a study of women with HRT given by oestradiol implants, it was found that vasomotor symptoms were related to falling oestradiol levels, but psychological symptoms were more closely related to minor stresses or hassles.[57]

Cross-sectional studies of large samples of the general population have found a small increase in depressive disorder.[38,48,52,58] In a cross-sectional study, McKinlay et al[58] found a slight increase in depression in the perimenopause and subsequent 12 months, but other studies have found conflicting results. A study of psychiatric morbidity in women attending a menopause clinic found high levels of psychiatric morbidity.[2] Seventy-eight women had had a natural menopause, and 35 (45%) had a current depressive disorder assessed using the Montgomery–Asberg Depression Rating Scale (MADRS).[59] Twenty-nine of those depressed at the clinic had been depressed previously. These levels seem high, and while clearly not representative of all menopausal women and of all clinics, indicate that gynaecologists should be prepared to find depression in their patients and perhaps refer women for psychiatric help.

In Hunter's longitudinal study,[53] most

women reported relief from the cessation of menstruation and the possibility of becoming pregnant. Those that expressed negative beliefs and expectations before the menopause were more likely to be depressed and report symptoms when they reached the menopause. Psychological problems had greater association with psychosocial factors than with menopausal status. In a study in general practice in London,[27] it was found that 57% agreed that 'hormonal changes at menopause can cause depression', although an equal number (58%) also agreed that 'menopause can mark the beginning of a new and fulfilling stage of a woman's life'. Women who believed that they were susceptible to menopause-related problems had a more negative attitude towards menopause and were more likely to believe in the ability of powerful others (measured by the Multi-dimensional Health Locus of Control (MHLC))[60] to modify their experience of menopause. In general, longitudinal studies have found little or no significant increase in depressive disorders during the perimenopause.[41,51,53,52,61] These studies and others have been discussed in recent reviews.[56,62] This has led the reviewers to the conclusion that psychosocial events contribute more to psychological changes than the timing of the menopause. Recent research publications are discussed below.

Recent research studies on depression in the perimenopause

Nicol-Smith published a critical review of the evidence for maintaining that the menopause causes depression.[50] Forty-three epidemiological primary research papers were identified and classified according to sample and measures and the researcher's own conclusion as to whether or not an association had been found. She found 24 review articles on Medline, and

although in 10 the authors concluded that depression was related to menopause, the reviews were not considered rigorous and were dismissed as 'informative but inconclusive'. In 17 research studies an association was found, and these papers were examined using Hill's criteria.[63] She argues that all the studies reported are essentially cross-sectional in design and, of course, the menopause is a universal occurrence rather than a disease that occurs in one group rather than another. The studies reviewed are very different. The sample size ranges from 36 to 5568; the assessment of depression varies from one depressive symptom to clinical depression; and the samples are from clinical and non-clinical populations. She concludes that there is no substantial evidence that either a natural menopause with its accompanying changes in hormone concentrations or psychosocial factors exclusive to middle age puts women at an increased risk of depression. She suggests that this has the implication for clinicians that women suffering from depression in middle age should not be treated differently from those attending at other ages. The description of the review as systematic and critical was subsequently challenged.[64] Pettigrew pointed out that those papers that found no association were not included, and that the methodology of the studies was not critically reviewed. Studd and Smith comment that oestrogen therapy has been found only to help women in the premenopause and that many women feel well for the first time in many years when the menopause relieves them from premenstrual syndrome, heavy painful periods, menstrual migraine and chronic cyclical depression.[65] They have also suggested that some women may be vulnerable to a depression which is responsive to hormones, and that markers can identify these women. These markers include a history of having a good affect during pregnancy, a history of postnatal depression, a history or premenstrual depression with a cyclical pattern of depressive symptoms, and menstrual migraine.[66] There is little evidence for this but it has some biological foundation and it has been argued that some women may be more vulnerable to changes in hormones than others.[67,68] Data from a longitudinal study of women enrolled at birth give some interesting insights.[69] The Medical Research Council (MRC) National Survey of health and development is a socially stratified cohort of 2548 women and 2814 men in the UK which has been followed up since their birth in 1946. In 1993, when they were 47, they were sent a postal questionnaire asking about common health problems (84% response rate). At the age of 36 years, they had been given the Present State Examination and a checklist of health problems. At 47 years of age, 24% were perimenopausal. The most bothersome health complaints were aches and pains in the joints, anxiety or depression, irritability, trouble in sleeping, forgetfulness, frequent severe headaches and breast tenderness. These severely affected the lives of at least one in ten women and were reported by around half the population. They increased significantly with each stage of the natural menopause even after adjusting for previous psychological and physical ill-health, smoking, educational background, or current life stress. A factor analysis revealed five factors, including 'symptoms of psychological ill-health', which explained 25% of the variance. Psychological symptoms were not related to the natural menopause except for a slight rise in irritability among perimenopausal women. The reporting of psychological symptoms at age 47 was very strongly related to current family and work stress, and related to higher levels of anxiety and depression and self-reported health problems at 36 years. Women who had had a hysterectomy and HRT users showed an increased risk of anxiety and depression over women in all stages of natural menopause. Data from the first 4 years of the Melbourne Women's Midlife Health Project have shown that positive affect was significantly lower in the 2-year postmenopausal group but this effect did not remain when controlled for hot flushes.[70] Affect was measured by a scale of wellbeing.[71] Whether or not there is a relationship between health status and endocrine status, it is clear that there is a high level of health problems in mid-life. Women who have had a previous history of psychological problems may be at risk during the perimenopause and are likely to come to the attention of clinicians.

Management

HRT and its effect on mood

The use of HRT seems to be rising, partly because of more knowledge and understanding of the menopause, partly because of advances in the development of different ways of delivery and marketing, and partly because of renewed evidence of benefits to health.

The contribution of oestrogens to psychological health is controversial, but detailed discussion of the effects of HRT on psychological and sexual problems is beyond the scope of this chapter. Early studies had many methodological problems,[31,56] but there have been well-designed studies which have shown a positive effect of oestrogen therapy in oophorectomized women.[72] The numerous clinical studies on mood have shown benefits of oestrogen therapy on a variety of symptoms.[73] Little is known about the effect of the addition of progestogen. In a placebo-controlled study it was found that women who had received conjugated oestrogen plus medroxyprogesterone experienced more negative moods and greater psychological symptomatology than those receiving conjugated oestrogen and placebo. The picture is not entirely clear. In a cross-sectional study we found that circulating levels of oestrogen were not related to symptom reporting in women who had requested replacement oestradiol implants.[74] In a study of the effects of discontinuation of HRT, it was found that women who received an active replacement implant were no different in psychological or psychiatric symptoms from women who received a placebo implant, even though the active group had higher oestradiol levels. The only effect of HRT was on vasomotor symptoms.[75]

The effects of hormone replacement on psychological symptoms may be mainly due to the domino effect. If this is so, then any therapy that alleviates vasomotor symptoms will have beneficial effects on mood.

Non-hormonal treatments

Many women do not wish to take HRT, or it may be contraindicated. Depression in middle-aged women may be unrelated to the perimenopause and can be treated by conventional psychotherapy or psychotropic drugs. There are a number of practical steps that women can take to help them cope with hot flushes and night sweats.[76] The use of natural fibres for bedsheets and clothes, reducing intake of stimulants and the development of positive attitudes have all been recommended. Relaxation has been found to help many women. Low self-esteem may be both a cause and a consequence of hot flushes, and therapy that enhances self-esteem and increases the woman's feelings of personal control will be effective. There may also be local self-help groups for menopausal women. Although there is little evidence for the effectiveness of herbal remedies, individual women may benefit. There has recently been an interest in the effect of soy on menopausal symptoms.[77] Soy may have weak oestrogenic effects, and this is supported by epidemiological evidence.

Conclusions

The perimenopause is associated with a time of psychological and endocrinological change but the relationships are unclear. The biological definition of the perimenopause is based on endocrinological status, but this may have little relationship to mood changes. The menopause occurs at around the age of 50, and for men and women this is a time which has particular demands. These may be no more nor less than those at other times of life, such as adolescence, or early parenthood.[78] The predominant symptoms of the perimenopause are vasomotor symptoms of hot flushes and night sweats and vaginal dryness. Psychological complaints are also reported. There is little evidence that these are related to endocrine events.

Many women seek help for these symptoms during the menopause and may report that they have increased since they experienced menstrual irregularities and vasomotor symptoms. These symptoms may respond to treatment with HRT, naturally leading the women and their doctors to believe that the psychological problems have been a consequence of the hormone changes. Women who attend menopause clinics are not representative of menopausal women in general. It has been suggested that they are either predisposed to psychological dysfunction because of previous history[69] or that there are some women who are particularly vulnerable to changes in levels of hormones.[2,66]

HRT has been shown to benefit women in a number of studies but this may be partly because of the alleviation of vasomotor symptoms. Psychological dysfunction in the perimenopause in the absence of any vasomotor symptoms is unlikely to respond to HRT, although there is a powerful placebo effect.

References

1. Utian WH, Overview on menopause, *Am J Obstet Gynecol* 1987; **156**:1280–3.

2. Hay AG, Bancroft J, Bancroft J, Johnstone EC, Affective symptoms in women attending a menopause clinic, *Br J Psychiatry* 1994; **164**:513–16.

3. Ussher J, *Misogyny and Madness* (Harvester Wheatsheaf: London, 1991).

4. Greer G, *The Change. Women, Ageing and the Menopause* (Hamish Hamilton: London, 1991) 11–35.

5. Alder B, *The Psychology of Health: Applications of Psychology for Health Professionals* (Harwood Academic Publishers: Luxembourg, 1995) 208.

6. Sarafino EP, *Health Psychology. Biopsychosocial Interactions*, 3rd edn (John Wiley: New York, 1998).

7. World Health Organization, *Research on the Menopause* (WHO: Geneva, 1981).

8. Wich BK, Carnes M, Menopause and the aging female reproductive system, *Endocrinol Metab Clin North Am* 1995; **24**:273–95.

9. McKinlay SM, Brambilla DJ, Posner JG, The normal menopause transition, *Maturitas* 1992; **14**:103–15.

10. Torgerson DJ, Avenell A, Russell IT, Reid DM, Factors associated with onset of menopause in women aged 45–49 *Maturitas* 1994; **19**:83–92.

11. Pokras R, Hufnagel VG, Hysterectomy in the United States, 1965–84, *Am J Public Health* 1988; **78**:852–3.

12. Soon TE, Teoh KLK, *Over 45 Feeling Fabulous* (Times Books International: Singapore, 1991).

13. Wilson RA, *Feminine Forever* (Evans: New York, 1966).

14. Payer L, The menopause in various cultures. In: Berger H, Boulet M, eds, *A Portrait of the Menopause* (Parthenon: London, 1991).

15. Martin MC, Block JE, Sanchez SD et al, Menopause without symptoms: the endocrinology of menopause among rural Mayan Indians, *Am J Obstet Gynecol* 1993; **168**:1839–43.

16. Llewlyn S, Osborne K, *Women's Lives* (Routledge: London, 1990) 221–52.

17. Lowenthal MF, Chiriboga D, Transition to the empty nest. Crisis, challenge or relief, *Arch Gen Psychiatry* 1972; **26**:8–14.

18. Datan N, Midas and other mid life crises. In: Norman WH, Scaramella TJ, eds, *Mid-life: Developmental and Clinical Issues* (Bruner/Mazel: New York, 1980).

19. Greene JG, *The Social and Psychological Origins of the Climacteric Syndrome* (Gower: Aldershot, 1984).

20. Ginsburg J, Hardiman P, O'Reilly B, Peripheral blood flow in menopausal women who have hot flushes and in those who do not, *Br Med J* 1989; **298**:1488–90.

21. Bakker IPM, Everaerd W, Measurement of menopausal hot flushes: validation and cross-validation, *Maturitas* 1966; **25**:87–98.

22. Pennebaker J, *The Psychology of Physical Symptoms* (Springer-Verlag: New York, 1982).

23. Genazzani AR, Petraglia F, Gambad O et al, Neuroendocrinology of the menstrual cycle, *Ann NY Acad Sci*, 1997; **816**:143–50.

24. Gannon L, Hansel S, Goodwin J, Correlates of menopausal hot flashes, *J Behav Med* 1987; **10**:277–85.

25. Slade P, Amaer S, The role of anxiety and temperature in the experience of menopausal hot flushes, *J Reprod Infant Psychol* 1995; **13**:127–34.

26. Liao K, Hunter MS, White P, Beliefs about menopause of general practitioners and mid-aged women, *Fam Pract* 1994; **11**:408–12.

27. Liao KL-M, Knowledge and beliefs about menopause in a general population sample of mid-aged women, *J Reprod Infant Psychol* 1995; **13**:101–14.

28. Blatt MH, Weisbader H, Kupperman HS, Vitamin E and climacteric syndrome, *Arch Intern Med* 1953; **91**:792–9.

29. Kupperman HS, Wetchler BB, Blatt MH, Contemporary therapy of the menopausal syndrome, *JAMA* 1959; **171**: 1627–37.

30. Ballinger CB, Psychiatric aspects of the menopause, *Br J Psychiatry* 1990; **156**:773–87.

31. Ross LA, Alder EM, Tibolone and climacteric symptoms, *Maturitas* 1995; **21**:127–36.

32. Alder EM, The Blatt Kupperman Menopausal Index: a critique, Maturitas 1998; **29**:19–24.

33. Neugarten BL, Kraines RJ, 'Menopausal symptoms' in women of various ages, *Psychosom Med* 1965; **27**:266–73.

34. Utian WH, Serr D, The climacteric syndrome. In: van Keep PA, Greenblatt RB, Fernett A, eds, *Consensus on Menopause Research* (University Park Press: Lancaster, 1976) 1–4.

35. Greene JG, *Guide to the Greene Climacteric Scale* (Glasgow University: Glasgow, 1991).

36. Kaufert PA, Gilbert P, Hassard T, Researching the symptoms of the menopause: an exercise in methodology, *Maturitas* 1988; **10**:17–31.

37. Mikkelsen A, Holte A, A factor-analytic study of 'climacteric symptoms', *Psychiatry Social Sci* 1982; **2**:266–73.

38. Hunter M, Battersby R, Whitehead M, Relationships between psychological symptoms, somatic complaints and menopausal status, *Maturitas* 1986; **8**:217–28.

39. Holte A, Mikkelsen A, The menopausal syndrome: a factor analytic replication, *Maturitas* 1991; **13**:193–203.

40. Perz JM, Development of the menopause symptom list: a factor analytic study of menopause associated symptoms, *Women Health* 1997; **25**:53–69.

41. Avis NE, Brambilla D, McKinlay SM et al, A longitudinal analysis of the association between menopause and depression. Results from the Massachusetts Women's Health Study, *Ann Epidemiol* 1994; **4**:214–20.

42. Furuhjelm M, Karlgren E, Carlstrom K, The effect of estrogen therapy on somatic and psychical symptoms in postmenopausal women, *Acta Obstet Scand Gynecol* 1984; **63**:655–61.

43. Zuckerman M, Lubin B, Rinck CM Construction of new scales for the Multiple Affect Adjective Check List, *J Behav Assessment* 1983; **5**:19–29.

44. Cawood EH, Bancroft J, Steroid hormones, the menopause, sexuality and well-being of women, *Psychol Med* 1996; **26**:925–36.

45. Barret L, Subcommittee of the Medical Women's Federation. An investigation of the menopause in one thousand women, *Lancet* 1933; **i**:106–8.

46. Thompson B, Hart SA, Durno D, Menopausal age and symptomatology in a general practice, *J Biosocial Sci* 1973; **5**:71–82.

47. Hagstad A, Jansen PO, The epidemiology of climacteric symptoms, *Acta Obstet Scand Suppl* 1986; **134**:59–65.

48. Kaufert PA, Gilbert P, Tate R, The Manitoba Project: a re-examination of the link between menopause and depression, *Maturitas* 1992; **14**:143–55.

49. O'Connor VM, Del Mar CB, Sheenan M et al, Do psycho-social factors contribute more to symptoms reporting by middle aged women than hormonal status? *Maturitas* 1995; **20**:63–9.

50. Nicol-Smith L, Causality, menopause, and depression: a critical review of the literature, *Br Med J* 1996; **313**:1229–32.

51. Matthews KA, Wing RR, Kuller LH et al, Influences of natural menopause on psychological characteristics and symptoms of middle-aged healthy women, *J Consult Clin Psychol* 1990; **58**:345–51.

52. Holte A, Influences of natural menopause on health complaints: a prospective study of healthy Norwegian women, *Maturitas* 1992; **14**:127–41.

53. Hunter M, The south-east England longitudinal study of the climacteric and postmenopause, *Maturitas* 1992; **14**:117–26.

54. Ballinger CB, Psychiatric morbidity and the menopause: survey of a gynaecological outpatient clinic, *Br J Psychiatry* 1977; **131**:83–9.

55. Ballinger CB, Browning MC, Smith AH, Hormone profiles and psychological symptoms in peri-menopausal women, *Maturitas* 1987; **9**:235–51.

56. Pearce J, Hawton K, Blake F, Psychological and sexual symptoms associated with the menopause and the effects of hormone replacement therapy, *Br J Psychiatry* 1995; **167**:163–73.

57. Alder E, The effects of hormone replacement therapy on psychological symptoms. In: Wijma K, von Schoultz B, eds, *Reproductive Life* (The Parthenon Publishing Group: Carnforth, 1992) 359–64.

58. McKinlay JB, McKinlay SM, Brambilla D, The relative contributions of endocrine changes and social circumstances to depression in mid-aged women, *J Health Social Behav* 1987; **28**:345–63.

59. Montgomery SA, Asberg M, A new depression scale designed to be sensitive to change, *Br J Psychiatry* 1979; **134**:382–9.

60. Wallston KA, Wallston BS, Devillis R, Development of the Multidimensional Health

Locus of Control (MHLC) scales, *Health Educ Monogr* 1978; **6**:160–70.

61. Hallstrom T, Samuelsson S, Mental health in the climacteric. The longitudinal study of women in Gothenberg, *Acta Obstet Scand Suppl* 1985; **130**:13–18.

62. Panay N, Studd JWW, Menopause and the central nervous system, *Eur Menopause J* 1996; **3**: 242–9.

63. Hill AB, The environment and disease: association or causality, *Proc R Soc Med* 1965; **58**:295–300.

64. Pettigrew M, Review did not fully examine the evidence, *Br Med J* 1997; **314**:608.

65. Studd JWW, Smith RNJ, Oestrogens and depression, *Menopause* 1994; **1**:18–23.

66. Studd J, Depression and the menopause. Oestrogens improve symptoms in some middle aged women, *Br Med J* 1997; **314**:977–8.

67. Bancroft J, *Human Sexuality and its Problems*, 2nd edn (Churchill Livingstone: Edinburgh, 1989) 119–22.

68. Barlow DH, Who understands the menopause? *Br J Obstet Gynaecol* 1997; **104**:879–80.

69. Kuh DL, Hardy R, Wadsworth M, Women's health in midlife: the influence of the menopause, social factors and health in earlier life, *Br J Obstet Gynaecol* 1997; **104**:1419.

70. Dennerstein L, Dudley E, Burger H, Well-being and the menopausal transition, *J Psychosom Obstet Gynecol* 1997; **18**:95–101.

71. Kammann R, Flett R, Affectometer 2: a scale to measure current levels of happiness, *Aust J Psychol* 1983; **35**:259–65.

72. Sherwin BB, Gelfand MM, Sex steroids and affect in the surgical menopause: a double-blind, crossover study, *Psychoneuroendocrinology* 1985; **10**:325–35.

73. Sherwin BB, Hormones, mood and cognitive functioning in postmenopausal women, *Obstet Gynecol* 1996; **87**:20S–6S.

74. Alder EM, Bancroft J, Livingstone J, Estradiol implants, and reported symptoms, *J Psychosom Obstet Gynaecol* 1992; **13**:223–35.

75. Pearce J, Mauton K, Blake T et al, Psychological effects of continuation versus discontinuation of hormone replacement therapy by estrogen implants: a placebo-controlled study, *J Psychosom Res* 1997; **42**:177–86.

76. Hunter M, *Your Menopause* (Pandora: London, 1990) 120–33.

77. Wilcox G, The effect of soy on menopausal symptoms. In: *Abstracts 8th International Congress on the Menopause*. (The Parthenon Publishing Group: Sydney, 1996).

78. Alder B, Reproductive and obstetric issues. In: Johnston M, Johnston D, eds, *Health Psychology* (Elsevier: New York, 1998) 383–407.

23

Personality disorders

Lisa Ekselius and Lars von Knorring

Introduction

The introduction of a separate Axis II and operationalized criteria for specific personality disorders in the DSM-III[1] have had a dramatic effect on interest in the personality disorders among clinicians and researchers in the field of psychiatry. Standardized methods for assessment, both structured interviews and self-report questionnaires, have been developed, resulting in improved diagnostic reliability for the different personality disorder categories.

In the DSM-IV[2] the separate axis for personality disorder (Axis II) is maintained. In the ICD-10, introduced by the World Health Organization,[3] no separate axis is used for the personality disorders but there is a separate chapter (F60–F69). Diagnostic Criteria for Research[4] also exist. DSM-IV covers 10 personality disorders, while ICD-10 Diagnostic Criteria for Research cover 9 personality disorders. Narcissistic personality disorder is not specified in the ICD-10. Furthermore, the DSM-IV schizotypal personality disorder is classified under schizophrenia spectrum disorders in the ICD-10.

In DSM-IV[2] the personality disorders are defined by means of general diagnostic criteria and specific criteria for the separate personality disorders. The general criteria include an enduring pattern of inner experiences and behaviours that deviate markedly from the expectations of the individual's culture. The pattern is to be manifested in at least two of the following areas: cognition, affectivity, interpersonal functioning or impulse control. Furthermore, the enduring pattern has to be inflexible and pervasive across a broad range of personal and social situations, lead to clinically significant distress or impairment in social or occupational functioning, and stable over time, and the onset should be traceable to adolescence or early childhood. Also in the ICD-10, there is a similar set of 'general criteria' that have to be met, in addition to the diagnostic criteria for each personality disorder. In short, the general criteria require that dysfunction or subjective distress be present.

Each category of personality disorder consists of 5–10 criteria, and the presence of 3–5 is required for diagnosis. The only exception from this polythetic principle, that is, the patient must fulfil only a certain number of non-specified criteria, is the impulsive type of the emotionally unstable personality disorder, where one specific criterion is obligatory. In the DSM-IV the personality disorders are divided into three clusters, A, B and C. Although the ICD-10 does not have the cluster subdivision, the personality disorders are listed in an equivalent order, beginning with the 'odd' or 'eccentric' personality disorders, followed by the 'dramatic' or 'erratic' personality disorders, and finally the 'anxious' personality disorders.

Many studies have focused on the frequency of personality disorders in different populations, and the results obtained indicate that personality disorders are prevalent in the general population. The frequencies tend to range from 10% to 13.5%.[5,6] However, more individuals fulfil the criteria for separate personality disorders. In a study by Reich et al,[7] 28.9% of the subjects in the general population met the criteria for a separate personality disorder. However, when the criteria for subjective distress or occupational functioning were added, the prevalence decreased to 11.1%, more in line with other reports from the general population. In our own study,[8] 21.2% of the women and 15.3% of the men fulfilled criteria for a personality disorder according to SCID screen with adjusted cut-off. However, no general function or distress criteria were assessed. In psychiatric settings, an even higher prevalence has been reported.[8–10] In the study by Bodlund et al,[8] a typical outpatient department population in a medium-sized university town in Sweden was investigated. The overall prevalence of personality disorders according to the SCID screen with adjusted cut-off was 61.5%. The results confirmed the previous findings,[9,11,12] where the prevalence rates in psychiatric outpatients varied between 48.8% and 81% when structured interviews or self-reports

were used. For psychiatric patients, we have reported that personality disorders tend to be more frequent among male than among female patients.[13] This observation was also made in a Norwegian study[9] and in a study by Reich.[12] One reason may be that men do not seek help until they have more severe problems, whereas women are more prone to seek advice.

Personality disorders, regardless of subtype, have been found to be significantly related to poor outcome, regardless of treatment, in a wide range of psychiatric disorders, especially in patients with major depression, panic disorder and obsessive-compulsive disorder. The relationship seems to be robust both in inpatients and outpatients.[14,15] In a study by Sato et al,[16] comprising inpatients with major depression, cluster A personality disorder, especially schizoid personality disorder, worsened the short-term outcome in the patients treated with antidepressants. Furthermore, research data indicate that personality disorders may frequently predispose to or complicate the clinical picture of various Axis I disorders.[17]

Personality disorders as categorical or dimensional

At present, personality disorders in the DSM-IV and the ICD-10 are organized as categories with defined cut-off points. The categorical approach is mainly based on clinical tradition in medicine and psychiatry and is favoured by clinicians, as it is consistent with clinical conventions and practice, while there is more empirical support for the dimensional approach.[18–21]

The dimensional model has psychometric advantages, increases the reliability, and to some extent explains the problem of diagnostic overlap between personality disorders.[22]

Furthermore, the dimensional model better demonstrates the relationship of traits occurring in the normal population with personality disorders. Thus, it is often reasonable to report not only the frequency of patients with certain personality disorders but also the number of fulfilled criteria for separate personality disorders.

Sex bias in diagnostic criteria

A prevailing view about psychopathology is that the actual content or manifestations of a disorder should be culture-free or universal. In the theory of psychopathology (the DSM system in particular, but also relevant to the ICD system), general descriptors of the person (demographic and cultural) play a comparatively minor role in the stipulation of the manifestations of psychiatric illness. Among socially and culturally oriented psychiatrists, on the other hand, such descriptors are considered to be important clues to the origins of psychopathology. However, in such an analysis, socio-cultural is usually equated with altogether symbolic/language traditions, although reports exist of sex differences in symptom expression within Western societies. Feminist critics assert that even within the socio-cultural tradition linked to the Anglo-American society, a bias exists with respect to how psychopathology is shaped, defined and handled.[23] As concerns personality disorders, Funtowicz and Widiger[24] have suggested several important reasons for a sex bias (Table 23.1).

The criticism has been taken into account and several changes have been made in the diagnostic criteria from DSM-III[1] to DSM-III R[25] and DSM-IV.[2] However, there are still unsolved questions. In the DSM-IV manual[2] it is concluded that certain personality disorders (e.g. antisocial personality disorder) are diag-

nosed more frequently in men, while others (e.g. borderline, histrionic and dependent personality disorders) are diagnosed more frequently in women. It is concluded that although these differences in prevalence rates probably reflect real gender differences in the presence of such patterns, clinicians and researchers must be careful not to overdiagnose or underdiagnose certain personality disorders in females or in males because of social stereotypes concerning typical gender roles and behaviours.

Diagnosing personality disorders

Clinical assessment of personality disorders involves systematic observations and collection of information from the patient, relatives, staff members, etc. Beyond the demand of specific criteria, the basic features, that is, early onset, persistence, pervasiveness, interpersonal focus and impairment in functioning or subjective distress, have to be present.

Diagnostic criteria make diagnoses more reliable by providing rules for summarizing clinical data into a diagnosis.[26] Since the publication of the DSM-III,[1] a number of assessment instruments for personality disorders have been developed, resulting in improved interrater reliability. However, it has been pointed out by Perry[27] that current methods for making personality disorder diagnoses yield diagnoses that are not significantly comparable across methods. He suggested that the lack of concordance between methods was due to variations in raters, interview occasions, sources of information, availability of historical clinical data, sensitivity to state effects and the formats of the different methods. Validation of personality disorder assessment procedures is complicated by the fact that there are no clear

Table 23.1 Sex biases in the diagnosis of personality disorders suggested by Funtowicz and Widiger.[24]

Reasons for bias	Examples
1. Biased diagnostic constructs	Dependent personality disorder and histrionic personality disorder. Both disorders are most commonly diagnosed in females
2. Biased application of diagnostic criteria	When identical case histories are used, females are more often classified as having histrionic personality disorder, while males are classified as having antisocial personality disorder
3. Biased assessment instruments	Some items from narcissistic and antisocial personality disorder scales such as the MMPI narcissistic item 'I have no dread of going into a room by myself where other people have already gathered and are talking'
4. Biased thresholds for diagnosis	The point at which stereotypic or extreme femininity is classified as excessive or maladaptive is lower than the threshold for the classification of excessive, maladaptive masculinity
5. Biased diagnostic criteria	Avoidant, histrionic and antisocial personality disorders. In particular, the fact that women tend to be diagnosed as having histrionic personality disorder while men tend to be diagnosed as having antisocial personality disorder has been debated

validity standards against which the diagnosis or the results of the procedure can be compared. In the absence of a true validity criterion or 'gold standard' for diagnoses, Spitzer et al[28] suggested what has come to be known as the LEAD standard, that is 'longitudinal expert evaluation using all data'.

Structured interviews provide a systematic and comprehensive personality profile for guiding differential diagnoses and treatment. However, in clinical practice, structured interviews are time-consuming and not feasible in every patient as a routine method. Self-administered questionnaires are less time-consuming than interviews and can be used as screening instruments to identify individuals who need further investigations. Inventories may also be helpful in epidemiological studies.

In our earlier studies, we used a modified version of the SCID II screen questionnaire.[29] The questions are very similar to the questions used in the SCID II interview.[30] In our[9,29] studies, we demonstrated that adjusting the cut-off level, by including one more criterion for all diagnoses, yields good agreement between the SCID screen and SCID II interviews and clinical diagnoses, respectively.

Based on our previous experiences from the SCID screen, and analyses of ICD-10 and DSM-IV diagnostic criteria, a new self-report inventory was developed, the DSM-IV and ICD-10 Personality Disorder Questionnaire (DIP-Q).[31] Out of the 140 items on the self-report questionnaire, 135 items reflect diagnostic criteria of the DSM-IV and the ICD-10 personality disorders, whereas five items cover the impairment in functioning/subjective distress criteria. In a validation study, agreement was tested between the DIP-Q and a structured clinical interview (the DSM-IV and ICD-10 Personality Disorder Interview—DIP-I) in a clinical sample.[32] Sensitivity, specificity and Cohen's kappa coefficient were in the acceptable range for most of the specific personality disorders. Later studies have confirmed that DIP-Q is a useful screening instrument for personality disorders in clinical practice and can be used as a diagnostic tool in epidemiological research.

Sex differences in the prevalence of personality disorders

In the DSM classification system, sex differences in the prevalence of certain personality disorders are suggested. In particular, DSM-IV[2] postulates that antisocial personality disorder is diagnosed more frequently in men, and that borderline, histrionic and dependent personality disorders are diagnosed more frequently in women.

In several studies, using the DSM-III and DSM-III-R criteria,[1,25] diagnoses of antisocial personality disorder have been documented as being more common among men than among women.[33–36]

The prevalence of obsessive-compulsive personality disorder in epidemiological surveys varies between 1.7% and 6.4%,[37] depending on the method of assessment used. In a study by Nestadt et al,[38] the rate among men was about five times higher than the rate among women.

Evidence also exists that men are more likely to be given a diagnosis of paranoid personality disorder.[9,12]

Data concerning sex differences in borderline personality disorder are contradictory. Swartz et al[39] found that a significantly higher proportion of women were diagnosed as having borderline personality disorder in a community sample, while Reich[12] and Kass et al[35] failed to find sex differences in clinical settings.

In a study by Nestadt et al,[40] the prevalence of histrionic personality disorder in the general population was found to be almost equal in men and women.

In an attempt to elucidate sex differences, we investigated a fairly large sample comprising subjects from the general population and psychiatric patients using the DSM-III-R criteria.[41] Fewer sex differences were found than those postulated by the authors of DSM-III/DSM-III-R. We were only able to demonstrate significant sex differences on a categorical level as concerns obsessive-compulsive personality disorder, borderline personality disorder and schizoid personality disorder (Table 23.2).

When sex differences were analysed dimensionally, borderline personality disorder still

Table 23.2 Frequency of personality disorders according to SCID screen questionnaire with adjusted cut-off in healthy volunteers and psychiatric patients divided according to sex, $N = 531$.

	Males (N = 231)		Females (N = 300)		P	
	n	%	n	%		
Avoidant	26	11.3	44	14.7	$\chi^2 = 1.33$	NS
Dependent	9	3.9	17	5.7	$\chi^2 = 0.88$	NS
Obsessive–compulsive	31	13.4	21	7.0	$\chi^2 = 6.09$	<0.02
Passive–aggressive	12	5.2	7	2.3	$\chi^2 = 3.10$	NS
Self-defeating	6	2.6	10	3.3	$\chi^2 = 0.24$	NS
Paranoid	31	13.4	32	10.7	$\chi^2 = 0.95$	NS
Schizotypal	3	1.3	5	1.7	$\chi^2 = 0.12$	NS
Schizoid	7	3.0	0	0	$\chi^2 = 7.03$	<0.01
Histrionic	7	3.0	12	4.0	$\chi^2 = 0.36$	NS
Narcissistic	26	11.3	20	6.7	$\chi^2 = 3.47$	NS
Borderline	19	8.2	46	15.3	$\chi^2 = 6.14$	<0.02
Antisocial	6	2.6	1	0.3	$\chi^2 = 3.53$	NS
Any personality disorder	81	35.1	98	31.7	$\chi^2 = 0.34$	NS

NS, not significant.

showed differences between sexes, while there were no differences for obsessive-compulsive and schizoid personality disorders. On the other hand, a different distribution was found between the sexes as concerns self-defeating personality disorder and antisocial personality disorders. A significantly higher proportion of fulfilled criteria for self-defeating personality disorder were obtained by women, while men had a higher proportion of fulfilled criteria for antisocial personality disorder.

Thus, the most robust finding was for borderline personality disorder. It has been suggested that clinicians might be overdiagnosing this disorder in women.[42] An earlier contrast analysis indicated that studies using semistruc-

tured interviews obtained a significantly higher percentage of women with borderline personality disorder than did studies using an unstructured interview.[43] In our study, a self-report questionnaire was used and thus the subjects' answers could not be biased by an interviewer. When the different criteria for borderline personality disorder were analysed, it was found that men had a significantly higher proportion of fulfilled criteria as concerns suicidal behaviour and feelings of emptiness, while women scored higher on unstable relationships, affective instability, anger or lack of control, and frantic efforts to avoid abandonment.

Diagnoses of antisocial personality disorder have been documented as being more common among men in a long series of studies.[33–36] We were unable to find significant sex differences on a categorical level for antisocial personality disorder, probably due to the small number of individuals with the disorder in the sample.[41] Dimensional differences between sexes were reflected in six criteria before the age of 15 years and four criteria after the age of 15 years; all were fulfilled in a higher proportion by men than by women. The separate criteria were: often to initiate physical fights, engage in physical cruelty against animals, deliberately destroy others' property, deliberately engage in firesetting, lie often, and steal. Furthermore, males were more prone to be irritable and aggressive, repeatedly fail to honour financial obligations, fail to plan ahead, and be reckless regarding their own personal safety.

The study reinforced the impressions from previous smaller studies that there are true sex differences concerning some personality disorders. However, when self-report questionnaires are used, the sex differences seem to be less pronounced than earlier reported. Thus it is possible that some of the sex differences earlier reported are artefacts, introduced by means of observer bias.

Sex differences in the prevalence of personality disorders in DSM-IV and ICD-10

The DSM-IV and ICD-10 Personality Questionnaire (DIP-Q)[31] have been constructed to measure self-evaluated personality disorder characteristics. In a validation study, agreement was tested between the DIP-Q and a structured clinical interview (the DSM-IV and ICD-10 Personality Interview (DIP-I)).[32] In total, 126 psychiatric patients were interviewed by means of this structured interview. The series comprised 71 females and 55 males. The sex differences as concerns the prevalence of personality disorders as well as the number of fulfilled criteria for separate personality disorders are presented in Tables 23.3 and 23.4.

In the DSM-IV system, the antisocial personality disorder was significantly more common among males, while the borderline personality disorder was significantly more common among females. In the same way, dissocial personality disorder was significantly more common in males, and unstable borderline personality disorder and unstable impulsive personality disorder were more common in females in the ICD-10 system (Table 23.3).

When the number of fulfilled criteria for the separate personality disorders were considered, antisocial/dissocial personality disorders were more common in males, and borderline, unstable borderline and unstable impulsive personality disorders were more common in females, in the same way as when the categorical diagnoses were considered. However, the female patients also fulfilled significantly more criteria for the dependent personality disorder in both the DSM-IV and the ICD-10 systems (Table 23.4).

The results are mainly in accordance with the opinions presented in the Manual of the DSM-IV. In the Manual, it is concluded that certain personality disorders (e.g. antisocial personality disorder) are diagnosed more frequently in men, while others (e.g. borderline, histrionic and dependent personality disorders) are diagnosed more frequently in women. It is also concluded that although these differences in prevalence probably reflect true gender differences, clinicians must be careful not to overdiagnose certain personality disorders in females because of social stereotypes concerning typical gender roles and behaviours.

Table 23.3 Prevalence and gender distribution of personality disorders among 71 female and 55 male psychiatric patients diagnosed with a structured clinical interview (DIP-I).

	DSM-IV				ICD-10			
	n	Male	Female	χ^2	*n*	Male	Female	χ^2
Paranoid	28	12 (22%)	16 (23%)	0.01	27	14 (25%)	13 (18%)	0.94
Schizotypal	12	4 (7%)	8 (11%)	0.57	17	7 (13%)	10 (14%)	0.05
Schizoid	6	3 (5%)	3 (4%)	0.10	21	10 (18%)	11 (15%)	0.16
Antisocial/Dissocial	11	9 (16%)	2 (3%)	7.14**	10	9 (16%)	1 (1%)	9.50**
Borderline	41	12 (22%)	29 (41%)	5.11*				
Unstable borderline					33	8 (15%)	25 (35%)	6.85**
Unstable impulsive					22	5 (9%)	17 (24%)	4.74*
Narcissistic	6	4 (7%)	2 (3%)	1.36				
Histrionic	7	1 (2%)	6 (8%)	2.60	8	2 (4%)	6 (8%)	1.21
Avoidant/anxious	45	17 (31%)	28 (39%)	0.98	41	17 (31%)	24 (34%)	0.12
Obsessive–compulsive anancastic	34	15 (27%)	19 (27%)	0.00	35	15 (27%)	20 (25%)	0.01
Dependent	13	3 (6%)	10 (14%)	2.50	16	4 (7%)	12 (17%)	2.59

* $P < 0.05$, ** $P < 0.01$.

Comorbidity between personality disorders and mood disorders

Studies reporting the prevalence of personality disorders in depressed patients generally suggest a 20–50% comorbidity rate in inpatients and a 50–85% comorbidity rate in outpatients.[44] There are several possible explanations for this high comorbidity:[45–48]

1. The personality disorder predisposes the person to depressive reactions.
2. The personality disorder may be a complication of a depressive disorder or result from it.
3. The personality disorder is an attenuated or alternative expression of the disease process which underlies the depressive disorder.
4. Both diagnoses may be independent manifestations of a common third factor.

Table 23.4 Number of fulfilled criteria of personality disorders among 71 female and 55 male psychiatric patients diagnosed with a structured clinical interview (DIP-I).

	DSM-IV					ICD-10				
	Sex				Frequency	Sex				Frequency
	Male		Female			Male		Female		
	Mean	SD	Mean	SD		Mean	SD	Mean	SD	
Paranoid	1.9	1.8	2.1	1.8	0.54	1.9	1.7	2.1	1.5	0.20
Schizotypal	1.8	2.0	1.9	1.7	0.11	1.6	1.9	1.8	1.6	0.43
Schizoid	1.4	1.7	1.1	1.4	1.36	1.8	1.9	1.0	1.8	0.31
Antisocial/dissocial	1.4	1.7	0.4	0.7	18.8***	0.9	1.4	0.4	0.7	8.39**
Borderline	2.3	2.3	3.7	2.8	9.06**					
Unstable Borderline						1.0	1.3	1.8	1.6	8.99**
Unstable Impulsive						1.4	1.4	2.1	1.7	5.06*
Narcissistic	1.4	1.7	1.4	1.4	0.03					
Histrionic	1.3	1.4	1.7	1.8	1.43	1.0	1.1	1.3	1.4	1.59
Avoidant/anxious	2.3	2.5	2.9	2.4	2.00	2.2	2.1	2.6	1.9	1.32
Obsessive–compulsive anancastic	2.1	1.8	2.5	1.7	1.40	2.3	1.8	2.6	1.9	0.75
Dependent	1.3	1.6	2.1	2.1	5.85*	1.1	1.4	1.8	1.8	5.59*

$* P < 0.05$, $** P < 0.01$, $*** P < 0.001$ (one way ANOVA).

5. The personality disorder contributes to the occurrence of events in life that often result from a depressive disorder.
6. The disorders are independent entities, but are frequently observed as occurring together, as they are both common.
7. The comorbidity of personality disorder and depression is largely an artefact of overlapping diagnostic criteria.

It has been pointed out that shared symptoms between borderline personality disorder and depression have resulted in inherent difficulties in evaluating the relationships between these disorders. Some theorists have argued that depression in patients with borderline personality disorder is qualitatively distinct from depression in non-borderline patients. There are also results in favour of such a hypothesis.[49]

Table 23.5 Frequency of personality disorders according to SCID screen questionnaire with adjusted cut-off in depressed outpatients treated by general practitioners, divided according to sex, N = 400.[51]

	Males $n = 112$	Females $n = 288$		
Paranoid	35 (31.3%)	78 (27.1%)	$\chi^2 = 0.69$	NS
Schizotypal	6 (5.4%)	5 (1.7%)	$\chi^2 = 3.95$	$P < 0.05$
Schizoid	4 (3.6%)	4 (1.4%)	$\chi^2 = 1.96$	NS
Cluster A	39 (34.8%)	82 (28.5%)	$\chi^2 = 1.54$	NS
Histrionic	8 (7.1%)	17 (5.9%)	$\chi^2 = 0.21$	NS
Narcissistic	28 (25.0%)	29 (10.1%)	$\chi^2 = 14.71$	$P < 0.0001$
Borderline	21 (18.8%)	61 (21.2%)	$\chi^2 = 0.29$	NS
Cluster B	38 (33.9%)	81 (28.1%)	$\chi^2 = 1.30$	NS
Avoidant	48 (42.9%)	103 (35.8%)	$\chi^2 = 1.73$	NS
Dependent	27 (24.1%)	50 (17.4%)	$\chi^2 = 2.36$	NS
Obsessive–compulsive	28 (25.0%)	69 (24.0%)	$\chi^2 = 0.05$	NS
Passive–aggressive	25 (22.3%)	22 (7.6%)	$\chi^2 = 16.77$	$P < 0.0001$
Cluster C	63 (56.3%)	145 (50.3%)	$\chi^2 = 1.13$	NS
Any personality disorder	76 (67.9%)	113 (60.1%)	$\chi^2 = 2.08$	NS

NS, not significant.

Depression associated with borderline personality disorder pathology appears to be in some respects unique, as well as distinct from non-borderline depression.

Substantial covariation has also been observed between individual borderline personality disorder items and dysthymia symptoms. In a study by Trull and Widiger,[50] four borderline personality disorder items (affective instability, suicidal threats/gestures/behaviour/ self-mutilating behaviour, chronic feelings of emptiness/boredom, and frantic attempts to avoid real/imagined abandonment) were significantly associated with both the number of dysthymia symptoms and a diagnosis of dysthymia.

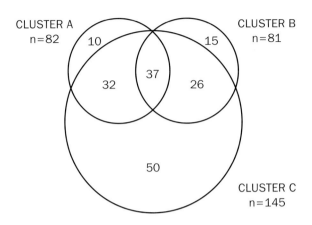

CLUSTER A
n=82

CLUSTER B
n=81

CLUSTER C
n=145

Figure 23.1 Comorbidity between personality disorders in female depressed outpatients (*N* = 288).[51]

In a large series of depressed outpatients treated by general practitioners, examined by Ekselius et al,[51] it could be demonstrated that 60% of the depressed females had a personality disorder (Table 23.5). The most common personality disorders were within cluster C, (50%) while clusters A and B were about equally common, 29% versus 28%, respectively.

Most of the personality disorders were equally common in males and females. However, schizotypal, narcissistic and passive-aggressive personality disorders were significantly more frequently diagnosed in males than in females (Table 23.5). We also found a very high comorbidity between personality disorders, as well as between the separate personality disorder clusters (Figure 23.1).

In a later study (Ekselius et al, unpublished work), depressed outpatients seen by psychiatrists were examined. The frequencies of personality disorders were even higher in this population (Table 23.6). Sixty-seven per cent of the female depressed patients seen by the psychiatrists had a personality disorder. However, also in this sample the frequencies of personality disorders were about as high in the males as in the females (Table 23.6).

Sex differences in precipitating life events

By means of a new scale, the Scale for Stressful Life Events (SSLE), it has been demonstrated[52] that women tend to perceive most stressful life events as more distressing than men, particularly regarding events implicating aggression and withdrawal. It is reasonable to believe that events of this kind have a more negative impact on women than on men. Thus, as effects of sex and culture on the experience of life events cannot be ignored, it is possible that these differences may also explain the sex differences in the prevalence of personality disorders.

In a study by Perris[53] it was hypothesized that women would need fewer stressful life events to develop a depression. The assumption was tested in a series of 204 consecutively admitted depressed patients, 77 men and 127 women, treated as in- or outpatients at the Department of Psychiatry, Umeå University. The results did not support the hypothesis that a lower number of events could be expected in women. In fact, there were no significant differences in the mean number of events experienced by patients of the two sexes in the different periods preceding the onset of depression. On the other hand, a closer analysis of the types of life event experienced by the patients revealed that significantly more events independent of depression had occurred in female than in male patients in the year preceding the onset of the depression.

Table 23.6 Frequency of personality disorders in depressed outpatients treated within general psychiatry, divided according to sex, $N = 290$ (Ekselius et al, unpublished work).

	Males $n = 93$	Females $n = 197$		
Paranoid	26 (28.0%)	52 (26.4%)	$\chi^2 = 0.08$	NS
Schizotypal	1 (1.1%)	10 (5.1%)	$\chi^2 = 2.77$	NS
Schizoid	1 (1.1%)	5 (2.5%)	$\chi^2 = 0.67$	NS
Cluster A	27 (29.0%)	59 (30.0%)	$\chi^2 = 0.03$	NS
Histrionic	8 (8.6%)	10 (5.1%)	$\chi^2 = 1.35$	NS
Narcissistic	14 (15.1%)	29 (14.7%)	$\chi^2 = 0.01$	NS
Borderline	23 (24.7%)	55 (27.9%)	$\chi^2 = 0.33$	NS
Cluster B	27 (29.0%)	73 (37.1%)	$\chi^2 = 1.80$	NS
Avoidant	32 (34.1%)	81 (41.1%)	$\chi^2 = 1.20$	NS
Dependent	24 (25.8%)	40 (20.3%)	$\chi^2 = 1.11$	NS
Obsessive–compulsive	35 (37.6%)	44 (22.3%)	$\chi^2 = 7.46$	$P < 0.01$
Passive–aggressive	20 (21.5%)	20 (10.2%)	$\chi^2 = 6.85$	$P < 0.01$
Cluster C	55 (59.1%)	103 (52.3%)	$\chi^2 = 1.20$	NS
Any personality disorder	59 (63.4%)	132 (67.0%)	$\chi^2 = 0.36$	NS

NS, not significant.

Treatment outcome in mood disorders with a comorbid personality disorder

Personality disorders, regardless of subtype, have been found to be significantly related to poor outcome, regardless of treatment, in a wide range of psychiatric disorders, especially in patients with major depression, panic disorders and obsessive-compulsive disorder.[14,15] However, an increasing number of studies are showing that the presence of a personality disorder does not impair clinical outcomes of specific treatments.[54–56] For example, Fava et al[55] reported a better response to treatment with the selective serotonin reuptake inhibitor (SSRI), fluoxetine, in their depressive patients with a coexisting cluster B personality disorder.

In a recent study[51] (Ekselius et al, unpublished work), where depressed outpatients were treated with the SSRIs sertraline or citalopram in a double-blind randomized trial, no differences in depression score reduction were found between patients with a personality disorder and patients without a personality disorder. It was also demonstrated that treatment of women with either of the two SSRIs reduced the number of fulfilled criteria for most of the separate personality disorders (Figure 23.2). Patients participating in the study did not receive any other systematic treatment for

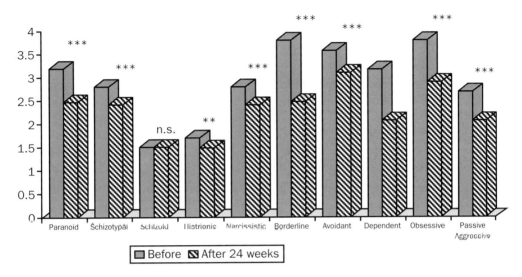

Figure 23.2 Changes in number of fulfilled criteria for separate personality disorders in depressed females treated with sertraline or citalopram in a double-blind randomized trial. No significant differences were seen between the effects of the two drugs. Significant changes from before to after treatment, t-test for dependent samples, ** $P < 0.01$, ***$P < 0.001$.[51]

depression. Investigators were asked to follow National Institute of Mental Health (NIMH) study guidelines. These included instructions, education and information about the illness and the medication, but no systematic psychotherapy.

It can, of course, be questioned as to what extent the changes in depressive symptomatology may have been of importance in the diminishing frequency of fulfilled criteria for separate personality disorders. However, in a series of stepwise multiple regressions, it was demonstrated that the changes in depressive symptomatology never explained more than 10% of the observed changes in the number of fulfilled personality disorder criteria.

In an earlier study by Perris et al,[57] it was demonstrated that personality traits as determined by means of the Karolinska Scales of Personality (KSP) were fairly stable when investigated during depression and after recovery. At that time, the patients were predominantly treated with tricyclic antidepressants or electroconvulsive therapy (ECT). However, in the present series,[51] when the patients were treated with SSRIs (sertraline or citalopram) (Figure 23.3), significant changes were seen in most of the scales of the KSP. Thus, it seems reasonable to believe that the SSRIs have an effect on symptoms attributed to personality disorders, such as 'affective instability', 'irritability' and so on.

Conclusions

It has been suggested[24] that there may be a sex bias in the diagnostic criteria or in the methods used for diagnosing personality disorders. In particular, the discussion has focused on biased

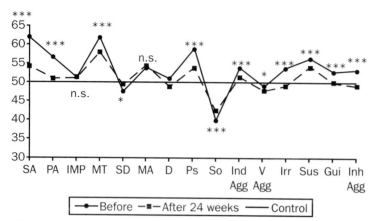

Figure 23.3 Changes in personality traits determined by means of the Karolinska Scales of Personality (KSP) in female depressed outpatients treated for 24 weeks with sertraline or citalopram. No significant differences between the two treatment groups, t-test for dependent samples, * $P < 0.05$, ***$P < 0.001$.[51]

SA, somatic anxiety; PA, psychic anxiety; IMP, impulsiveness; MT, muscular tension; SD, social desirability; MA, monotony avoidance; D, detachment; Ps, psychosthenia; So, socialization; Ind Agg, indirect aggression; V Agg, verbal aggression; Irr, irritability; Sus, suspicion; Gui, guilt; Inh Agg, inhibition of aggression.

diagnostic constructs, biased application of diagnostic criteria, biased assessment instruments, biased thresholds for diagnosis and biased diagnostic criteria. The criticism has been taken into account and several changes have been made in the diagnostic criteria from DSM-III[1] to DSM-III-R[25] and DSM-IV.[2] However, there are still unsolved questions.

In the DSM classification system, sex differences are suggested in the prevalence of certain personality disorders. In particular, DSM-IV[2] postulates that antisocial personality disorder is diagnosed more frequently in men, and that borderline, histrionic and dependent personality disorders are diagnosed more frequently in women.

In our own study,[41] fewer sex differences were found than those postulated by the authors of DSM-III/DSM-III-R/DSM-IV. We were only able to demonstrate significant sex differences on a categorical level as concerns

obsessive-compulsive personality disorder, borderline personality disorder and schizoid personality disorder. When sex differences were analysed dimensionally, borderline personality disorder still showed differences between sexes, while there were no differences for obsessive-compulsive and schizoid personality disorders. On the other hand, a different distribution was found between the sexes as concerns self-defeating personality disorder and antisocial personality disorder. A significantly higher proportion of fulfilled criteria for self-defeating personality disorder was obtained by women, while men had a higher proportion of fulfilled criteria for antisocial personality disorder. The study reinforced the impressions from previous smaller studies that there are true sex differences concerning some personality disorders. However, when self-report questionnaires are used, the sex differences seem to be less pronounced. Thus it is possible that some of the sex differences earlier reported are artefacts, introduced by means of observer bias.

In a later study,[32] a structured clinical interview (DIP-I) was used. In the DSM-IV system, the antisocial personality disorder was significantly more common among males, while the borderline personality disorder was significantly more common among females. In the same way, dissocial personality disorder was significantly more common in males, and unstable borderline personality disorder and unstable impulsive personality disorder were more common in females in the ICD-10 system. When the numbers of fulfilled criteria for the separate personality disorders were considered, antisocial/dissocial personality disorders were more common in males, and borderline, unstable borderline and unstable impulsive personality disorders were more common in females, in the same way as when the categorical diagnoses were considered. However, the female patients also fulfilled significantly more criteria for the dependent personality disorder, in both the DSM-IV and ICD-10 systems.

Thus, some sex differences in the presence of personality disorders seem to exist either when self-report questionnaires or structured clinical interviews are used and regardless of whether the DSM-III, the DSM-III-R, the DSM-IV or the ICD-10 criteria are used.

Studies reporting the prevalence of personality disorders in depressed patients generally suggest a 20–50% comorbidity rate in inpatients and a 50–85% comorbidity rate in outpatients.[44] In a large series of depressed outpatients studied by Ekselius et al,[51] it could be demonstrated that 60% of the depressed females had a personality disorder. The most common personality disorders were within cluster C (50%), while clusters A and B were about equally common, 29% versus 28%, respectively. In a later study (Ekselius et al, unpublished work), depressed outpatients seen by psychiatrists were examined. The frequencies of personality disorders were even higher in this population. Sixty-seven per cent of the female depressed patients seen by the psychiatrists had a personality disorder.

In a study by Caballo and Cardena,[52] it was demonstrated that women tend to perceive most stressful life events as more distressing than men. Thus, as effects of sex and culture on the experience of life events cannot be ignored, it is possible that differences of this kind may explain why sex differences are sometimes found in the frequencies of personality disorders.

Personality disorders, regardless of subtype, have been found to be significantly related to poor outcome, regardless of treatment, in a wide range of psychiatric disorders.[14,15] However, an increasing number of studies are showing that the presence of a personality disorder does not impair clinical outcomes of specific treatments.[54,56] For example, Fava et al[55] reported a better response to treatment with the SSRI fluoxetine in their depressive patients with a coexisting cluster B personality disorder. In a recent study,[51] where depressed outpatients were treated with the SSRIs sertraline or citalopram in a double-blind randomized trial, no differences in depression score reduction were found between patients with a personality disorder and patients without a personality disorder. It was also demonstrated that treatment of women with either of the two SSRIs reduced the number of fulfilled criteria for most of the separate personality disorders. Thus, it is possible that the SSRIs might also be useful when the patients have a comorbid personality disorder combined with a depressive disorder. It is also possible that the SSRIs have a beneficial effect on symptoms attributed to personality disorders, such as 'affective instability', 'irritability' and so on.

References

1. American Psychiatric Association, *Diagnostic and Statistical Manual of Mental Disorders*, 3rd edn (APA: Washington DC, 1980).

2. American Psychiatric Association, *Diagnostic and Statistical Manual of Mental Disorders*, 4th edn (APA: Washington DC, 1994) 629–74.

3. WHO, *International Statistical Classification of Diseases and Related Health Problems*, 10th revision, ICD-10 (World Health Organization: Geneva, 1992) 357–69.

4. WHO, *The ICD-10 Classification of Mental and Behavioural Disorders. Diagnostic Criteria for Research* (World Health Organization: Geneva, 1993) 123–39.

5. Maier W, Lichtermann D, Klinger T, Heun R, Prevalences of personality disorders (DSM-III-R) in the community, *J Pers Disord* 1992; **6:** 187–96.

6. Zimmerman M, Coryell WH, Diagnosing personality disorders in the community. A comparison of self-report and interview measures. *Arch Gen Psychiatry* 1990; **47:**527–31.

7. Reich J, Yates W, Nduaguba M, Prevalence of DSM-III personality disorders in the community, *Soc Psychiatr Epidemiol* 1989; **24:**12–16.

8. Bodlund O, Ekselius L, Lindström E, Personality traits and disorders among psychiatric outpatients and normal subjects on the basis of the SCID screen questionnaire, *Nord J Psychiatry* 1993; **47:**425–33.

9. Alnaes R, Torgersen S, DSM-III symptom disorders (Axis I) and personality disorders (Axis II) in an outpatient population, *Acta Psychiatr Scand* 1988; **78:**348–55.

10. Kullgren G, Personality disorders among psychiatric inpatients, *Nord J Psychiatry* 1992; **46:**27–32.

11. Kass F, Skodol AE, Charles E et al, Scaled ratings of DSM-III personality disorders, *Am J Psychiatry* 1985; **142:**627–30.

12. Reich J, Sex distribution of DSM-III personality disorders in psychiatric outpatients, *Am J Psychiatry* 1987; **144:**485–8.

13. Ekselius L, *Personality Disorders in the DSM-III-R* (Uppsala University, Faculty of Medicine: Uppsala, 1994).

14. Reich JH, Green AI, Effect of personality disorders on outcome of treatment, *J Nerv Ment Dis* 1991; **179:**74–82.

15. Reich JH, Vasile RG, Effect of personality disorders on the treatment outcome of axis I conditions: an update, *J Nerv Ment Dis* 1993; **181:**475–84.

16. Sato T, Sakado K, Sato S, Is there any specific personality disorder or personality disorder cluster that worsens the short-term treatment outcome of major depression? *Acta Psychiatr Scand* 1993; **88:**342–9.

17. McGlashan TH, The borderline syndrome. II. Is it a variant of schizophrenia or affective disorder? *Arch Gen Psychiatry* 1983; **40:** 1319–23.

18. Costa PT, McCrae RR, Personality disorders and five factormodels of personality, *J Pers Disord* 1990; **4:**362–71.

19. Eysenck HJ, Wakefield JA Jr, Friedman AF, Diagnosis and clinical assessment: the DSM-III, *Annu Rev Psychol* 1983; **34:**167–93.

20. Ekselius L, Lindström E, von Knorring L et al, Personality disorders in DSM-III-R as categorical or dimensional, *Acta Psychiatr Scand* 1993; **88:**183–7.

21. Ekselius L, Lindström E, von Knorring L et al, A principal component analysis of the DSM-III-R Axis II personality disorders, *J Pers Disord* 1994; **8:**140–8.

22. Gunderson JG, Links PS, Reich JH, Competing models of personality disorders, *J Pers Disord* 1991; **5:**60–8.

23. Fabrega H Jr, Mezzich J, Ulrich R, Benjamin L, Females and males in an intake psychiatric setting, *Psychiatry* 1990; **53:**1–16.

24. Funtowicz MN, Widiger TA, Sex bias in the diagnosis of personality disorders. A different approach, *J Psychopathol Behav Assess* 1995; **17:**145–65.

25. American Psychiatric Association, *Diagnostic and Statistical Manual of Mental Disorders*, 3rd edn revised (APA: Washington DC, 1987) 335–58.

26. Skodol AE, Spitzer RL, The development of reliable diagnostic criteria in psychiatry, *Annu Rev Med* 1982; **33:**317–26.

27. Perry JC, Problems and considerations in the valid assessment of personality disorders, *Am J Psychiatry* 1992; **149:**1645–53.

28. Spitzer RL, Psychiatric diagnosis: are clinicians still necessary? *Comp Psychiatry* 1983; **24:** 399–411.

29. Ekselius L, Lindström E, von Knorring L et al, Comorbidity among the personality disorders in the DSM-III-R. *Pers Individ Diff* 1994; 17:155–60.

30. Spitzer RL, Williams JBW, Gibbon M, *Structured Clinical Interview for DSM-III-R Personality Disorders (SCID-II)* (New York State Psychiatric Institute, Biometrics Research: New York, 1987).

31. Ottosson H, Bodlund O, Ekselius L et al, The DSM-IV and ICD-10 personality questionnaire (DIP-QW): construction and preliminary validation, *Nord J Psychiatry* 1995; **49:**285–91.

32. Ottosson H, Bodlund O, Ekselius L et al, DSM-IV and ICD-10 Personality Disorders: a comparison of a self-report questionnaire (DIP-Q) with a structured interview, *Eur Psychiatry* 1998; 13:246–53.

33. Robins LN, Helzer JE, Weissman MM et al, Lifetime prevalence of specific psychiatric disorders in three sites, *Arch Gen Psychiatry* 1984; **41:**949–58.

34. Dahl AA, Some aspects of DSM-III personality disorders illustrated by a consecutive sample of hospitalized patients, *Acta Psychiatr Scand (Suppl)* 1986; **328:**61–7.

35. Kass F, Spitzer RL, Williams JBW, An empirical study of the issue of sex bias in the diagnostic criteria of DSM-III Axis II personality disorders, *Am Psychologist* 1983; **38:**799–803.

36. Golomb M, Fava M, Abraham M, Rosenbaum JF, Gender differences in personality disorders, *Am J Psychiatry* 1995; **152:**579–82.

37. Weissman MM, The epidemiology of personality disorders: a 1990 update, *J Pers Disord* 1993; 7(suppl 1):44–62.

38. Nestadt G, Romanoski AJ, Brown CH et al, DSM-III compulsive personality disorder: an epidemiological survey, *Psychol Med* 1991; 21:461–71.

39. Swartz M, Blazer D, George L, Winfield I, Estimating the prevalence of borderline personality disorder in the community, *J Pers Disord* 1990; 4:257–72.

40. Nestadt G, Romanoski AJ, Cahal R et al, An epidemiological study of histrionic personality disorder, *Psychol Med* 1990; **20:**413–22.

41. Ekselius L, Bodlund O, von Knorring L et al, Sex differences in DSM-III-R, Axis II personality disorders, *Pers Individ Diff* 1996; **20:** 457–61.

42. Henry KA, Cohen CI, The role of labeling processes in diagnosing borderline personality disorder, *Am J Psychiatry* 1983; **140:**1527–9.

43. Widiger TA, Trull JT, Borderline and narcissistic personality disorders. In: Sutker PB, Adams HE, eds, *Comprehensive Handbook of Psychopathology*, 2nd edn (Plenum Press: New York, 1993) 371–94.

44. Corruble E, Ginestet D, Guelfi JD, Comorbidity of personality disorders and unipolar major depression: a review, *J Affect Disord* 1996; 37:157–70.

45. Akiskal HS, Hirschfeld, RM, Yerevanian BI, The relationship of personality to affective disorders, *Arch Gen Psychiatry* 1983; **40:**801–10.

46. Docherty JP, Fiester SJ, Shea T, Syndrome diagnosis and personality disorder, *Am Psychiatr Assoc Annu Rev* 1986; **5:**315–55.

47. Gunderson JG, Elliott GR, The interface between borderline personality disorder and affective disorder, *Am J Psychiatry* 1985; **142:**277–88.

48. Widiger TA, The categorical distinction between personality and affective disorders, *J Pers Disord* 1989; **3:**77–91.

49. Rogers JH, Widiger TA, Krupp A, Aspects of depression associated with borderline personality disorder, *Am J Psychiatry* 1995; **152:** 268–70.

50. Trull TJ, Widiger TA, The relationship between borderline personality disorder criteria and dysthymia symptoms, *J Psychopathol Behav Assess* 1991; **13:**91–105.

51. Ekselius L, von Knorring L, Eberhard G, A double-blind multicenter trial comparing sertraline and citalopram in patients with major depression treated in general practice, *Int J Clin Psychopharmacol* 1997; **12:**323–31.

52. Caballo VE, Cardena E, Sex differences in the perception of stressful life events in a Spanish sample: some implications for the Axis IV of the DSM-IV, *Pers Individ Diff* 1997; **23:**353–9.

53. Perris H, *A Multifactorial Study of Life Events in Depressed Patients*, Umeå University Medical Dissertations, New series No. 78 (Umeå University: Umeå, 1982).

54. Patience DA, McGuire RJ, Scott AI, Freeman CP, The Edinburgh primary care depression study: personality disorder and outcome, *Br J Psychiatry* 1995; **167**:324–30.

55. Fava M, Bouffides E, Pava JA et al, Personality disorder comorbidity with major depression and response to fluoxetine treatment, *Psychother Psychosom* 1994; **62**:160–7.

56. Fava M, Uebelacker LA, Alpert JE et al, Major depressive subtypes and treatment response, *Biol Psychiatry* 1997; **42**:568–76.

57. Perris C, Eisemann M, Eriksson U et al, Variations in self-assessment of personality characteristics in depressed patients, with special reference to aspects of aggression, *Psychiatr Clin* 1979; **12**:209–15.

24

Anorexia nervosa and bulimia nervosa

Claire V Wiseman, Suzanne R Sunday, Leslie Born and Katherine A Halmi

Introduction

Eating disorders is a general term that usually refers to anorexia nervosa and bulimia nervosa. The former was first called *anorexia hysterique* by Lasegue in 1873.[1] He conceptualized the illness as an extreme loss of weight resulting from emotional difficulties, intra-psychic turmoil and disturbed relationships. The connection between mood disturbances and anorexia has been noted by numerous twentieth-century researchers.[2] Similarly, when bulimia was first described in the third edition of the *Diagnostic and Statistical Manual of Mental Disorders* (DSM-III),[3] one of the main diagnostic criteria was depressed mood following binge-eating episodes. Clearly, mood disturbances have been a significant component of eating disorders since they were initially described; eating disorders are frequently comorbid with other psychiatric (axis I and axis II) disorders. Over the past two decades, these behavioural syndromes have been the object of numerous systematic studies. Anorexia nervosa and bulimia nervosa are best understood using a multidimensional model which encompasses medical, psychological, and socio-cultural factors. This chapter will present an overview of these eating disorders, with particular attention to gender differences in epidemiology, comorbidity, and clinical management strategies.

Clinical description

Anorexia nervosa

Anorexia nervosa (AN) is a disorder that is characterized by severe weight loss (a loss of 15% or more from expected weight), intense fear of weight gain, severely disturbed body image and, in women, amenorrhoea for a period of at least 3 consecutive months or, in prepubertal girls, primary amenorrhoea. These four diagnostic criteria, which appear in the fourth edition of the *Diagnostic and Statistical Manual of Mental Disorders* (DSM-IV),[4] stem directly from the original three core features of anorexia first described by Russell and Beardwood in 1970.[5] More than 90% of cases occur in females.[4]

Intense fear of weight gain is at times difficult to understand in the face of the anorectic's intense denial of such fear. This fear, however, may be most evident as the anorectic recovers and begins to gain weight. The fear is at times so intense that the anorectic may be in emotional distress for hours after discovering a slight weight increase.

Anorectics have a severe disturbance in the way that they experience their bodies and cannot see themselves as they truly are. When looking at themselves in the mirror, they will focus on specific parts of their bodies and find them disproportionately large. This distorted image produces much distress and, in turn, has undue influence upon the individual's self-evaluation. The anorectic will deny the level of seriousness of the extremely low weight. Accompanying the distorted body image is an obsessional style of thinking about weight and shape. Preoccupation with food that might lead to weight gain is common.

There are two distinct types of anorexia nervosa: restricting and binge-eating/purging types. The restricting anorectic (AN-R) simply reduces intake of food to an extremely low caloric intake which leads to the severe reduction in weight. The AN-R may also engage in excessive amounts of exercise which contribute to the weight loss. The binge-eating/purging type (AN-BP) binges and purges but remains extremely underweight; AN-BP behaviour is similar to bulimic behaviour described in the following section.

The medical consequences of AN can be severe and life-threatening. It is important to mention a few of the more extreme problems associated with the weight loss and malnutrition. Anorectics are at risk for cardiac arrest resulting from electrolyte disturbances, especially if they purge. The starvation state produces endocrine aberrations which may reinforce the dieting behaviour.[6] The decreased oestrogen secretion contributes to early-onset osteoporosis.[5] The most severe complication of AN is death, which occurs in approximately 7.4% of diagnosed cases according to a 10-year follow-up study;[7] 15–30 years following diagnosis, this rate climbs to 15–18%.[8]

Bulimia nervosa

As with AN, more than 90% of those with bulimia nervosa (BN) are female.[4] BN patients, however, are not extremely underweight and are within 10–15% of the normal weight range for their height. The bulimic will engage in discrete eating episodes in which they will consume considerably more food than would be considered normal for that situation. This large amount of food is consumed in a relatively short amount of time (e.g. 2 h). Finally, the episode of overeating is 'out of control' meaning that the person cannot or does not feel as though they can stop eating or prevent the binge from occurring altogether. The binge episode usually causes distress. Critical to the diagnosis of BN is the compensatory behaviour that follows a binge-eating episode; this may include one or more of self-induced vomiting, laxative abuse, diuretic abuse, diet medications, fasting or extremely vigorous exercise.

The bulimic will generally participate in purging behaviours shortly after the binge-eating episode. The bulimic may go to extremes in order to induce purging by using ipecac. Taking large doses of the laxatives or diuretics is also a common occurrence. To meet DSM-IV criteria for a diagnosis of BN, the binge-eating and purging behaviours must occur on average at least two times a week for a period of 3 months.[4]

In addition to the pattern of bingeing and purging, bulimics place great emphasis on their body shape and weight[9] for assessing their self-worth. Similar to anorectics, bulimics become distraught when seeing their bodies in the mirror, and they may also distort their body image towards a heavier and more distasteful shape.

There are two subtypes of BN: purging and non-purging types. The bulimic who engages in the purging behaviour (vomiting, laxative abuse, diuretic abuse) on a regular basis is considered to be a purging type (BN-P). The bulimic who fasts or over-exercises but does not engage in any purging behaviours in order to compensate for the overeating episode is considered to be a non-purging type (BN-NP).

The BN-P and the AN-BP types are also at risk for significant medical complications from repeated purging. These may include increased risk of dental cavities due to enamel erosion on the teeth from vomiting, swollen parotid glands and tears in the oesophagus.[10] The vomiting and overuse of laxatives can lead to gastric complications, as well as a dependence on laxatives. The bulimic is also at risk for cardiac arrest from electrolyte imbalance or from high levels of ipecac if the latter substance is used to initiate vomiting. A crude mortality rate for BN is 2.4%.[7]

Epidemiology

In the past 30 years, eating disorders have become a significant health problem. Apart from those women who meet criteria for AN or BN, countless others suffer from one or more of the numerous symptoms of eating disorders without actually meeting criteria for a full diagnosis. In addition, changes in diagnostic criteria and the number of cases each year which are not formally assessed make it difficult to determine the exact numbers of people suffering from eating disorders.

Incidence

Despite difficulties with diagnosis and identification, there is significant evidence of a sharp rise in the number of cases of AN in the past 50 years. A recent study showed a six-fold increase of anorexia between 1965 and 1991 in Scotland.[11] Other studies have shown that the incidence of eating disorders increased during 1960–69 and 1970–76 in females 15–24 years of age.[12]

Using primary care visits as a method of determining incidence, recent studies have demonstrated that the incidence of AN in The Netherlands increased from 6.3 to 8.1 per year per 100 000 population between 1985 and 1989 (with the highest incidence for females in the 15–19 age group: 79.6 per year per 100 000 females).[13,14] A large-scale community survey in London found that the 1-year prevalence of AN among females aged 15–29 was 19.2 cases per 100 000 (0.1%).[15]

Bulimia was only identified as a specific disorder in 1979.[16] Unfortunately, there are few studies on the incidence of bulimia. Hoek found the incidence of bulimia in The Netherlands to be 9.9 per year per 100 000 population during 1985–86;[13] during 1985–89, the incidence increased to 11.5 per year per 100 000 population (with the highest incidence rate in females in the 20–24 age group: 82.1 per year per 100 000 females).[14]

Gender differences

Overall, eating disorders are fairly rare among males.[17] In general, in community-based samples, the literature supports a 5–10% prevalence rate of males among those with anorexia[18] and a 10–15% rate of males among those with bulimia.[19]

A community sample of US high school students found that 32.1% of the females compared with 22.8% of the males were at risk for eating disorders.[20] One possible explanation for relatively high levels of risk but low levels of illness among males is that women are under extreme pressure to achieve a thin ideal, which is not as true for males. Another explanation is that women have increased feelings of depression (29%) following a binge and males do not.[21]

Clinically, there is little difference in the presentation of symptoms between the male and the female anorectics. Men and women share features, including age of onset, dieting method, attitudes about the eating disorder, rates of comorbid diagnoses, and body dissatisfaction.[22–24]

There is some controversy concerning possible differences in age of onset of eating disorder and dieting methods used. While some did not find such differences,[22] others reported that males had a later onset than females and were less likely to use diet pills as a weight loss strategy.[23] In a recent Australian study, the differences in incidence of eating disorders between sexes were largely accounted for by the high rates of earlier dieting and psychiatric morbidity in females.[25]

Andersen and Holman[17] have noted that with the influence of social learning, gender differences concerning body shape usually emerge between the third and sixth grades: girls direct their (critical) attention to the lower body, while males focus on their upper body. Further, males use dieting to achieve specific external goals[17] such as performance in a sport or occupation which requires weight control,[23] or in potentially high-risk occupations such as modelling or acting, jobs traditionally held by women, or food-related jobs.[24] In addition, Carlat et al[24] found that 42% of the male bulimic patients were either homosexual or bisexual and 58% of the anorectic males were asexual.

Men were found to seek out treatment less often than women.[22] This may contribute, in part, to the documented low rate of eating disorders in males. Thus, the less severe cases of eating disorders in men may go undetected.

The impact of pregnancy on BN has been prospectively studied, and, in general, bulimic symptoms improved throughout pregnancy; following parturition, however, recurrence of bulimic symptoms and significant risk for postnatal depression were observed.[26]

Precipitating factors

The aetiology of AN and BN is not yet fully understood, but is likely to be due to multiple factors. The overarching precipitant of eating disorders is some form of dieting behaviour.[27] Other risk factors may include cultural factors, socio-economic status and age, biological vulnerability, and family issues.[28,29] Some societal pressures may be inescapable and therefore may always exert an influence on women. Interestingly, millions of people are continually exposed to negative images regarding diet and body ideals in the media, yet few develop eating disorders. A possible explanation for this may lie in the influence of other precipitating factors, including biological vulnerability (e.g. genetic factors), as well as developmental, personality, family and environmental factors. In a recent comparative study using female subjects, investigators found that premorbid perfectionism and negative self-evaluation distinguished eating disorder cases from general psychiatric controls; in addition, the subjects with BN had a significantly earlier menarche and greater exposure to parental obesity than the other groups.[30] Previous episode(s) of AN are significantly more frequent among BN-NP than among BN-P patients.[31]

Biological markers

While a detailed description of the biological factors underlying eating disorders is beyond the scope of this chapter, a number of review articles have been written on this topic.[32–36]

Abnormalities have been reported—for both anorectics and bulimics—in neurotransmitters, neuropeptides, metabolism, the hypothalamic–pituitary–adrenal axis, the hypothalamic–pituitary–gonadal axis, and growth hormone. Thus far, these abnormalities have not been found to be primary aetiological factors in eating disorders, but rather there is some evidence to suggest that some (e.g. growth hormone) may contribute to the course and maintenance of the illness.[36]

Few studies have measured these hormones in recovered eating disorder patients. Halmi et al[37] found normal follicle-stimulating hormone (FSH) and luteinizing hormone (LH) responses to gonadotropin-releasing hormone at a 10-year follow-up of anorectics, regardless of current menstrual status. Cerebrospinal fluid (CSF) corticotrophin-releasing hormone levels were correlated with depression in weight-restored, but not in emaciated, anorectic patients.[38]

In another recent study, investigators found that 13 of 15 children and adolescents with AN showed reduced regional cerebral bloodflow; this abnormality persisted after weight restoration, suggesting an underlying biological substrate.[39]

Of the neurotransmitters, serotonin has been studied more extensively in eating disorders. Evidence for the role of serotonin stems from multiple lines of investigation and, in general, suggests central serotonin (5-HT) system dysregulation. Elevated concentrations of CSF 5-hydroxyindoleacetic acid (5-HIAA) have been found in recovered AN and BN women; this suggests an association with the cluster of behaviours typically found in recovered AN and BN women (i.e. obsessions with order and symmetry, perfectionism, and negative affect).[40] Clinically recovered women with BN experienced relapse of bulimic symptoms (lowering of mood, increases in body image concern, loss of control of eating) following acute dietary tryptophan depletion, suggesting that diminished 5-HT activity may trigger some of the cognitive and mood disturbances associated with BN.[41] There is accumulating evidence of the efficacy of the selective serotonin reuptake inhibitors (SSRIs) in the treatment of eating disorder symptomatology (BN; AN after weight restoration) and in significantly reducing the high rate of relapse normally seen in AN,[42] further endorsing disturbance of 5-HT activity.

Genetic factors

The investigation of the role of genetic factors in eating disorders is hampered by the difficulties in conducting prospective studies. Because of the relatively low incidence of eating disorders, genetic–family studies require multicentre collaborations. Nonetheless, there seem to be significant genetic factors that influence the onset of the disorders. In one study, there was a significantly higher rate of concordance for AN-R among monozygotic twins (66%) than dizygotic twins (10%).[43] Similarly, a higher rate of concordance for bulimia has been found among monozygotic twins (83%) as compared with dizygotic twins (26.7%).[44] In a recent, controlled family study (n = 458) using direct interviews, a very strong familial aggregation of a broad spectrum of eating disorders was found among female (and very few male) relatives of women with BN: 43% of the sisters and 26% of the mothers of BN probands had a lifetime diagnosis of eating disorder, most often the 'not otherwise specified' type.[45]

Family environment

There may be some influence from the family environment on the development and/or maintenance of eating disorders. In a review of the literature, eating-disordered patients had families that were less cohesive, less expressive, in greater conflict, emphasizing control, and placing more focus on achievement compared with families of healthy controls.[20,46]

Social attitudes

In the past 30 years, significant evidence has accumulated concerning societal pressures for a thin body type as the standard of beauty.[47,48] This pursuit of thinness transcends cultures within the westernized world. Several studies have shown that people who have moved to a Western culture from a non-Western culture tended to have higher rates of eating disorders compared to those in their homeland. For example, Fichter et al[49] found that twice the number of girls from Greece and Turkey had eating disorders if they were living in Germany than those who lived in either Turkey or Greece.

Comorbidity

Clinicians have long recognized that AN and BN rarely present without other comorbid psychiatric problems. Researchers have been systematically investigating such comorbidity for the past 10–15 years. Most studies are in agreement that there is considerable evidence of a significant comorbidity among eating disorder patients, especially major depression, and anxiety disorders. The emaciated or malnourished state has been discussed as leading to depression and anxiety, but several studies have demonstrated that there is significant lifetime comorbidity which cannot be accounted for by weight and nutritional status.

Braun et al[50] found that 81.9% of their inpatient anorectic and bulimic patients had another axis I diagnosis which was not accounted for by their eating disorder. Halmi et al[2] reported high levels of comorbidity during a 10-year period following treatment for

AN. In fact, 65% of these patients had lifetime diagnoses of anxiety disorders and 68% had major depression. Two-thirds of the bulimic sample was found to have had another axis I disorder which pre-dated the bulimia.

The high rate of comorbidity will probably influence the presentation of the eating disorder and will need to be considered in treatment. For example, Heebink et al,[51] in a study of 250 female inpatients with AN or BN, found that severity of depressive and anxiety symptoms was associated with eating disorder type *and* age of onset: less severe mood symptomatology was seen in patients younger than age 14 with AN-R.

Axis I comorbidity

Mood disorders

Affective disorder, particularly major depression, is the most commonly occurring comorbid diagnosis for both anorectics and bulimics. Several carefully conducted studies have documented this using structured clinical interviews. For example, Braun et al,[50] using the Structured Clinical Interview for DSM-III-R (SCID), reported that 62.9% of their eating disorder sample had an affective disorder and 50.5% had major depression. Other studies have documented similar rates of between 43% and 55% of eating disorder comorbid with major depression.[52,53]

The relationship between affective disorders and eating disorders is not completely understood. Affective disorders can occur prior to,[50] during or after the onset of an eating disorder.[2,50] Since few studies have focused on chronology, it remains to be seen if the order of comorbidity affects clinical presentation or treatment response in these patients. In a recent review of the literature on depression and eating disorders, Casper[54] has suggested that—in spite of the high frequency of depressive disorders (in particular major depression and dysthymia) with eating disorders—the evidence to date for a shared aetiology is sparse.

Both current and lifetime diagnoses of affective disorders (major depression, bipolar and dysthymic disorders) were found to strongly influence the severity of the eating disorder symptomatology and of general psychiatric symptoms in bulimic patients, while borderline personality traits had little influence.[55] Patients with a current or past history of an affective disorder displayed greater levels of psychopathology, including general psychiatric symptoms such as anxiety, ineffectiveness, and interpersonal distrust, as well as symptoms more specific to eating disorders, such as body dissatisfaction and interoceptive awareness. These findings emphasize the importance of assessing affective history when assessing the severity of all eating disorder symptoms.

Differences between anorectic and bulimic patients have been reported with respect to comorbid affective disorders. AN-R patients had lower rates of affective disorders than other eating disorder patients, whereas AN-BP patients and bulimics with a past history of anorexia had the highest incidence of major depression.[50] Other researchers have reported similar findings.[56,57] Dancyger et al[58] used the Minnesota Multiphasic Personality Inventory (MMPI) and the Beck Depression Inventory (BDI) as indicators of psychopathology and showed that the AN-R patients had lower ratings compared to the other eating disorder subgroups. Overall, the AN-R patients in this study were less depressed, immature, impulsive and anxious than bulimics, and most of the differences in MMPI scores between the eating disorder groups (AN-R, AN-BP and BN) were dependent upon the patient's level of depression rather than their eating disorder subtype.

Just as high levels of affective disorders have been found in patients with eating disorders, patients diagnosed primarily with a mood disorder have higher than expected rates of eating disorders. In a recent study, Gruber et al[59] found that 25.5% of those meeting criteria for seasonal affective disorder also had a comorbid eating disorder.

Anxiety disorders

Higher rates of anxiety disorders have also been reported among patients with AN or BN. Toner et al[60] found rates of 60% for comorbid anxiety disorders and, more specifically, 29% for comorbid social phobia. Halmi et al[2] reported that 34% of the AN patients followed for 10 years after eating disorder treatment had social phobia, and 26% met criteria for obsessive-compulsive disorder (OCD). In a subsequent study, OCD and social phobia were also found to be frequent comorbid disorders, although less frequently in AN-R patients.[50] In contrast to these data, Lilenfeld et al[53] found that 31% of AN-R patients and 15% of the bulimics had a history of social phobia, and 62% of the AN-R and 21% of the BN patients had a history of OCD. A high rate of current post-traumatic stress disorder (PTSD) symptomatology has also been documented in women with eating disorders (AN, BN, eating disorders not otherwise specified); the severity of the PTSD symptoms was significantly associated with depression, anxiety, and dissociative experiences, but were not related to either the type or the severity of eating disorder.[61]

In the Braun et al[50] study, while less than 3% of AN-R patients had social phobia, 14% of AN-BP and 20% of BN patients had social phobia. These levels of social phobia far exceed those found in the general population[62] or in psychiatric control subjects.[2] For most of the patients in the Braun et al[50] study, the social phobia preceded the eating disorder. These results are consistent with other findings.[62,63] It may be that early onset of social phobia is a risk factor for developing bulimia. Lilenfeld et al[64] separated their bulimic subjects into those with and without lifetime alcohol or substance dependence: social phobia was found almost exclusively in those with comorbid substance dependence (30% versus 4% respectively).

Many of the obsessional and compulsive symptoms of eating disorders appear to be similar to those of the thoughts and behaviours of OCD. For example, the eating disorder patients' obsessive thinking about their body weight and shape or the fat content of food, the compulsive need to chew each mouthful of food a certain number of times or to count calories, and the bingeing and purging rituals, all seem reminiscent of OCD.[65,66] However, these are actually core eating disorder symptoms and are not associated with OCD. Additionally, few patients with eating disorders view such thoughts and behaviours as excessive or nonsensical. The extreme ego syntonicity of these OCD-like symptoms distinguish the eating disorders from OCD.

Comorbid OCD is quite common in patients with eating disorders. For example, Braun et al[50] reported that 20% of AN-R, 18% of AN-BP and 16% of BN patients met criteria for OCD. Thornton and Russell,[67] on the other hand, found comorbid OCD in 37% of the anorectics (subtype was unspecified) but only in 3% of their bulimic patients. Kaye et al[68] also found high rates of obsessive-compulsive behaviours in anorectic patients using the Yale–Brown Obsessive-Compulsive Scale (Y-BOCS). They reported that all of their 19 patients endorsed individual obsessive and/or compulsive symptoms (excluding all eating disorder-related symptoms), and that their Y-BOCS scores were similar to those of OCD patients; the extent and type of the OCD symptoms were unrelated to current weight or nutritional state. A subsequent study found that while OCD patients endorsed a wide variety of obsessions and compulsions, anorectics tended to endorse symptoms that were related to symmetry and order.[69]

Such high levels of comorbidity have led some researchers to even suggest that eating disorders may be a form of OCD.[70] However, most researchers believe that the two are distinct, but often comorbid, and may share a common aetiology or neurochemical deficit. For example, Hsu et al[71] have suggested that serotonergic deficits underlie both disorders.

Others have suggested a relationship between the severity of the eating disorder and the number of OCD symptoms.[72] For patients with comorbidity, the more symptomatic they are with respect to their eating disorder, the more OCD symptoms they demonstrate. Our group has found that eating disorder patients with comorbid OCD and/or comorbid depression displayed higher levels of eating disorder severity (Halmi and Sunday, unpublished data). Pollice et al[73] found that elevated scores on the Y-BOCS for underweight anorectics (a mix of AN-R and AN-BP patients) did not significantly decline after a short-term partial weight restoration and were significantly higher than those of long-term recovered AN patients.

Finally, a history of AN has been reported at a higher than expected rate of up to 13% among female OCD patients;[74,75] interestingly, prevalence rates for AN were slightly—albeit not significantly—higher for the male versus the female OCD patients.[76]

Substance abuse and dependency

Numerous studies have concluded that there is a significant relationship between eating disorders and substance abuse. Many authors suggest that the incidence of substance abuse is more prevalent among bulimics than among anorectics, people with other psychiatric disorders, or the general population. In a review of 51 studies,[77] it was found that about

20–25% of bulimic women had a history of alcohol or drug abuse. Braun et al[50] reported that 47% of their inpatient bulimics had a history of alcohol or substance dependency, while only 11.8% of their AN-R patients had such a history; similar findings have been reported by others.[53,78]

Conversely, Schuckit et al[79] examined over 3000 subjects with alcohol abuse or dependence and found a higher rate of bulimia than anorexia among this group; more specifically, they found that of those who met criteria for an eating disorder, 93% had BN. Goldbloom et al[80] found that 30.1% of those meeting criteria for alcoholism also had an eating disorder. This rate is higher than the norm for the population at large. A more recent study confirmed that a diagnosis of eating disorder seems to be more likely when a person has a substance use disorder.[81] Moreover, bulimic women who also had alcohol dependence had higher rates of depression, borderline personality disorder, theft and suicide attempts, and a faster progression of alcohol dependence from habitual to problem drinking, compared with women with only bulimia.[82–84] Likewise, Lilenfeld et al[64] found higher levels of social phobia, conduct disorder and personality disorders in bulimics with comorbid substance dependence than in bulimics with no substance dependence. In a comparative study of eating disorder subtypes, Deep et al[85] reported that 65% of their (all female) subjects with comorbid BN and substance dependence also had a history of sexual abuse.

Some differences in clinical presentation (symptoms, weight history, personality) may be observed if a comorbid diagnosis of substance dependence is made. For example, those diagnosed with alcohol dependence had a significantly higher weight history than bulimics not diagnosed with alcohol dependence.[86] Recent work by the authors[87] suggests that the impact of substance dependency in eating disorder patients may reflect, in part, the chronology of the disorders. Eating disorder patients who developed their eating disorder *before* their substance dependency had higher rates of social phobia and OCD than either eating disorder patients with no substance dependency or those whose substance dependency predated their eating disorder.

Schizophrenia and other psychotic disorders

To date, there is little literature on concurrent eating disorder and psychotic illness. Hugo and Lacey[88] described four case studies of women (aged 17–26), two with transient psychotic illness and a history of eating disorder, and two with the diagnosis of schizophrenia in conjunction with an eating disorder. In all cases, improvement in eating precipitated or exacerbated the psychotic symptoms, suggesting that the eating disorder serves as a defence against psychosis.

Axis II comorbidity: Personality disorders

The studies on personality disorders are somewhat controversial, and incidence varies greatly between studies. For example, the prevalence of personality disorders in BN patients ranges from 28% to 77%[64,89,90] and in anorectics from 23% to 80%.[56,90] Methodological limitations of these studies include small numbers of subjects and differences in methods of diagnosing personality disorder.

Among studies which used more rigorous diagnostic procedures (e.g. the SCID), several patterns of personality disorders have emerged among eating disorder subgroups.[91] For example, Braun et al[50] found significantly higher levels of histrionic, narcissistic, antisocial and especially borderline (known as 'Cluster B') personality disorder in bulimic subgroups than in AN-R patients; 25% of BN and AN-BP but none of the AN-R patients met criteria for borderline personality disorder. Further, the presence of a personality disorder was associated with lower overall functioning and greater chronicity of the eating disorder.[92]

Avoidant, dependent, passive-aggressive, obsessive-compulsive (known as 'Cluster C') personality disorders were common in all eating disorder subgroups, with nearly 30% of patients having a personality disorder within this cluster.[50] Herzog et al[57] found high rates of Cluster C personality disorders only in AN subjects but not in bulimics. Some researchers have recently reported higher levels of obsessive-compulsive personality disorder in anorectic subjects than in bulimic subjects.[53,67]

The risk factors for comorbid personality disorder and eating disorder are not yet known. For example, we do not know if having an eating disorder makes one more likely to develop a personality disorder, or vice versa. Prospective studies may answer this question.

Treatment

Of considerable importance in the treatment of eating disorders is simultaneous treatment of the comorbid diagnosis. Treating an eating disorder alone might temporarily alleviate the symptoms, but there is a risk of relapse if the comorbid illness is ignored. As assessed in a prospective, large-scale, longitudinal study, approximately one-third of both women with AN and women with BN relapse after full recovery, yet no significant predictors of relapse emerged.[93] Facilitating detailed assessment of both eating disorders and general psychopathology, the Structured Interview for Anorexic and Bulimic Disorders (SIAB) has been recently modified—incorporating the diagnostic criteria of both DSM-IV[4] and ICD-10.[94,95]

The primary and most successful treatment, cognitive-behavioural therapy (CBT), has been adapted from the treatment of depression. Most of the pharmacological treatments are also adapted from treatments for other disorders such as depression or OCD. The goals of treating the eating disorder patient are: (1) to re-establish and maintain a weight within a normal range for height; (2) to eliminate any bulimic and compensatory behaviours such as purging or over-exercise; (3) to establish a reasonable nutritional meal schedule; and (4) to re-establish a non-distorted body image consistent with reality.

The current consensus is that the best way to achieve these goals is to use a multidimensional treatment programme. The degree of intensity of the programme varies, based on the level of acuity of the individual. In general, the criterion for inpatient treatment is the presence of a dangerous and unstable medical condition. In anorectic patients, this is often a weight 20% or more below the expected weight.

Multidimensional treatment includes the following: a cognitive behavioural-based therapy, medical management (including medications as needed) and nutritional counselling. Family counselling in patients aged 18 and under is essential. This combination of treatment can be offered on an outpatient, day hospital or inpatient basis, the level of care depending on acuity. Medical monitoring is of particular importance in both the inpatient and outpatient settings. Treatment should be conducted by an experienced team, which may consist of a psychiatrist, an internist, a psychologist or social worker skilled in cognitive therapy or CBT, and a nutritionist. For all levels of care, the therapy will follow the same basic pattern.

Psychotherapy

The original form of CBT was designed by

Beck et al[96] for depression. Its basic premise is that people have automatic thoughts, cognitive distortions and underlying assumptions which shape the emotional and behavioural reactions of the individual. CBT uses a variety of techniques designed to increase awareness and ultimately change the undesired emotions or behaviours.

For anorectic patients, the therapy combines cognitive therapy as first adapted for eating disorders by Garner and Bemis[97] and behavioural interventions designed to normalize weight and eating. An outpatient programme utilizing CBT for AN has been developed, with foci on confronting fears and avoidance behaviours, and developing new problem-solving skills.[98] CBT can help to increase the patient's understanding and awareness of how thinking contributes to the eating disorder and provides tools with which to change distorted thoughts. Examples of distorted thinking include: all-or-none thinking, catastrophic thinking, and judgmental thinking. The therapist utilizes cognitive restructuring to change these distorted thoughts. For the extremely low-weight anorectic, weight restoration is critical and is the initial focus of inpatient treatment. To date, however, there is only limited evidence of the efficacy of CBT for AN.[99]

For bulimic patients, on the other hand, manual-based CBT[100] is the first-line treatment of choice.[99] The therapist can target both eating and depressive symptoms at the same time. The behavioural component is designed to break the pattern of bingeing and purging. Some of the techniques include: food records, thought records, and regular meals. Several CBT protocols include a more didactic component in order to eliminate the ever-present myths about dieting and weight loss.

A recent study has shown that frequency of bingeing at baseline and higher (character) self-directedness are associated with a rapid (eight sessions) and sustained response (abstinence from bingeing and purging for 1 year following treatment) to CBT for BN.[101] Despite the demonstrated benefits of CBT, in a recent telephone survey investigators found that the bulk (96.7%) of eating disorder patients ($n = 581$) had received some type of psychotherapy, but rarely CBT (6.9%).[102]

For both anorectic and bulimic patients, eating regular meals is critical. Depending on admission weight, the anorectic might benefit from a supplemental diet in order to restore weight. For extremely underweight anorectics, weight restoration is initially achieved through supplemental liquid feedings with a progression towards eating of meals of regular food. Following weight restoration, the anorectic would be on a similar plan as the bulimic, eating planned and nutritionally balanced meals, and then practising choosing their own foods in order to maintain a weight within the normal range.

Pharmacotherapy

As with many psychiatric disorders, there is growing evidence that pharmacotherapy can be effectively used in conjunction with CBT.[103] The medications used to treat the eating disorder are also, in many cases, effective ways to treat the underlying comorbid psychopathology.

Anorexia nervosa

Because of the high levels of comorbidity between AN, depression and OCD, antidepressants are frequently used. To date, however, there have been relatively few randomized controlled studies of psychotropic medication for AN, as well as few longer-term follow-up studies. Tricyclic antidepressants have been reported to have mixed results in the treatment of depression and eating disorders. In a double-blind placebo-controlled study ($n = 16$), clomipramine was significantly associated with increased hunger, appetite and energy intake; moreover, clomipramine was associated with more stable appetite and better weight maintenance following the trial end.[104] Yet, in a 5-week double-blind placebo-controlled study ($n = 43$) comparing amitriptyline, placebo, and psychosocial treatment, all three groups manifested little benefit from treatment.[105] Cyproheptadine, a 5-HT antagonist, was found to have significant benefit in reducing depressive symptoms while promoting weight gain in AN-R patients.[106]

There is some evidence from two open trials that the SSRI fluoxetine[107,108] may promote weight gain and maintenance of body weight, reduce AN and depressive symptomatology, and significantly lower the rate of relapse. It must be emphasized that fluoxetine has been found to be most effective *following* weight restoration.[38,41] In a recent 7-week controlled trial ($n = 31$), in which fluoxetine (60 mg/day) was initiated when subjects had reached 65% of their ideal body weight and maintained this weight until the end of the trial, researchers found no significant differences in clinical outcome measures between the fluoxetine and placebo groups.[109] Investigators also found little difference in post-hospital course and outcome (remaining at target weight, eating disorder symptomatology, mood ratings) between patients receiving adjunctive fluoxetine (initiated 1 month after hospital intake and continued for 24 months after discharge; maximum dose 60 mg/day) and a historical control group.[110]

Of the other medications, lithium has been found to reduce depressive symptoms but to have little effect on weight gain.[111] Of significant concern are the risks inherent in the use of lithium: it is not recommended for use with people who are already dehydrated or who are purging, because of the risk of sudden toxicity.

Bulimia nervosa

For bulimia, antidepressants in general have been found to be moderately effective. Over a dozen double-blind, placebo-controlled trials of various antidepressants have been conducted with bulimic patients.[41] In almost all of these studies, antidepressant therapy was associated with reduced eating disorder symptoms (such as bingeing frequency, preoccupations with weight, shape, and food) as well as improved mood. These findings are especially important given the high degree of comorbidity of depression with eating disorders. However, the majority of patients have not shown long-term decreases in bingeing frequency.

The most promising findings to date have been those involving the SSRIs such as fluoxetine. The therapeutic benefit of fluoxetine (60-mg dose) has been demonstrated in 8-week and 16-week large-scale, multicentre, double-blind placebo-controlled studies.[112,113] The fluoxetine groups demonstrated significant decreases in vomiting and binge-eating episodes per week; in addition, these subjects also experienced greater rates of improvement and a higher percentage experienced remission. Fluvoxamine has also been shown to have a significant effect compared with placebo in relapse prevention (in particular, severity of illness and obsessive-compulsive symptoms) following inpatient behavioural psychotherapy treatment for BN.[114]

SSRIs have also been used effectively in OCD patients,[71] so the use of these medications in the treatment of eating disorders appears to be highly advantageous not only for treating the depression and OCD but also for reducing the core eating disorder behaviours and psychopathology.

Conclusion

Eating disorders are complex disorders that have high comorbidity with mood and anxiety disorders. There is accumulating evidence from both twin and family studies of eating disorders that AN and BN are independently transmitted familial liabilities with a unique pathophysiology.[115] These findings, in turn, will contribute to new, more specific treatment strategies for AN and BN. At present, the treatments of choice for eating disorders and many of the comorbid disorders are one and the

same. CBT alone or in combination with antidepressant medications—especially the SSRIs—has been shown to be effective for treating BN, as well as the frequent comorbid conditions. To date, there is limited evidence of the efficacy of these treatments for AN. Further investigation of treatment strategies to reduce longer-term risk of relapse and recurrence of these disorders is required.

References

1. Bell RM, *Holy Anorexia* (University of Chicago Press: Chicago, 1985) 7.
2. Halmi KA, Eckert E, Marchi P et al, Comorbidity of psychiatric diagnoses in anorexia nervosa, *Arch Gen Psychiatry* 1991; **48**:712–18.
3. American Psychiatric Association, *Diagnostic and Statistical Manual of Mental Disorders*, 3rd edn (American Psychiatric Association Press: Washington, DC, 1980) 67–71.
4. American Psychiatric Association, *Diagnostic and Statistical Manual of Mental Disorders*, 4th edn (American Psychiatric Association Press: Washington, DC, 1994) 539–45.
5. Russell GM, Beardwood C, Amenorrhea in the feeding disorders: anorexia nervosa and obesity, *Psychother Psychosom* 1970; **18**:358–64.
6. Newman MM, Halmi KA, The endocrinology of anorexia nervosa and bulimia nervosa, *Endocrinol Metab Clin North Am* 1988; **17**:195–212.
7. Crow S, Praus B, Thuras P, Mortality from eating disorders: a 5- to 10-year record linkage study, *Int J Eat Disord* 1999; **26**:97–101.
8. Theander S, Outcome and prognosis in anorexia nervosa and bulimia: some results of previous investigations, compared with those of a Swedish long-term study, *J Psychiatr Res* 1985; **19**:493–508.
9. Wilson GT, Smith D, Assessment of bulimia nervosa: an evaluation of the eating disorders examination, *Int J Eat Disord* 1989; **8**:173–9.
10. Halmi KA, Eating disorders: anorexia nervosa, bulimia nervosa, and obesity. In: Hales

KE, Yudofsky SC, Talbott J, eds, *American Psychiatric Press Textbook of Psychiatry*, 2nd edn (American Psychiatric Association Press: Washington, DC, 1997) 857–75.
11. Eagles JM, Johnston MI, Hunter D et al, Increasing incidence of anorexia nervosa in the female population of northeast Scotland, *Am J Psychiatry* 1995; **152**:1266–71.
12. Jones DJ, Fox MM, Babigian HM, Hutton HE, Epidemiology of anorexia nervosa in Monroe County, New York: 1960–1976, *Psychosom Med* 1980; **42**:551–8.
13. Hoek HW, The incidence and prevalence of anorexia nervosa and bulimia nervosa in primary care, *Psychol Med* 1991; **21**:455–60.
14. Hoek HW, Bartelds AIM, Bosveld JJF et al, Impact of urbanization on detection rates of eating disorders, *Am J Psychiatry* 1995; **152**:1272–8.
15. Rooney B, McClelland L, Crisp AH, Sedgewick PM, The incidence and prevalence of anorexia nervosa in three suburban health districts in South West London, UK, *Int J Eat Disord* 1995; **18**:299–307.
16. Russell GM, Bulimia nervosa: an ominous variant of anorexia nervosa, *Psychol Med* 1979; **9**:429–48.
17. Andersen AE, Holman JE, Males with eating disorders: challenges for treatment and research, *Psychopharmacol Bull* 1997; **33**: 391–7.
18. Sharp CW, Clark SA, Dunan JR et al, Clinical presentation of anorexia nervosa in males: 24 new cases, *Int J Eat Disord* 1994; **15**:125–34.
19. Garfinkel P, Goering L, Spegg C et al, Bulimia

nervosa in a Canadian community sample: prevalence and comparison of subgroups, *Am J Psychiatry* 1995; **52**:1052–8.

20. Felker KR, Stivers C, The relationship of gender and family environment to eating disorder risk in adolescents, *Adolescence* 1994; **29**: 821–34.

21. Hawkings R, Clement P, Development and construct validation of a self-report measure of binge-eating tendencies, *Addict Behav* 1980; **7**:435–9.

22. Olivardia R, Pope HG, Mangweth B, Hudson JI, Eating disorders in college men, *Am J Psychiatry* 1995; **152**:1279–85.

23. Braun DL, Sunday SR, Huang A, Halmi KA, More males seek treatment for eating disorders, *Int J Eat Disord* 1999; **25**:415–24.

24. Carlat DJ, Camargo CA, Herzog DB, Eating disorders in males: a report on 135 patients, *Am J Psychiatry* 1997; **154**:1127–32.

25. Geist R, Heinmaa M, Katzman D, Stephens D, A comparison of male and female adolescents referred to an eating disorder program, *Can J Psychiatry* 1999; **44**:374–8.

26. Morgan JF, Lacey JH, Sedgwick PM, Impact of pregnancy on bulimia nervosa, *Br J Psychiatry* 1999; **174**:135–40.

27. Patton GC, Selzer R, Coffey C et al, Onset of adolescent eating disorders: population based cohort study over 3 years, *Br Med J* 1999; **318**:765–8.

28. Striegel-Moore RH, Silberstein LR, Rodin J, Toward an understanding of risk factors for bulimia, *Am Psychol* 1986; **41**:246–63.

29. Halmi KA, Eating disorder research in the past decade, *Ann NY Acad Sci* 1996; **789**:67–77.

30. Fairburn CG, Cooper Z, Doll HA, Welch SL, Risk factors for anorexia nervosa: three integrated case-control comparisons, *Arch Gen Psychiatry* 1999; **56**:468–76.

31. Santonastaso P, Ferrara S, Favaro A, Differences between binge eating disorder and nonpurging bulimia nervosa, *Int J Eat Disord* 1999; **25**:215–18.

32. Heebink DM, Halmi KA, Eating disorders. In: Gorman J, ed., *Annual Review of Psychiatry*, Vol. 13 (APPI Press: Washington, DC, 1994) 227–51.

33. Mauri MC, Rudelli R, Somaschini E et al, Neurobiological and psychopharmacological basis in the therapy of bulimia and anorexia, *Prog Neuropsychopharmacol Biol Psychiatry* 1996; **20**:207–40.

34. Ericsson M, Poston WS 2nd, Foreyt JP, Common biological pathways in eating disorders and obesity, *Addict Behav* 1996; **21**: 733–43.

35. Davis C, Eating disorders and hyperactivity: a psychobiological perspective, *Can J Psychiatry* 1997; **42**:168–75.

36. Stoving RK, Hangaard J, Hansen-Nord M, Hagen C, A review of endocrine changes in anorexia nervosa, *J Psychiatr Res* 1999; **33**: 139–52.

37. Halmi KA, Stokes P, Eckert E, Sunday S, FSH and LH responses to GnRH in anorexia nervosa patients at a ten-year follow-up, *Biol Psychiatry* 1991; **2**:305–7.

38. Kaye WH, Gwirtsman HE, George DT et al, Elevated cerebrospinal fluid levels of immunoreactive corticotropin-releasing hormone in anorexia nervosa: relation to state of nutrition, adrenal function, and intensity of depression, *J Clin Endocrinol Metab* 1987; **64**:203–8.

39. Gordon I, Lask B, Bryant-Waugh R et al, Childhood-onset anorexia nervosa: towards identifying a biological substrate, *Int J Eat Disord* 1997; **22**:159–65.

40. Kaye W, Gendall K, Strober M, Serotonin neuronal function and selective serotonin reuptake inhibitor treatment in anorexia and bulimia nervosa, *Biol Psychiatry* 1998; **44**: 825–38.

41. Smith KA, Fairburn CG, Cowen PJ, Symptomatic relapse in bulimia nervosa following acute tryptophan depletion, *Arch Gen Psychiatry* 1999; **56**:171–6.

42. Mayer LES, Walsh BT, The use of selective serotonin reuptake inhibitors in eating disorders, *J Clin Psychiatry* 1998; **59**:28–34.

43. Treasure J, Holland AJ, Genetic vulnerability to eating disorders: evidence from twin and family studies. In: Remschmidt H, Schmidt MH, eds, *Child and Youth Psychiatry: European Perspectives* (Hogrefe and Hubert: New York, 1989) 59–68.

44. Fichter MN, Noegel R, Concordance for bulimia nervosa in twins, *Int J Eat Disord*

1990; **9:**255–63.

45. Stein D, Lilenfeld LR, Plotnicov K et al, Familial aggregation of eating disorders: results from a controlled family study of bulimia nervosa, *Int J Eat Disord* 1999; **26:**211–15.

46. Strober M, Humphrey LL, Familial contributions to the etiology and course of anorexia nervosa and bulimia, *J Consult Clin Psychol* 1987; **55:**654–9.

47. Garner DM, Garfinkel PE, Schwartz D, Thompson M, Cultural expectations of thinness in women, *Psychol Rep* 1980; **47:** 483–91.

48. Wiseman CV, Gray J, Mosimann J, Ahrens A, Cultural expectations of thinness in women: an update, *Int J Eat Disord* 1992; **11:**85–9.

49. Fichter MM, Elton M, Sourdi L et al, Anorexia nervosa in Greek and Turkish adolescents, *Eur Arch Psychiatry Neurol Sci* 1988; **237:**200–8.

50. Braun DL, Sunday SR, Halmi KA, Psychiatric comorbidity in patients with eating disorders, *Psychol Med* 1994; **24:**859–67.

51. Heebink DM, Sunday SR, Halmi KA, Anorexia nervosa and bulimia nervosa in adolescence: effects of age and menstrual status on psychological variables, *J Am Acad Child Adolesc Psychiatry* 1995; **34:**378–82.

52. Kennedy SH, Kaplan AS, Garfinkel PE et al, Depression in anorexia nervosa and bulimia nervosa: discriminating depressive symptoms and episodes, *J Psychosom Res* 1994; **38:** 773–82.

53. Lilenfeld LR, Kaye WH, Greeno CG et al, A controlled family study of anorexia nervosa and bulimia nervosa, *Arch Gen Psychiatry* 1998; **55:**603–10.

54. Casper RC, Depression and eating disorders, *Depress Anxiety* 1998; **8:**96–104.

55. Sunday SR, Levey CM, Halmi KA, Effects of depression and borderline personality traits on psychological state and eating disorder symptomatology, *Comp Psychiatry* 1993; **34:**70–4.

56. Fornari V, Kaplan M, Sandberg DE et al, Depressive and anxiety disorders in anorexia nervosa and bulimia nervosa, *Int J Eat Disord* 1992; **12:**21–9.

57. Herzog DB, Keller MB, Lavori PW et al, The prevalence of personality disorders in 210

women with eating disorders, *J Clin Psychiatry* 1992; **48:**712–18.

58. Dancyger IF, Sunday SR, Halmi KA, Depression modulates non-eating disordered psychopathology in eating disordered patients, *Eat Disord: Treatment Prevention* 1997; **5:** 59–68.

59. Gruber NP, Dilsaver SC, Bulimia and anorexia nervosa in winter depression: lifetime rates in a clinical sample, *J Psychiatry Neurosci* 1996; **21:**9–12.

60. Toner BB, Garfinkel PE, Garner DM, Affective and anxiety disorders in the long-term follow-up of anorexia nervosa, *Int J Psychiatry Med* 1988; **18:**357–64.

61. Gleaves DH, Eberenz KP, May MC, Scope and significance of posttraumatic symptomatology among women hospitalized for an eating disorder, *Int J Eat Disord* 1998; **24:** 147–56.

62. Schneier FR, Johnson J, Hornig CD et al, Social phobia: comorbidity and morbidity in an epidemiologic sample, *Arch Gen Psychiatry* 1992; **49:**282–8.

63. Brewerton TD, Lydiard RB, Herzog DB et al, Comorbidity of axis I psychiatry disorders in bulimia nervosa, *J Clin Psychiatry* 1995; **56:**77–80.

64. Lilenfeld LR, Kaye WH, Greeno CG et al, Psychiatric disorders in women with bulimia nervosa and their first degree relatives: effects of comorbid substance dependence, *Int J Eat Disord* 1997; **22:**253–64.

65. Mazure CM, Halmi KA, Sunday SR et al, The Yale–Brown–Cornell Eating Disorder Scale: development, use, reliability, and validity, *J Psychiatry Res* 1994; **28:**425–45.

66. Sunday SR, Halmi KA, Einhorn A, The Yale–Brown–Cornell Eating Disorders Scale: a new scale to assess eating disorder symptomatology, *Int J Eat Disord* 1995; **18:**237–45.

67. Thornton C, Russell J, Obsessive compulsive comorbidity in the dieting disorders, *Int J Eat Disord* 1997; **21:**83–7.

68. Kaye WH, Weltzin TE, Hsu LKG et al, Patients with anorexia nervosa have elevated scores on the Yale–Brown Obsessive-Compulsive Scale, *Int J Eat Disord* 1992; **12:**57–62.

69. Bastiani AM, Altemus M, Pigott TA et al,

Comparison of obsessions and compulsions in patients with anorexia nervosa and obsessive compulsive disorder, *Biol Psychiatry* 1996; 39:966–9.

70. Rothenberg A, Eating disorder as a modern obsessive-compulsive syndrome, *Psychiatry* 1986; 49:45–53.

71. Hsu LKG, Kaye W, Weltzin T, Are the eating disorders related to obsessive compulsive disorder? *Int J Eat Disord* 1993; 14:305–18.

72. Thiel A, Broocks A, Ohlmeier M et al, Obsessive-compulsive disorder among patients with anorexia nervosa and bulimia nervosa, *Am J Psychiatry* 1995; 152:72–5.

73. Pollice C, Kaye WH, Greeno CG, Weltzin TE, Relationship of depression, anxiety, and obsessionality to state of illness in anorexia nervosa, *Int J Eat Disord* 1997; 21:367–76.

74. Kasvikis YG, Tsakiris F, Marks IM et al, Past history of anorexia nervosa in women with obsessive-compulsive disorder, *Int J Eat Disord* 1986; 6:1069–75.

75. Fahy TA, Osacar A, Marks I, History of eating disorders in female patients with obsessive-compulsive disorder, *Int J Eat Disord* 1993; 14:439–43.

76. Rubenstein CS, Pigott TA, L'Heureux F et al, A preliminary investigation of the lifetime prevalence of anorexia and bulimia nervosa in patients with obsessive-compulsive disorder, *J Clin Psychiatry* 1992; 53:309–14.

77. Holderness CC, Brooks-Gunn J, Warren MP, Comorbidity of eating disorders and substance abuse: review of the literature, *Int J Eat Disord* 1994; 16:1–34.

78. Bulik CM, Sullivan PF, Epstein LH et al, Characteristics of bulimic women with and without alcohol abuse, *Am J Drug Alcohol Abuse* 1992; 20:273–83.

79. Schuckit MA, Tipp JE, Anthenelli RM et al, Anorexia nervosa and bulimia nervosa in alcohol dependent men and women and their relatives, *Am J Psychiatry* 1996; 153:74–82.

80. Goldbloom DS, Naranjo CA, Bremner KE, Hicks LK, Eating disorders and alcohol abuse in women, *Br J Addictions* 1992; 87:913–19.

81. Grilo CM, Levy KN, Becker DF et al, Eating disorders in female inpatients with versus without substance use disorders, *Addictive Behav* 1995; 20:255–60.

82. Hatsukami D, Mitchell JE, Eckert ED, Pyle R, Characteristics of patients with bulimia only, bulimia with affective disorder, and bulimia with substance abuse problems, *Addictive Behav* 1986; 11:399–406.

83. Suzuki K, Higuchi S, Yamada K et al, Bulimia nervosa with and without alcoholism: a comparative study in Japan, *Int J Eat Disord* 1994; 16:137–46.

84. Suzuki K, Higuchi S, Yamada K et al, Young female alcoholics with and without eating disorders: a comparative study in Japan, *Am J Psychiatry* 1993; 150:1053–8.

85. Deep AL, Lilenfeld LR, Plotnicov KH et al, Sexual abuse in eating disorder subtypes and control women: the role of comorbid substance dependence in bulimia nervosa, *Int J Eat Disord* 1999; 25:1–10.

86. Bulik CM, Sullivan PF, McKee M et al, Characteristics of bulimic women with and without alcohol abuse, *Am J Drug Alcohol Abuse* 1994; 20:273–83.

87. Wiseman CV, Sunday SR, Halligan P et al, Substance dependence and eating disorders: impact of sequence and comorbidity, *Compr Psychiatry* 1999: 40:332–6.

88. Hugo PH, Lacey JH, Disordered eating: a defense against psychosis? *Int J Eat Disord* 1998; 24:329–33.

89. Powers PS, Coovert DL, Brightwell DR, Stevens BA, Other psychiatric disorders among bulimic patients, *Compr Psychiatry* 1988; 29:503–8.

90. Schmidt NB, Telch MJ, Prevalence of personality disorders among bulimics, nonbulimic binge eaters, and normal controls, *J Psychopathol Behav Assess* 1990; 12:170–85.

91. Wonderlich SA, Swift WJ, Slotnick HB, Goodman S, DSM-III-R personality disorders in eating-disorder subtypes, *Int J Eat Disord* 1990; 9:607–16.

92. Skodol AE, Oldham JM, Hyler SE et al, Comorbidity of DSM-III-R eating disorders and personality disorders, *Int J Eat Disord* 1993; 14:403–16.

93. Herzog DB, Dorer DJ, Keel PK et al, Recovery and relapse in anorexia and bulimia nervosa: a 7.5-year follow-up study, *J Am Acad Child Adolesc Psychiatry* 1999; 38:829–37.

94. World Health Organization, Mental, behav-

ioural and developmental disorders. In: *Tenth Revision of the International Classification of Diseases (ICD-10)* (WHO: Geneva, 1996).

95. Fichter MM, Herpertz S, Quadflieg N, Herpertz-Dahlmann B, Structured interview for anorexic and bulimic disorders for DSM-IV and ICD-10: updated (third) revision, *Int J Eat Disord* 1998; **24**:227–49.

96. Beck AT, Rush AJ, Shaw BF, Emery G, *Cognitive Therapy of Depression* (Guilford: New York, 1979).

97. Garner DM, Bemis KM, A cognitive-behavioral approach to anorexia nervosa, *Cognitive Ther Res* 1982; **6**:1223–50.

98. Kleifield EI, Wagner S, Halmi KA, Cognitive-behavioral treatment of anorexia nervosa, *Psychiatr Clin North Am* 1996; **19**:715–37.

99. Wilson GT, Cognitive behavior therapy for eating disorders: progress and problems, *Behav Res Ther* 1999; **37**:S79–95.

100. Fairburn CG, Marcus MD, Wilson GT, Cognitive-behavioral therapy for binge eating and bulimia nervosa: a comprehensive treatment manual. In: Fairburn CG, Wilson GT, eds, *Binge Eating: Nature, Assessment, and Treatment* (Guilford: New York, 1995) 270–86.

101. Bulik CM, Sullivan PF, Carter FA et al, Predictors of rapid and sustained response to cognitive-behavioral therapy for bulimia nervosa, *Int J Eat Disord* 1999; **26**:137–44.

102. Crow S, Mussell MP, Peterson C et al, Prior treatment received by patients with bulimia nervosa, *Int J Eat Disord* 1999; **25**:39–44.

103. Peterson CB, Mitchell JE, Psychosocial and pharmacological treatment of eating disorders: a review of research findings, *J Clin Psychol* 1999; **55**:685–97.

104. Lacey JH, Crisp AH, Hunger, food intake and weight: the impact of clomipramine on a refeeding anorexia nervosa population, *Postgrad Med J* 1980; **56**:79–85.

105. Biederman J, Herzog DB, Rivinus TM et al, Amytriptyline in the treatment of anorexia nervosa: a double-blind, placebo-controlled study, *J Clin Psychopharmacol* 1985;

5:10–16.

106. Halmi KA, Eckert E, LaDu TJ, Cohen J, Anorexia nervosa: treatment efficacy of cyproheptadine and amitriptyline, *Arch Gen Psychiatry* 1986; **43**:177–81.

107. Gwirtsman HE, Guze BH, Yager J, Gainsley B, Fluoxetine treatment of anorexia nervosa: an open trial, *J Clin Psychiatry* 1990; **51**:378–82.

108. Kaye WH, Weltzin TE, Hsu LG, Bulik CM, An open trial of fluoxetine in patients with anorexia nervosa, *J Clin Psychiatry* 1991; **52**:464–71.

109. Attia E, Haiman C, Walsh BT, Flater SR, Does fluoxetine augment the inpatient treatment of anorexia nervosa? *Am J Psychiatry* 1998; **155**:548–51.

110. Strober M, Freeman R, DeAntonio M et al, Does adjunctive fluoxetine influence the post-hospital course of restrictor-type anorexia nervosa? A 24-month prospective, longitudinal followup and comparison with historical controls, *Psychopharmacol Bull* 1997; **33**:425–31.

111. Gross HA, Ebert MH, Faben VB et al, A double-blind controlled trial of lithium carbonate in primary anorexia nervosa, *J Clin Psychopharmacol* 1981; **1**:376–81.

112. Fluoxetine Bulimia Nervosa Collaborative Study Group, Fluoxetine in the treatment of bulimia nervosa: a multicenter, placebo-controlled, double-blind trial, *Arch Gen Psychiatry* 1992; **49**:139–47.

113. Goldstein DJ, Wilson MG, Thompson VL et al, Long-term fluoxetine treatment of bulimia nervosa, *Br J Psychiatry* 1995; **166**:660–6.

114. Fichter MM, Leibl C, Kruger R, Reif W, Effects of fluvoxamine on depression, anxiety, and other areas of general psychopathology in bulimia nervosa, *Pharmacopsychiatry* 1997; **30**:85–92.

115. Kaye W, Strober M, Stein D, Gendell K, New directions in treatment research of anorexia and bulimia nervosa, *Biol Psychiatry* 1999; **45**:1285–92.

25

Obesity, weight gain and dieting
Judith J Wurtman

Background

Failure to maintain weight loss after successful dieting is so commonplace that it barely needs mention. In fact, it is so unusual that a study was recently published showing that, indeed, some people are capable of maintaining their weight loss for an average of 5 years.[1] As this study points out, much more is known about weight loss failures than successes, and often what is known does not lead to therapeutic interventions transforming the former into the latter.

Despite the many past and current theories about the aetiology of obesity, its primary cause is obvious. Hamburger stated in 1951 that overeating always underlies obesity, regardless of theories concerning energy utilization and storage.[2] Although conceding that inactivity contributed to the imbalance between energy intake and outflow, he stated that it was the consumption of calories in excess of need that always produced and sustained weight gain. Moreover, along with his colleagues of that decade such as Bruch,[3] he emphasized that

the reason why people overeat was not that they were unable to regulate their food intake in response to hunger, that is, the physiological need for energy, but that they were unable to control a psychological need to eat. He called this psychological hunger 'appetite', and stated that it was the sum of many social, aesthetic and emotional factors. The emotional component of this psychological appetite was emphasized by Freed in 1947, when he reported that a significant number of obese patients overeat when nervous, tired, idle or bored.[4] Hamburger pursued these findings with his own detailed investigation of the emotional factors behind the hyperphagia of obese patients. Persistent cravings for carbohydrate-rich foods, especially sweets, eating in response to depressed mood or frustration and helplessness, and increased appetite when tense and upset, were some of the most frequently reported factors associated with an inability to control food intake among his patient population.[2] More than 45 years later, his observations are still true and relevant to the understanding and treatment of obesity, as will be seen in the rest of this chapter.

Many obese individuals hold mood perturbations responsible for their inability to control their eating behaviour. The inability to control food intake when experiencing negative effect is called disinhibition, and includes the impulsive excessive eating not only of many obese individuals but also of women suffering from premenstrual syndrome, patients with seasonal affective disorder (SAD) and individuals undergoing nicotine withdrawal. Most of our information on eating behaviour under these conditions is derived indirectly from self-reports; that is, individuals are asked to rate their control over eating while experiencing emotional distress and, if possible, to record what they have just consumed. However, in studies carried out in the MIT Clinical Research Center over the past 15 years, we have been able to measure actual food intake from snacks as well as meals among individuals who experience episodic periods of disinhibited eating. As will be described below, our observations confirmed that excessive food intake occurred in association with negative mood, and the foods selected for consumption were, as noted so many years earlier by Hamburger, sweet and/or starchy carbohydrates. Moreover, when affect was normalized, so too was food intake.

When we began our studies, the general view concerning those who were eating sweet and starchy foods in excess was that these individuals were seeking love, affection and comfort and found their symbolic representation in foods. One of our early subjects told us that her doctor interpreted her excessive need for sweet snacks as lack of maturity and regression to childhood, when her mother used to feed her cookies after school. Although the choice of food made by the disinhibited eater may be based on past associations, we have now shown through extensive laboratory and clinical studies that choosing to eat a carbohydrate-rich food in association with a dysphoric state has a neurochemical basis.[5] The emotional overeater is seeking carbohydrate-rich foods because, when they are eaten, they can act like an edible tranquillizer. They bring about an improvement in mood because their consumption is followed by an increased synthesis of brain serotonin, a neurotransmitter involved in the regulation of mood state.

Serotonin synthesis and release increase after carbohydrate is eaten, as a result of an insulin-mediated increase in the brain levels of tryptophan, the amino acid precursor of serotonin. Insulin causes an increase in the ratio of plasma tryptophan to that of five large neutral amino acids that normally compete with circulating tryptophan for uptake into the brain, and, as tryptophan levels increase, so does serotonin synthesis.[6] Assessment of behaviour prior to and 30–60 min after carbohydrate ingestion demonstrates significant improvement in mood which may last as long as 3 h.[5] Thus it appears that the disinhibited obese eater is seeking to ameliorate anger, depression, tension or fatigue by consuming a sweet or starchy food. Unfortunately, this eating often promotes weight gain or an inability to remain on a diet. The foods sought by the distressed impulsive eater are rarely low in fat and restricted in portion size. Rather than rice cakes or dry toast, the foods chosen are high-fat snack foods such as cookies, doughnuts, french fries, crackers, chips, chocolate or ice cream, or carbohydrate foods that serve as a vehicle for a layer of fat, such as crackers and cheese, or peanut butter and bread. The rapidity of consumption and quantity eaten by the disinhibited eater can contribute an excessive number of calories to the daily food intake. In studies of obese individuals who found themselves unable to control their carbohydrate intake at specific times of the day or evening because they experienced a dysphoric state, the number of calories consumed as snacks was as high as 800–900 a day.[5] If the dysphoria lasts for several months, as would be the case in a patient suffering from SAD or the early months of nicotine withdrawal, or occurs every month, as with a woman suffering from premenstrual syndrome (PMS), a considerable amount of weight may be gained.

Interestingly, dietary interventions which lower serotoninergic function have confirmed this relationship between serotonin activity and mood, and suggest that dieting itself may alter serotoninergic function so as to leave the dieter vulnerable to post-diet weight gain. Protein intake prevents brain tryptophan uptake and subsequent serotonin synthesis[6] because the tryptophan content of all protein foods is considerably smaller than that of the five neutral amino acids with which it competes for uptake into the brain. Plasma measurements of the tryptophan/neutral amino acid ratio following a protein meal demonstrate a significant decrease from baseline. Thus it is possible that dietary regimens which eliminate or minimize the possibility of consuming sufficient amounts of carbohydrate-rich, protein-poor foods might affect brain serotonin levels, and with them functions such as mood regulation and satiety that are regulated by this neurotransmitter. Cowen et al tested this possibility by measuring the sensitivity of the 5-HT$_{2c}$ receptors before and following a 3-week calorie-deficient, carbohydrate-deficient diet.[7] They tested this hypothesis by challenging their female subjects with m-chlorophenypiperazine and comparing baseline and post-diet plasma prolactin levels. The post-diet increase in plasma prolactin levels following treatment with the receptor agonist was interpreted as indicative of increased receptor sensitivity due to inadequate serotonin availability. The authors speculate that the putative decrease in brain serotonin synthesis following this brief period of dieting

may be due to a diet-induced decrease in plasma tryptophan availability demonstrated in earlier studies by this group.[8–10] Indeed, this observation of diminished tryptophan availability was confirmed in a recent report that measured plasma tryptophan/large neutral amino acid ratios among women who followed a 4-week weight loss regimen.[11] Future measurements of post-diet mood and eating behaviours among individuals with diminished serotonin activity will be needed to establish this as a causative factor in post-diet weight gain. However, the present findings do suggest an explanation as to why recidivism is as high as 95% after a diet is concluded. If weight was gained initially because of excessive consumption of carbohydrates in association with a negative mood state, such eating is even more likely to occur after a diet that may have impaired serotonin synthesis and release.

The role of mood disturbances in the aetiology of obesity

It is curious that the obese individual has been stereotyped as being jolly, the life of the party, and good-humoured when for many their obesity is a consequence of chronic emotional distress. Indeed, psychological stress may promote excessive food intake not only among the obese but among those with normal weight as well. If such stress is chronic, sufficient weight will be gained to transform a formerly thin individual into someone who is now obese. An example of overeating and weight gain in response to chronic psychological stress among initially normal-weight individuals was described by Vitaliano et al.[12] They questioned over 80 spouse caregivers of individuals with Alzheimer's disease who had cared for their husbands or wives for more than 3.5 years. The survey asked them how their weight had changed during that time and to rate their current levels of anger, distress and lack of control in their role as caregiver. Their responses were compared with matched controls for age and duration of marriage. Weight gain among women caregivers was related to their perceived inability to control their anger, and a similar relationship between weight gain and the perception of having no control over any aspect of their lives was seen among the male caregivers. The psychological correlates of weight gain were also seen among a population of obese individuals seeking professional weight loss treatment in a hospital-based programme. This group had significantly higher psychopathology and were more likely to overeat in association with negative emotional states than were obese people who did not feel that their problem was sufficiently severe to require a hospital-based weight loss programme.[13]

Psychological stress may promote extremely rapid weight gain if it results in binge eating. Binging is best described as acute periods of excessive calorie consumption during which the binger feels unable to control food intake. Usually, eating continues until the eater is physically uncomfortable or interrupted by the presence of others. According to a study by Arnow et al,[14] 100% of 19 obese binge-eating women claimed to feel negative emotions before and after binging. The pre-binge moods included anger/frustration, anxiety/agitation, sadness/depression and regret. The mood following the binge was predominantly guilt.[14]

It is often difficult to obtain accurate records of the foods selected for a binge. Much of the eating is done covertly, and individuals in the throes of this impulsive type of food intake are rarely able to remember and record what they have consumed. However, in one such study that was able to account for the food choices made during binge episodes, food choices of obese bingers were found to be similar to those of obese non-bingers. The only difference between the two groups was the amount of food consumed; subjects who binged ate significantly more than the non-bingers. However, both groups preferred sweet and starchy carbohydrate-rich foods such as cake, ice cream, chips and rice, and none preferred protein-rich foods.[15] What is not yet understood is whether the obese non-binger differs from the obese binger only in the frequency and amount of foods consumed at one time, and in the intensity or types of emotional state preceding the binge, or whether there are additional neurochemical and behavioural impairments that account for binging itself. That bingers may be suffering from a comorbid condition is suggested by the prevalence of major depressive disorders in this population[16–20] and their response to treatment with serotonin reuptake blockers such as fluoxetine. The efficacy of such treatment implicates serotonin in the pathology of this eating behaviour; what is not known at present is whether the binger is consuming excessive amounts of food in an attempt to ameliorate dysphoric symptoms, as may be occurring with the disinhibited eater, or suffers from another clinical disorder that may share similar behaviours but has different aetiologies.

Despite the many studies examining the behavioural correlates of weight gain and obesity, the extent to which disinhibited eating prevents successful weight loss and maintenance in the population at large is not yet known. The oft repeated statement that healthy lifestyle changes must be made before obesity is conquered is well known; however, no one knows the effect of disinhibited eating on preventing these changes from becoming permanent. Moreover, since many studies have been carried out only among women and only among those women who volunteer for such research, there is little knowledge of the role that disinhibited eating plays among the population in general. The reliability of the information collected is also a problem, as the data are derived from self-reports of food intake and emotional state usually made in the midst of an emotionally charged eating situation or retrospectively. Thus it is impossible to validate their accuracy and inclusiveness.

Nevertheless, several recent studies using relatively large samples confirm the influence of disinhibition on promoting overeating and weight gain. In one such study, 230 obese women were asked to record over a 2-week period their food intake and social, environmental and emotional factors present when they ate.[21] The eating behaviours of the women resolved into five groups. Two groups were characterized by overeating in response to negative emotions such as depression and boredom; these groups also reported significantly higher consumption of carbohydrate-rich food, especially sweets, than the other groups. These two emotional overeating groups differed from each other in that one group alternated between periods of restrained eating and bouts of excessive food intake, whereas the other group showed little restraint or ability to restrict food intake in response to negative emotions at all times. The eating behaviour of the other groups indicated the ability to show restraint, that is, an absence of overeating in response to emotional changes or overeating in general.

The excessive intake of food, especially sweet carbohydrates, among obese subjects in response to emotional cues was also described by Lindroos et al.[22] In this study, obese and non-obese Swedish women were asked to report their dietary intake over 3 months; the questionnaire used was specific for Swedish meal and snack foods, and special attention was given to recording foods eaten as snacks.

The obese women obtained significantly more of their total energy from chocolates/candies and cakes/cookies than the non-obese, and ate disproportionately larger portion sizes of potatoes/rice at meals. The obese as a group demonstrated a significantly greater likelihood of overeating in response to emotional cues (disinhibition) than the non-obese and were unlikely to use restraint under such circumstances.[22]

The effect of disinhibited eating on repetitive weight gain was examined by Bartlett et al.[23] They studied individuals who completed weight loss programmes that attempt to improve eating and exercise patterns. The subjects were classified as mild, moderate and severe weight cyclers based on the number of previous dieting attempts, and the response of the subjects to stress-induced overeating was assessed. They found that mild cyclers had significantly less disinhibition than moderate and severe gainers and losers, suggesting that the inability to alter eating behaviour in order to maintain weight loss was compromised by the need to eat in response to emotional changes.

Similar results based on actual measurements of weight change after dieting were reported in a study of Swedish women who were followed for 16 months after the completion of an 8-month weight-reducing diet. Baseline measurements of disinhibition were predictive of long-term weight maintenance; subjects with the greatest difficulty in resisting emotional eating cues were more likely to regain weight after the diet was concluded.[24] These observations were confirmed by Carmody et al in their study of normal-weight and obese males and females.[25] Self-reported disinhibition prior to a weight loss programme was significantly related to subsequent weight cycling. Gender may have affected outcome as well; women scored significantly higher than men in their self-reports of responding to emotional cues by overeating. However, this study was not designed to test whether males are less likely to respond to stress by overeating, or conversely not notice that they are overeating when stressed.

Obese and non-obese people may differ significantly in their tendency to overeat in response to emotional distress. Using a self-report on snacking behaviour when stressed, we asked about 120 obese women applying for a weight loss study to describe how stress affected their snacking behaviour and to list the emotions that triggered their overeating. Over 70% of them reported that stress caused them to start snacking, and that when they did so, their snacking tended to be out of control and they found themselves unable to continue on a diet. The predominant precipitants of snacking identified by these women were anger, depression, frustration, tension, worry, boredom and exhaustion. Sixty-two non-obese women applying for a study on cognition at the research centre were also surveyed and their responses differed significantly. They were unlikely to snack when stressed, and did not have difficulty in controlling their snack intake or find it hard to stay on a diet. Fewer than 15% claimed that any emotional state promoted snacking, with the exception of boredom; 24% reported that they snacked in response to that mood (personal communication). Of interest in this regard are findings from a study of normal and obese female college students who tracked their emotional state prior to eating at meal-times and snacking. Psychological tests indicated that the obese students were no more emotionally distraught than normal-weight subjects but, unlike their normal-weight counterparts, were significantly more likely to snack when experiencing emotional distress.[26]

Most of the studies on the effects of mood on uncontrolled overeating describe female eating behaviour. That women are more likely to participate in research studies, especially those concerned with weight, may be an explanation for this gender disparity in the composition of the study samples. However, the possibility must be considered that gender differences in the prevalence of pathological eating behaviour may be generated by gender differences in brain serotonin metabolism, synthesis or turnover.[27] Evidence for a gender discrepancy in brain serotonin has been obtained by examining synthesis of serotonin during a period of relative serotonin depletion. It is now possible to decrease acutely serotonin synthesis by limiting the availability of its amino acid precursor, tryptophan. Subjects are fed a tryptophan-free diet (an amino acid mixture that contains no tryptophan) and approximately 5 h later exhibit an 80–90% decrease in plasma tryptophan levels.[28–31] This results in a decrease in brain tryptophan uptake and subsequent reduction in the rate of serotonin synthesis. The behavioural consequences of such a reduction have been examined in several studies. At the conclusion of the test period, serotonin synthesis is restored by administering a 1-g tryptophan tablet along with a high-protein snack.

Recently, Nishizawa et al[32] used this technique to measure serotonin synthesis in the brains of healthy volunteers. Using positron emission tomography (PET) and a tracer which accumulates in serotonin neurons, they examined rates of serotonin synthesis at baseline and after acute tryptophan depletion. Eight males and seven female subjects participated in the study. Significant differences in the rates of serotonin synthesis were found between males and females: the rate in males after acute tryptophan depletion was decreased by a factor of about 9.5 and that in females by a factor of about 40. Interestingly, the levels of tryptophan in the plasma did not correlate with brain serotonin synthesis in either group.

As the authors suggest, the higher incidence

of major depressive disorders among women may be related to their rate of serotonin synthesis. Stressful situations which may increase serotonin utilization could result in a more rapid decline in serotonin stores in women. One consequence would be an increased vulnerability to affective disorders; another, intense cravings for carbohydrate-rich foods and the inability to control food intake. Subjects were not allowed to eat during the test period and nor was there any measurement of changes in hunger, food cravings or desire to eat impulsively, so that the possibility of appetitive changes is still speculative. (Indeed, it may not be possible to carry out these measurements, as nausea is a common side-effect following consumption of the amino acid mixture.) However, these results do suggest that the seemingly greater prevalence of disinhibited eating among females may be the result of their greater susceptibility to increased serotonin activity when experiencing emotional distress.

Although Hamburger and his contemporaries noted the preference for sweet and starchy foods among their obese patients, and this observation was confirmed in many other studies of disinhibited eating behaviour, it is possible to challenge its significance. Aside from the unreliability of self-reports of food intake, especially those made during a period of some emotional distress, it is easy to explain the choice of carbohydrate-rich foods when the psychological need to eat arises. Sweet and starchy foods are more widely available as snacks than any other type of food; they are cheap, do not require preparation, and, by and large, appeal to a large variety of tastes. Thus, before claiming a neurochemical or even psychological basis for the choice of such foods, it is important to show that they will be preferentially eaten instead of other foods which are similarly convenient, tasty and accessible.

We developed a method for directly measuring snack choices of obese subjects who claimed to have an excessive appetite for sweet and starchy foods. Inpatient studies were conducted at the Massachusetts Institute of Technology's Clinical Research Center using a computerized vending machine to record 24-h snack consumption. The machine was stocked with isocaloric snacks that were high in either protein or carbohydrate. The protein snacks included miniature hot dogs, cold cuts, and cheese; the carbohydrate snacks included crackers, cookies, and tiny candy bars. Subjects had access to the vending machine at all times except during meals.[33-35] Meal foods were presented in preweighed containers containing only carbohydrate-rich or protein-rich foods. The measurement period lasted for 3 days and subjects had to eat only foods available in the research centre. Although the subjects' mealtime food intake was similar to that of eaters without self-described appetite for carbohydrate-rich foods, they all snacked at a time of day or evening specific for each individual and at that time consumed 800 or more calories. Moreover, almost all of the snacks consumed were carbohydrates; more than half of the subjects ate none of the protein snacks and the others ate only one or two, even though they were as accessible as the carbohydrate foods.

The results negated the possibility that carbohydrate foods are preferred only for logistical reasons, since protein-rich foods were similarly accessible and not eaten. In contrast, the appetite for carbohydrate-rich foods appeared to be under neurochemical regulation. When the subjects were treated with dexfenfluramine[33,34] and fluoxetine,[35] drugs that increase intrasynaptic serotonin, their consumption of carbohydrate snack foods decreased significantly, presumably because the brain was fooled into thinking that carbohydrates had already been eaten. Further studies examining mood changes prior to and following consumption of a carbohydrate-rich beverage provided evidence that the increase in serotonin availability following such consumption had behavioural consequences.[36] The obese subjects who claimed to have a carbohydrate appetite reported themselves as feeling less depressed and fatigued and more alert after consuming a carbohydrate-rich beverage. It appears, therefore, that the obese individual who is eating carbohydrate-rich foods from psychological rather than physiological hunger is doing so in order to effect a serotonin-mediated improvement in mood.

Although research techniques do not yet enable brain serotonin levels to be measured concurrently with carbohydrate-associated mood changes, one study has shown an association between peripheral serotonin levels and carbohydrate cravings among males. Blum et al measured platelet-poor plasma serotonin levels (PPP serotonin) and the macronutrient preferences of obese individuals[37] to see whether carbohydrate cravings of non-obese and obese individuals might correlate with peripheral serotonin levels. Both obese and lean males who craved carbohydrates had lower PPP serotonin than lean and obese males who craved protein. PPP serotonin levels and carbohydrate appetite did not correlate among females, however. No differences were found between carbohydrate and protein cravings of lean females, and since all the obese females craved only carbohydrates, there were no obese protein cravers with whom a comparison could be made. Information is limited at this time as to whether these peripheral serotonin measurements reflect levels in the brain.

Before assuming that the carbohydrate appetite of the disinhibited eater is due primarily to abnormal availability of serotonin, more studies must be carried out to test whether increasing serotonin synthesis or availability will minimize uncontrolled eating in response to emotional cues. Should this association explain the inability of some obese individuals to control their food intake, then specific interventions targeted at increasing serotonin availability can be developed, and those which might decrease serotonin levels can be avoided.

Premenstrual syndrome, seasonal affective disorder and excessive carbohydrate intake

Emotional precipitants of overeating may be associated with more than situational stress. The individual who fails to maintain weight despite repeated weight loss attempts may be sensitive to episodic changes in appetite caused by PMS or SAD. PMS and SAD generate intense cravings for carbohydrate-rich foods that may last through the post-ovulatory weeks of each menstrual cycle or from late autumn until early spring each year respectively. It has been postulated that some of these adverse affective and appetitive symptoms, that is, dysphoria and carbohydrate cravings, are due to deficiencies in serotonin-mediated neurotransmission, and the consumption of large quantities of carbohydrate has been explained as an attempt to alleviate the symptoms by raising brain serotonin synthesis. As in the obese individual whose disinhibited eating is linked to situational stress, such eating behaviour may also increase weight.

Typically, the PMS sufferer will complain of fatigue, depression, anger, agitation, tension and an inability to control the consumption of carbohydrate-rich foods during the luteal phase of the menstrual cycle. The mood and appetite disturbances resolve only when menses begins.

In 1969, Smith and Sauder[38] described intense cravings for sweet carbohydrates among nurses who self-reported premenstrual increases in tension, agitation, anger and depression. In a more recent study, the dietary intakes of eight women over 60 days were obtained by daily interviews and analysed for calorie and macronutrient contents. Carbohydrate was the only macronutrient whose consumption fluctuated with the menstrual cycle. Post-ovulatory consumption was more than twice as high as pre-ovulatory intake; no changes were seen in the consumption of fat- or protein-rich foods.[39] Direct measurements of food and macronutrient intake were made for non-obese women suffering from premenstrual mood changes and for controls by our MIT research group. Using the methodology that was used previously to characterize the eating behaviours of carbohydrate-craving obese subjects, calorie and macronutrient intakes were measured among the participants during the follicular and luteal (pre- and post-ovulatory) phases of their cycles. Non-PMS sufferers showed no alteration in food intake throughout the cycle, whereas those with premenstrual mood changes ate 500 or more calories daily when they were in their luteal phase. Moreover, this increased calorie intake was due to a specific increase in carbohydrate consumption.[40]

The drive to consume excessive amounts of carbohydrate-rich foods by women when they suffer from PMS is apparently due in part to alterations in serotonin activity during this phase of the cycle. Serotonin-activating drugs such as dexfenfluramine[41] and the selective serotonin reuptake blockers (SSRIs)[42–46] have brought about normalization of food intake[41] and premenstrual mood changes.

Because of the responsiveness of women with PMS to pharmacological therapy which increased serotonin availability, we hypothesized that the premenstrual appetite for carbohydrate was yet another example of individuals attempting to cope with negative moods by consuming sweet and starchy foods. This was tested in two studies in which women with well-defined premenstrual mood and appetite changes were treated with a food or drink that increased the plasma tryptophan/large neutral amino acid ratio relatively soon after eating. Mood, appetite and, in the second study, cognitive function were measured prior to and following consumption of the test food or a placebo which did not increase tryptophan/large neutral amino acid ratio. Significant improvements in anger, tension, fatigue and depressed mood followed consumption of the carbohydrate[40] as well as a decrease in carbohydrate appetite and improvement in attentiveness.[47]

PMS-generated overeating may not be of sufficient duration to cause serious weight gain. However, those individuals whose control over eating is impaired for several days each month may view PMS as an obstacle to sustained weight loss or weight maintenance efforts. It would be of interest to see whether the threshold to disinhibited eating is lowered during the premenstrual phase of the cycle; if so, dietary and pharmacological interventions might be tried to diminish the emotional fluctuations that lead to excessive food intake.

SAD, which shares with PMS many similarities in the affective and appetitive symptoms, does persist for long enough each year to result in substantial weight gain. Its appearance coincides with the decreased length of daylight characterizing the late autumn and winter months, and the symptoms of this disorder usually disappear in late spring, when the hours of daylight are significantly increased. Although depression is one of the symptoms, the earliest signs of SAD are usually fatigue and an excessive appetite for sweet and starchy foods. Weight gain secondary to the decreased energy output and increase in energy intake is often inevitable. Until very recently, the weight gain that many people experience in the winter was mistakenly attributed to 'holiday eating' and 'holiday blues', even though changes in activity and appetite along with mood were evident weeks before Christmas and persisted well into the spring. Moreover, people may suffer from a milder variant of SAD, subsyndromal SAD, without realizing it, since often the only symptoms are increased food intake and lethargy.[48–51]

When the disorder remits in the spring, the individual often feels sufficiently energetic and disinterested in eating that weight loss becomes easy; theoretically, dieting during the spring and summer should compensate for autumn and winter weight gain. Unfortunately, this is not always the case, and the remnant of weight gained in a previous winter may persist until the following year, eventually adding up to considerable obesity. Phototherapy has been used as a treatment for SAD with some success, and even exposure to environmental light can bring about an improvement in mood.[52]

Although the connection is unclear, a Swiss study was able to predict the therapeutic response to phototherapy by the intensity of craving for sweet carbohydrates in the afternoon.[53] As in PMS and emotional overeating, the intense craving for carbohydrate-rich foods suggests that abnormalities in serotonergic function may underlie these seasonal mood and appetitive changes. In an early study examining this possible relationship, patients meeting the diagnostic criteria for SAD were treated with dexfenfluramine or placebo for 4 weeks in a double-blind, placebo-controlled crossover study. The study was carried out over two consecutive winter seasons with the same group of patients. Dexfenfluramine treatment brought about complete remission of psychiatric symptoms in the majority of patients along with

weight loss,[54] and in a follow-up study during the third winter, treatment with dexfenfluramine over the entire 3 months of winter was effective in sustaining normal mood and appetite.

The role of serotonin in the aetiology of SAD has been shown in other studies using 1-tryptophan and SSRIs.[55] However, a comparison of the effects of citalopram, a SSRI, and light therapy found light to act considerably faster in reversing both the mood and appetitive disorders than the antidepressant, without the side-effects of the latter. Although the treatment did not last long enough to allow the assessment of weight change, the suppression of food intake by light treatment would have the additional advantage of minimizing weight gain.[56]

The unrelenting urge to consume excessive calories in the form of sweet and starchy carbohydrates throughout the late autumn, winter and, in some localities, early spring does function as a readily available means of improving mood. That carbohydrate consumption acting via increased serotonin synthesis brings about an amelioration of dysphoric state was shown by Rosenthal et al with patients suffering from SAD.[57] Unfortunately, the improvement in mood resulting from eating a carbohydrate-rich diet comes at a cost of substantial weight gain. The typical SAD patient is rarely sensitive to the fat content of the carbohydrate foods being eaten, and does not restrict the size of what is being eaten to adjust for his SAD-associated decrease in physical activity. Many weeks of increased energy intake and negligible voluntary physical activity leave the SAD patient with an excess of weight at the end of each winter. The result after several years may be considerable obesity.

Therapeutic interventions

If one accepts the involvement of a neuro-chemical factor, that is, abnormal serotonergic transmission, in the excessive consumption of carbohydrates associated with dysphoric state, then it follows that such behaviour will not be normalized without normalizing serotoninergic function as well. Although the scientific and commercial literature is replete with dietary and behavioural interventions that purport to change and control food intake, these interventions work only as long as the individual is able to exercise a relatively rigid control over food intake. As this chapter has shown, such control may fail when serotonin-mediated alterations in mood provoke an excessive appetite for sweet and starchy foods. The cessation of dieting and weight gain that follows is ample evidence that novel therapies must be developed to prevent or minimize this eating pathology. At present, no such interventions are available. The serotonin-enhancing drug dexfenfluramine (Redux) is suspended pending investigation into a new risk factor.

This drug, by enhancing serotonin activity, was able to restrain overeating in women with seasonal premenstrual appetitive changes, and in obese, 'carbohydrate cravers', who overeat daily in response to negative mood changes.

No other weight loss drugs with similar effects on serotonin function are entering the weight loss market; the SSRIs have not been shown to be effective in promoting long-term weight loss, nor has the so-called natural anti-depressant, St John's Wort, been shown to have any affect on food intake.

It is hoped that focusing on abnormalities in serotoninergic activity as underlying the mood and appetitive problems of many obese individuals will promote research into developing new pharmacological interventions. Obviously, weight loss efforts must include more than treatment with weight loss agents. On the other hand, it is unrealistic to expect an individual whose control of overeating is susceptible to periodic changes in mood to adhere successfully to a weight loss programme without pharmacological support as well.

References

1. Klem ML, Wing RR, McGuire MT et al, A descriptive study of individuals successful at long-term maintenance of substantial weight loss, *Am J Clin Nutr* 1997; **66**:239–46.
2. Hamburger W, Emotional aspects of obesity, *Med Clin North Am* 1951; **35**:483–99.
3. Bruch HH, Psychological aspects of overeating and obesity, *Psychosomatics* 1964; **5**:269–74.
4. Freed S, Psychic factors in the development and treatment of obesity, *JAMA* 1947; **133**:369–71.
5. Wurtman R, Wurtman J, Brain serotonin, carbohydrate-craving, obesity and depression. In: Graziella A, Allegri I, Filippini E et al, eds, *Recent Advances in Tryptophan Research* (Plenum Press: New York, 1996) 35–41.
6. Fernstrom JD, Wurtman RJ, Brain serotonin content: increase following ingestion of carbohydrate diet, *Science* 1971; **174**:1023–5.
7. Cowen PJ, Clifford EM, Walsh AE et al, Moderate dieting causes 5-HT2c receptor supersensitivity, *Psychol Med* 1996; **26**:1155–9.
8. Anderson IM, Crook WS, Gartside SE et al, Effect of moderate weight loss on prolactin secretion in normal female volunteers, *Psychiatry Res* 1989; **29**:161–7.
9. Goodwin GM, Cowen PJ, Fairburn CG et al, Plasma concentrations of tryptophan and dieting, *Br Med J* 1990; **300**:1499–500.
10. Walsh AE, Oldman AD, Franklin M et al, Dieting decreases plasma tryptophan and

increases the prolactin response to d-fenfluramine in women not men, *J Affect Disord* 1995; **33**:89–97.

11. Wolfe BE, Metzger ED, Stollar C, The effects of dieting on plasma tryptophan concentration and food intake in healthy women, *Physiol Behav* 1997; **61**:537–41.

12. Vitaliano PP, Russo J, Scanlan JM et al, Weight changes in caregivers of Alzheimer's care recipients: psychobehavioral predictors, *Psychol Aging* 1996; **11**:155–63.

13. Fitzgibbon ML, Stolley MR, Kirschenbaum DS, Obese people who seek treatment have different characteristics than those who do not seek treatment? *Health Psychol* 1993; **12**:342–5.

14. Arnow B, Kenardy J, Agras WS, Binge eating among the obese: a descriptive study, *J Behav Med* 1992; **15**:155–70.

15. Yanovski SZ, Leet M, Yanovski JA et al, Food selection and intake of obese women with binge-eating disorder, *Am J Clin Nutr* 1992; **56**:975–80.

16. Yanovski SZ, Nelson JE, Dubbert BK, Spitzer RL, Association of binge eating disorder and psychiatric comorbidity in obese subjects, *Am J Psychiatry* 1993; **150**:1472–9.

17. Hudson JI, Pope HG Jr, Wurtman J et al, Bulimia in obese individuals. Relationship to normal-weight bulimia, *J Nerv Ment Dis* 1988; **176**:144–52.

18. Marcus M, Wing R, Ewing L, Psychiatric disorders among obese binge eaters, *Int J Eat Disord* 1994; **9**:69–77.

19. Hudson JI, Carter WP, Pope HG, Antidepressant treatment of binge-eating disorder: research findings and clinical guidelines. *J Clin Psychiatry* 1996; **57** (suppl 8):73–9.

20. Specker S, de Zwaan M, Raymond N et al, Psychopathology in subgroups of obese women with and without binge eating disorder, *Comp Psychiatry* 1994; **35**:185–90.

21. Schlundt DG, Taylor D, Hill JO et al, A behavioral taxonomy of obese female participants in a weight-loss program, *Am J Clin Nutr* 1991; **53**:1151–8.

22. Lindroos A-K, Lissner L, Mathiassen ME et al, Dietary intake in relation to restrained eating, disinhibition and hunger in obese and nonobese Swedish women, *Obesity Res* 1997; **5**:175–82.

23. Bartlett SJ, Wadden TA, Vogt RA, Psychosocial consequences of weight cycling, *J Consult Clin Psychol* 1996; **64**:587–92.

24. Karlsson J, Hallgren P, Kral J et al, Predictors and effects of long-term dieting on mental well-being and weight loss in obese women, *Appetite* 1994; **23**:15–26.

25. Carmody TP, Brunner RL, St Jeor ST, Dietary helplessness and disinhibition in weight cyclers and maintainers, *Int J Eat Disord* 1995; **18**:247–56.

26. Lowe MR, Fisher EB Jr, Emotional reactivity, emotional eating, and obesity: a naturalistic study, *J Behav Med* 1983; **6**:135–49.

27. Steiner M, Lepage P, Dunn E, Serotonin and gender specific psychiatric disorders, *Int J Psychiatry* 1997; **1**:3–13.

28. Benkelfat C, Ellenbogen MA, Dean P et al, Mood-lowering effect of tryptophan depletion. Enhanced susceptibility in young men at genetic risk for major affective disorders, *Arch Gen Psychiatry* 1994; **51**:687–97.

29. Delgado PL, Charney DS, Price LH et al, Serotonin function and the mechanism of antidepressant action. Reversal of antidepressant-induced remission by rapid depletion of plasma tryptophan, *Arch Gen Psychiatry* 1990; **47**:411–18.

30. Moja EA, Antinoro E, Cesa-Bianchi M et al, Increases in stage 4 sleep after ingestion of a tryptophan-free diet in humans, *Pharmacol Res Commun* 1984; **16**:909–14.

31. Young SN, Gauthier S, Effect of tryptophan administration on tryptophan, 5-hydroxyindoleacetic acid and indoleacetic acid in human lumbar and cisternal cerebrospinal fluid, *J Neurol Neurosurg Psychiatry* 1981; **44**:323–7.

32. Nishizawa S, Benkelfat C, Young SN et al, Differences between males and females in rates of serotonin synthesis in human brain, *Proc Natl Acad Sci USA* 1997; **94**:5308–13.

33. Wurtman J, Wurtman R, Mark S et al, Dextrofenfluramine selectively suppresses carbohydrate snacking by obese subjects, *Int J Eat Disord* 1985; **4**:89–99.

34. Wurtman J, Wurtman R, Reynolds S et al, d-Fenfluramine suppresses snack intake among carbohydrate cravers but not among noncarbohydrate cravers, *Int J Eat Disord* 1987; **6**:687–99.

35. Wurtman J, Wurtman R, Berry E et al, Dexfenfluramine, fluoxetine and weight loss among female carbohydrate cravers, *Neuropsychopharmacology* 1993; **9**:201–10.

36. Lieberman HR, Wurtman JJ, Chew B, Changes in mood after carbohydrate consumption among obese individuals, *Am J Clin Nutr* 1986; **44**:772–8.

37. Blum I, Nessiel L, Graff E et al, Food preferences, body weight, and platelet-poor plasma serotonin and catecholamines, *Am J Clin Nutr* 1993; **57**:486–9.

38. Smith SL, Sauder C, Food cravings, depression, premenstrual problems, *Psychosom Med* 1969; **31**:281–7.

39. Dalvit-McPhillips SP, The effect of the human menstrual cycle on nutrient intake, *Physiol Behav* 1983; **31**:209–12.

40. Wurtman JJ, Brzezinski A, Wurtman RJ, Laferrere B, Effect of nutrient intake on premenstrual depression, *Am J Obstet Gynecol* 1989; **161**:1228–34.

41. Brzezinski AA, Wurtman JJ, Wurtman RJ et al, D-Fenfluramine suppresses the increased calorie and carbohydrate intakes and improves the mood of women with premenstrual depression, *Obstet Gynecol* 1990; **76**:296–301.

42. Elkin M, Open trial of fluoxetine therapy for premenstrual syndrome, *South Med J* 1993; **86**:503–7.

43. Stone AB, Pearlstein TB, Brown WA, Fluoxetine in the treatment of late luteal phase dyphoric disorder, *J Clin Psychiatry* 1991; **52**:290–3.

44. Steiner M, Steinberg S, Stewart D et al, Fluoxetine in the treatment of premenstrual dysphoria, *N Engl J Med* 1995; **332**:1529–34.

45. Rickels K, Freedman EW, Sondheimer S et al, Fluoxetine in the treatment of premenstrual syndrome, *Curr Ther Res* 1990; **48**:161–6.

46. Eriksson E, Hedberg MA, Andersch B et al, The serotonin reuptake inhibitor paroxetine is superior to the noradrenaline reuptake inhibitor maprotiline in the treatment of premenstrual syndrome, *Neuropsychopharmacology* 1995; **12**:167–76.

47. Sayegh R, Schiff I, Wurtman J et al, The effect of a carbohydrate-rich beverage on mood, appetite, and cognitive function in women with premenstrual syndrome, *Obstet Gynecol* 1995; **86**:520–8.

48. Rosenthal NE, Sack DA, Gillin JC et al, Seasonal affective disorder. A description of the syndrome and peliminary findings with light therapy, *Arch Gen Psychiatry* 1984; **41**:72–80.

49. Wehr TA, Rosenthal NE, Seasonality and affective illness, *Am J Psychiatry* 1989; **146**:829–39.

50. Judd LL, Rapaport MH, Paulus M et al, Subsyndromal symptomatic depression: a new mood disorder? *J Clin Psychiatry (Suppl)* 1994; **55**:18–28.

51. Rosenthal NE, Genhart FM, Jacobsen FM, Disturbances of appetite and weight regulation in seasonal affective disorder, *Ann NY Acad Sci* 1987; **499**:216–30.

52. Wirz-Justice A, Graw P, Krauchi K et al, 'Natural' light treatment of seasonal affective disorder, *J Affect Disord* 1996; **37**:109–20.

53. Krauchi K, Wirz-Justice A, Graw P, High intake of sweets late in the day predicts a rapid and persistent response to light therapy in winter depression, *Psychiatry Res* 1993; **46**:107–17.

54. O'Rourke D, Wurtman JJ, Wurtman RJ et al, Treatment of seasonal depression with d-fenfluramine, *J Clin Psychiatry* 1989; **50**:343–7.

55. Terman M, Terman J, *Seasonal Affective Disorder and Light Therapy: Report to the Depression Guidelines Panel* (PHS Agency for Health Care Policy and Research NYS Psychiatric Institute: New York, 1991).

56. Wirz-Justice A, van der Velde P, Bucher A et al, Comparison of light treatment with citalopram in winter depression: a longitudinal single case study, *Int Clin Psychopharmacology* 1992; **7**:109–16.

57. Rosenthal NE, Genhart MJ, Caballero B et al, Psychobiological effects of carbohydrate- and protein-rich meals in patients with seasonal affective disorder and normal controls, *Biol Psychiatry* 1989; **25**:1029–40.

26

Alcohol and drug abuse in women
Shirley Y Hill

Introduction

The purpose of this chapter is to bring together diverse literatures concerning substance dependence in women, with a focus on the possible role of mood disorders in the aetiology and treatment of substance dependence disorders in women. A number of myths concerning substance dependence in women have altered the research questions that have been asked and the treatment strategies that have been adopted for women. One of these myths is that substance dependence in women is more often a secondary consequence of another psychiatric disorder than in men. A corollary to this myth is the notion that substance dependence in women is less severe and for the most part is a reaction to environmental stressors (e.g. divorce, empty nest syndrome when children leave home).

This chapter will argue that the high rate of depression reported for substance-abusing women may be an artefact of the varying definitions used (e.g. depressed mood rather than a clinical syndrome) and the fact that depression is a greater motivating force for women to seek treatment than it is for men. Accordingly, this chapter will include data concerning depression and its effect on substance abuse outcome, evidence for genetic mediation of a more severe early-onset form of alcohol dependence in women, and evidence that neurobiological markers may make it possible to identify those individuals at highest risk for intensive intervention and/or treatment. Finally, the sociocultural and familial environmental factors that alter the likelihood that a woman will use alcohol or drugs in sufficient quantity to become addicted will be reviewed. This latter portion of the chapter will illustrate how our understanding of the factors leading to substance dependence and its outcome for the individual woman will be determined not only by her familial/genetic diathesis for substance dependence disorders and mood disorders, but by the sociocultural environment that promotes or prevents excessive exposure to alcohol and drugs.

Depression: the varying definitions used with substance-dependent persons

Depression has variously been noted in reference to substance-abusing populations as a symptom, syndrome or diagnosis. It should be noted that the presence of depressive symptoms does not necessarily mean that a depressive disorder is present.[1] Some studies that discuss depression among substance abusers have utilized depression rating scales (Beck Depression Inventory, Hamilton Rating Scale), whereas others have utilized syndromal definitions usually following DSM-III, DSM-IIIR, or DSM-IV. The diagnosis of depression in chronic alcohol abusers can be quite difficult because alcohol use can produce a dysphoric mood that lifts following a period of being dried out. Similar findings have been reported for cocaine, marihuana and other drugs of abuse. The important pharmacological effects of chronic alcohol consumption on mood were first demonstrated by Tamerin and Mendelson in 1969.[2] This research team hospitalized alcoholics on a research ward for several weeks and administered intoxicating doses of alcohol on a daily basis, simultaneously recording changes in mood before, during and after the alcohol administration phase. They noted a dramatic increase in dysphoric mood brought about by administration of alcohol.

A number of reports are now available documenting this phenomenon among alcoholics admitted to inpatient programmes for alcohol treatment. For example, among newly admitted alcoholic patients to a veteran's hospital, Brown and Schuckit[3] found that 40% qualified for a diagnosis of depression by the Hamilton Depression Rating Scale. After 4 weeks of abstinence, this figure dropped to only 6%. Other studies[4,5] support this trend in observing significant drops in the percentage of cases continuing to meet criteria for depression following detoxification. For example, Nakumura et al[4] found that 72 of 88 patients had Hamilton depression ratings within the normal range after 4 weeks of inpatient hospitalization.

However, one early report indicated no improvement in depressive symptoms at 1-year follow-up.[6] It is interesting that, at the time this study was published, depressive symptoms were less often treated with antidepressant medications in inpatient AA-oriented substance dependence treatment programmes, a trend that appears to have been reversed in the past 20 years. For example, in a recent survey of women treated in facilities in a three-county area in Pennsylvania, we find that over a third of women are on antidepressant medication either at discharge or within 6 months of discharge.[7] Is this a positive trend? If re-evaluation of these women occurs to determine if they are clinically depressed at varying intervals after discharge, then medication may ameliorate symptoms of depression that could increase the risk for relapse. However, indiscriminate use of antidepressants could have a negative impact on alcohol and drug use behaviour in women who are primary alcoholics with secondary depression, and who, with a sufficient period of drying out, will be free of depressive symptoms. For women whose depressive symptoms are an outgrowth of drinking, medication may merely serve to increase their belief that they must use pills or substances to feel normal.

Two independent disorders: separate aetiology?

The association between substance dependence and depression has been considered from the perspective of two independent disorders with separate aetiologies co-occurring in the same individual. More commonly, each disorder has been seen as having consequential effects on the likelihood of the other occurring (for example, depression leads to self-medication with alcohol or drugs, or, alternatively, chronic use of substances leads to depression). Evidence for alcohol dependence and depression being two independent clinical disorders comes from several family studies conducted at Washington University in St Louis in the late 1960s, 1970s and early 1980s.[8–11] The last three studies compared rates of depression in relatives of probands with primary alcoholism, relatives of probands with primary alcoholism and secondary depression and relatives of probands with depression only. Clearly, the rates of depression observed in relatives of probands who were only alcoholic were lower than they were among relatives of probands with both alcoholism and depression. While the classic study of Pitts and Winokur[8] did find elevated rates of depression among female relatives of proband alcoholics, the probands were not diagnosed with respect to presence of affective disorder. These data, along with both twin and adoption data, appear to suggest independent transmission of alcohol dependence and affective disorder.[12–16] Why, then, do we continue to observe associations between alcohol dependence and depression in the same patient?

The pharmacological effects of chronic heavy use of alcohol and, probably, many abused drugs promote depressive symptoms. For those predisposed to depressive illness, alcohol initially acts as a self-medication, improving mood and initiating sleep. However, with continued heavy use, dysphoria and sleep disruption occur, further exacerbating the depressed mood. Polysomnographic recordings of alcoholics show that sleep parameters can be disrupted for up to 2 years following abstinence.[17]

The self-medication concept has been most commonly discussed with respect to women substance abusers. More often, women have been thought to become depressed before they become substance dependent, while men are thought to become substance dependent and then subsequently develop a mood disorder.[18,19] Schutte et al[20] recently modelled the reciprocal relationship between depression and alcohol use and problems in men and women followed over a 3-year period. Structural equation modelling revealed that more baseline depression was associated with less alcohol consumption at 1-year follow-up in both men and women. However, later in the follow-up, increased levels of depressive symptoms predicted increased drinking, but only in women. However, they found that heavier drinking predicted increased depressive symptoms in both men and women. Thus, it would appear that the dysphoric mood produced by heavy use of alcohol is a pharmacological one that is equally likely to occur in women as in men. However, depressed mood may have more salience as an aetiological factor for heavy drinking in women than it does in men. Interestingly, because the Schutte et al study[20] involved 414 individuals from multiple treatment sites, the authors did not have access to individual medical records that would have contained diagnostic status and medication history. These variables might be quite useful for determining which individuals respond to depressive symptoms by drinking. Possibly this is not a gender difference but reflects the fact that more of the women in treatment suffered from independent diagnosable clinical depression.

At any rate, for those individuals who initially meet criteria for major depressive disorder, we know that alcohol dependence complicates the treatment course. Ten-year follow-up data from the NIMH Collaborative study of depression, in which 78% of the original 955 probands (some with and some without alcohol dependence) were followed, illustrate that having a diagnosis of alcohol dependence leads to poorer treatment outcome for these individuals.[21]

Gender and the relative likelihood of developing substance dependence and depressive disorders

Alcohol dependence and major depression in population surveys

The most common psychiatric disorders found in the recent National Comorbidity Survey (NCS) were major depressive episode and alcohol dependence.[22] Consistent with numerous previous reports, the NCS found that women had elevated rates of affective and anxiety disorders.[22] Based on the data obtained from the NCS, the ratio of affected cases (lifetime diagnosis) among women for any affective disorder is approximately 1.5 times higher than it is for men (23.9% versus 14.7%). In contrast, substance dependence (17.9% versus 35.4%) and alcohol dependence (8.2% versus 20.1%) are approximately 0.5 times lower in women. One large-scale multi-site survey, the Epidemiological Catchment Area (ECA) programmes[23] also found male rates of drug abuse/dependence to be higher than in females (7.8% versus 4.8%), as was the case for alcohol abuse/alcohol dependence (23.8% versus 4.6%).

There is a general consensus between the two national epidemiological surveys (ECA and NCS) that comorbidity for a number of psychiatric disorders is common among substance-dependent individuals. The ECA found that of the respondents having at least one DSM-III lifetime disorder, over 60% had two or more disorders. Similarly, the NCS survey found that of the respondents with one lifetime disorder, 56% met DSM-IIIR criteria for two or more other disorders.

Comorbidity rates in clinical populations

Numerous studies of clinical populations have pointed to elevated rates of depressive symptoms among alcoholics.[24–26] Ross et al,[25] studying 260 men and 241 women seeking treatment for alcohol and drug dependence, evaluated the rates of comorbidity for other psychiatric disorders, and found exceptionally high rates of other psychiatric disorders. Among persons seeking treatment for either alcohol or drug dependence, 78% were found to have a lifetime diagnosis of another psychiatric disorder, with 65% currently having another disorder. Those individuals meeting criteria for both alcohol and drug dependence had the highest rates of comorbidity. The affective disorders were among the most common, with 24% of the sample meeting lifetime criteria for major depression. Even higher rates of major depression have been reported for treatment-seeking opiate-dependent individuals.[27]

Examining the patterns of comorbidity, particularly by gender, is useful with regard to aetiology and treatment. If substance-dependent women show greatly elevated rates of depression compared to substance-dependent men, then the aetiology of substance dependence in women can be said to be more clearly based on an affective diathesis. This would suggest, perhaps, a better treatment response to antidepressant medication for women. On the other hand, the excess cases of depression seen in women alcoholics may merely reflect the gender ratio observed in the general population. In this case, the greater likelihood that alcoholic women will carry a diagnosis of depression compared to alcoholic men is noteworthy, but suggests little about aetiology or treatment of the underlying substance dependence. Data from the ECA survey suggest that substance abusing women are more often depressed than substance abusing men, because of the gender ratio for depression seen in the general population. Every psychiatric disorder examined in the ECA survey was found to have higher rates in alcoholics than in non-alcoholics.[18] However, when the prevalence ratios by gender for the co-occurrence of major depression and alcoholism are calculated, quite similar ratios, 2.7 (female) to 2.4 (male), are found.[28] Thus, the study authors further concluded that while the associations between antisocial personality disorder (ASPD), other substance abuse and mania were quite strong, the association between alcoholism and depressive disorder though positive, was not very strong.

Thus, rates of major depression are elevated among both male and female alcoholics relative to non-alcoholics when found as cases in population surveys. This trend is not nearly as impressive as it is in clinical samples, however. Investigations of clinical samples tend to report much higher rates of depression among alcoholics than among non-alcoholics,[29] and particularly so for women. Further examination of clinical samples reveals, however, that women treated for alcohol dependence who carry a lifetime diagnosis of major depression may actually be represented in the proportion that one would expect in the general population. For example, Hesselbrock[29] studied the admission and 1-year follow-up diagnosis of 197 male and 69 female alcoholics admitted to three inpatient treatment centres in the greater Hartford, Connecticut area. Approximately one-third of the males had an admission diagnosis of major depression with or without ASPD, while one-half of the women alcoholics carried a depression diagnosis (with or without ASPD). Thus, 1.5 times as many women as men carried an admission diagnosis of depression. This is the rate one sees in the general population, 15% and 23% for males and females, respectively.[22] In other words, though the process of having alcoholism elevates rates of depression, it would appear that the relative risk for developing depression by gender is not altered by this process. Moreover, even in clinical samples, the increased risk which alcoholics have for carrying a diagnosis of depression, if the alcoholic is female, is the risk that all women share, that is, approximately 1.5 times the relative risk seen in men.

Effects of depression on treatment outcome in women

Several studies have examined the effects of comorbid depression on the outcome of alcohol dependence treatment, though few have specifically evaluated the effect of drug abuse or dependence other than alcohol. Also, many have included only male alcoholics.[11,30,31] Those that have included women provide conflicting results.[18,29,32-34] The early work of Schuckit and Winokur[32] suggested that for female alcoholics the presence of an affective disorder predicted better outcomes in drinking-related measures at 3-year follow-up. These results stand in direct contrast to the findings of Kranzler et al,[34] who found a protective effect of having a depressive disorder in a mixed sample of men and women alcoholics with concurrent drug abuse (42%) at the time of admission to an inpatient facility. An overlap between alcohol dependence and depression occurred in 38%, and in those cases no deleterious effect on drinking measures was seen. In fact, these authors reported decreased drinking intensity for both men and women. Therefore, whether depression has a negative influence on treatment outcome in substance-abusing women is currently unclear.

Rounsaville et al[33] found that gender conferred differential effects on alcoholism treatment outcome. For alcoholic men, having an additional diagnosis of major depression, ASPD or drug abuse was associated with poorer treatment outcome. However, for alcoholic women, having major depression was associated with better outcome in drinking-related measures. These authors did note poorer outcome in alcoholic women with drug abuse and ASPD. Similarly, Hesselbrock[29] found that women alcoholics were no more likely to relapse if they met criteria for comorbid depression, unlike their male counterparts. In fact, the lowest rates of relapse reported for women alcoholics at 1-year follow-up were in the comorbid depression and antisocial personality groups.

While the data are conflicting with regard to whether comorbid depression prevents or promotes substance dependence relapse, or whether it affects the time required to achieve remission following treatment, it is clear that depressive symptoms promote treatment seeking. Helzer and Pryzbeck[18] report that women alcoholics are significantly more likely to use treatment services than are men. Comorbidity, as well as gender, was found to increase the likelihood of treatment seeking. However, treatment seeking does not always indicate an amelioration of alcohol- or drug-seeking behaviour following treatment. Hasin et al[35] found that alcohol dependence indicators, including previous chronicity, predicted poorer outcome (longer time to remission). During a 5-year observation period, they found that outcome was unrelated to receiving alcohol-specific treatments. The results of another study involving 581 late-life problem drinkers underscore the importance of severity at diagnosis as a predictor of outcome at follow-up.[36] This study found the most salient predictors of drinking-related outcome measures at 4-year

follow-up were being male, being an early-onset problem drinker, and having friends who approved of drinking. Several predictors were found for being depressed at follow-up, including being female, being unmarried, having early-onset status, and using more emotional rather than cognitive coping strategies to deal with life events. However, an independent role for depression in drinking-related measures was not reported.

In summary, while the effect of having comorbid depression may or may not facilitate remission once a woman comes to treatment, we do know that having a depressive disorder increases the chance that she will seek some form of treatment. Further work is needed to separate those women who meet lifetime criteria for major depressive disorder and enter treatment in an episode from those who simply show evidence of dysphoria or depressed mood that remits within 4 weeks. In addition to the importance of distinguishing between depressed mood and major depressive disorder is the need to adequately address the woman's medication history and response to antidepressant medication. Some promising results have been reported for fluoxetine-treated patients who met criteria for major depression at entry to an alcoholism treatment facility.[37] Similar findings have been reported for imipramine treatment.[38] Obtaining the family history for both substance dependence and major depression may be instructive regarding the likelihood that the individual may have a familial diathesis for clinical depression and would be a good candidate for antidepressant therapy if she has not previously been medicated. Obtaining a family history for substance dependence to determine the relative loading for substance dependence disorders in the family along with determining the pattern of disorders for the individual can be instructive. As the following section discusses, one form of alcohol dependence in women may be more severe and determined by genetic factors. This form currently has a poorer prognosis, as it is less responsive to a positive environment (e.g. higher socio-economic status, intact family). New treatments for these women appear to be urgently needed. Possibly the move towards greater utilization of outpatient treatment in the present climate of cost control may be detrimental to these women. In the past, 4-week inpatient care was common and allowed clinicians the opportunity to observe patients after they had dried out, to determine if there was residual depression. With the greater observation window, women could be prescribed antidepressant medication with more informed judgment than can occur with discharge after only 1–2 weeks for detoxification.

Aetiology of alcohol dependence in women: evidence for genetic mediation

Adoption data

Transmission of alcoholism within families appears to occur with a higher probability than most psychiatric disorders, including the affective disorders.[39] The now classic adoption study concerning aetiology in males[12] suggested that such transmission can occur even in the absence of exposure to the alcoholic parent. Fewer adoption data are available for women, so the conclusions that can be reached are somewhat tentative.[40,41] However, to summarize, three adoption studies have been conducted in Sweden,[42] and one each in Denmark[13] and the USA.[43] The Swedish and Danish studies had too few alcoholic women to draw firm conclusions. However, Cadoret et al employed a reasonable sample size and sophisticated data-analysis techniques, and concluded that genetic factors operate in the aetiology of alcoholism in both men and women.

Twin data

Further evidence for genetic mediation of alcoholism in women can be gained from studies that have utilized adult twin pairs. Concordance for drinking,[44] and concordance for alcohol dependence[45–49] have been studied. While some studies[45–47] did not find monozygotic (MZ)/dizygotic (DZ) rates suggestive of genetic mediation in female twin pairs, recent publications[48,49] are quite convincing. Pickens and Svikis,[48] studying 114 male and 55 female twin pairs, concluded that a genetic component was operating in female alcoholism as well. Finally, Kendler et al,[49] studying 1030 MZ and DZ twin pairs, found substantially higher correlations in MZ than in DZ twins, with over 50% of the variance in alcoholism risk being explained by genetic factors.

In summary, we have previously noted that the aetiology of alcoholism has as much likelihood of being mediated through genetic factors in women as it does in men.[41] The evidence includes two persuasive twin studies of female alcoholism[48,49] and the adoption study of Cadoret et al.[43] Moreover, alcoholism appears to be heterogeneous in women, with one form being more clearly mediated by genetic factors. Studies by Glenn and Nixon[50] and Lex et al[51] give evidence for greater severity of symptoms in the early-onset groups of women, along with greater familial density of alcoholism in the severe form. Preliminary results from our own laboratory suggest a very early onset of alcoholism for female alcoholics who had multigenerational alcoholism in their families. This programme of research has been designed around ascertainment criteria that ensure obtaining women and their families who have more severe alcoholism. Specifically, a pair of alcoholic sisters, at least one of whom is currently in treatment, is required for entry of the family into our studies. This strategy results in an early-onset disorder in these women with multiple affected first-degree relatives (median = 4.0). The median age of onset for alcoholic women ascertained by familial alcoholism density was 16 years.[52]

Are there two types of alcoholism?

Cloninger et al[53] have described male type I alcoholics, in contrast to type II alcoholics, as those whose likelihood of drinking depends much more heavily on the environmental milieu in which the individual resides. Type II males tend to be of the familial form and display earlier onset. Previously we have noted[40] that, quite possibly, there are two forms of alcoholism in women: one that is largely the result of environmental pressures and the tendency for heavy drinking to peak between the ages of 35 and 49, and another early-onset form that occurs between the ages of 18 and 24,[23] which is much more likely to be genetically mediated. While many young women drink heavily, often with problems that would allow them to meet criteria for alcohol dependence, many will 'mature out'. However, one subgroup of women has been identified which shows excessive drinking in young adulthood but does not appear to change its pattern of drinking and persists in this abusive style of drinking. This subgroup is the type that has a familial diathesis with presumably greater genetic loading.

Thus, at least two types of alcoholism have been identified in men,[53,54] based largely on the severity exhibited, and also on the proportion of genetic variance explaining the emergent behaviour. It is very likely that there are two types of alcohol abuse/dependence in women as well. A less severe form appears to exist that often arises during middle age in response to environmental change (e.g. divorce, loss of parental role). However, this form has the potential for better outcome because it is responsive to positive environmental change. The other type, arising at a much earlier age (18–24 years), is not simply part of a youthful rebellion that 'matures out' with the individual acquiring new responsibilities of young adulthood (career, marriage, child-rearing). This form is not as responsive to environmental pressures. In contrast, it is proposed that this form is most often a part of a familial alcoholism diathesis, often being part of an intergenerational pattern of substance abuse that reappears in multiple generations. Accordingly, this form has greater severity, and is present even in families where the environment is relatively propitious (the family has a higher socioeconomic status, is intact, and subscribes to traditional values), as we have seen in our ongoing family study of male alcoholic probands.[54]

Further evidence for two types of alcoholism comes from studies by Glenn and Nixon[50] and Lex et al.[51] Glenn and Nixon[50] showed that when women were classified by age of onset, several significant differences emerged with respect to the severity of alcoholism exhibited. In general, the early-onset group displayed greater severity of symptoms and more affected relatives. Lex et al[51] studying women with more severe alcohol problems who came to the attention of the courts because of their drinking (driving while intoxicated [DWI] offences), found that these women exhibited a greater density of familial alcoholism than those who did not.

Evidence for genetic mediation of the early-onset form

Early-onset female alcoholism, though much less common in the population, may be a more severe form, with greater genetic mediation. It is suggested that the familial form of alcoholism seen in women may resemble that seen in men (e.g. early onset, multiple affected relatives, relative independence from environmental antecedents). The question arises, however, as to whether the familial transmission seen in families of women with the more severe form could be genetically mediated. With the promising results from the twin studies in women,[49] it should be possible to find genes responsible for increasing the likelihood that a woman will become alcohol dependent. If the aetiologies are somewhat different in men and women, or in early- and late-onset alcoholism, different genes may possibly be found. To date, we have examined a number of candidate genes in collective samples of men and women, including the dopamine D2 receptor.[55] With enlarged samples, we plan to test for genetic linkage and association separately by gender. In addition, we have pursued neurobiological markers for over 10 years now, markers that have been shown to be heritable.

Promising neurobiological risk markers for susceptibility to alcohol dependence

Several research efforts have been initiated in the past 20 years in an attempt to identify reliable and valid markers for alcoholism risk. Broadly defined, these appear to belong within the domains of personality or temperament, on the one hand, and neurocognition on the other. The notion of an 'alcoholic personality' has been a common theme in discussions both by clinicians and researchers. However, whether temperament/personality factors have aetiological significance is dependent on the research designs used to test these personality theories. Studying alcoholics does not allow one to separate cause from consequence. Chronic alcohol consumption leads to neuropathological consequences that can be reflected in personality changes. Neurocognitive and neurobehavioural theories have also been plentiful among the aetiological models proposed for alcoholism.

These capacities for processing information may prove to be relevant to why one individual is more suited or motivated to pursue intellectual pursuits, endeavours that may be incompatible with long-term abusive drinking. The neurobehavioural characteristics deserve mention because they reflect both the 'neurological health' of the brain and the 'final common pathway' for the behavioural expression of this capacity. For example, it has long been known that children with 'minimal brain dysfunction' have problems related to motoric inhibition and have been variously described as 'hyperactive' or 'attentionally deficient', or both—attention deficit hyperactivity disorder as currently outlined in DSM-IV. If high-risk individuals are born with a subtle neurological 'wiring' handicap, this may be expressed as motoric hyperactivity and impulsivity and may additionally be reflected in higher levels of tonic autonomic arousal, or increased response to environmental stressors, than are found in individuals who are at low risk for developing alcoholism.

Alcohol metabolism may play a role in the development of alcoholism. Theoretically, any living organism can be addicted to alcohol if sufficient quantities are ingested over a period of time. In fact, passive dependence on alcohol can easily be achieved in laboratory rats by restricting their fluid to alcohol-adulterated water.[56] Whether some individuals are born with greater or lesser capacities to metabolize alcohol, a tendency that might be enhanced by being from a high-risk family, is currently unknown. Some groups of individuals who are low consumers of alcohol (e.g. those with an Asian background) may actually have altered alcohol metabolism. However, it is necessary to show that high-risk groups (alcoholics or their relatives) from the same ethnic background have elevated rates of metabolism compared with their low-risk (no family or personal history of alcoholism) counterparts, in order for the observed difference to be of major aetiological significance. Also it is possible that high- and low-risk groups have similar rates of metabolism but differ in their innate tissue tolerance for alcohol, or differ in the rate at which they develop acute tolerance. Women may be at greater risk for developing alcohol dependence than men because, at the same level of consumption (corrected for body weight), they exhibit reduced levels of alcohol dehydrogenase (ADH) in the gastrointestinal tract relative to men.[57]

Of course, within the neurocognitive/neurobehavioural domain, one must include possible differences in subjective, behavioural and motoric responses to alcohol as a function of the individual's familial risk for alcoholism and information-processing capacities. However, the individual's response to alcohol will also be conditioned by the person's unique metabolism of alcohol, state of alcohol tolerance, and beliefs about alcohol effects. These beliefs are derived from the culture he or she lives in, and are also dependent on whether the individual grew up in a family in which an alcoholic(s) resided. Additionally, the individual's personality/temperament will determine his or her response to alcohol (for example, is the subject in the test environment cooperative and compliant, or disbelieving and difficult?). For these reasons, it may be very difficult to learn about the unique characteristics of high-risk individuals that predispose them to becoming alcoholic

by using only those tests that involve alcohol administration.

As part of a programme designed to uncover neurobiological factors contributing to alcoholism vulnerability in alcoholic women, we have investigated potential markers from the neurocognitive/neurobehavioural domains. We have uncovered a number of differences between alcoholic women and their children when compared with control women and their children. We speculate that at least some of these differences may contribute to higher risk for alcoholism, and, specifically, early-onset female alcoholism. Whether or not these risk markers will be found to differentiate women whose primary drug of choice is not alcohol is currently unknown. The women and their families who have been included in the Program on the Genetics of Alcoholism and have been studied in our laboratory are primary alcoholics. Primary alcoholics are those who have a lifetime diagnosis of alcohol dependence that precedes any other coexisting Axis I disorder (e.g. drug dependence, major depressive disorder).

Neurobiological characteristics

The primary areas of inquiry have been with respect to event-related potential characteristics of adults[58,59] and children,[60–62] cardiovascular responding,[63] and body sway (static ataxia) in children.[64,65] Event-related potential (ERP) characteristics, including particular components of the waveform (e.g. P300, N250), are of interest for several reasons. The N250 component is a negative wave occurring approximately 250 ms after the onset of a stimulus and is thought to become less negative during a child's development. P300 is a scalp-positive wave that occurs after an informative event occurs. These components are of particular interest because, first, long-latency components of ERPs, including P300, are associated with particular sensory and cognitive aspects of information processing.[66,67] Second, the ERP waveform appears to be under genetic control,[68–71] and third, the P300 component of the event-related potential has received considerable attention as a possible neurophysiological risk marker for the development of alcoholism, both in our own laboratory and in others.

Event-related potentials and risk for developing alcohol dependence

Although there has been some controversy concerning whether P300 is a risk marker for later development of alcoholism, it should be noted that there are now several laboratories, besides our own,[60,61,62] showing consistent results.[72,73] Decrements in P300 are usually seen when high-risk minor children are tested with sufficiently difficult paradigms, and when the density of the alcoholism in the high-risk group is sufficient to allow the variation between high-risk and low-risk groups to be explored (see Hill and Steinhauer[61] and Steinhauer and Hill[62] for discussion). We have reserved the use of the term 'high-risk' to denote cases where the familial constellation is of sufficient density to produce a lifetime risk of 50% or greater for young males, a more stringent requirement than the family history positive (FHP) designation used by many.[74] For an individual to have a predicted recurrence risk of this magnitude, multiple relatives must be alcoholic.[75]

Risk to children of female alcoholics versus children of male alcoholics

Our laboratory has been in a unique position to compare children from male and children from female alcoholic families. As part of a large-scale family study of alcoholism in which families are identified through multi-

generational alcoholism and the presence of at least two alcoholic brothers per family, we are studying children of male alcoholics prospectively. We have observed remarkable consistency in our findings of reduced P300 in these high-risk children, using an auditory oddball paradigm. Two studies have been published utilizing two different samples of children ascertained through male alcoholic probands which found P300 amplitude reduction using an auditory task.[60,62] P300 amplitude reduction in high-risk children from families of male alcoholics have also been found when a visual paradigm was utilized.[61]

Using a similar ascertainment scheme requiring multiple alcoholic family members, we have been studying families of alcoholic women. We have chosen this design because we believe that in those families where female alcoholism is multigenerational, with multiple affected relatives, one might expect an early onset of the problem. These families are much more likely to transmit alcoholism to the next generation, thereby increasing the risk to the offspring. Also, because this subtype is more severe, a minority of affected individuals will achieve remission simply as part of a 'maturing out' process.

Analysis of data obtained from the offspring of female proband alcoholism families indicated, once again, that the amplitude of the P300 component is smaller in high-risk children ($P = 0.016$) when compared with control children.[76] Non-parametric analysis of data supports this result; 9 of 28 high-risk children were one or more standard deviations below the mean of age- and gender-matched controls, while only 3 of 28 controls were this deviant. Because of the importance of these findings, we looked for other explanations for why children from female alcoholism families would show reduced P300. The variables we considered were: (1) drinking during pregnancy; (2) presence of 'other psychopathology' in mothers, especially ASPD, which has been linked to P300 reduction by some, though not all, laboratories; and (3) lower socio-economic status. None of these explanations could explain our data, leading us to conclude that a diathesis for alcoholism was a strong predictor of P300 reduction in children from these female alcoholism families.

Even in families with an extremely high density of alcoholism, the recurrence risk for alcoholism in offspring will be less than 1.0; that is, only some offspring will become alcoholic. Therefore, one would not expect every child from a high-risk family to carry the marker (reduced P300 amplitude), even if the marker was perfectly correlated with affection status. Therefore, it is not surprising that one-third of high-risk boys and one-fifth of high-risk girls show P300 reductions that place them one or more standard deviations below the mean of an age- and gender-matched control group (these proportions are based on visual data for children from the male alcoholism families).[61]

Although this was only a preliminary analysis, we were intrigued by the fact that a greater proportion of girls from high-risk female alcoholism families (30%) than girls from the high-risk males alcoholism families (20%) showed P300 reduction (one or more SDs < mean). In view of the more frequent female-to-female transmission than cross-gender transmission reported in the Swedish adoption study,[42] we speculate that more girls from these high-risk for female alcoholism families may carry a neurobiological diathesis for alcoholism than do girls from similarly matched high-risk for male alcoholism families.

Establishing that P300 deficits occur in female alcoholics is another important step. Our laboratory has an extensive database on adult relatives of male proband alcoholics (both alcoholic and non-alcoholic) and low-risk subjects.[58,59,77] A more modest data set of high-risk women has enabled us to determine that those who develop alcoholism exhibit a 50% reduction in the amplitude of P300 in comparison to their non-alcoholic sisters and to controls in response to information-processing demands.[59] A recent history of drinking (past 7 and past 30 days) was entered into these analyses as a covariate without significant effect. Thus, we can ask whether the absence of a P300 decrement is protective for the high-risk non-alcoholic sister?

Integration of neurobiological and sociocultural perspectives

Any model of alcoholism vulnerability that supports a purely neurobiological–genetic perspective without taking into account the sociocultural factors that mitigate against drinking, and heavy drinking in particular, is incomplete. Moreover, a 'process' model may be a more accurate representation of the waxing and waning, episodic nature of alcoholism through the life course than a 'static' one.[78,79] According to this view, the alcoholic is thought to have certain neurobiological characteristics at birth that may predispose her to becoming alcoholic. The likelihood of that happening will be determined by the consequences of drinking (both biological and psychosocial), which in turn become antecedent conditions for maintenance of abusive drinking.

Substance dependence from a sociocultural perspective

The socio-cultural perspective will be discussed from the point of view of a woman beginning to drink alcohol regularly. Alcohol is a good 'model' drug because it is legal, relatively inexpensive and readily available in most societies. In order for women to become alcoholic they must make a decision to drink alcohol, a decision to continue using alcohol, and a decision to either moderate their ongoing use of alcohol or drink as often or as much as they wish. As seemingly simplistic as this statement may seem, it summarizes the enormous variability in drinking patterns between men and women, particularly in some cultures. Socio-cultural factors determine the likelihood that women will drink and the manner in which they drink. The following review will highlight some of the sociocultural aspects of women's drinking that alter their vulnerability to becoming alcoholic. These include familial environmental factors, the cultural tradition with which they identify, and secular trends in alcohol use.

Familial–environmental factors and use of alcohol and other drugs

Although environmental effects are usually not thought of as 'markers' for substance dependence risk, nevertheless, the effects of environment, if they are non-random and occur at a developmentally critical stage, may endure beyond childhood. Therefore, certain kinds of environmental exposures may be thought of as markers of risk. For example, suppose that the same behavioural characteristic shows up in all children whose drug-dependent mothers failed to achieve remission during their preschool years. This behavioural trait might be thought of as aetiological if these children have higher rates of drug or alcohol dependence as adults than they would by virtue of having a family history without environmental exposure. Currently, we know very little about the effects of early experience on later development of alcoholism or substance abuse. However, it is interesting to note that even laboratory rats, when differentially reared (impoverished versus enriched), show differences in drug preference as adults.[80] Specifically, rats reared in enriched

environments display a greater preference for cocaine solutions when offered a choice between plain water and cocaine-adulterated water than do rats reared in impoverished environments. These results are intriguing in view of reported differences in brain neurochemistry in rats[81] differentially reared in environments similar to those employed in the preference study.[80] Extrapolating to the human condition, one could argue that the immature brain may be open to 'tuning' by environmental stimuli such that those reared in highly stimulating environments (good or bad) may seek similar levels of stimulation. The change of state which alcohol or drug intoxication provides may satisfy this craving for excessive stimulation. This need for excessive stimulation is embodied in the concept of 'sensation-seeking' frequently described for substance-dependent individuals.[82]

In addition to possible environmental effects on neurobiological 'fine-tuning', there is also the clear possibility that expectations concerning the effects of alcohol or other drugs may be transmitted within families. There is a growing body of evidence suggesting that expectancies are learned early in life and are predictive of later development of alcohol use patterns.[83,84] Johnson et al[85] studied members of families of college students living in Hawaii, and found moderate to high correlations between parents and their offspring with respect to the expected physiological and subjective effects of alcohol. Whether these expectancy effects are as salient for girls and young women is unclear. Beliefs about the substantive effects of alcohol were correlated for pairs of family members to reflect resemblance in beliefs. The data presented indicate that the father–son and mother–son correlations were higher than the father–daughter or mother–daughter correlations. Thus, expectancy effects may be transmitted within families but to a lesser degree among females.

Cross-cultural variation in alcohol use among women

Cross-cultural variation will be examined with respect to alcohol use because availability across cultures is probably more similar than the patterns for specific drugs of abuse. Those cultures that have a low availability of particular drugs because of more intense policing of drug trafficking will often have alcohol readily available because of locally made alcohol products. In fact, women are often involved in the manufacture of alcohol products in Third World countries.[86]

Examining cross-cultural variation in rates of drinking, abuse of alcohol and alcohol dependence is not only instructive with respect to understanding how cultural variation influences the likelihood that individuals will develop alcoholism, but also elucidates those factors influencing vulnerability to alcoholism in women compared with those found in men.

The fact that more men than women become alcoholic in most cultures has led to a number of misconceptions about women's drinking. One of these is the notion that women traditionally have not had as much freedom with regard to access to alcohol. Child et al,[87] examined records concerning drinking in 139 societies, and found adequate data for analysis from 113, only four of which did not allow women to drink. Only in one society was drunkenness forbidden in women. Moreover, in some cultures women actually have greater access to alcohol than do men. As noted by Heath[88] in Latin America and parts of Africa, women are the primary producers and distributors of grain- or vegetable-based home brews that are used as both foods and intoxicants. In some of these societies women own and operate public drinking establishments where they market the alcohol they produce. In some tribal societies the home brew business is the focus of the economy.

Because a greater proportion of men than women become alcoholic in most societies, much of the current thinking that presupposes a greater genetic (biological) vulnerability to alcoholism for men than for women[89] may have been influenced by this observation. Yet, formal tests of heterogeneity among women alcoholics have not been performed in any of the family studies of women undertaken to date,[89] so it is not possible to rule out the possibility of two (perhaps more) types of alcoholism in women. We suspect that there may be an equal number of more genetically determined cases of male and female alcoholism in the population, but the higher rates seen overall in men are largely due to the fact that environmental pressures to drink heavily are much greater for males. This conclusion is, in part, based on analysis of our high-density families selected through male alcoholic probands. In these families the age of onset for females who become alcoholic is as early as it is for brothers who become alcoholic.[40] Also, families selected through female probands for their high density of alcoholism and multigenerational affectation show that female alcoholism can be as severe as the most familial form identified in men. As will be recalled, we have found the median age of onset for alcoholism in these women to be 16 years.

If the discrepancy between alcoholism rates among men and women is largely due to variations in environmental pressures to not drink heavily in the first place, one should find widely varying ratios between male and female rates from society to society. This is exactly what one sees in reviewing the ratio of male to female alcoholism across those societies that permit women to drink, which, as noted previously, include the majority of societies. For example, reanalysis of data provided by epidemiological surveys in Israel and the USA[90] reveals a 6-month prevalence male/female ratio for alcoholism of approximately 6 : 1 in the USA, versus 14 : 1 in Israel. Another cross-national study using the Diagnostic Interview Schedule (DIS), the instrument originally developed for the US ECA study, compared the lifetime prevalence of alcohol abuse and alcohol dependence in the USA, Canada, Puerto Rico, Taiwan, and South Korea.[91] This study found ratios of 5.4 : 1, 4.7 : 1, 9.8 : 1, 29 : 1 and 20 : 1, respectively. Clearly, cultural variation changes the likelihood that individuals will become alcoholic. This variation is not equally effective by gender. This observation is further illustrated in an intriguing study in which the Korean version of the DIS was administered to Korean men and women living in two sites, Kangwha, Korea and Yanbian, China.[92] All were native Koreans who lived in different socio-cultural environments, with those living in China being subject to more traditional and conservative attitudes towards drinking. A significant difference in lifetime prevalence of alcohol abuse and alcohol dependence was reported by the authors. What is of interest with respect to socio-cultural influences on female drinking and alcoholism is the widely varying male/female ratios in alcohol abuse. For Kangwha, the ratio was 17.5 : 1, whereas the ratio for Yanbian, China, where traditional societal values are more salient, was 115 : 1!

In contrast, in those societies that are more permissive of drinking, the male/female ratio is much less discrepant. Brown et al[93] have examined alcoholism in Southern Cheyenne Indians, and found a ratio of 1.7 : 1. Moreover, the majority of both male and female alcoholics had an early onset (<25 years) of the disorder. In fact, there are cases where females drink more than males, as noted by Weibel-Orlando.[94] She found that Sioux women drank more frequently than Sioux men, and appeared to consume more alcohol per occasion than did the men.

Finally, mention should be made of the possibility that there are different mechanisms involved in alcohol use and alcohol dependence. Societies that have undergone rapid changes in attitudes and behaviours related to substance use provide the opportunity to evaluate whether alcohol dependence and alcohol abuse are equally influenced by societal changes. Hwu et al[95] have reported that the prevalence of alcohol abuse is five times greater than that of alcohol dependence in current (post-World War II) Taiwanese society, suggesting that alcohol abuse may be more responsive to changes in societal norms than is alcohol dependence.

Because alcohol use is culturally, and, in many societies, legally controlled, it is not surprising that women are less likely to drink abusively, and consume less alcohol overall, than men. However, if some alcoholism is genetically mediated (perhaps a greater proportion of female than male alcoholics), then one might expect that the manifestations of alcoholism would be equivalent in men and women once they become alcoholic. Several recent studies would appear to support this conclusion. The World Health collaborative project has been collecting data concerning the prevalence of harmful levels of alcohol consumption in six countries: Australia, Bulgaria, Kenya, Mexico, Norway, and the USA. For all national groups, the level of consumption for men is significantly higher than that for women. However, among alcoholics the average daily intake for women was 74% of the intake for men (176 g for women and 200 g for men). Correcting for body weight differences indicates that women alcoholics may be drinking more in terms of gram per kilogram intake than are alcoholic men.

Furthermore, Kawakami et al[96] found that, among a sample of over 2500 employees of a computer factory in Tokyo, 15% of the men and 6% of the women could be classified as having alcohol problems using an alcoholism screening test (Kurihama Alcoholism Screening Test) designed for use among Japanese, and embodying similar concepts to those used in DSM-III definitions of alcoholism. Importantly, there was no significant gender difference in the prevalence of alcohol-related problems for a given amount of alcohol consumption. These results support the conclusions reached by Edwards et al[97] that women have the same susceptibility to alcohol-related problems when they drink the same amount as males.

Summary of findings and implications for treatment and prevention

Review of the current US epidemiological survey data suggests that while women have a greater risk for developing major depression, they have lower risks for developing alcohol and drug abuse problems. If the disorders each have moderately high heritability and are transmitted independently, one should be able to determine the potential risk for carrying both disorders by gender by multiplying the independent probabilities for each disorder. This exercise results in quite comparable rates of comorbid alcohol dependence and depression in women and men (2% versus 3%). Perhaps it is not surprising, then, that the alcoholic to non-alcoholic ratio for depression is similar by gender in the ECA data. As may be recalled, Helzer et al reported ratios of 2.4 for men and 2.7 for women. The elevation in depression in women relative to men that is commonly found in treated samples is most probably due to the well-known Berk effect—women with depres-

sion are more likely to seek treatment. Whether the presence of depression alters treatment outcome positively or adversely is currently unknown. We do know that treatment outcome is adversely affected by having a more severe (usually early-onset) form of the disorder.

There is as much evidence that at least one form of alcoholism in women is genetically mediated as there is for men. For women with the more severe form of alcoholism, onset of the disorder is as early as it is in men. Identification of children at risk for developing this form of alcohol dependence is needed to target appropriate candidates for more intense prevention efforts. Similarly, the early-onset alcohol-dependent (or drug-dependent) woman may require new treatment modalities. Finally, it has been noted that gender differences in rates of alcoholism probably have more to do with cultural variations that have greater impact on women than on men, preventing them from becoming heavy drinkers. Once they become heavy drinkers, their chances of developing alcohol problems are equivalent to that of men. Neurobiological risk factors identified in very high-risk men appear to apply equally well to women and girls who are at very high risk for becoming alcoholic by virtue of the high-density, multigenerational nature of the alcoholism running in their families.

Acknowledgments

Preparation of this manuscript was supported in part by awards from the National Institute on Alcohol Abuse and Alcoholism AA005909-14, AA05808-08 and AA11304-01.

References

1. Willengbring ML, Measurement of depression in alcoholics, *J Stud Alcohol* 1986; **47**:367–72.
2. Tamerin JS, Mendelson JH, The psychodynamics of chronic inebriation: observations of alcoholics during the process of drinking in an experimental group setting, *Am J Psychiatry* 1969; **125**:886–99.
3. Brown SA, Schuckit MA, Changes in depression among abstinent alcoholics, *J Stud Alcohol* 1988; **49**:412–17.
4. Nakamura MM, Overall JE, Hollister LE, Radcliffe E, Factors affecting outcome of depressive symptoms in alcoholics, *Alcohol Clin Exp Res* 1983; **7**:188–93.
5. Overall JE, Reilly EL, Kelley JT, Hollister LE, Persistence of depression in detoxified alcoholics, *Alcohol Clin Exp Res* 1985; **9**:331–3.
6. Pottenger M, McKernon J, Patrie LE et al, The frequency and persistence of depressive symptoms in the alcohol abuser, *J Nerv Ment Dis* 1978; **166**:562–70.
7. Hill SY, Lowers L, Antidepressant medication use in women recently treated for alcohol dependence, unpublished.
8. Pitts FN, Winokur G, Affective disorder—VII: Alcoholism and affective disorder, *J Psychiatr Res* 1966; **4**:37–50.
9. Winokur G, Rimmer J, Reich T, Alcoholism IV. Is there more than one type of alcoholism? *Br J Psychiatry* 1971; **118**:525–31.
10. Cloninger CR, Reich T, Wetzel R, Alcoholism and affective disorders: familial association and genetic models. In: Goodwin DW, Erickson CK, eds, *Alcoholism and Affective Disorders: Clinical, Genetic, and Biochemical Studies* (SP Medical and Scientific Books: New York, 1979) 57–86.
11. Schuckit MA, The clinical implications of primary diagnostic groups among alcoholics, *Arch Gen Psychiatry* 1985; **42**:1043–9.
12. Goodwin DW, Schulsinger F, Hermansen L et al, Alcohol problems in adoptees raised apart from alcoholic biological parents, *Arch Gen Psychiatry* 1973; **28**:238–43.
13. Goodwin DW, Schulsinger F, Knop J et al, Alcoholism and depression in adopted-out daughters of alcoholics, *Arch Gen Psychiatry* 1977; **34**:751–5.

14. Kaij L, *Alcoholism in Twins: Studies on the Etiology and Sequels of Abuse of Alcohol* (Almquist and Wiksell: Stockholm, 1960).
15. Mullan MJ, Gurling HM, Oppenheim BE, Murray RM, The relationship between alcoholism and neurosis: evidence from a twin study, *Br J Psychiatry* 1986; **148**:435–41.
16. Kendler KS, Walters EE, Neale MC et al, The structure of the genetic and environmental risk factors for six major psychiatric disorders in women. Phobia, generalized anxiety disorder, panic disorder, bulimia, major depression, and alcoholism, *Arch Gen Psychiatry* 1995; **52**:374–83.
17. Adamson J, Burdick JA, Sleep of dry alcoholics, *Arch Gen Psychiatry* 1973; **28**:146–9.
18. Helzer JE, Pryzbeck TR, The co-occurrence of alcoholism with other psychiatric disorders in the general population and its impact on treatment, *J Stud Alcohol* 1988; **49**:219–24.
19. Bedi AR, Halikas JA, Alcoholism and affective disorder, *Alcohol Clin Exp Res* 1985; **9**:133–4.
20. Schutte KK, Hearst J, Moos RH, Gender differences in the relations between depressive symptoms and drinking behavior among problem drinkers: a three-wave study, *J Consult Clin Psychol* 1997; **65**:392–404.
21. Mueller TI, Lavori PW, Keller MB et al, Prognostic effect of the variable course of alcoholism on the 10 year course of depression, *Am J Psychiatry* 1994; **151**:701–6.
22. Kessler RC, McGonagle KA, Zhao S et al, Lifetime and 12-month prevalence of DSM-III-R psychiatric disorders in the United States. Results from the National Comorbidity Survey, *Arch Gen Psychiatry* 1994; **51**:8–19.
23. Robins LN, Helzer JE, Pryzbeck TR, Regier DA, Alcohol disorders in the community: a report from the Epidemiological Catchment Area. In: Rose RM, Barrett JE, eds, *Alcoholism: Origins and Outcome* (Raven Press: New York, 1988) 15–30.
24. Schuckit M, Alcoholic patients with secondary depression, *Am J Psychiatry* 1983; **140**:711–14.
25. Ross HE, Glaser FB, Germanson T, The prevalence of psychiatric disorders in patients with alcohol and other drug problems, *Arch Gen Psychiatry* 1988; **45**:1023–31.
26. Merikangas KR, Gelernter CS, Comorbidity for

alcoholism and depression, *Psychiatr Clin North Am* 1990; **13**:613–32.

27. Rounsaville BJ, Kleber HD, Untreated opiate addicts. How do they differ from those seeking treatment? *Arch Gen Psychiatry* 1985; **42**: 1072–7.

28. Helzer JE, Burnam A, McEvoy LT, Alcohol abuse and dependence. In: Robins LN, Regier DA, eds, *Psychiatric Disorders in America: The Epidemiologic Catchment Area Study* (The Free Press: New York, 1991) 81–115.

29. Hesselbrock MN, Gender comparison of antisocial personality disorder and depression in alcoholism, *J Subst Abuse* 1991; **3**:205–19.

30. Schuckit MA, The clinical implications of primary diagnostic groups among alcoholics, *Arch Gen Psychiatry* 1985; **42**:1043–9.

31. Powell BJ, Penick EC, Nickel EJ et al, Outcomes of co-morbid alcoholic men: a 1-year follow-up, *Alcohol Clin Exp Res* 1992; **16**: 131–8.

32. Schuckit MA, Winokur G, A short term follow up of women alcoholics, *Dis Nerv Syst* 1972; **33**:672–8.

33. Rounsaville BJ, Dolinsky ZS, Babor TF et al, Psychopathology as a predictor of treatment outcome in alcoholics, *Arch Gen Psychiatry* 1987; **44**:505–13.

34. Kranzler HR, Del Boca FK, Rounsaville BJ, Comorbid psychiatric diagnosis predicts three-year outcomes in alcoholics: a posttreatment natural history study, *J Study Alcohol* 1996; **57**:619–26.

35. Hasin DS, Endicott J, Keller MB, Alcohol problems in psychiatric patients: 5-year course, *Comp Psychiatry* 1991; **32**:303–16.

36. Brennan PL, Moos RH, Late-life problem drinking: personal and environmental risk factors for 4-year functioning outcomes and treatment seeking, *J Subst Abuse* 1996; **8**:167–80.

37. Kranzler HR, Burleson JA, Korner P et al, Placebo-controlled trial of fluoxetine as an adjunct to relapse prevention in alcoholics, *Am J Psychiatry* 1995; **152**:391–7.

38. Mason BJ, Kocsis JH, Desipramine treatment of alcoholism, *Psychopharmacol Bull* 1991; **27**:155–61.

39. Merikangas KR, Leckman JF, Prusoff BA et al, Familial transmission of depression and alcoholism, *Arch Gen Psychiatry* 1985; **42**:367–72.

40. Hill SY, Smith TR, Evidence for genetic mediation of alcoholism in women, *J Subst Abuse* 1991; **3**:159–74.

41. Hill SY, Genetic vulnerability to alcoholism in women. In: Gomberg E, Nirenberg TD, eds, *Women and Substance Abuse* (Ablex Publishing Corp.: Norwood, 1993) 42–61.

42. Bohman M, Sigvardsson S, Cloninger CR, Maternal inheritance of alcohol abuse. Cross-fostering analysis of adopted women, *Arch Gen Psychiatry* 1981; **38**:965–9.

43. Cadoret RJ, O'Gorman TW, Troughton E et al, Alcoholism and antisocial personality. Interrelationships, genetic and environmental factors, *Arch Gen Psychiatry* 1985; **42**:161–7.

44. Heath AC, Jardine R, Martin NG, Interactive effects of genotype and social environment on alcohol consumption in female twins, *J Stud Alcohol* 1989; **50**:38–48.

45. Gurling HMD, Murray RM, Clifford CA, Investigations into the genetics of alcohol dependence and into its effects on brain function. In: Gedda L, Parisi P, Nance WE, eds, *Twin Research 3: Epidemiological and Clinical Studies* (Alan R Liss, Inc.: New York, 1981) 77–87.

46. McGue M, Pickens RW, Svikis DS, Sex and age effects on the inheritance of alcohol problems: a twin study, *J Abnorm Psychol* 1992; **101**:3–17.

47. Pickens RW, Svikis DS, McGue M et al, Heterogeneity in the inheritance of alcoholism. A study of male and female twins, *Arch Gen Psychiatry* 1991; **48**:19–28.

48. Pickens RW, Svikis DS, The twin method in the study of vulnerability to drug abuse, *NIDA Res Monogr* 1988; **89**:41–51.

49. Kendler KS, Heath AC, Neale MC et al, A population-based twin study of alcoholism in women, *JAMA* 1992; **268**:1877–82.

50. Glenn SW, Nixon SJ, Applications of Cloninger's subtypes in a female alcoholic sample, *Alcohol Clin Exp Res* 1991; **15**:851–7.

51. Lex BW, Sholar JW, Bower T et al, Putative type II alcoholism characteristics in female third DUI offenders in Massachusetts: a pilot study, *Alcohol* 1991; **8**:283–7.

52. Hill SY, Familial risk for alcoholism in women: is P300 a marker? *Proc Am College Neuropharmacol* 1993; **32**:39.

53. Cloninger CR, Bohman M, Sigvardsson S, Inheritance of alcohol abuse. Cross-fostering

analysis of adopted men, *Arch Gen Psychiatry* 1981; **38**:861–8.

54. Hill SY, Absence of paternal sociopathy in the etiology of severe alcoholism: is there a type III alcoholism? *J Stud Alcohol* 1992; **53**:161–9.

55. Neiswanger K, Hill SY, Kaplan BB, Association and linkage studies of the TAQ1 A1 allele at the dopamine D2 receptor gene in samples of female and male alcoholics, *Am J Med Genet* 1995; **60**:267–71.

56. Hill SY, Addiction liability of Tryon rats: independent transmission of morphine and alcohol consumption, *Pharmacol Biochem Behav* 1978; **9**:107–10.

57. Frezza M, di Padova C, Pozzato G et al, High blood alcohol levels in women. The role of decreased gastric alcohol dehydrogenase activity and first-pass metabolism, *N Engl J Med* 1990; **322**:95–9.

58. Hill SY, Steinhauer SR, Zubin J et al, Event-related potentials as markers for alcoholism risk in high density families, *Alcohol Clin Exp Res* 1988; **12**:545–54.

59. Hill SY, Steinhauer SR, Event-related potentials in women at risk for alcoholism, *Alcohol* 1993; **10**:349–54.

60. Hill SY, Steinhauer S, Park J et al, Event-related potential characteristics in children of alcoholics from high density families, *Alcohol Clin Exp Res* 1990; **14**:6–16.

61. Hill SY, Steinhauer SR, Assessment of pre-pubertal and postpubertal boys and girls at risk for developing alcoholism with P300 from a visual discrimination task, *J Stud Alcohol* 1993; **54**:350–8.

62. Steinhauer SR, Hill SY, Auditory event-related potentials in children at high risk for alcoholism, *J Stud Alcohol* 1993; **54**:408–21.

63. Hill SY, Steinhauer SR, Zubin J, Cardiac responsivity in individuals at high risk for alcoholism, *J Stud Alcohol* 1992; **53**:378–88.

64. Hill SY, Armstrong J, Steinhauer SR et al, Static ataxia as a psychobiological marker for alcoholism, *Alcohol Clin Exp Res* 1987; **11**:345–8.

65. Hill SY, Steinhauer SR, Postural sway in children from pedigrees exhibiting a high density of alcoholism, *Biol Psychiatry* 1993; **33**:313–25.

66. Sutton S, Braren M, John ER et al, Evoked potential correlates of stimulus uncertainty, *Science* 1965; **150**:1187–8.

67. Surwillo WW, Cortical evoked potentials in monozygotic twins and unrelated subjects: comparisons of exogenous and endogenous components, *Behav Genet* 1980; **10**:201–9.

68. Polich J, Burns T, P300 from identical twins, *Neuropsychologia* 1987; **25**:299–304.

69. Aston CE, Hill SY, A segregation analysis of the P300 component of the event-related potential, *Am J Hum Genet* 1990; **47** (suppl):A127.

70. Rogers TD, Deary I, The P300 component of the auditory event-related potential in monozygotic and dizygotic twins, *Acta Psychiatr Scand* 1991; **83**:412–16.

71. van Beijsterveldt CEM, *The Genetics of Electrophysiological Indices of Brain Activity: An EEG Study in Adolescent Twins* (University of Amsterdam: Amsterdam, 1996).

72. Begleiter H, Porjesz B, Bihari B et al, Event-related brain potentials in boys at risk for alcoholism, *Science* 1984; **225**:1493–6.

73. Berman SM, Whipple SC, Fitch RJ et al, P3 in young boys as a predictor of adolescent substance use, *Alcohol* 1993; **10**:69–76.

74. Polich J, Bloom FE, Event-related brain potentials in individuals at high and low risk for developing alcoholism: failure to replicate, *Alcohol Clin Exp Res* 1988; **12**:368–73.

75. Aston CE, Hill SY, Segregation analysis of alcoholism in families ascertained through a pair of male alcoholics, *Am J Hum Genet* 1990; **46**:879–87.

76. Hill SY, Muka D, Steinhauer S, Locke J, P300 amplitude decrements in children from families of alcoholic female probands, *Biol Psychiatry* 1995; **38**:622–32.

77. Hill SY, Steinhauer S, Locke J, Event-related potentials in alcoholic men, their high-risk male relatives and low-risk male controls, *Alcohol Clin Exp Res* 1995; **19**:567–76.

78. Hill SY, A vulnerability model for alcoholism in women, *Focus Women: J Addict Health* 1981; **2**:68–91.

79. Hill SY, Biological consequences of alcoholism and alcohol-related problems among women. In: *Alcohol and Health Monograph No. 4, Special Population Issues* DHHS Pub. No. (ADM)82-1193 (US Department of Health and Human Services, National Institute on Alcohol Abuse and Alcoholism: Rockville, 1982) 43–73.

80. Hill SY, Powell BJ, Cocaine and morphine self-administration: effects of differential rearing, *Pharmacol Biochem Behav* 1976; **5**:701–4.

81. Krech D, Rosenzweig MR, Bennett EL, Effects of environmental complexity and training on brain chemistry, *J Comp Physiol Psychol* 1960; **53**:509–19.

82. Zuckerman M, Sensation seeking and the endogenous deficit theory of drug abuse, *NIDA Res Monogr* 1986; **74**:59–70.

83. Christiansen BA, Smith GT, Roehling PV et al, Using alcohol expectancies to predict adolescent drinking behavior after one year, *J Consult Clin Psychol* 1989; **57**:93–9.

84. Miller PM, Smith GT, Goldman MS, Emergence of alcohol expectancies in childhood: a possible critical period, *J Stud Alcohol* 1990; **51**:343–9.

85. Johnson RC, Nagoshi CT, Danko GP et al, Familial transmission of alcohol use norms and expectancies and reported alcohol use, *Alcohol Clin Exp Res* 1990; **14**:216–20.

86. World Health Organization, *Women and Substance Abuse: A Gender Analysis and Review of Health and Policy Implications* (WHO: Geneva, 1993) 41.

87. Child IL, Barry H, Bacon MK, A cross-cultural study of drinking: III. Sex differences, *Q J Stud Alcohol* 1965; **3**:49–61.

88. Heath DB, Women and alcohol: cross-cultural perspectives, *J Subst Abuse* 1991; **3**:175–85.

89. Gilligan SB, Reich T, Cloninger CR, Etiologic heterogeneity in alcoholism, *Genet Epidemiol* 1987; **4**:395–414.

90. Levav I, Kohn R, Dohrenwend BP et al, An epidemiological study of mental disorders in a 10-year cohort of young adults in Israel, *Psychol Med* 1993; **23**:691–707.

91. Helzer JE, Canino GJ, Yeh EK et al, Alcoholism—North America and Asia. A comparison of population surveys with the diagnostic interview schedule, *Arch Gen Psychiatry* 1990; **47**:313–19.

92. Namkoong K, Lee HY, Lee MH et al, Cross-cultural study of alcoholism: comparison between Kangwha, Korea and Yanbian, China, *Yonsei Med J* 1991; **32**:319–25.

93. Brown GL, Albaugh BJ, Robin RW et al, Alcoholism and substance abuse among selected Southern Cheyenne Indians, *Cult Med Psychiatry* 1993; **16**:531–42.

94. Weibel-Orlando J, Women and alcohol: special populations and cross-cultural variations. In: National Institute on Alcohol Abuse and Alcoholism, ed., *Women and Alcohol: Health Related Issues* (National Institute on Alcohol Abuse and Alcoholism: Rockville, 1986) 161–87.

95. Hwu HG, Yeh EK, Yeh YL, Risk factors of alcoholism in Taiwan Chinese: an epidemiological approach, *Acta Psychiatr Scand* 1990; **82**:295–8.

96. Kawakami N, Haratani T, Hemmi T et al, Prevalence and demographic correlates of alcohol-related problems in Japanese employees, *Soc Psychiatry Psychiatr Epidemiol* 1992; **27**:198–202.

97. Edwards G, Chandler J, Hensman C et al, Drinking in a London suburb. II. Correlates of trouble with drinking among men, *Q J Stud Alcohol* 1972; **6** (suppl):94–119.

27

Pain: adding to the affective burden
Marta Meana and Donna E Stewart

Introduction

The gender differential in the prevalence of mood disorders has been the focus of much attention recently. With depression and anxiety being grossly overrepresented in women, research has turned to the identification of biopsychosocial aetiological factors that might explain the gender difference. At its most expansive, the literature points to societal norms that may place women at risk for mood disturbances. The more modest hope has been that a greater understanding of potential contributing factors may result in a more effective clinical management of these debilitating disorders.

It appears that, in addition to the mood disorder burden on women, there is a higher prevalence of pain complaints and pain disorders. First, women are more likely than men to experience pain associated with normal physiological events that pose no significant threat. Menstruation and childbirth result in pain for many women, even when devoid of any pathological process or complication.

Second, pathological processes associated with reproductive cycles and function, such as ovarian cysts, uterine fibroids, and endometriosis, represent another set of potential pain sources that do not affect men. Third, there is a marked preponderance of women over men in a significant number of chronic pain syndromes. Among these are migraines, temporomandibular joint disorder, fibromyalgia, rheumatoid arthritis, osteoarthritis, interstitial cystitis, and burning mouth syndrome. Many of these pain syndromes also happen to be idiopathic.

Is there a relationship between the higher prevalences of mood disorders and pain reports in women? The answer is equivocal. Our current understanding of the relationship between pain and mood disorders in women is limited both by a lack of attention to gender in much pain research to date and by methodological problems endemic to pain research in general. More often than not, gender is left unexamined in pain study outcomes and is considered a sociodemographic variable not expected to moderate results. The lack of epidemiologically sound research also complicates matters. The majority of studies on the comorbidity of pain and mood disturbances have been conducted on clinical samples, possibly inflating the prevalence of psychological problems. Cross-study comparisons are also difficult because of the wide range of conditions under which these studies were undertaken. Another methodological conundrum that plagues the gender and pain literature is the problem of distinguishing between sensory differences and response-style differences. As pain studies rely heavily on self-report, differences in the cognitive and emotional responses to pain continue to be candidates for, at least part of, the explanation of gender differences in pain reporting. Finally, studies linking pain and mood disorders have focused almost exclusively on depression. There are only a handful of studies on the relationship between anxiety and persistent pain, although interest in the role of anxiety is growing.

Limitations in the existing literature notwithstanding, gender differences in pain are finally starting to receive significant research attention. No longer considered a curiosity, gender differences in this and other areas are increasingly considered to have the potential to: (1) uncover basic mechanisms of disease in both men and women; and (2) inform clinical management efforts about the relative risks and benefits of differentiated treatment strategies. It is in light of this important potential that this chapter critically reviews the relationships among gender, pain and mood disturbance, from empirical, theoretical and clinical perspectives. Because almost all of the research in this area has focused on the relationship between pain and depression, the focus of this chapter is necessarily the same.

Gender differences in pain

Experimentally induced pain

One strategy in the attempt to determine whether men and women differ in their experience of pain has been to deliver noxious stimuli to volunteers, under controlled experimental circumstances. These psychophysical studies, many of which have been carried out with undergraduate students, have focused on gender differences in three pain variables: thresholds, intensity, and tolerance. Overall, the results seem to indicate that sex differences in pain reports exist. Under experimental conditions, women report lower thresholds, higher intensity ratings, and less tolerance of pain than men.[1-3] However, the differences are small and their presence and direction seem to be influenced by specific experimental conditions and subject characteristics.

Gender differences in experimental pain are not consistently found for all types of stimuli. Women seem to be most reactive to electrical and pressure stimuli.[4] Pain-rating variations have also been linked to menstrual phase and reproductive status in women, although these findings have been inconsistent.[5-8] Dysmenorrheic women report lower pressure pain ratings during the follicular phase of their cycle and high pain sensitivity premenstrually.[5] Women with bulimia nervosa have higher pain thresholds for pressure pain stimuli.[9] Thus, it seems that women with specific pain or other disorders do not respond to pain in the same way as women without health problems. Age, class and ethnicity are additional variables that have not received much attention in the experimental study of pain and gender.[10]

Further complicating the issue of sex differences in the experience of experimentally induced pain is the difficulty in distinguishing sensory from response factors. Are women more willing to report pain? Can these small gender differences in pain perception be explained by different response styles rather than by differing sensory experiences? In one study, male subjects reported much less pain when the experimenter was an attractive woman.[11] Although other studies have not found significant effects of experimenter gender,[2,12] there is good theoretical support for the idea that sex role expectations may have an impact on pain report.

Few experimental studies, however, can claim to have separated response style from sensory experience. Ellermeier and Westphal isolated an objective indicator of pain intensity by way of pupillomotor behaviour in response to a pressure stimulus.[13] A significant correlation was found between pupil dilation and subjective pain ratings. At high levels of stimulation, women reported more intense pain than men and their pupils confirmed the sex difference as belonging to the realm of sensation rather than expression. Women also seem to discriminate among heat intensities better than men, which also indicates that at least some of the gender differences may be more sensory than response related.[2]

Thus, with small and inconsistent differences that seem to be mediated by stimulus, experimenter and subject characteristics, it is difficult to be confident in the reliability of the small pain perception gender differences found under experimental conditions.[14]

Clinical pain

Women in North America have higher rates of illness and health-care utilization,[15-18] have a higher incidence of both temporary and chronic pain,[19,20] and report pain in more multiple sites than do men.[21] However, if the empirical support for gender differences in experimentally induced pain is complicated by multiple mediating factors, the literature on gender differences in clinical pain is even more difficult to interpret. First, there is the inescapable reality that research with clinical populations is generally less controlled and scientifically rigorous than experimental research. Second, there are significant differences between experimental and clinical pain. Clinical pain is generally longer in duration and greater in intensity. Unlike experimentally induced pain, clinical pain often has consequences. It may impact on self-concept, mood, function and relationships. Any and all of these may differentially affect both the experience of pain and its expression in men and women.

One of the ways in which these variables have been accounted for has been through the expansion of outcomes from the simple pain report ratings used in experimental studies to more ecological measures such as quality of life, functional impact of pain and psychosocial adjustment. Although clearly important, the inclusion of these outcome measures in clinical pain studies remains unsuccessful in distinguishing between sensory factors and attitudinal ones. Adding to potential attitudinal gender differences in clinical pain is the influence of health-care practitioner attitudes about gender and pain, as well as gender-linked diagnostic biases.[22]

The relatively voluminous literature on clinical pain and gender is thus somewhat confusing, although Unruh's review is enormously helpful in organizing the often conflicting results.[23] Discussions of gender differences in clinical pain are generally divided into: (1) gender-specific pain that is limited to anatomical differences between men and women; and (2) pain conditions that are more prevalent in one gender than in the other. A review of both of these is necessary to provide a comprehensive picture of the gender-differential burden of pain.

Gender-specific pain

Women are much more likely than men to experience pain that has no obvious or hypothesized pathological basis. Normal menstruation, ovulation, pregnancy and childbirth are sources of recurrent pain for many women. By late adolescence, 81% of all girls have menstrual pain and, although the severity of the pain seems to wane with age, the prevalence of menstrual pain is still high, at 45% of women aged 35–49 years.[24] Uncomplicated childbirth is also accompanied by pain reported as being more intense than many other acute pains associated with serious pathology, such as cancer.[25] In addition to these non-pathological pains, women also suffer from a host of gynaecological and obstetrical problems. These include persistent pain disorders such as chronic pelvic pain, uterine fibroids, endometriosis and vulvodynia, in addition to the acute pain from common complications such as miscarriage, ectopic pregnancy, rupture of ovarian cysts, and pelvic inflammatory disease.[26–28] Episiotomies performed to facilitate delivery can also result in chronic genital pain.[29]

Much of the higher morbidity of pain in women can probably be accounted for by these gynaecological and obstetrical problems.[30] Although men also suffer from gender-specific pains, it is more often the case that these conditions are consequent to injury and disease and more amenable to resolution through treatment.[23] Chronic pain conditions are more common in female-specific anatomy.

Pain disorders more prevalent in women

In the International Association for the Study of Pain's Classification of Chronic Pain, there are approximately twice as many pain disorders with a higher female prevalence than disorders with a higher male prevalence. Among the most common of these are headaches, orofacial pain and musculoskeletal pain. In addition to these, women are diagnosed with irritable bowel syndrome, interstitial cystitis and psychogenic pains much more often than are men.[31]

The higher prevalence of migraines and chronic tension headaches in women has been demonstrated in numerous epidemiological studies across the world (see Unruh[23] for a list of these studies). The headaches reported by women are also more severe, more frequent, and longer in duration. While menopause seems to bring some relief and the prevalence drops with age, postmenopausal women continue to have higher rates of migraine than age-matched men.

The most common type of orofacial pain is temporomandibular disorder (TMD). Its primary clinical sign is tenderness on palpation of the joint and related masticatory muscles. This chronic pain disorder has a female/male ratio that ranges from 2 : 1 to 9 : 1, and women describe their symptoms as more severe than those reported by men with TMD.[32,33] Another type of orofacial pain that predominates in women is burning mouth syndrome, a chronic burning pain in the tongue and other mucous membranes. Patients with this disorder are mostly over 50 years of age, and the female/male ratio is 3 : 1. The prevalence in postmenopausal women has been estimated at 18–33% and, despite theories about hormonal influences, the aetiology of burning mouth syndrome remains unknown.[34,35]

The majority of epidemiological studies find that women report more musculoskeletal pain than do men.[23] Much of this difference could probably be accounted for by the higher female prevalence rates of fibromyalgia, rheumatoid arthritis and osteoarthritis.[36] Fibromyalgia is characterized by generalized muscle aching, stiffness and fatigue. It is estimated to affect 15% of the general population, and the female/male ratio is 6 : 1.[31,37] One study reported no gender differences in threshold responses when pressure was applied to trigger points, but female fibromyalgia patients reported more pain than male fibromyalgia patients.[38] Rheumatoid arthritis disproportionately affects women of all ages, and osteoarthritis disproportionately affects women over 45 years compared to age-matched men.[31]

In terms of lower body pains, irritable bowel syndrome is also diagnosed more often in women and it is described as 'chronic abdominal pain with no apparent cause associated with alteration in bowel habit'.[31] The often excruciating bladder pain of interstitial cystitis has only recently started to become recognized as a pain syndrome, and 90% of sufferers are women.[39]

Prevalence rates for clusters of multiple coexisting idiopathic pains are generally higher in women; these fall into the category of somatization disorders. Although the general prevalence of somatization disorder is low, at 1% of the general population, women account for almost all occurrences.[40,41] Prior to the recognition that tissue damage is not a prerequisite for the experience of pain, there was a tendency to attribute any idiopathic pain disorder to psychological causes and psychiatric disorders. Despite the lack of explanatory mechanisms for purely hysterical pains and the perils of diagnosis by exclusion, the concept of psychogenic pain has not entirely disappeared. Considering the preponderance of women with idiopathic pain disorders now and in the past, this dualistic categorization of pain is worrisome and might constitute a gender-linked diagnostic bias.

Functional impact of pain

The fact that women suffer from more temporary and persistent pain that men and report their pain as being more severe does not directly establish the extent to which the pain interferes with their lives. Do women in pain suffer more disability and invalidism than do men in pain? The results of studies comparing the functional impact of pain on men and women are inconsistent. Some studies have found similar rates of impairment in activities of daily living for both sexes,[42,43] while others report higher rates of disability for women.[44,45] In terms of work absences or sick leave, the literature remains equivocal, with results ranging from no statistically significant gender differences, to women missing work more often, to men having higher work absences attributable to pain.[23] Thus, despite women's reports of more severe and frequent pain experiences, there is no strong evidence that this gender difference results in increased disability and invalidism.

Coping strategies

The lack of strong gender differences in the functional impact of pain may be attributable, in part, to the possibility that men and women use different strategies for coping with pain. Women tend to have a greater variety of coping strategies than do men for dealing with health problems in general. They more often avail themselves of social support and use relaxation and distraction techniques, while men are more action and problem focused.[40] In the case of chronic pain, women have reported more information-seeking and more use of cognitive-restructuring strategies than have men, and have been more frequently classified as active copers.[46,47] The implication is that women may cope better with severe pain than do men. However, women have also been found to be more prone to catastrophizing.[48] Cross-study comparisons in the research on coping and gender in pain are complicated by the fact that type and severity of pain differ across studies. Gender-specific coping strategies may vary with pain characteristics, making the relationship between gender and coping in chronic pain more complex than the current literature reflects.

Gender differences in the comorbidity of pain and depression

The higher prevalence of depression and of pain in women does not, in and of itself, confirm that there is a direct and meaningful relationship between the two. With the prevalences of both depression and pain in the general population being so elevated, the association could be coincidental. Establishing the exact nature of the relationship between pain and depression has proved somewhat elusive, but there seems to be little question that there is a high degree of comorbidity.

Prevalence of pain and depression

Without analysing for gender differences, a strong relationship between chronic pain and depression has been reported consistently. However, estimates of the prevalence of depression in chronic pain patients have varied greatly, from 31% to 100%.[49] Studies on the prevalence of pain complaints in patients with depression are not as numerous, and the estimated prevalence found therein ranges from 34% to 66%.[50] Attempts to further analyse the specific aspects of the pain experience that correlate with the experience of depression have been inconclusive. The degree of association between measures of pain and depressive symptomatology is not clear. Several studies have reported strong associations between pain intensity and depressive symptomatology, whereas other studies have found no association between these measures.[51] Yet others have

found duration of pain, rather than intensity, to be related to depressive symptomatology.[52]

There are some thorny methodological issues that may account for some of the inconsistencies in the prevalence rates reported. Chief among these is the cross-study variability in the diagnosis of depression and chronic pain, in addition to the distinction between these major disorders and milder variants, often referred to as depressive symptomatology and pain complaints. Another measurement problem in all studies of depression and in pain is the somatic content of depression measures. Physical symptoms associated with depression, such as fatigue, sleep disturbance, decreased energy and libido, may be secondary to pain and unrelated to depression. This symptomatological overlap thus raises some concern about a possible overestimation of the prevalence of depression in chronic pain patients.[53]

Is the comorbidity of pain and depression more prevalent in women?

Although the literature on the association between pain and depression is voluminous, only a handful of studies have focused specifically on gender differences in the comorbidity of pain and depression. A review of this limited research effort yields equivocal results.

In three different studies consisting of chronic pain samples with heterogeneous pain sites, men and women were equally likely to meet criteria for major depression.[54–56] Buckelew et al actually found higher rates of somatization, depression, anxiety and psychoticism in men.[46] However, a larger number of clinical pain studies have found higher prevalence rates for depression in women.[57–60] In one of the rare prospective studies of pain and depression, Magni et al found a strong association between female sex and depression in the development of chronic musculoskeletal pain.[58] When depression was controlled in their analyses of pain predictors in a sample of 2324 chronic pain patients, male sex was a more powerful predictor of pain than female sex, which was a stronger predictor of depression. Yet another study found an age–gender interaction in a sample of 254 chronic pain patients, with younger women and older men reporting more depression.[52]

The characteristics of the pain may be also differentially related to depression in men and women. In a prospective study, Haley et al found that although depression occurred equally for women and men with chronic pain, the reported severity of the pain was related to depression in women, whereas functional impairment was related to depression in men.[54] The presence of multiple symptoms may also be more strongly related to depression than regional pain, and women consistently report more multiple pain sites than do men.[61] Finally, in female gender-specific pains and in pain syndromes that disproportionately affect women, there are higher rates of depression than in the general female population. Chronic pelvic pain has been consistently associated with a history of prolonged sexual abuse, health-related quality of life, health-care utilization, and depression.[62–64] In their studies on the medical/ surgical treatment of chronic pelvic pain, Steege and Stout repeatedly note the influence of 'psychosocial compromise' on resolution of the pain problem.[65,66] In one fibromyalgia study, current and past diagnoses of depression were found in 71% of fibromyalgia patients.[67] Women with TMD have higher rates of depression than do similarly afflicted men.[68] Patients with rheumatoid arthritis, burning mouth syndrome, interstitial cystitis and vulvodynia also have significantly elevated rates of depression.[39,69–71]

Although more research is needed to determine conclusively that pain and depression co-occur more often in women than in men, most of the existing research suggests that this might be the case.

Explanatory models of the relationship between pain and depression

More elusive than establishing the comorbidity of pain and depression has been an understanding of the nature of the relationship. Does pain cause depression or does depression cause pain? Do they develop in tandem? Or, alternatively, are they mediated by altogether different variables? And, finally, are the answers to these questions the same for men as they are for women? The difficulty in discovering the nature of the pain–depression relationship lies primarily in the fact that most of the research is cross-sectional and cannot claim to uncover cause-and-effect relationships.

A handful of prospective and causal modelling studies have addressed the issue of cause and effect, and there seems to be support for causality in both directions. Brown demonstrated that pain episodes preceded increases in depressive symptomatology in rheumatoid arthritis patients, most of whom were women.[51] On the other hand, Leino and Magni's longitudinal study of metal industry workers found that depressive symptoms predicted the development of musculoskeletal pain in both men and women.[72] In another longitudinal study of a large sample from the National Health and Nutrition Examination Surveys, Magni et al found support for a bi-directional relationship between pain and depression in chronic musculoskeletal pain.[58]

Without the benefit of strong empirical

support for any one causal direction, much of the discussion has centred on theoretical models, a number of which have been postulated to explain the relationship between pain and depression. These fall under the general categories of biogenic, psychogenic, and sociogenic. Each of these models has been invoked, singly and in combination, to support differing views about the nature of the relationship. Dworkin and Gitlin caution about the pitfalls of both empirical and theoretical attempts to determine causation, by emphasizing that medical disorders and the various medications prescribed to pain patients can both cause symptoms that are generally associated with depression. They further warn about the inevitable problem of cases in which the pain and the depression are completely unrelated.[73]

Biogenic models

The earliest formulations of a biological explanation for the relationship between pain and depression hypothesized that individuals with mood disorders might be more sensitive to pain. The responses of mood-disordered individuals to nociceptive stimuli were experimentally tested in a large number of studies. Unexpectedly, the near consensus seemed to be that patients with mood disorders were *less* responsive to experimental pain than were control subjects. This paradoxical finding was retrospectively explained by attributing results to the difference between clinical and experimental pain and by invoking compensatory processes in which one pain 'weakened' the experience of another.[74]

Currently, there seems to be a general agreement that depression and pain may share a common pathophysiology. Pain pathways are known to involve the reticulolimbic structures of the brain, which also regulate emotionality.[75] Serotonin and noradrenaline have been implicated in both the perception of pain and the pathogenesis of depression, and the neurotransmission of pain has been observed to be mediated, in part, through serotonergic mechanisms.[76] In addition, both tricyclic antidepressants and selective serotonin reuptake inhibitors have been shown to relieve pain in some groups of chronic pain patients.[77]

If pain and depression share common neuroanatomical pathways, could gender differences in brain chemistry, metabolism, physical structures and hormonal influences affect depression, pain transmission/perception, and their relationship? The available research is insufficient to answer the question, but there is solid theoretical reasoning and some data in the pain literature to suggest that the answer may be yes. From a deductive analysis of the available literature (including animal studies), pain and gender researcher Berkley posits that there are important factors that could operate differently to affect pain in men and women. First, she considers the vaginal canal to be a gateway for pathological agents that, through neural mechanisms of sensitization, can give rise to referred hyperalgesia in regions removed from the initial source of the trauma. Second, she posits that both the composition and temporal patterns of sex hormones may explain sex differences in how pain is learned and interpreted, as well in differential responses to both opioid and non-opioid mechanisms of analgesia.[14] The recent finding that kappa-opiate analgesics produced significantly greater analgesia in women than in men lends support to Berkley's hypotheses.[78]

Biological differences may predispose women to have more pain in general and more pain without evidence of peripheral pathology. Together with the evidence of gender-specific biological mechanisms of depression, there is reason to hypothesize that biology (cross-gender and female-specific) can account for some of the suspected higher prevalence of pain–depression comorbidity in women.

Psychogenic model

Perhaps the most intuitive model of the pain–depression relationship is the one positing that depression develops as a consequence of pain. Chronic pain disturbs psychologically reinforcing activities, such as work, play and social interactions, and consequently depression develops and persists.[79] Research that demonstrates a correlation between depression and functional impairment, rather than pain intensity, provides support for this model.[80] However, in terms of gender differences, there is no evidence regarding the ways in which this process might differentially affect men and women. There is even some support for the idea that severity of the pain rather than functional impact is more strongly related to depression in women. It could be that women who suffer from pain and depression maintain high levels of activity despite pain severity, because of their multiple primary role responsibilities.

Another important psychological mechanism that has been invoked as being central to the pain–depression relationship is the cognitive appraisal of pain. Cognitive appraisals refer to interpretations of the pain: 'What does this pain mean?' 'Should I worry?' One study found that depressed chronic pain patients had a high level of cognitive distortion for pain-related situations only. In contrast, depressed patients without pain had equal levels of cognitive distortion for both pain-related and non-pain-related situations.[81] These data support the idea that there may be some situational specificity to the cognitive distortions of depressed chronic pain patients; they see pain as their problem. There is also evidence that women may engage in a greater variety of cognitive distortions than

do men. Novy et al found that female depressed chronic pain patients more often endorsed body image distortion items on depression questionnaires.[82] As previously reported, Jensen et al found that women catastrophized more in response to pain,[48] and catastrophizing has been linked to depression and chronic pain.[83] This finding is interesting in relation to the popular belief held by both men and women that women cope better with pain than do men.[10] Perhaps men's reports of pain to doctors and in clinical studies differ significantly from their expressions of pain to spouses and family members.

A related theory posits that depressed patients have an increased somatic focus which, coupled with negative interpretations, activates pain receptors.[84] In general, women pay more attention to illness and worry more about pain.[21,85] Perhaps because of their roles as caregivers, a somatic focus may be more sociobiologically adaptive for women than for men, but it may also make them more vulnerable to depression and pain. Perhaps women attend to pain sooner in an effort to minimize its disruption of their multiple primary role responsibilities. In any case, because of the differences in pain experiences that men and women undergo over a lifespan, it is probable that they have constructed different meanings around the experience of pain. One example of this is women's perception that emotion has a great impact on pain; this view is not shared by men.[10]

Whether one espouses the theory that pain causes depression or depression causes pain, there is little doubt that psychological factors play a major role in the perception and expression of pain. Gender differences in role expectations, cognitive appraisals and general pain beliefs are certainly theoretically credible as potential influences on the relationship between pain and depression.

Sociogenic model

A discussion of gender differences cannot escape the inevitable influence of societal norms, stereotypes and institutions on both the diagnosis and the experience of both pain and depression, singly or in tandem. The most glaring example of this is a recognized propensity on the part of health-care practitioners to attribute both idiopathic pain and women's pain to psychological causes.[86–88] Physicians may have a lower threshold for diagnosing psychiatric illness in pain patients without obvious organicity. Bilkey presented four psychiatrists with a sample of chronic pain patients and asked that they separately determine what percentage of the patients had an identifiable personality disorder. Each psychiatrist indicated that 90% of the sample had a personality disorder. Bilkey reminds us that, incidentally, personality-disordered patients are generally considered difficult to manage clinically.[88] It is possible that this bias towards psychogenic causation may result in the overdiagnosis of depression in all chronic pain patients. It is even more probable that the overdiagnosis affects women even more, as they have the higher prevalence of idiopathic pain syndromes and thus constitute a larger proportion of 'difficult patients'. Weir et al speculate that women may delay getting medical help because they feel, more than men do, that they need to prove the existence of their painful condition.[18] This may result in women presenting with more severe pain and more depression.

Thus, psychiatric diagnoses and psychological attributions made by health professionals can be perceived by patients as efforts on the part of health-care professionals to avoid dealing with the pain, which most depressed chronic pain patients still perceive as their primary problem. Even a well-intentioned focus on the psychological aspects of their pain condition can be interpreted as a lack of validation of their pain, in turn adding to iatrogenically worsened feelings of hopelessness and depression.

Another theory that may explain, in part, the higher prevalence of comorbid depression and pain in women is that depression is a more socially acceptable reaction to pain for women than for men. The reasoning behind this theory emanates from the depression literature and claims that women learn to turn their distress inwards because it is more socially reinforced than externalization, which is the more acceptable option for men.[89,90] The result may be an increase in learned helplessness, a decrease in self-esteem, and negative cognitions that centre on personal undesirability, such as in the case of female chronic pain patients who endorse body image distortion items disproportionately when compared to men. None of these help in the timely attention to health problems.

The disadvantaged socio-economic status of women also clearly places them at risk for a variety of health problems, including depression and pain. Poverty is among the life circumstances that have been consistently associated with depression and health problems.[91] Although it is often treated as a sociodemographic variable, socio-economic status continues to be the most powerful predictor of health status, and women continue to be much poorer than men. Victimization in interpersonal relationships is also a significant risk factor for both depression and chronic pain. Survey research in non-clinical populations has found rates of childhood sexual assault ranging from 21% to 37% among women, and chronic pelvic pain has been consistently associated with sexual abuse.[63,91] Domestic violence can also result in chronic pain and depression. Women in these situations fail to seek medical care after beatings that often involve head injuries, and learned helplessness and depression are central components of prolonged victimization.[91]

Integrative model

With two phenomena as complex as depression and pain, it is unlikely that any single causal pathway would be sufficient to explain the relationship between them in either men or women. Although it does not render research any easier, the biopsychosocial model is the most promising candidate for understanding the nature of the relationship. Biological, psychological and social factors are at work in different ways in every individual. Rather than one causal pathway being accurate, each is probably accurate, at times, for different patients in different combinations. This is a complicated proposition for research, which attempts to profile large groups of patients. However, the task is not as daunting for the clinician who treats one patient at a time and can carefully consider the individual's unique configuration of factors contributing to pain and depression.

Clinical management of pain and depression

The co-occurrence of pain and depression clearly has treatment implications. Non-depressed pain patients have been found to benefit more from pain treatment than do depressed pain patients.[92] This is not surprising, as pain treatment typically involves physical therapy and exercise, and depressed patients are less likely to engage in these. On the other hand, pain patients have reported improvements with antidepressant medications. However, in the absence of clinical trials for the treatment of comorbid pain and depression in either men or women, recommendations

have to emanate from a cobbling together of the available evidence and some sound theoretical reasoning.

The current reality is that there is little evidence of the relationship between pain and depression being unidirectional, in either direction. Even if the origins of either the pain or the depression were identifiable the factors that initiated the pain and/or depression may not be the ones maintaining them. The recommended strategy is thus to assess and treat both simultaneously.

This bifurcated approach does not highlight the importance of one disorder over another. The diagnosis of depression should not lead to inadequate evaluation and treatment of the pain, as has often been the case in the past. Explaining this approach to the patient is crucial, so that they do not assume that, because depression is being assessed, the implication is that the pain 'is all in their head'. They have probably already had a number of such experiences to sensitize them to even the faintest suggestion of psychogenicity. It is important that both the somatic and psychological aspects of their experience be validated, so as not to engage in any further iatrogenic harm.

After a comprehensive medical and psychological assessment, both physician and patient should engage in the process of treatment planning. This involves the determination of appropriate treatment goals. Many patients and physicians fail to distinguish between acute and chronic pain, and both feel frustrated when a full resolution of the pain does not occur as expected. At a minimum, appropriate goals include improving adjustment to the pain condition, increasing function in activities of daily living, improving mood, and reducing dependence on the health-care system for pain control. Once these goals have been achieved, there can then be a re-evaluation of objectives, if needed.

Fortunately, there is a significant degree of overlap in the treatment of both pain and depression. Both tricyclic antidepressants and selective serotonin reuptake inhibitors have shown impressive results in the treatment of depression and moderate results in the treatment of certain types of pain. In addition, cognitive-behavioural therapy consistently performs as well as antidepressants in the treatment of mild to moderate depression and happens to be a key component of multidisciplinary pain treatment programmes.

Pain treatment programmes have a number of goals that they have been fairly successful in attaining with the majority of pain patients. Some of these are to: (1) reduce pain; (2) reduce medication intake; (3) reduce psychological impairment; (4) correct range of motion abnormalities; (5) educate patients in the roles that emotions, behaviour and attitudes play in the experience of pain; (6) reinforce health behaviour; and (7) improve function.[93,94] Clearly, the overall goal of pain treatment programmes is rehabilitative. Chronic pain is not treated as acute pain.

The treatment implications of gender differences in pain and depression are somewhat more contentious. Part of the problem is that, without any empirical evidence, women and men in pain are already being treated differently. There is strong evidence that they have been receiving differential pharmacological care for their pain problems. Women are given less opioid analgesics than are men after appendectomies with no complications and after coronary artery bypass graft.[95,96] In a recent multicentre study of pain management in cancer, women were given significantly less medication than were men, whereas in a study of pain clinics men were prescribed more opioids than were women.[97,98] The general explanation for these differences seems to be that nurses and physicians may perceive women to express pain more freely, and women are thus taken less seriously than men. Nurses believe that there are significant gender differences in sensitivity to pain, pain tolerance, pain distress, willingness to report pain, exaggeration of pain, and the non-verbal expressions of pain, as well as that female patients should be given smaller amounts of narcotic analgesics.[99,100]

Beliefs in gender differences about pain generally have not helped women. More often than not, they have resulted in women being undertreated. Considering this and the fact that the gender differences found in the experience and report of pain are inconsistent and small, there seems to be little reason to recommend gender-tailored treatment strategies for women with pain and depression. Perhaps when we have more and clearer evidence of gender differences and what they mean, this customized treatment approach will be warranted. For the moment, it would be a great improvement if women received the same treatment as men. The only current gender difference that seems relevant in the context of pain and depression is that more women than men appear to suffer from both. In light of this difference, the best scientific and clinical service we can do is to continue researching potential aetiological factors and not allow the high prevalence of these disorders in women to lead to attributions (e.g. psychogenic pain) that result in impoverished assessment and treatment efforts.

References

1. Lander J, Fowler-Kerry S, Hill A, Comparison of pain perceptions among males and females, *Can J Nurs Res* 1990; **22**:39–49.

2. Feine JS, Bushnell MC, Miron D, Duncan GH, Sex differences in the perception of noxious heat stimuli, *Pain* 1991; **44**:255–62.

3. Fillingim RB, Maixner W, Gender differences in response to noxious stimuli, *Pain Forum* 1995; **4**:209–21.

4. Lautenbacher S, Rollman GB, Sex differences in responsiveness to painful and non-painful stimuli are dependent upon the stimulation method, *Pain* 1993; **53**:255–64.

5. Hapidou EG, De Catanzaro D, Sensitivity to cold pressor pain in dysmenorrheic and non-dysmenorrheic women as a function of menstrual cycle phase, *Pain* 1988; **34**:277–83.

6. Goolkasian P, Phase and sex effects in pain perception: a critical review, *Psychol Women Q* 1985; **9**:15–28.

7. Whipple B, Josimovich JB, Komisaruk BR, Sensory thresholds during the antepartum, intrapartum and postpartum periods, *Int J Nurs Stud* 1990; **27**:213–21.

8. Procacci P, Chronobiological studies on pain threshold, *Pain* 1993; **55**:277.

9. Faris PL, Raymond NC, DeZwaan M et al, Nociceptive, but not tactile, thresholds are elevated in bulimia nervosa, *Biol Psychiatry* 1992; **32**:462–6.

10. Bendelow G, Pain perceptions, emotions and gender, *Soc Health Illness* 1993; **15**:273–94.

11. Levine FM, DeSimone LL, The effects of experimenter gender on pain report in male and female subjects, *Pain* 1991; **44**:69–72.

12. Otto MW, Dougher MJ, Sex differences and personality factors in responsivity to pain, *Percept Mot Skills* 1985; **61**:383–90.

13. Ellermeier W, Westphal W, Gender differences in pain ratings and pupil reactions to painful pressure stimuli, *Pain* 1995; **61**:435–9.

14. Berkley K, Sex differences in pain, *Behav Brain Sci* 1997; **20**:371–80.

15. Verbrugge LM, Sex differences in complaints and diagnosis, *J Behav Med* 1980; **3**:327–55.

16. Ministry of Industry, Science and Technology, *Health Status of Canadians: Report of the 1991 General Social Survey* (Ministry of Industry, Science and Technology: Ontario, 1994).

17. Dawson DA, Adams PF, *Current Estimates from the National Health Interview Survey: United States, 1986* (National Center for Health Statistics: Hyattsville, MD, 1987).

18. Weir R, Browne G, Tunks E et al, Gender differences in psychosocial adjustment to chronic pain and expenditures for health care services used, *Clin J Pain* 1996; **12**:277–90.

19. Crook J, Rideout E, Browne G, The prevalence of pain complaints in a general population, *Pain* 1984; **18**:299–314.

20. Von Korff M, Dworkin SF, Le Resche L, Kruger A, An epidemiological comparison of pain complaints, *Pain* 1988; **32**:173–83.

21. Klonoff EA, Landrine H, Brown M, Appraisal and response to pain may be a function of its bodily location, *J Psychosom Res* 1993; **37**:661–70.

22. Vallerand AH, Gender differences in pain, *Image: J Nurs Scholarship* 1995; **27**:235–7.

23. Unruh AM, Gender variations in clinical pain experience, *Pain* 1996; **65**:123–67.

24. Taylor H, Curran NM, *The Nuprin Pain Report* (Louis Harris and Associates Inc.: New York, 1985).

25. Melzack R, The myth of painless childbirth: The John J. Bonica Lecture, *Pain* 1984; **19**:321–37.

26. Guzinski GM, Gynecological pain. In: Bonica JJ, ed., *The Management of Pain*, Vol. 2 (Lea & Febiger: Philadelphia, 1990) 1344–67.

27. Beard RW, Gangar K, Pearce S, Chronic gynecological pain. In: Wall PD, Melzack R, eds, *Textbook of Pain*, 2nd edn (Churchill Livingstone: Edinburgh, 1989) 597–614.

28. McKay M, Vulvodynia: diagnostic patterns, *Derm Clin* 1992; **10**:423–33.

29. Kitzinger S, Episiotomy pain. In: Wall PD, Melzack R, eds, *Textbook of Pain* (Churchill Livingstone: Edinburgh, 1984) 293–303.

30. Gijsbers van Wijk CM, Kolk AM, van den Bosch WJ, van den Hoogen HJ, Male and female morbidity in general practice: the nature of sex differences, *Soc Sci Med* 1992; **35**:665–78.

31. Merskey H, Bogduk N, eds, *Classification of Chronic Pain: Descriptions of Chronic Pain Syndromes and Definitions of Pain Terms*, 2nd edn (IASP Press: Seattle, 1994).

32. Bush FM, Harkins SW, Harrington WG, Price DD, Analysis of gender effects on pain perception and symptom presentation in temporomandibular pain, *Pain* 1993; **53**:73–80.

33. Pullinger AG, Monteiro AA, Functional impairment in TMJ patient and non-patient groups according to a disability index and symptom profile, *Cranio Pract* 1988; **6**:156–64.

34. Grushka M, Clinical features of burning mouth syndrome, *Oral Surg Oral Med Oral Pathol* 1987; **63**:30–6.

35. Zakrzewska JM, The burning mouth syndrome remains an enigma, *Pain* 1995; **62**:253–7.

36. Verbrugge LM, Lepkowski JM, Konkol LL, Levels of disability among US adults with arthritis, *J Gerontol* 1991; **46**:S71–83.

37. McCain GA, Fibromyalgia and myofascial pain syndromes. In: Wall PD, Melzack R, eds, *Textbook of Pain*, 3rd edn (Churchill Livingstone: Edinburgh, 1994) 475–93.

38. Tunks E, Crook J, Norman G, Kalaher S, Tenderpoints in fibromyalgia, *Pain* 1988; **34**:11–19.

39. Ratner V, Slade D, Whitmore KE, Interstitial cystitis: a bladder disease finds legitimacy, *J Women Health* 1992; **1**:63–8.

40. Vingerhoets AJ, Van Heck GL, Gender, coping and psychosomatic symptoms, *Psychol Med* 1990; **20**:125–35.

41. Katon W, Lin E, Von Korff M et al, Somatization: a spectrum of severity, *Am J Psychiatry* 1991; **148**:34–40.

42. Deyo RA, Tsui-Wu YJ, Descriptive epidemiology of low-back pain and its related medical care in the United States, *Spine* 1987; **12**:264–8.

43. Heliovaara M, Sievers K, Impivaara O et al, Descriptive epidemiology and public health aspects of low back pain, *Ann Med* 1989; **21**:327–33.

44. Walsh K, Cruddas M, Coggon D, Low back pain in eight areas of Britain, *J Epidemiol Commun Health* 1992; **46**:227–30.

45. Makela M, Heliovaara M, Sievers K et al, Musculoskeletal disorders as determinants of disability in Finns aged 30 years or more, *J Clin Epidemiol* 1993; **46**:549–59.

46. Buckelew SP, Shutty MS Jr, Hewett J et al, Health locus of control, gender differences and adjustment to persistent pain, *Pain* 1990; **42**:287–94.

47. Strong J, Ashton R, Stewart A, Chronic low back pain: towards an integrated psychosocial assessment model, *J Consult Clin Psychol* 1994; **62**:1058–63.

48. Jensen I, Nygren A, Gamberale F et al, Coping with long-term musculoskeletal pain and its consequences: is gender a factor? *Pain* 1994; **57**:167–72.

49. Romano JM, Turner JA, Chronic pain and depression: does the evidence support a relationship? *Psychol Bull* 1985; **97**:18–34.

50. Smith GR, The epidemiology and treatment of depression when it co-exists with somatoform disorders, somatization, or pain, *Gen Hosp Psychiatry* 1992; **14**:265–72.

51. Brown GK, A causal analysis of chronic pain and depression, *J Abnormal Psychol* 1990; **99**:127–37.

52. Averill PM, Novy DM, Nelson DV, Berry LA, Correlates of depression in chronic pain patients: a comprehensive examination, *Pain* 1996; **65**:93–100.

53. Estlander AM, Takala EP, Verkasalo M, Assessment of depression in chronic musculoskeletal pain patients, *Clin J Pain* 1995; **11**:194–200.

54. Haley WE, Turner JA, Romano JM, Depression in chronic pain patients: relation to pain, activity, and sex differences, *Pain* 1985; **23**:337–43.

55. Haythornwaite JA, Sieber WJ, Kerns RD, Depression and the chronic pain experience, *Pain* 1991; **46**:177–84.

56. Kramlinger KG, Swanson DW, Maruta T, Are patients with chronic pain depressed? *Am J Psychiatry* 1983; **140**:747–9.

57. Fishbain DA, Goldberg M, Meagher BR et al, Male and female chronic pain patients categorized by DSM-III psychiatric diagnostic criteria, *Pain* 1986; **26**:181–97.

58. Magni G, Moreschi C, Rigatti-Luchini S, Merskey H, Prospective study on the relationship between depressive symptoms and chronic musculoskeletal pain, *Pain* 1994; **56**:289–97.

59. Von Knorring L, Perris C, Eisemann M et al, Pain as a symptom in depressive disorders. 1. Relationship to diagnostic subgroup and depressive symptomatology, *Pain* 1983; **15**:19–26.

60. Keefe FJ, Wilkins RH, Cook WA Jr et al, Depression, pain and pain behavior, *J Consult Clin Psychol* 1986; **54**:665–9.

61. Dworkin SF, Von Korff M, Le Resche L, Multiple pains and psychiatric disturbance. An epidemiologic investigation. *Arch Gen Psychiatry* 1990; **47**:239–44.

62. Nolan TE, Metheny WP, Smith RP, Unrecognized association of sleep disorders and depression with chronic pelvic pain, *South Med J* 1992; **85**:1181–3.

63. Jamieson DJ, Steege JF, The association of sexual abuse with pelvic pain complaints in a primary care population, *Am J Obstet Gynecol* 1997; **177**:1408–12.

64. Matthias SD, Kupperman M, Liberman RF, Lipschutz RC, Steege JF, Chronic pelvic pain: prevalence, health-related quality of life, and economic correlates, *Obstet Gynecol* 1996; **87**:321–7.

65. Steege JF, Stout AL, Resolution of chronic pelvic pain after laparoscopic lysis of adhesions, *Am J Obstet Gynecol* 1991; **165**:278–81.

66. Stout AL, Steege JF, Dodson WC, Hughes CL, Relationship of laparoscopic findings to self-report of pelvic pain, *Am J Obstet Gynecol* 1991; **164**:73–9.

67. Hudson JI, Hudson MS, Pliner LF et al, Fibromyalgia and major affective disorder: a controlled phenomenology and family history study, *Am J Psychiatry* 1985; **142**:441–6.

68. Vimpari SS, Knuuttila ML, Sakki TK, Kivela SL, Depressive symptoms associated with symptoms of the temporomandibular joint pain and dysfunction syndrome, *Psychosom Med* 1995; **57**:439–44.

69. Creed F, Murphy S, Jayson MV, Measurement of psychiatric disorder in rheumatoid arthritis, *J Psychosom Res* 1990; **34**:79–87.

70. Stewart DE, Whelan CI, Fong IW, Tessler KM, Psychosocial aspects of chronic, clinically unconfirmed vulvovaginitis, *Obstet Gynecol* 1990; **76**:852–6.

71. Rojo L, Silvestre FJ, Bagan JV et al, Psychiatric morbidity in burning mouth syndrome, *Oral Surg Oral Med Oral Pathol* 1993; **75**:308–11.

72. Leino P, Magni G, Depressive and distress symptoms as predictors of low back pain, neck–shoulder pain, and other musculoskeletal morbidity: a 10-year follow-up of metal industry employees, *Pain* 1993; **53**:89–94.

73. Dworkin RH, Gitlin MJ, Clinical aspects of depression in chronic pain patients, *Clin J Pain* 1991; **7**:79–94.

74. Dworkin RH, Clark WC, Lipsitz JD, Pain responsivity in major depression and bipolar disorder, *Psychiatr Res* 1995; **56**:173–81.

75. Parker JC, Wright GE, The implications of depression for pain and disability in rheumatoid arthritis, *Arthritis Care Res* 1995; **8**:279–83.

76. Ruoff GE, Depression in the patient with chronic pain, *J Fam Pract* 1996; **43**:S25–33.

77. Magni G, The use of antidepressants in the treatment of chronic pain. A review of the current evidence, *Drugs* 1991; **42**:730–48.

78. Gear RW, Miaskowski C, Gordon NC et al, Kappa-opioids produce significantly greater analgesia in women than in men, *Nature Med* 1996; **2**:1248–50.

79. Fordyce WE, *Behavioral Methods for Chronic Pain and Illness* (Mosby: St Louis, 1976).

80. Rudy TE, Kerns RD, Turk DC, Chronic pain and depression: toward a cognitive-behavioral mediation model, *Pain* 1988; **35**:129–40.

81. Smith TW, O'Keeffe JL, Christensen AJ, Cognitive distortion and depression in chronic pain: association with diagnosed disorders, *J Consult Clin Psychol* 1994; **62**:195–8.

82. Novy DM, Nelson DV, Averill PM, Berry LA, Gender differences in the expression of depressive symptoms among chronic pain patients, *Clin J Pain* 1996; **12**:23–9.

83. Geisser ME, Robinson ME, Keefe FJ, Weiner ML, Catastrophizing, depression and the sensory, affective and evaluative aspects of chronic pain, *Pain* 1994; **59**:79–83.

84. Fields H, Depression and pain: a neurobiological model, *Neuropsychiatr Neuropsychol Behav Neurol* 1991; **4**:83–92.

85. Crook J, Women and chronic pain. In: Roy R, Tunks E, eds, *Chronic Pain: Psychosocial Factors in Rehabilitation* (Williams & Wilkins: Baltimore, 1982) 68–78.

86. Bernstein B, Kane R, Physicians' attitudes toward female patients, *Med Care* 1981; **XIX:**600–8.

87. Colameco S, Becker LA, Simpson M, Sex bias in the assessment of patient complaints, *J Fam Pract* 1983; **16:**1117–21.

88. Bilkey WJ, Confusion, fear, and chauvinism: perspectives on the medical sociology of chronic pain, *Perspect Biol Med* 1996; **39:**270–80.

89. Warren LW, Male intolerance of depression: a review with implications for psychotherapy, *Clin Psychol Rev* 1983; **3:**147–56.

90. Nolen-Hoeksema S, Sex differences in unipolar depression: evidence and theory, *Psychol Bull* 1987; **101:**259–82.

91. McGrath E, Keita GP, Strickland BR, Russo NF, *Women and Depression: Risk Factors and Treatment Issues: Final Report of the American Psychological Association's National Task Force on Women and Depression* (American Psychological Association: Washington DC, 1991) 28–32.

92. Weickgenant AL, Slater MA, Patterson TL et al, Coping activities in chronic low back pain: relationship with depression, *Pain* 1993; **53:**95–103.

93. Deathe AB, Helmes E, Evaluation of a chronic pain programme by referring physicians, *Pain* 1993; **52:**113–21.

94. Fishbain DA, Rosomoff HL, Goldberg M et al, The prediction of return to the workplace after multidisciplinary pain center treatment, *Clin J Pain* 1993; **9:**3–15.

95. McDonald DD, Gender and ethnic stereotyping and narcotic analgesic administration, *Res Nurs Health* 1994; **17:**45–9.

96. Calderone K, The influence of gender on the frequency of pain and sedative medication administered to post-operative patients, *Sex Roles* 1990; **23:**713–25.

97. Cleeland CS, Gonin R, Hatfield AK et al, Pain and its treatment in outpatients with metastatic cancer, *N Engl J Med* 1994; **330:**592–6.

98. Lack DZ, Women and pain: another feminist issue, *Women Ther* 1982; **1:**55–64.

99. Cohen FL, Post-surgical pain relief: patient's status and nurse's medication choices, *Pain* 1980; **9:**265–74.

100. McCaffery M, Ferrell BR, Does the gender gap affect your pain-control decisions? *Nursing* 1992; **22:**48–51.

28

Psychoneuroimmunology: implications for mood disorders
Malcolm P Rogers

Introduction

Interactions between the immune system, brain, mind and experience are complex and intriguing. Our curiosity about these interactions is rooted in clinical observation. Consider, for example, a clinical situation in which a 48-year-old married woman becomes strongly attracted to her boss, who is single. The attraction is mutual but never explicitly expressed until the woman in question, her husband and young child move away, in pursuit of a new job opportunity. She and her former boss both feel bereaved, but must work through their grief and conflicts in private, with little social support. Neither one can accept that their relationship with one another, which feels more intense and important than any other prior relationship, is over. She becomes significantly impaired at work, unable to concentrate or feel pleasure in it. The rest of her life also seems devoid of pleasure and meaning. She has trouble falling asleep and wakes up early in the morning. She feels tired, and develops a persistent upper respiratory infection

which lingers, in spite of antibiotic therapy. She blames herself for not having expressed her feelings earlier. She feels trapped by her circumstances, including a long-standing and now intensified dissatisfaction with her marriage. Eventually, she seeks psychiatric intervention, feeling unable to go on. Her doctor recommends both antidepressant medication and psychotherapy.

This brief example immediately highlights a number of interesting questions. Has this loss led into a major depression and, if so, what distinguishes it from a normal grief reaction? Could the persistent respiratory symptoms be a result of a weakened immune response? Is she at increased risk for developing any other illnesses? If so, what are the underlying physiological changes which might account for these vulnerabilities?

I would answer most of these questions in the affirmative, but we are only beginning to understand some of the specific mechanisms involved. Hopefully, this chapter will help to provide a framework by laying out some of the research investigations which have been sparked by the sort of questions raised by this clinical example.

The rapidly developing field of psychoneuroimmunology encompasses these interactions, and has given rise to an enormous amount of research and even to its own journals, e.g. *Advances in Neuroimmunology* and *Journal of Neuroimmunology*.

The immune system is generally divided into humoral (antibody) or cellular components. Most psychophysiological studies of immune system function have focused on the cellular immune system, which involves T or thymus-dependent lymphocytes. T-cell measures have focused on their quantity, their functional activity, and their subsets, such as so-called suppressor or helper cells, or natural killer (NK) cells. Another immune cell or immunocyte, the macrophage, which plays a pivotal role, has been the focus of particular attention.[1,2] Cytokines, such as interleukin-1 (IL-1), are proteins released by activated lymphocytes which have potent regulatory effects on other lymphocytes and surrounding and even distant tissue sites.

From the outset, the field of psychoneuroimmunology has been driven by probing questions about the role of psychological factors in the onset and course of diseases such as rheumatoid arthritis (RA) and viral infections. As knowledge of the underlying immunological mechanisms in autoimmune disorders grew, more attention was directed at the possible links between the immune system and psychological states, and, in turn, between the immune and central nervous systems. There have been many excellent reviews of the field of psychoneuroimmunology.[3–6]

Animal models of immunologically mediated diseases have provided a particularly useful window on complex psychoneuroimmunological interactions. Animal studies have shown that the immune response is affected by lesions

in key brain areas such as the hypothalamus, which may influence neurotransmitter physiology. Observations on the effect of stress on the onset and course of infections and autoimmune and other medical disorders has added to our understanding of psychoneuroimmunological interactions. We now know that these interactions are bi-directional—from brain to immune system and from immune system back to brain. Environmental stressors and modifiers such as social support, long-familiar concepts in psychosomatic research, influence the underlying biology of immunity. Identifying the precise role of various neurotransmitters and neuromodulators in these interactions may also have important therapeutic implications not only for immunologically mediated medical disorders but also for mood disorders.

Recently, the study of immunocyte behaviour in certain clinical conditions associated with a stress response has helped to flesh out details of the neuroendocrine–neuroimmune stress response system. Stress, defined as a state of disharmony or threatened homeostasis, remains an important dynamic concept in both normal and pathological mechanisms of adaptation.[7] Various concomitants of stress influence a number of disease processes.[8] These concomitants include biochemical (neurotransmitters, steroids, peptides), physiological (heart rate, blood pressure), and behavioural (anxiety, depression) elements. Depression has received particular attention in relation to immune system changes, and thus is appropriate for inclusion in this book.

The two major arms of the stress response system are the limbic–hypothalamic–pituitary–adrenal axis and the sympathetic nervous system. Evidence indicates that one stimulates and modulates the other.[7] There are similar neurotransmitter effects on both systems. Serotonin and acetylcholine stimulate both systems, while GABAergic, opioid and glucocorticoid substances inhibit them. The importance of serotonin in depression can hardly be overstated.

Immune activation resulting in the secretion of corticotrophin-releasing hormone (CRH) leads to a series of events which affect inflammatory processes. These effects are mediated by a range of factors, including eicosanoids, platelet-activating factor, serotonin, and cytokines such as interleukin-1 (IL-1), interleukin-6 (IL-6), and tumor necrosis factor (TNF).[7,9] As we shall see, major depression is itself associated with a chain of metabolic events, including the activation and regulation of immune responses.

The psychoneuroendocrine–immune response proposed by Evans et al[10] emphasizes the concept that depression and stress can result in alterations in both endocrine and immune system function. There are sound experimental data in support of both these phenomena. Fricchione and Stefano[11] have helped to pull together the evidence supporting a bi-directional neuroimmune hypothesis, drawing on a variety of previous publications.[7,10,12–15] Such bi-directional communication between the brain and the immune system may be of critical importance in the development and perpetuation of various diseases. A stress system marked by prolonged CRH hyperactivity is associated with the development of melancholic depression and immunosuppression. On the other hand, a stress system marked by CRH hyporeactivity may be associated with autoimmune diseases such as RA and systemic lupus erythematosus (SLE). If such linkages can be clearly established, we will be better able to understand the pathogenesis of diseases which involve both the nervous and immune systems, depression among them.

However, I will begin by reviewing some of the more important findings produced by the last two decades of psychoneuroimmunological research.

Stress studies

Many different naturalistic stresses have been shown to influence immunological activity. Bereavement,[16,17] women experiencing marital separation, marital dissatisfaction and divorce,[18,19] the strain on family members caring for relatives afflicted with Alzheimer's disease,[20] job loss and chronic unemployment[21] and examination stress[22–24] have all been shown to be associated with diminished immunological functioning. Widowers more than widows appear to be at risk for higher morbidity and mortality following bereavement.[25] Differences in gender responses have also been noted among caregivers,[26] and many investigators have explored gender differences in coping style and adaptation to stress.[27] All of these stresses, except for examination stress, are associated with chronic stress, and, in many cases, secondary depression. Linn's work[28] supported the notion that depression was the dimension of most stress situations which actually led to suppression of the immune response, and, as discussed below, there is now considerable evidence for depression-related immunological changes.

Natural disasters

Natural disasters have been taken as extreme instances of stress, which may simultaneously disrupt social support networks. Several studies have taken advantage of the occurrence of natural disasters to learn more about the potential health consequences of such events for both mental and physical function. Solomon[29] investigated the psychological and immunological consequences of the North Ridge earthquake. He and his investigators found that those with the highest levels of distress showed the highest levels of CD3$^+$ (helper) and CD8$^+$ (suppressor) T-lymphocytes.

The short-term and long-term effects of such stress are quite different, a finding supported by many animal studies. Ironson[30] found that the survivors of Hurricane Andrew showed a high frequency of post-traumatic stress disorder (PTSD). Those with PTSD and negative intrusive thoughts had lower NK cell cytotoxicity (NKCC). NK cells are thought to be important in the surveillance against cancer cells.

Depression

Building on the earlier work on bereavement, Schleifer et al[31] found suppressed lymphocyte reactivity and abnormalities in some subpopulations of T-lymphocytes in severely depressed patients. The more severely depressed the subjects, the more impaired the immunological function.[32] The work of other investigators[33,34] provided further evidence for immunological changes in depression. Some investigators, however, found no depression-related differences in measures of lymphocytes, subsets of T-cells, or NK cells.[35,36] On further analysis, after controlling for the effects of age, Schleifer's previous findings were more qualified. There were no immunological differences between 91 subjects with unipolar depression and their matched controls.[37] Only the elderly subjects with severe depression still showed decreased lymphocyte responsivity to mitogen stimulation. The latter is an in vitro measure of cell division elicited by stimuli referred to as mitogens. In effect, it is one measure of the functional vigour of lymphocytes. The effect of age on immune changes in depression continues to be an area of research. In a more recent study, younger adults with major depressive disorder had more circulating leukocytes and granulocytes but fewer NK cells and less NK activity compared to normal age-matched controls.[38] Response to mitogen

stimulation was similar between the two groups.

Gender is clearly an important differentiating factor in the prevalence of major depression. It may also be an important variable in depression-related immune change. Evans et al[10] found that NK cell activity was reduced in men but not in women with major depression. In addition to gender and age, alcohol may also play a role in the impact of depression on immunity. Irwin[39] found that depressed subjects with comorbid alcoholism had significantly lower levels of NK cell activity. In a further observation, reduction in NK cell activity in depression seemed to be specifically related to sleep disturbance and psychomotor retardation.[40] Others have noted that smoking[41] and malnutrition[42] are associated with immunosuppression, in particular with diminished NK cell activity. Comorbid panic disorder also appears to be associated with immunological changes in major depression, both in numbers of T-cells and in responsivity to mitogen stimulation.[43] Thus, there are a number of confounding variables which need to be controlled when assessing the impact of depression on immunity.

Disruption in normal circadian rhythms is often cited as another important physiological dimension of major depression. The regulation of the immune system is quite sensitive to diurnal variations and disruptions. Petitto[44] has noted an abnormal diurnal variation of B-lymphocyte circulation patterns in major depression. Not surprisingly, in her recent review of the interconnections between depression and the immune system, Anderson[45] calls for careful circadian and ultradian observations of immune system organization.

Overall, despite some inconsistencies, Herbert's careful meta-analysis of methodologically sound studies of the relationship between depression and immune function concluded that there are reliable, reproducible correlations: lowered proliferative response to mitogens, lowered NK cell activity, and several white blood cell populations.[46] The intensity of depressive affect also appeared to be linked with these immune changes. One needs also to consider some of the confounding variables, including sleep deprivation, malnutrition, alcohol, smoking, advanced age, circadian rhythms and other psychiatric disorders, such as panic disorder, which may all have additional effects on the immune system in their own right.

Lesserman et al[47] investigated a group of HIV-infected men, and noted that depression combined with stress was associated with decreased numbers of NK cells and CD8 T-lymphocytes. They point out that comorbid depression may have significant clinical implications in the course of HIV infection.

Maes et al[48] have taken some of these observations a step further. Rather than simply viewing these immune changes as a result of depression, he has developed a more integrated hypothesis, in which the immune changes are seen as an integral part of the biology of the depressive response. We shall explore the evidence for this hypothesis below.

Coping, social support and relaxation

Helplessness in the face of stressful stimuli characterizes depression. On the other hand, coping with stress implies a very different mental and physiological state, with implications for immune function. There is a significant literature differentiating coping into problem-solving focused or emotion focused.[49] Subjects in the former mode of coping seem to have better adjustment and affective balance. Some studies, like Locke's,[50] have measured coping indirectly. His subjects with high stress but low psychological distress were defined as good copers, whereas poor copers had low stress but

a high level of symptoms. Good copers had significantly higher NK cell activity.

There is much evidence in the psychosomatic literature that social support buffers the adverse physiological effects of stress.[51] The functioning of the immune system also seems to benefit from social support.[52] Spouses of cancer patients who had high levels of social support showed more cell activity and lymphocyte responsivity to mitogens. Experimental animal work provides further support for the beneficial effects of social support of immunity. Boccia et al,[53] in investigating the effects of separation of bonnet macaque infants from their mothers, found that those infants for whom alternative juvenile attachment figures were available had stronger NK cell activity and lymphocyte responsivity to mitogens.

Conditioned immunosuppression

In an intriguing line of research, Ader and Cohen[54] demonstrated a conditioning effect on the immune response. Using a taste aversion paradigm in rats, Ader showed that a conditioned stimulus, such as a novel saccharin-flavoured solution, when paired with an unconditioned stimulus, such as cyclophosphamide (an immunosuppressive and emetic agent) could produce a subsequent conditioned immunosuppressive response in a rat. This phenomenon has been observed repeatedly in carefully controlled studies, not only by Ader but also by several other investigators.[55] Subsequent research using a similar conditioning paradigm has shown specific effects of this conditioning on T- and B-cells separately, as well as both augmentation and diminution of the immune response in laboratory animals. Although the magnitude of the effect is small, it has been shown to modify the degree of kidney involvement in a mouse model of SLE.[56] The mechanism accounting for the conditioned immunosuppressive or immunoenhancing effect remains one of the more intriguing mysteries in psychosomatic research.

The phenomenon of conditioned immunosuppression may also have some implications for human patients receiving chemotherapy. Clinical experience suggests that many patients receiving chemotherapy develop some conditioned responses, such as nausea, to neutral stimuli associated with the setting of the chemotherapy. Fredrikson et al[57] noted that women with breast cancer, especially those with high trait anxiety, had reduced numbers of monocytes and NK cell activity in anticipation of receiving adjuvant chemotherapy. This anticipatory immunosuppression was felt to be consistent with the phenomenon of conditioned immunosuppression.

Disease-related studies

Immune system dysfunction is central to the aetiology of autoimmune disorders. This fact becomes even more interesting when taken together with evidence of the role of psychological states in the onset of these disorders (e.g. RA), and in mental changes which seem to be a result of the disorder (e.g. SLE). Accordingly, we will discuss both of these disorders in detail, as well as summarizing some of the data from other autoimmune and medical disorders which seem to arise from disturbances in immune function.

Autoimmune disorders

Gender differences

Elevated autoimmune reactions in females in both human disease and animal models have been recognized for years.[58,59] Gender and sex hormones have a clear effect on various hetero- and autoimmune responses. Androgens and progesterone may have a protective effect, while oestrogens have a mixed effect, protective in RA but harmful in SLE. Although the details are yet to be fully worked out, oestrogens appear to have a dual effect on immunity, suppressing antigen-specific T-cell-dependent reactions while enhancing B-cell activities.[60] Sex hormones also appear to alter the regulation of cytokines, for example interferon-γ (IFN-γ).[61] One study, looking at the prevalence of autoimmunity in women with premature ovarian failure and thus oestrogen decreases, found a 77% level of autoreactivity of at least one identified class of autoantibodies.[62] Pregnancy also has effects on the course of autoimmune diseases, frequently suppressive, although exacerbating in the case of multiple sclerosis,[63] and sometimes associated with postpartum exacerbations. Further gender differences for specific disorders involving the immune system will be described below.

Rheumatoid arthritis

For centuries, clinicians have been impressed by the role of psychological and emotional factors in RA, an autoimmune disorder which affects women four times as commonly as it does men. Women generally develop more aggressive disease with a worse long-term outcome, yet men more frequently die from its extra-articular complications. Menopausal hormonal changes appear to be related to the fact that the peak time of onset in women is in the mid-forties, while in men the peak time of onset comes later in life.

In the 1950s and 1960s, RA came to be viewed as one of the classical psychosomatic diseases. Over time, however, the view that RA was caused or triggered by a unique and specific conflict or personality style has not held up. Instead, the focus shifted to a non-specific stressor which might trigger or exacerbate the course of RA, at least in a subset of patients. There are continuing observations about personality features common to patients with RA and other autoimmune disorders,[64] such as hyperconformability and excessive kindness, although it seems more plausible that these are the result rather than the cause of these chronic diseases. There is an extensive literature on the effects of psychological stress on the onset and course of RA.

The principal methodological difficulty in all of these efforts has been the retrospective nature of the analysis. Patients also tend to attribute the cause of their arthritis or flare-ups to psychological stress, excessive physical activity, or fluctuations in the weather.[65] Not surprisingly, patients have difficulty with the uncertainty and sense of helplessness often associated with this disease, and look for reasons to explain their disease, a process which often distorts retrospective memory of stress.

Nevertheless, some interesting data lend support to the role of stress in RA. Meyerowitz et al[66] studied eight sets of twins discordant for RA. They found convincing evidence in the majority of the twin sets that the arthritic twin experienced an increase in life stress prior to the onset of arthritis. One example was the twin who remained home to care for a psychotic stepfather (and became ill) while the other left home (and did not become ill).

Two studies used a quantitative measure of stress by having subjects list life events over the 6 months prior to the onset of RA. Both found an increase in such events compared to the controls prior to the onset of arthritis.[67,68] However, another study[69] did not support these later observations. More recently, Wallace and Metzger[70] have suggested that flare-ups in RA and SLE were triggered by the San Francisco

earthquake, a finding of particular interest in light of the other studies documenting the impact of disasters on immune function.

A few investigators have attempted to measure fluctuations in disease activity over the course of weeks in relation to fluctuations in immune and psychological measures. Rimon et al[71] looked for changes in viral antibody levels in patients with juvenile RA in relation to life stress. He divided patients into low- and high-conflict groups. Patients in the high-conflict group tended to have higher antibody titres, although this was not statistically significant Parker et al[72] attempted to correlate immunological factors with psychological factors and disease activity in 80 male patients with RA. Severity of joint involvement was related to measures of depression, and a sense of helplessness was associated with changes in subsets of lymphocytes. Harrington et al[73] found that changes in soluble IL-2 receptor levels covaried with joint inflammation and mood disturbances.

To this point, there have been studies of coping styles in RA,[74] but no studies which combine measures of coping with immune measures. This may happen in the near future, as there is an accumulating literature on the effects of induced emotions—positive and negative—on immune function.[75–77]

Some studies have attempted to examine the role of stress in a more prospective, longitudinal approach. In one study,[78] 67 RA patients completed questionnaires daily for 75 days concerning mood, emotionally significant events and symptoms. They also underwent joint and tender point examinations every 2 weeks. When joint tenderness was controlled for, point tenderness correlated significantly with degree of daily stress.

Both Crown et al[79] and Rimon[80] proposed that the importance of stress in RA might vary according to different subtypes of patients.

They suggested that patients without rheumatoid factor (and perhaps a lower genetic predisposition to the disease) might have a greater degree of stress preceding the onset, a more acute onset, and a greater tendency for course exacerbation due to stress. Rimon's view has received support from more recent work by Stewart et al,[81] which showed a greater role for stress effects on disease onset and continuing activity in the seronegative subgroup of RA patients.

Both the rate of disease progression[82] and level of functional limitation disproportionate to objective measures of disease activity[83] have been associated with maladaptive defences. A 15-year follow-up[84] of Rimon's earlier study[80] confirmed the importance of psychological stress for disease course over time. As in the original study, the so-called 'major conflict group' characterized by acute onset, absence of family history, and a lower incidence of rheumatoid factor, was more vulnerable to these stress effects. Slightly more than half of the 74 patients in the follow-up were in this major conflict group.

When McFarlane et al[85] followed a group of 30 patients with RA over a 3-year period, they were surprised to find that symptoms of depression and anxiety actually predicted a better outcome, whereas externalized hostility predicted a poorer outcome. Moreover, patients who denied the emotional significance of their illness seemed to fare worse over time. In evaluating patients' course, it also needs to be kept in mind that the degree of disability cannot be explained fully by the severity of RA.[86]

Intervention studies have included stress management and support groups. One such study,[87] in which 105 RA patients were randomly assigned to either a stress management group, a support group or a control group, showed that patients in the intervention groups had greater improvement in joint tenderness.

The evidence that altered immunity is at the root of RA and other autoimmune disorders is convincing.[88] The extravascular immune complex hypothesis holds that an interaction between antigens and antibodies occurs in the synovial tissues, and in the synovial fluid around the cartilage. These antigens are thought to be constituents of articular tissue or byproducts of the inflammatory process, such as collagen, cartilage, fibrinogen, and fibrin. The antigen–antibody interaction in the joint tissues mediated by the macrophage in turn activates the complement sequence, increases vascular permeability, and causes an accumulation of cellular blood elements. Polymorphonuclear leukocytes, attracted by complement-derived chemotactic factors, then release enzymes that cause synovial inflammation and joint damage.

An alternative hypothesis focuses on the cellular arm of the immune system.[88] The presence of activated T-lymphocytes in rheumatoid synovium and of soluble factors derived from T-cells (lymphokines or cytokines) in the synovial fluid supports this hypothesis. In addition, the removal of T-lymphocytes by thoracic duct drainage[89] and total nodal irradiation are both associated with clinical improvement. Some investigators have proposed an imbalance in the immune system, consisting of a relative lack of suppressor T-lymphocytes able to control helper T-lymphocytes, as a mechanism in this and other autoimmune diseases.[90]

Solomon[91] was one of the pioneers in suggesting that psychological factors might influence the immune system, which in turn could mediate the pathophysiology of RA and other diseases caused by altered immune reactions. He found that experimental stress could alter the level of antibody response to immunization in rats. Other work[92,93] has demonstrated that stress can affect the level of joint inflammation in animal models of arthritis. Chrousos and Gold[7] have presented an animal model of autoimmune inflammatory arthritis involving the Lewis rat. A hypofunctional CRH neuron in this rat model allows for the development of a RA-like syndrome and other autoimmune inflammatory phenomena. A generalized CRH neuron gene defect in Lewis rats makes them CRH-hyporesponsive to noxious stimuli. They also display behavioural hypoarousal and a hyperimmune profile. These phenomena are of particular interest in contrast to the CRH hyperarousal evident in major depression.

Systemic lupus erythematosus

SLE is an autoimmune disease which affects women 10–15 times more frequently than it does men. There has long been interest in the role of stress and other psychological issues surrounding this disease. A few earlier uncontrolled and retrospective studies suggested that high levels of life stress preceded disease flare-ups in patients with SLE.[94] More recent approaches have used prospective study designs. Utilizing prolonged neuropsychological testing as a convenient induced stress, Hinrichsen et al[95] observed that SLE patients had reduced CD19[+] T-cell mobilization compared to normal controls, despite normal hormonal responses.

In another careful prospective study of the relationship between daily stress and SLE activity, Adams et al[96] studied 41 patients with SLE. Much like Rimon[97] with RA patients, Adams et al found that some individuals appeared to be stress responders, while others did not. While there was no clear evidence that in these susceptible individuals stress exacerbated underlying disease activity, stress, anxiety, depression and anger were all associated with self-reported symptomatology. Wekking et al[98] prospectively compared groups of

patients with SLE and RA in terms of the relationship between disease activity and daily stress. They found that there was a stronger correlation between level of daily stress and physical and psychosocial status in SLE patients.

Probably more than half of the patients with SLE experience some form of neuropsychiatric symptomatology, ranging from seizures, headaches, psychosis and mood disorders to cognitive impairment.[99] The latter is probably the most prevalent neuropsychiatric symptom.[100] Most observers agree that cognitive change and psychosis are generally secondary to a more diffuse process involving both alterations in small blood vessels in the brain and antibodies directed to neuronal tissue.[101] It also appears likely that circulating cytokines may have a role in the fatigue, cognitive impairment, and other neuropsychiatric manifestations of SLE. There is also some evidence that different antibodies are associated with different patterns of neuropsychiatric symptoms. For example, elevated titres of lymphocytotoxic antibody (LCA) are associated with specific visuospatial cognitive impairment.[102]

Insulin-dependent diabetes mellitus

Insulin-dependent diabetes mellitus is caused by β-cell destruction, which probably results from a cell-mediated autoimmune process in genetically susceptible individuals. A variety of triggering mechanisms have been suggested, including psychological stress, fetal viral exposure, early exposure to cows' milk proteins, and a high exposure level to nitrosamines.[103] Factors such as high rate of growth, infection or psychological stress may increase the demand for insulin and thus accelerate or highlight β-cell destruction. One group of investigators followed up this hypothesis by looking at changes in T-cell subsets in relation to re-experiencing grief at the loss of a loved one.[104] Diabetics who had experienced a recent loss had a marked increase in helper T-cell percentages after viewing a film about the loss of a love affair, presumably resonating with their earlier loss. The recruitment of additional helper T-cells could augment the ongoing immune attack on β-cells.

One of the strongest pieces of evidence comes from observations on the effect of stress on an animal model of diabetes.[105] In this group of bio-breeding (BB) rats, which serve as an animal model for autoimmune insulin-dependent diabetes mellitus, a significantly higher rate of disease developed in the rats exposed to a chronic moderate stress over a 14-week period.

Multiple sclerosis and experimental allergic encephalomyelitis

Experimental allergic encephalomyelitis (EAE) is widely used as an animal model for multiple sclerosis, an autoimmune, demyelinating disease of the central nervous system. There are data to suggest that stressful experiences can suppress the clinical expression of this disorder in rats and that they do so by altering immune responses.[106–109]

Griffin et al had noted that female Lewis rats exhibited significantly higher basal circadian levels of corticosterone than their male counterparts. They then explored the possible differential effects of restraint stress on male and female expression of EAE. Indeed, they found that both clinical and histopathological changes of EAE were more suppressed in female than in male Lewis rats. Stress seemed to affect presentation or processing of the myelin basic protein (MBP) and to decrease IL-2 and IFN-γ production. AEA appears to be mediated via Th1 cells, the mediation involving at least one of its cytokines, IL-2, the produc-

tion of which can be reduced by stress.[108] Stress may act through not only glucocorticoid but also opioid receptors, which have been found on some lymphoid cells.[110]

Cytokines, in particular TNF, have also been implicated in the myelin damage which is the hallmark of multiple sclerosis.[111] The relationship between stress and disease activity is less clear than in other autoimmune disorders such as RA, perhaps because of the time lag between immune changes and neurological symptom manifestation.[112–114]

Other autoimmune disorders

There are numerous other autoimmune disorders in which cognitive status may change, including animal models of autoimmune dementia,[115] developmental learning disabilities,[116] and reading disabilities and left-handedness.[117,118] Investigators have also speculated about autoimmunity as the aetiology of schizophrenia.[119–121]

Although SLE is the most prominent example of neuropsychiatric complications of a systemic autoimmune disorder, other examples have been cited. For example, psychosis has been described in three cases of myasthenia gravis and thymoma.[122]

Following up on Geschwind's hypothesis[117] about autoimmunity and left-handedness, Searleman and Fugagli[123] found a significantly higher incidence of left-handedness in males with type I diabetes mellitus, as well as in patients with two other autoimmune disorders, Crohn's disease and ulcerative colitis.

There has long been speculation that psychological factors play a role in the onset and course of Crohn's disease and ulcerative colitis.[124] A more recent study[125] showed that patients with ulcerative colitis who experience more recent life events show evidence of increased mucosal damage, even if they remain asymptomatic. Recent studies in psychoneuroimmunology have helped to establish a rationale for such an effect. There are, after all, lymphoid cells in the intestinal mucosa which are regulated by neuropeptides, such as substance P, vasoactive intestinal protein, and somastatin. Sympathetic and parasympathetic pathways link the central nervous system to these lymphoid cells.[126]

Psychogenic purpura (autoerythrocyte sensitization) is a condition of inflammatory bruises primarily in adult women thought to be caused by sensitization of patients to the stroma of their own erythrocytes. One investigator has noted that most cases occur within a short period of time after severe emotional stress.[127] Injury and surgical procedures were also noted to be probable precipitating events.

Hetzel[128] and Kung[129] have shown that stress may play a significant role in the pathogenesis of thyrotoxicosis and Grave's disease.

Infectious disease

Acquired immunodeficiency syndrome

HIV is one of several viruses to infect immune cells and neurons, making it of particular interest in the study of psychoneuroimmunology. Our concept of HIV infection has changed considerably in recent years. It is now understood to be a long struggle in which the immune system combats the HIV virus, and the rate of disease progression can vary widely. Vigorous treatments early on which tip the balance in favour of the host have received considerable attention and have been associated with newer and far more effective treatment strategies. Some psychological and social factors seem to correlate with the rates of progression of the disease. For example, a study by Temoshok[130]

found that one factor influencing survival in AIDS patients was the degree of control that patients experienced over their lives. Those who felt they had more control survived longer. Depressive symptoms have been associated with more rapid progression of HIV infection as well as recurrence of herpes simplex virus (HSV) infection.[131] Both depressive symptoms[47] and stressors[132] have been associated with immune function, in particular with diminished NK cell and other cytotoxic T-cell populations. There is also evidence that psychosocial intervention, in the form of stress management, might also influence the course of disease. A combination of focused relaxation training, group support and cognitive therapy has been shown to increase CD4 cell counts in both seropositive and seronegative subjects.[133]

Other infectious diseases

There is considerable evidence from animal studies of the role of stress on the timing and pathophysiology of infection.[134] Restraint stress in mice increases mycobacterial infection,[135] at least in part as a result of increased corticosterone production, but also as a result of suppression of TNF-α and nitric oxide, both potent microbicidal substances produced by macrophages. Another common pulmonary infection in humans, influenza, has also been shown in mouse models to be increased by restraint stress, through suppressed production of IFN[136] and IL-2.[137] Similar immobilization stress[138] and stress induced by mild electrical shock[139] in mice have been shown to worsen another viral infection, herpes simplex.

Tumours and metastasis

There has long been evidence that noise, handling and other stresses can differentially affect the rate of tumour growth in laboratory animals.[140] More recent studies have provided stronger evidence that such effects are mediated by immune mechanisms. For example, in a rat model of mammary adenocarcinoma, the stress of forced swimming caused increased lung metastases, apparently through diminished NK cell lysis.[141]

There have also been studies in human cancer linking psychological factors, immune function, and outcome. Spiegel et al[142] provided a structured group intervention in patients with metastatic breast cancer. Those who received the intervention had roughly twice the survival time (36 months versus 19 months) of control subjects. Gruber et al[143] provided a similar intervention in patients with a variety of metastatic tumours and found significant increases in some measures of immune function, including T-cell function, mixed lymphocyte responsiveness, and total levels of immunoglobulins G and M. Following up with a randomized controlled study in patients with stage 1 breast cancer, Gruber et al[144] noted that the intervention reduced anxiety levels and proportionately enhanced immune measures. A 6-year follow-up study of the effects of a focused psychological intervention in patients with metastatic melanoma provides perhaps the most comprehensive evidence to date.[145] Patients receiving the structured intervention early in their course had lower rates of recurrence and mortality, had greater NK cell activity, and showed more adaptive coping with lower levels of emotional distress.

Atherosclerosis

There is even some evidence that atherosclerosis may in part be mediated by immune activity. Decades of evidence support a role for certain kinds of stress and personality style in the pathogenesis of coronary artery disease. Sympathetic activation undoubtedly plays a role in this pathogenic process. Within atherosclerotic lesions one finds evidence of many immune components: immunoglobulins, complement, mononuclear phagocytes, activated T-cells, and numerous cytokines. Wick et al[146] and others have postulated that such immune elements, in conjunction with increased sympathetic activity, may play a role in atherosclerosis.

Communication between the immune and central nervous systems

Brain lesions in experimental animals, particularly in the anterior hypothalamus, have been noted to alter the immune response.[147] Pituitary hormones are known to affect immune responses. Prolactin can stimulate cytokine production and secretion by lymphocytes,[5] and growth hormone can also exert positive effects on the immune system, while the effect of adrenocorticotrophic hormone (ACTH) is inhibitory.[148,149] Clearly, environmental factors, stress and alterations in circadian rhythms can affect the regulation of these hormones via the limbic system and hypothalamic–pituitary–adrenal (HPA) axis. An important mediator in this is the CRH system, with neurons projecting from the lateral paraventricular nuclei (PVN). The release of CRH activates the pituitary gland, in turn releasing ACTH, β-endorphin and α-melanocyte stimulating hormone (α-MSH). ACTH and β-endorphin have a regulatory effect, inhibiting further release of corticotrophin-releasing factor (CRF).

Within the brain, the sympathetic nervous system is modulated by noradrenaline-containing fibres which arise in the locus coeruleus, a brainstem nucleus. Sympathetic fibres, originating in the nervous system, directly innervate the thymus, spleen, lymph nodes and bone marrow.[150] Lymphocytes, in turn, are known to have β-adrenergic receptors, and to respond to neurotransmitters. After sympathectomy, experimental animals have been shown to have a heightened antibody response to immunization.[151] An intact sympathetic nervous system, on the other hand, seems to dampen the immune response. Catecholamines released from the adrenal medulla and at autonomic nerve endings can result in leukocytosis and NK cell deactivation.[152]

During an immune response in experimental animals, brain recordings have revealed that certain areas of the brain increase their level of neuronal firing, in particular the ventromedial hypothalamus.[153] Glucocorticoid elevations also occur during immune responses, and may have a feedback modulating effect on the immune response.[154] IL-1 from the macrophage, which is known to increase CRH and ACTH release, is a likely mediator for this feedback communication between the immune response and the brain. IL-1 may also stimulate noradrenergic and serotonergic turnover, exciting both the CRH system and the sympathetic nervous system.

Cells of the immune system have surface receptors for a wide variety of neurotransmitters, neuropeptides, and hormones. Whether or not immune cells generate their own neurotransmitters or hormones is a matter of debate. However, what is clear is that they produce chemical messengers, cytokines such as interferons and interleukins, which are important in regulating immune system responses. We have already seen how important these cytokines are in the pathogenesis of various autoimmune disorders. Some of these hormones have direct effects on the nervous system.[155] Mammalian glial cells, such as astrocytes and microglia,

which are derived from macrophages which have migrated to the central nervous system,[156] are involved in neural growth and mediate various central nervous system immune responses.[157]

The macrophage is a protypical example of the bi-directional interaction between the immune and central nervous systems, responsive to both neuropeptide and cytokine signals. The macrophage plays a central role in the initiation of the acute-phase response, in which a wide variety of stressors such as trauma, burns, infection and inflammation initiate a cascade of events which destroy foreign agents and remove damaged tissue. One of the jobs of the macrophage is to present foreign antigens to other immune cells for production of antibodies. Macrophages may even enter areas of the brain following trauma and inflammation.[14] Numerous neuropeptides, including endogenous opioids,[158] TNF, ACTH, MSH and substance P,[159] modulate the activity of the macrophage and other immunocytes. In turn, macrophages release their own cytokines. Fricchione et al[160] have shown that psychological stress such as the anticipation of cardiac surgery can have effects on the shape and locomotion of such immunocytes, presumably through the modulatory effects of these neuropeptides. There is considerable evidence that these macrophage-derived microglial cells may have a role in some neuropsychiatric and psychophysiological disorders.[1]

There is also evidence for the impact of cytokines on specific locations in the brain. IL-1 can influence sleep patterns,[161] and can interact with the hypothalamus (whose medial region lacks the usual blood–brain barrier) to produce fever[162] and release CRF.[163] CRF causes the release of ACTH by the pituitary gland, and this in turn causes the release of cortisol from the adrenal gland. In this regard, it is interesting that astrocytes also make interleukins, and thus may interact with the pituitary–adrenal axis as well.

Gorman[164] has suggested a 'Darwinian explanation' for many of these connections, namely, that at one time the immune system and nervous system were one. Some immune cells, in the form of astrocytes, remain within the brain. Neurons continue to send axons to make connections with the spleen and lymph nodes. Both immune cells and neurons, as he and others have pointed out, are unique in their capacity for memory. It also follows from the Darwinian perspective that some of the receptors and interactions between the brain and immune system may be vestigial and no longer of clinical significance. On the other hand, some may still have important clinical implications. It is just this challenge, namely of deciphering which neuroimmunological connections are clinically significant, which is central to this emerging field.

The multiplicity of interconnections between the immune, endocrine and central nervous system accounts for the psychophysiological observations noted above in many disorders which are mediated by the immune system.

Psychoneuroimmunology in mood disorders—implications for the future

What are the implications of these psychoneuroimmunological findings for the future—especially with regard to our understanding of mood disorders? Special attention should probably be focused on the cytokines, because of their wide-ranging effects on the nervous system. As we have seen, IL-1 affects the sleep cycle, and also appetite, two important symptoms of depression. Such discoveries may help

to explain the fact that neuropsychiatric SLE, with its associated cytokine release, can present with major depression or schizophrenia-like symptoms.

Increased levels of certain cytokines have been observed in major depression. Maes et al[165] found that antinuclear antibodies (ANAs) and circulating soluble IL-2 receptors were found more frequently in depressed patients than in normal volunteers. They also noted that there seems to be a depression-related state of T-cell activation, characterized by a higher T-helper to T-suppressor-cytotoxic cell ratio.[166] In further investigations, Maes et al[167] found that plasma concentrations of IL-6, soluble IL-6 receptor (sIL-6R), soluble IL-2 receptor (sIL-2R) and transferrin receptor (TfR) were all elevated in major depression, whether active or in remission, suggesting that the coordinated and upregulated production of these cytokines may be a trait marker for major depression.

Interestingly, in more severe, melancholic depression, the same authors[168] noted that IL-6 production was increased, in conjunction with a failure to suppress cortisol production in response to dexamethasone, itself a well-described, though non-specific, marker for severe depression.[169] In another report, Maes et al[170] suggested that increased IL-1β production might account for the non-suppression of cortisol in response to dexamethasone. Levels of phytohaemagglutinin (PHA)-stimulated IL-1β produced from monocytes in 38 patients with major depression were correlated positively with post-dexamethasone cortisol levels.

One of the further pieces of evidence supporting the idea of chronic CRH hypersecretion and overactivation of the HPA axis in major depression is a finding of computerized tomographic evidence of adrenal hypertrophy.[171] Thus, the interleukins appear to increase the activation of the HPA axis. In major depression, glucocorticoid receptors both on lymphocytes[172] and in the hippocampus[173] are diminished.

Selye[174] was the first to suggest that severe chronic stress would lead to depression, loss of weight, reduced gonadal function, ulcer disease, and immunosuppression, producing many of the physiological changes known to occur with depression. Prolonged and elevated CRH production may be at the core of the physiology of depression.

It is interesting that cytokines have been focused on in connection with chronic fatigue syndrome (CFS), a mysterious disorder which has many symptoms in common with depression. CFS patients have subtle immune abnormalities such as decreased NK cell activity and decreased mitogen responsivity.[175] In addition, many patients with CFS also have major depression.[176] The exogenous administration of interleukins in the treatment of cancer has a variety of systemic side-effects, including fever, fatigue, and cognitive impairment.[177] When given to volunteers, cytokines such as IL-1 and TNF can cause symptoms of depression.[178]

These findings, taken in their entirety, led Maes et al to propose the monocyte T-lymphocyte hypothesis of major depression.[48] This hypothesis is rooted in the earlier observations of the activation of cell-mediated immunity in major depression, but extends them to encompass: cytokine activity at central brain regions, such as the hypothalamus, hippocampus and locus ceruleus; the interaction between cytokines and the HPA axis's neuroendocrine function and with monoamine neurotransmitters such as noradrenaline and serotonin; and finally the behavioural effects of cytokines. Noting the evidence for increases in depression following stroke, Maes et al speculate about the roles of macrophages and cytokines in that process. Brain tissue injury leads to a rapid local aggregation of macrophages and microglia along with an IL-2 titre elevation.

In a recent paper, Maes[179] summarizes the immune changes noted in depression. Stress or an activated immune process resulting from some medical condition may induce HPA-axis hyperactivity and the increased production of cytokines by macrophages. This hypersecretion of cytokines IL-1β and IL-6 in turn triggers an immune activation (T-cell activation, B-cell proliferation, and neutrophilia), the acute-phase response, prostaglandin secretion, and the neurovegetative symptoms and behavioural changes seen in major depression. By a feedback loop, serotonergic activity may be altered. HPA-axis hyperactivity may exert a negative feedback effect on various aspects of immunity, such as the numbers of T- and B-cells.

The acute-phase response, which is triggered by a wide variety of noxious stimuli, such as infection and trauma, is characterized by a sequence of metabolic, immune, neuroendocrine and behavioural changes. It is accompanied by a serum increase in so-called acute-phase proteins (APPs), including haptoglobin, α_1-acid glycoprotein, α_1-antichymotrypsin, C-reactive protein, and ceruloplasmin. There is clear evidence for an increase in these APPs in major depression.[180–183] Sluzewska et al[184] have also provided evidence for the presence of elevated APPs in patients with refractory depression treated with lithium potentiation. This provides further evidence of immune activation. Nonresponders to the lithium had higher pretreatment APP levels, suggesting more inflammatory patterns.

As noted, there is clear evidence for increased levels of IL-6 and IL-1 in patients with major depression.[167] These cytokines are the major mediators of the immune and acute-phase response in humans.[185] Sluzewska et al[186] have also provided evidence that after patients with major depression are treated with and respond to fluoxetine, their IL-6 levels decline.

One possibly related area of exploration has concerned the so-called G-proteins, which play an important role in post-receptor information transduction. They have also been implicated in mood disorders. In one study of patients with bipolar disorder,[187] levels of inhibitory and stimulatory G-proteins were found to be higher and were suspected of playing an aetiological role in the pathophysiology of bipolar disorder. In a more recent study, other investigators[188] have noted reduced levels and function of G-proteins in mononuclear leukocytes in patients with depression. Specifically, both the inhibitory and stimulatory G-proteins are reduced in function and quantity. Whether the changes in G-proteins are related to the overall immune activation process in major depression is unknown.

Summary

Taken as a whole, these studies provide strong evidence for the role of psychological factors such as stress, depression and social support in the regulation of immune functions and in the clinical expression of disorders mediated in part by the immune system—autoimmune disorders, cancer, and infection. Depression, stress and bereavement are all associated with immunological changes. What is less clear is whether such immunological changes are clinically significant. In animal studies they are, but in human studies the evidence is sparser. A study[145] of the effects of a focused psychological intervention in patients with metastatic melanoma provides perhaps the best evidence to date. In this study, structured interventions changed not only the course of the disease, but also some immunological parameters linked with psychological parameters. We need more studies which combine psychological measures with immune measures, and then actually link them to an important measurable clinical outcome.

We have also seen that some autoimmune disorders, such as SLE, provide compelling examples of immunological factors, in turn, influencing cognitive, affective and behavioural states. The indications of an acute-phase response and immune activation seen in SLE and RA are similar to what has been noted in depression.[189] Consequent on the research of Maes et al,[48] Smith[178] and Sluzewska et al[186] into its underlying biology, major depression has emerged as another condition in which immune activation and cytokine release may well help to explain the basic biology of the disorder. They certainly help to explain some of the observations on the impact of depression on the course and development of other medical disorders. These integrated immune, neuroendocrine and psychological responses may help to account for the manifestations of depression, both clinically and as seen in the laboratory. They may also provide important new markers and some new approaches for treatment in the future.

References

1. Perry VH, The role of macrophages in models of neurological and psychiatric disorder, *Psychol Med* 1992; **22**:551–5.
2. Adams DO, Molecular biology of macrophage activation: a pathway whereby psychosocial factors can potentially affect health, *Psychosom Med* 1994; **56**:316–27.
3. Ader R, Felten DL, Cohen N, eds, *Psychoneuroimmunology*, 2nd edn (Academic Press: San Diego, CA, 1991).
4. Stein M, Miller AH, Trestman RL, Depression, the immune system, and health and illness. Findings in search of meaning. *Arch Gen Psychiatry* 1991; **48**:171–7.
5. Reichlin S, Neuroendocrine–immune interactions, *N Engl J Med* 1993; **329**:1246–53.
6. Kiecolt-Glaser JK, Glaser R, Psychoneuroimmunology and health consequences: data and shared mechanisms, *Psychosom Med* 1995; **57**:269–74.
7. Chrousos GP, Gold PW, The concepts of stress and stress system disorders. Overview of physical and behavioral homeostasis, *JAMA* 1992; **267**:1244–52.
8. Vogel WH, Bower DB, Stress, immunity and cancer. In: Plotnikoff NP, Margo AJ, Faith RE, Wybran J, eds, *Stress and Immunity* (CRC Press: Boca Raton, 1991) 493–507.
9. Plata-Salaman CR, Immunomodulators and feeding regulation: a humoral link between the immune and nervous systems, *Brain Behav Immun* 1989; **3**:193–213.
10. Evans DL, Folds JD, Petitto JM et al, Circulating natural killer cell phenotypes in men and women with major depression. Relation to cytotoxic activity and severity of depression, *Arch Gen Psychiatry* 1992; **49**:388–95.
11. Fricchione GL, Stefano GB, The stress response and autoimmunoregulation, *Adv Neuroimmunol* 1994; **4**:13–27.
12. Perkins DO, Leserman J, Gilmore JH et al, Stress, depression, and immunity: research findings and clinical implications. In: Plotkinoff NP, Margo AJ, Faith RE, Wybran J, eds, *Stress and Immunity* (CRC Press: Boca Raton, 1991) 167–88.
13. Stefano GB, Role of opioid neuropeptides in immunoregulation, *Prog Neurobiol* 1989; **33**:149–59.
14. Stefano GB, Bilfinger TV, Fricchione GL, The immune-neurolink and the macrophage: postcardiotomy delirium, HIV-associated dementia and psychiatry, *Prog Neurobiol* 1994; **42**:475–88.
15. Scharrer B, Stefano GB, Neuropeptides and autoregulatory immune processes. In: Scharrer B, Smith EM, Stefano GB, eds, *Neuropeptides and Immunoregulation* (Springer-Verlag: New York, 1994) 1–13.
16. Bartrop RW, Luckhurst E, Lazarus L et al, Depressed lymphocyte function after bereavement, *Lancet* 1977; **1**:834–6.
17. Schleifer SJ, Keller SE, Camerino M et al, Suppression of lymphocyte stimulation following bereavement, *JAMA* 1983; **250**:374–7.
18. Kiecolt-Glaser JK, Fisher LD, Ogrocki P et al, Marital quality, marital disruption and immune function, *Psychosom Med* 1987; **49**:13–34.
19. Kiecolt-Glaser JK, Kennedy S, Malkoff S et al, Marital discord and immunity in males, *Psychosom Med* 1988; **50**:213–29.
20. Kiecolt-Glaser JK, Glaser R, Shuttleworth EC et al, Chronic stress and immunity in family caregivers of Alzheimer's disease victims, *Psychosom Med* 1987; **49**:523–35.
21. Arnetz BB, Wasserman J, Petrini B et al, Immune function in unemployed women, *Psychosom Med* 1987; **49**:3–12.
22. Dorian B, Garfinkel P, Brown G et al, Aberrations in lymphocyte subpopulations and function during psychological stress, *Clin Exp Immunol* 1982; **50**:132–8.
23. Glaser R, Kiecolt-Glaser JK, Stout JC et al, Stress-related impairments in cellular immunity, *Psychiatry Res* 1985; **16**:233–9.
24. Glaser R, Mehl VS, Penn G et al, Stress-associated changes in plasma immunoglobulin levels, *Int J Psychosom* 1986; **33**:41–2.
25. Stroebe MS, New directions in bereavement research: exploration of gender differences, *Palliat Med* 1998; **12**:5–12.
26. Good DM, Bower DA, Einsporn RL, Social support: gender differences in multiple sclerosis spousal caregivers, *J Neurosci Nurs* 1995; **27**:305–11.

27. King LA, Broyles SJ, Wishes, gender, personality, and well being, *J Pers* 1997; **65**:49–76.

28. Linn MW, Linn BS, Jensen J, Stressful events, dysphoric mood, and immune responsiveness, *Psychol Rep* 1984; **54**:219–22.

29. Solomon GF, Segerstrom SC, Grohr P et al, Shaking up immunity: psychological and immunologic changes after a natural disaster, *Psychosom Med* 1997; **59**:114–27.

30. Ironson G, Wynings C, Schneiderman N et al, Posttraumatic stress symptoms, intrusive thoughts, loss, and immune function after Hurricane Andrew, *Psychosom Med* 1997; **59**:128–41.

31. Schleifer SJ, Keller SE, Meyerson AT et al, Lymphocyte function in major depressive disorder, *Arch Gen Psychiatry* 1984; **41**:484–6.

32. Schleifer SJ, Keller SE, Siris SG et al, Depression and immunity. Lymphocyte function in ambulatory depressed patients, hospitalized schizophrenic patients, and patients hospitalized for herniorraphy, *Arch Gen Psychiatry* 1985; **42**:129–33.

33. Syvalahti E, Eskola J, Ruuskanen O et al, Nonsuppression of cortisol in depression and immune function, *Prog Neuropsychopharmacol Biol Psychiatry* 1985; **9**:413–22.

34. Irwin M, Daniels M, Bloom ET et al, Life events, depressive symptoms and immune function, *Am J Psychiatry* 1987; **144**:437–41.

35. Wahlin A, von Knorring L, Roos G, Altered distribution of T lymphocyte subsets in lithium-treated patients, *Neuropsychobiology* 1984; **11**:243–6.

36. Darko DF, Gillin JC, Risch SC et al, Immune cells and the hypothalamic–pituitary axis in major depression, *Psychiatry Res* 1988; **25**:173–9.

37. Schleifer SJ, Keller SE, Bond RN et al, Major depressive disorder and immunity. Roles of age, sex, severity, and hospitalization, *Arch Gen Psychiatry* 1989; **46**:81–7.

38. Schleifer SJ, Keller SE, Bartlett JA et al, Immunity in young adults with major depressive disorder, *Am J Psychiatry* 1996; **153**:477–82.

39. Irwin M, Caldwell C, Smith TL et al, Major depressive disorder, alcoholism and reduced natural killer cytotoxicity. Role of severity of depressive symptoms and alcohol consumption, *Arch Gen Psychiatry* 1990; **47**:713–19.

40. Cover H, Irwin M, Immunity and depression: insomnia, retardation, and reduction of natural killer cell activity, *J Behav Med* 1994; **17**:217–23.

41. Phillips B, Marshall ME, Brown S et al, Effect of smoking on human natural killer cell activity, *Cancer* 1985; **56**:2789–92.

42. Chandra RK, Nutrition and immunity: lessons from the past and new insights into the future, *Am J Clin Nutr* 1991; **53**:1087–101.

43. Andreoli A, Keller SE, Rabaeus M et al, Immunity, major depression, and panic disorder comorbidity, *Biol Psychiatry* 1992; **31**:896–908.

44. Petitto JM, Folds JD, Evans DL, Abnormal diurnal variation of B lymphocyte circulation patterns in major depression, *Biol Psychiatry* 1993; **34**:268–70.

45. Anderson JL, The immune system and major depression, *Adv Neuroimmunol* 1996; **6**:119–29.

46. Herbert TB, Cohen S, Depression and immunity: a meta-analytic review, *Psychol Bull* 1993; **113**:472–86.

47. Leserman J, Petitto JM, Perkins DO et al, Severe stress, depressive symptoms, and changes in lymphocyte subsets in human immunodeficiency virus-infected men. A 2-year follow-up study, *Arch Gen Psychiatry* 1997; **54**:279–85.

48. Maes M, Smith R, Scharpe S, The monocyte-T-lymphocyte hypothesis of major depression, *Psychoneuroendocrinology* 1995; **20**:111–16.

49. Lazarus RS, Folkman S, *Stress, Appraisal and Coping* (Springer: New York, 1984) 1–21.

50. Locke SE, Kraus L, Leserman L et al, Life change stress, psychiatric symptoms, and natural killer cell activity, *Psychosom Med* 1984; **46**:441–53.

51. Cobb S, Presidential Address – 1976. Social support as a moderator of life stress, *Psychosom Med* 1976; **38**:300–14.

52. Baron RS, Cutrona CE, Hicklin D et al, Social support and immune function among spouses of cancer patients, *J Pers Soc Psychol* 1990; **59**:344–52.

53. Boccia ML, Scanlan JM, Laudenslager ML et al, Juvenile friends, behavior, and immune

responses to separation in bonnet macaque infants, *Physiol Behav* 1997; **61**:191–8.

54. Ader R, Cohen N, Behaviorally conditioned immunosuppression, *Psychosom Med* 1975; **37**:333–40.

55. Rogers MP, Reich P, Strom TB, Carpenter CB, Behaviorally conditioned immunosuppression: replication of a recent study, *Psychosom Med* 1976; **38**:447–51.

56. Ader R, Conditioned immune responses and pharmacotherapy, *Arthritis Care Res* 1989; **2**:S58–64.

57. Fredrikson M, Furst CJ, Lekander M et al, Trait anxiety and anticipatory immune reactions in women receiving adjuvant chemotherapy for breast cancer, *Brain Behav Immun* 1993; **7**:79–90.

58. Schuurs AH, Verheul HA, Effects of gender and sex steroids on the immune response, *J Steroid Biochem* 1990; **35**:157–72.

59. Lahita RG, The basis for gender effects in the connective tissue diseases, *Ann Med Interne (Paris)* 1996; **147**:241–7.

60. Cuchacovich M, Gatica H, Tchernitchin AN, Role of sex hormones in autoimmune diseases, *Rev Med Chil* 1993; **121**:1045–52.

61. Sarvetnick N, Fox HS, Interferon-gamma and the sexual dimorphism of autoimmunity, *Mol Biol Med* 1990; **7**:323–31.

62. Blumenfeld Z, Halachmi S, Peretz BA et al, Premature ovarian failure—the prognostic application of autoimmunity on conception after ovulation induction, *Fertil Steril* 1993; **59**:750–5.

63. Grossman CJ, Roselle GA, Mendenhall CL, Sex steroid regulation of autoimmunity, *J Steroid Biochem Mol Biol* 1991; **40**:649–59.

64. Dupond JL, Humbert P, Taillard C, de Wazieres B, Vuitton D, Relationship between autoimmune diseases and personality traits in women, *Presse Med* 1990; **19**:2019–22.

65. Affleck G, Pfeiffer C, Tennen H, Fifield J, Attributional processes in rheumatoid arthritis patients, *Arthritis Rheum* 1987; **30**:927–31.

66. Meyerowitz S, Jacox RF, Hess DW, Monozygotic twins discordant for rheumatoid arthritis: a genetic, clinical and psychological study of 8 sets, *Arthritis Rheum* 1968; **11**:1–21.

67. Heisel JS, Life changes as etiologic factors in juvenile rheumatoid arthritis, *J Psychosom Res* 1972; **16**:411–20.

68. Baker GH, Life events before the onset of rheumatoid arthritis, *Psychother Psychosom* 1982; **38**:173–7.

69. Hendrie HC, Paraskevas F, Baragar FD, Adamson JD, Stress, immunoglobulin levels and early polyarthritis, *J Psychosom Res* 1971; **15**:337–42.

70. Wallace DJ, Metzger AL, Can an earthquake cause flares of rheumatoid arthritis or lupus nephritis? *Arthritis Rheum* 1994; **37**:1826–8.

71. Rimon R, Viukari M, Halonen P, Relationship between life stress factors and viral antibody levels in patients with juvenile rheumatoid arthritis, *Scand J Rheumatol* 1979; **8**:62–4.

72. Parker JC, Smarr KL, Angelone EO et al, Psychological factors, immunologic activation, and disease activity in rheumatoid arthritis, *Arthritis Care Res* 1992; **5**:196–201.

73. Harrington L, Affleck G, Urrows S et al, Temporal covariation of soluble interleukin-2 receptor levels, daily stress, and disease activity in rheumatoid arthritis, *Arthritis Rheum* 1993; **36**:199–203.

74. van Lankveld W, van't Pad Bosch P, van de Putte L et al, Disease-specific stressors in rheumatoid arthritis: coping and well-being, *Br J Rheumatol* 1994; **33**:1067–73.

75. Knapp PH, Levy EM, Giorgi RG et al, Short-term immunological effects of induced emotion, *Psychosom Med* 1992; **54**:133–48.

76. Esterling BA, Antoni MH, Fletcher MA et al, Emotional disclosure through writing or speaking modulates latent Epstein–Barr virus antibody titers, *J Consult Clin Psychol* 1994; **62**:130–40.

77. Futterman AD, Kemeny ME, Shapiro D, Fahey JL, Immunological and physiological changes associated with induced positive and negative mood, *Psychosom Med* 1994; **56**:499–511.

78. Urrows S, Affleck G, Tennen H, Higgins P, Unique clinical and psychological correlates of fibromyalgia tender points and joint tenderness in rheumatoid arthritis, *Arthritis Rheum* 1994; **37**:1513–20.

79. Crown S, Crown JM, Fleming A, Aspects of

the psychology and epidemiology of rheumatoid disease, *Psychol Med* 1975; 5:291–9.

80. Rimon R, Social and psychosomatic aspects of rheumatoid arthritis, *Acta Rheumatol Scand* 1969; **13** (suppl):1–154.

81. Stewart M, Knight R, Palmer D et al, Differential relationships between stress and disease activity for immunologically distinct subgroups of people with rheumatoid arthritis, *J Abnorm Psychology* 1994; **103**:251–8.

82. Feigenbaum SL, Masi AT, Kaplan SB, Prognosis in rheumatoid arthritis. A longitudinal study of newly diagnosed younger adult patients, *Am J Med* 1979; **66**:377–84.

83. Moos RM, Solomon GF, Personality correlates of the degree of functional incapacity of patients with physical disease, *J Chronic Dis* 1965; **18**:1019–38.

84. Rimon R, Laakso RL, Life stress and rheumatoid arthritis. A 15-year follow-up study, *Psychother Psychosom* 1985; **43**:38–43.

85. McFarlane AC, Kalucy RS, Brooks PM, Psychological predictors of disease course in rheumatoid arthritis, *J Psychosom Res* 1987; **31**:757–64.

86. Hagglund KJ, Haley WE, Reveille JD, Alarcon GS, Predicting individual differences in pain and functional impairment among patients with rheumatoid arthritis, *Arthritis Rheum* 1989; **32**:851–8.

87. Shearn MA, Fireman BH, Stress management and mutual support groups in rheumatoid arthritis, *Am J Med* 1985; **78**:771–5.

88. Trentham DE, Belli JA, Anderson RJ et al, Clinical and immunologic effects of fractionated total lymphoid irradiation in refractory rheumatoid arthritis, *N Engl J Med* 1981; **305**:976–82.

89. Pearson CM, Paulus HE, Machleder HI, The role of the lymphocyte and its products in the propagation of joint disease, *Ann NY Acad Sci* 1975; **256**:150–68.

90. Reinherz EL, Rubinstein A, Geha RS et al, Abnormalities of immunoregulatory T cells in disorders of immune function, *N Engl J Med* 1979; **301**:1018–22.

91. Solomon GF, Stress and antibody response in rats, *Int Arch Allergy Appl Immunol* 1969; **35**:97–104.

92. Amkraut AA, Solomon GF, Kraemer HC, Stress, early experience and adjuvant-induced arthritis in the rat, *Psychosom Med* 1971; **33**:203–14.

93. Rogers MP, Trentham DE, McCune WJ et al, Effect of psychological stress on the induction of arthritis in rats, *Arthritis Rheum* 1980; **23**:1337–42.

94. Kreindler S, Cancro R, An ego psychological approach to psychiatric manifestations in systemic lupus erythematosus, *Dis Nerv Syst* 1970; **31**:102–7.

95. Hinrichsen H, Barth J, Ruckemann M et al, Influence of prolonged neuropsychological testing on immunoregulatory cells and hormonal parameters in patients with systemic lupus erythematosus, *Rheumatol Int* 1992; **12**:47–51.

96. Adams SG Jr, Dammers PM, Saia TL et al, Stress, depression, and anxiety predict average symptom severity and daily symptom fluctuation in systemic lupus erythematosus, *J Behav Med* 1994; **17**:459–77.

97. Rimon RH, Connective tissue diseases. In: Cheren S, ed., *Psychosomatic Medicine: Theory, Physiology, and Practice*, Vol. 2 (International Universities Press: Madison CT, 1989) 565–609.

98. Wekking EM, Vingerhoets AJ, van Dam AP et al, Daily stressors and systemic lupus erythematosus: a longitudinal analysis—first findings, *Psychother Psychosom* 1991; **55**:108–13.

99. Kelly MJ, Rogers MP, Neuropsychiatric aspects of systemic lupus erythematosus. In: Stoudemire A, Fogel BS, eds, *Medical-Psychiatric Practice*, Vol. 3 (American Psychiatric Press: Washington, DC, 1991), 183–214.

100. Denburg SD, Denburg JA, Carbotte RM et al, Cognitive deficits in systemic lupus erythematosus, *Rheum Dis Clin North Am* 1993; **19**:815–31.

101. Denburg JA, Carbotte RM, Denburg SD, Neuronal antibodies and cognitive function in systemic lupus erythematosus, *Neurology* 1987; **37**:464–7.

102. Denburg SD, Behmann SA, Carbotte RM, Denburg JA, Lymphocyte antigens in neuropsychiatric systemic lupus erythematosus. Relationship of lymphocyte antibody specificities to clinical disease, *Arthritis Rheum* 1994; **37**:369–75.

103. Dahlquist G, Etiological aspects of insulin-dependent diabetes mellitus: an epidemiological perspective, *Autoimmunity* 1993; **15**:61–5.

104. McClelland DC, Patel V, Brown D, Kelner SP Jr, The role of affiliative loss in the recruitment of helper cells among insulin-dependent diabetics, *Behav Med* 1991; **17**:5–14.

105. Lehman CD, Rodin J, McEwen B, Brinton R, Impact of environmental stress on the expression of insulin-dependent diabetes mellitus, *Behav Neurosci* 1991; **105**:241–5.

106. Levine S, Strebel R, Wenk EJ et al, Suppression of experimental allergic encephalomyelitis by stress, *Proc Soc Exp Biol Med* 1962; **109**:294–8.

107. Bukilica M, Djordjevic S, Maric I et al, Stress-induced suppression of experimental allergic encephalomyelitis in the rat, *Int J Neurosci* 1991; **59**:167–75.

108. Griffin AC, Lo WD, Wolny AC et al, Suppression of experimental autoimmune encephalomyelitis by restraint stress: sex differences, *J Neuroimmunol* 1993; **44**:103–16.

109. Kuroda Y, Mori T, Hori T, Restraint stress suppresses experimental allergic encephalomyelitis in Lewis rats, *Brain Res Bull* 1994; **34**:15–17.

110. Bidlack JM, Saripalli LD, Lawrence DM, κ-Opioid binding sites on a murine lymphoma cell line, *Eur J Pharmacol* 1992; **227**:257–65.

111. Hartung HP, Immune-mediated demyelination, *Ann Neurol* 1993; **33**:563–7.

112. Grant I, Brown GW, Harris T et al, Severely threatening events and marked life difficulties preceding onset or exacerbation of multiple sclerosis, *J Neurol Neurosurg Psychiatry* 1989; **52**:8–13.

113. Sibley WA, Bamford CR, Clark K et al, A prospective study of physical trauma and multiple sclerosis, *J Neurol Neurosurg Psychiatry* 1991; **54**:584–9.

114. Franklin G, Nelson L, Heaton R et al, Stress and its relationship to acute exacerbations in multiple sclerosis, *J Neurol Rehab* 1992; **49**:238–44.

115. Michaelson DM, Alroy G, Goldstein D et al, Characterization of an experimental autoimmune dementia model in the rat, *Ann NY*

Acad Sci 1991; **640**:290–4.

116. Schrott LM, Denenberg VH, Sherman GF et al, Environmental enrichment, neocortical ectopias, and behavior in the autoimmune NZB mouse, *Brain Res Dev Brain Res* 1992; **67**:85–93.

117. Geschwind N, The biology of cerebral dominance: implications for cognition, *Cognition* 1984; **17**:193–208.

118. Gilger JW, Pennington BF, Green P et al, Reading disability, immune disorders and non-right-handedness: twin and family studies of their relations, *Neuropsychologia* 1992; **30**:209–27.

119. Kornhuber HH, Kornhuber J, A neuroimmunological challenge: schizophrenia as an autoimmune disease, *Arch Ital Biol* 1987; **125**:271–2.

120. Knight J, Knight A, Ungvari G, Can autoimmune mechanisms account for the genetic predisposition to schizophrenia? *Br J Psychiatry* 1992; **160**:533–40.

121. Yang ZW, Chengappa KN, Shurin G et al, An association between anti-hippocampal antibody concentration and lymphocyte production of IL-2 in patients with schizophrenia, *Psychol Med* 1994; **24**:449–55.

122. Musha M, Tanaka F, Ohuti M, Psychoses in three cases with myasthenia gravis and thymoma—proposal of a paraneoplastic autoimmune neuropsychiatric syndrome, *Tohoku J Exp Med* 1993; **169**:335–44.

123. Searleman A, Fugagli AK, Suspected autoimmune disorders and left-handedness: evidence from individuals with diabetes, Crohn's disease, and ulcerative colitis, *Neuropsychologia* 1987; **25**:367–74.

124. Knoflach P, Etiology and pathogenesis of Crohn's disease and ulcerative colitis, *Wien Klin Wochenschr* 1986; **98**:754–8.

125. Turnbull GK, Vallis TM, Quality of life in inflammatory bowel disease: the interaction of disease activity with psychosocial function, *Am J Gastroenterol* 1995; **90**:1450–4.

126. Ramchandani D, Schindler B, Katz J, Evolving concepts of psychopathology in inflammatory bowel disease. Implications for treatment, *Med Clin North Am* 1994; **78**: 1321–30.

127. Ratnoff OD, Psychogenic purpura (autoery-

throcyte sensitization): an unsolved dilemma, *Am J Med* 1989; 87:16N–21N.

128. Hetzel BS, The pathogenesis of thyrotoxicosis, *Med J Aust* 1970; 2:663–7.

129. Kung AW, Life events, daily stresses and coping in patients with Grave's disease, *Clin Endocrinol* 1995; 42:303–8.

130. Temoshok L, O'Leary A, Jenkins SR, Survival time in men with AIDS: relationships with psychological coping and autonomic arousal, *Int Conf AIDS* 1990; 6:435(abstract no. 3133).

131. Zorrilla EP, McKay JR, Luborsky L, Schmidt K, Relation of stressors and depressive symptoms to clinical progression of viral illness, *Am J Psychiatry* 1996; 153:626–35.

132. Evans DL, Leserman J, Perkins DO et al, Stress-associated reductions of cytotoxic T lymphocytes and natural killer cells in a symptomatic HIV infection, *Am J Psychiatry* 1995; 152:543–50.

133. LaPerriere A, Antoni M, Klimas N et al, Psychoimmunology and stress management in HIV-1 infection. In: Gorman JM, Kertzner RM, eds, *Psychoimmunology Update* (American Psychiatric Press: Washington DC, 1991) 81–112.

134. Moynihan JA, Ader R, Psychoneuroimmunology: animal models of disease, *Psychosom Med* 1996; 58:546–58.

135. Brown DH, Sheridan J, Pearl D et al, Regulation of mycobacterial growth by the hypothalamus–pituitary–adrenal axis: differential responses of *Mycobacterium bovis* BCG-resistant and -susceptible mice, *Infect Immun* 1993; 61:4793–800.

136. Chetverikova LK, Frolov BA, Kramskaya TA et al, Experimental influenza influence of stress, *Acta Virol* 1987; 31:424–33.

137. Hermann G, Tovar CA, Beck FM et al, Restraint stress differentially affects the pathogenesis of an experimental influenza viral infection in three inbred strains of mice, *J Neuroimmunol* 1993; 47:83–94.

138. Bonneau RH, Sheridan JF, Feng NG et al, Stress-induced effects on cell-mediated innate and adaptive memory components of the murine immune response to herpes simplex virus infection, *Brain Behav Immun* 1991; 5:274–95.

139. Kusnecov AV, Grota LJ, Schmidt SG et al, Decreased herpes simplex viral immunity and enhanced pathogenesis following stressor administration in mice, *J Neuroimmunol* 1992; 38:129–37.

140. Riley V, Psychoneuroendocrine influences on immunocompetence and neoplasia, *Science* 1981; 212:1100–9.

141. Ben-Eliyahu S, Yirmiya R, Liebeskind JC et al, Stress increases metastatic spread of a mammary tumor in rats: evidence for mediation by the immune system, *Brain Behav Immun* 1991; 5:193–205.

142. Spiegel D, Bloom JR, Kraemer HC, Gottheil E, Effect of psychosocial treatment on survival of patients with metastatic breast cancer, *Lancet* 1989; 2:888–91.

143. Gruber BL, Hall NR, Hersh SP, Dubois P, Immune system and psychological changes in metastatic cancer patients using relaxation and guided imagery: a pilot study, *Scand J Behav Ther* 1988; 17:25–46.

144. Gruber BL, Hersh SP, Hall NR et al, Immunological responses of breast cancer patients to behavioral interventions, *Biofeedback Self Regul* 1993; 18:1–22.

145. Fawzy FI, Fawzy NW, Hyun CS et al, Malignant melanoma. Effects of an early structured psychiatric intervention, coping, and affective state on recurrence and survival 6 years later, *Arch Gen Psychiatry* 1993; 50:681–9.

146. Wick G, Schett G, Amberger A et al, Is atherosclerosis an immunologically mediated disease? *Immunol Today* 1995; 16:27–33.

147. Stein M, Schleifer SJK, Keller SE, Psychoimmunology in clinical psychiatry. In: Hales RE, Frances AJ, eds, *Psychiatry Update*, Vol. 6 (American Psychiatric Press: Washington DC, 1987) 210–34.

148. Baroni CD, Fabris N, Bertoli G, Effects of hormones on development and function of lymphoid tissue. Synergistic action of thyroxin and somatotropic hormone in pituitary dwarf mice, *Immunology* 1969; 17:303–14.

149. Bernton EW, Meltzer MS, Holaday JW, Suppression of macrophage activation and T-lymphocyte function in hypoprolactinemic mice, *Science* 1988; 239:401–4.

150. Felten DL, Felten SY, Carlson SL et al, Noradrenergic and peptidergic innervation of lymphoid tissue, *J Immunol* 1985; **135**: 755s–65s.

151. Miles K, Quintans J, Chelmicka-Schorr E et al, The sympathetic nervous system modulates antibody response to thymus-independent antigens, *J Neuroimmunol* 1981; **1**:101–5.

152. Weiss JM, Sundar S, Effects of stress on cellular immune responses in animals, *Rev Psychiatry* 1992; **11**:145–80.

153. Besedovsky H, del Rey A, Sorkin E et al, The immune response evokes changes in brain noradrenergic neurons, *Science* 1983; **221**:564–6.

154. Besedovsky HO, del Rey A, Immune neuroendocrine network. In: Cinader B, Miller RG, eds, *Progress in Immunology VI* (Academic Press: New York, 1986) 578–87.

155. Stefano GB, Pharmacological and binding evidence for opioid receptors on vertebrate and invertebrate blood cells. In: Scharrer B, Smith EM, Stefano GB, eds, *Neuropeptides and Immunoregulation* (Springer-Verlag: New York, 1994) 139–51.

156. Thomas WE, Brain macrophages: evaluation of microglia and their functions, *Brain Res Rev* 1992; **17**:61–74.

157. Zajicek JP, Wing M, Scolding NJ, Compston DA, Interactions between oligodendrocytes and microglia. A major role for complement tumour necrosis factor in oligodendrocyte adherence and killing, *Brain* 1992; **115**: 1611–31.

158. Stefano GB, Cadet P, Dokun A, Scharrer B, A neuroimmunoregulatory-like mechanism responding to stress in the marine bivalve Mytilus edulis, *Brain Behav Immun* 1990; **4**:323–9.

159. Stefano GB, Kushnerik V, Rodriguez M, Bilfinger TV, Inhibitory effect of morphone on granulocyte stimulation by tumor necrosis factor and substance P, *Int J Immunopharmacol* 1994; **16**:329–34.

160. Fricchione G, Bilfinger TV, Jandorf L, Smith EM, Stefano GB, Surgical anticipatory stress manifests itself in immunocyte desensitization: evidence for autoimmunoregulatory involvement, *Int J Cardiol* 1996; **53** (suppl):S65–73.

161. Moldofsky H, Lue FA, Eisen J et al, The relationship of interleukin-1 and immune functions to sleep in humans, *Psychosom Med* 1986; **48**:309–18.

162. Dion DL, Blalock JE, Neuroendocrine properties of the immune system. In: Bridge TP, Mirsky AF, Goodwin FK, eds, *Psychological, Neuropsychiatric, and Substance Abuse Issues in AIDS* (Raven Press: New York, 1988) 15–20.

163. Sapolsky R, Rivier C, Yamamoto G et al, Interleukin-1 stimulates the secretion of hypothalamic corticotropin-releasing factor, *Science* 1987; **238**:522–4.

164. Gorman JM, Psychoimmunology: a Darwinian approach. In: Gorman JM, Kertzner RM, eds, *Psychoimmunology Update* (American Psychiatric Press: Washington DC, 1991) 1–8.

165. Maes M, Bosmans E, Suy E, Vandervorst C, Dejonckheere C, Raus J, Antiphospholipid, antinuclear, Epstein–Barr and cytomegalovirus antibodies, and soluble interleukin-2 receptors in depressive patients, *J Affect Disord* 1991; **21**:133–40.

166. Maes M, Stevens W, DeClerck L et al, Immune disorders in depression: higher T helper/T suppressor-cytotoxic cell ratio, *Acta Psychiatr Scand* 1992; **86**:423–31.

167. Maes M, Meltzer HY, Bosmans E et al, Increased plasma concentrations of interleukin-6, soluble interleukin-6, soluble interleukin-2 and transferrin receptor in major depression, *J Affect Disord* 1995; **34**:301–9.

168. Maes M, Scharpe S, Meltzer HY et al, Relationships between interleukin-6 activity, acute phase proteins, and function of the hypothalamic–pituitary–adrenal axis in severe depression, *Psychiatry Res* 1993; **49**:11–27.

169. APA Task Force on Laboratory Tests in Psychiatry, The dexamethasone suppression test: an overview of its current status in psychiatry, *Am J Psychiatry* 1987; **144**:1253–62.

170. Maes M, Bosmans E, Meltzer HY, Scharpe S, Suy E, Interleukin-Iβ: a putative mediator of HPA axis hyperactivity in major depression, *Am J Psychiatry* 1993; **150**:1189–93.

171. Nemeroff CB, Krishnan KR, Reed D et al, Adrenal gland enlargement in major depres-

sion. A computed tomographic study, *Arch Gen Psychiatry* 1992; **49**:384–7.

172. Lowry MT, Gormley GJ, Reder AT, Meltzer HY, Immune function, glucocorticoid receptor regulation, and depression. In: Miller AH, ed., *Depressive Disorders and Immunity* (American Psychiatric Press: Washington DC, 1989) 105–34.

173. Sapolsky RM, Krey LC, McEwen BS, The neuroendocrinology of stress and aging: the glucocorticoid cascade hypothesis, *Endocrine Rev* 1986; **7**:284–301.

174. Selye H, The evolution of the stress concept, *Am J Cardiol* 1970; **26**:289–99.

175. Barker E, Fujimara SF, Fadem M et al, Immunologic abnormalities associated with chronic fatigue syndrome, *Clin Infect Dis* 1994; **18**:S136–141.

176. Manu P, Lane TJ, Matthews DA, The pathophysiology of chronic fatigue syndrome: confirmation, contradictions and conjectures, *Int J Psychiatry Med* 1992; **22**:397–408.

177. Denicoff KD, Durkin TM, Lotze MT et al, The neuroendocrine effects of interleukin-2 treatment, *J Clin Endocrinol Metab* 1989; **69**: 402–10.

178. Smith RS, The macrophage theory of depression, *Med Hypoth* 1991; **35**:298–306.

179. Maes M, Evidence for an immune response in major depression: a review and hypothesis, *Prog Neuropsychopharmacol Biol Psychiatry* 1995; **19**:11–38.

180. Maes M, Scharpe S, Van Grootel L et al, Higher alpha-1-antitrypsin, haptoglobin, and ceruloplamin and lower retinol binding protein plasma levels during depression: further evidence for the existence of an inflammatory response during that illness, *J Affect Disord* 1992; **24**:183–92.

181. Joyce PR, Hawes CR, Mulder RT et al, Elevated levels of acute phase plasma proteins in major depression, *Biol Psychiatry* 1992; **32**:1035–41.

182. Song C, Dinan T, Leonard BE, Changes in immunoglobulin, complement and acute phase protein levels in the depressed patients and normal controls, *J Affect Disord* 1994; **30**:283–8.

183. Sluzewska A, Rybakowski JK, Sobieska M et al, Concentration and microheterogeneity glycophorms of alpha-1 acid glycoprotein in major depressive disorder, *J Affect Disord* 1996; **39**:149–55.

184. Sluzewska A, Sobieska M, Rybakowski JK, Changes in acute-phase proteins during lithium potentiation of antidepressants in refractory depression, *Neuropsychobiology* 1997; **35**:123–7.

185. Heinrich PC, Castell JV, Andus T, Review article: interleukin-6 and the acute phase response, *Biochem J* 1990; **265**:621–36.

186. Sluzewska A, Rybakowski JK, Laciak M et al, Interleukin-6 serum levels in depressed patients before and after treatment with fluoxetine, *Ann NY Acad Sci* 1995; **762**:474–6.

187. Young LT, Li PP, Kamble A, Siu KP, Warsh JJ, Mononuclear leukocyte levels of G proteins in depressed patients with bipolar disorder or major depressive disorder, *Am J Psychiatry* 1994; **151**:594–6.

188. Avissar S, Nechamkin Y, Roitman G, Schreiber G, Reduced G protein functions and immunoreactive levels in mononuclear leukocytes of patients with depression, *Am J Psychiatry* 1997; **154**:211–17.

189. Mackiewicz A, Pawlowski T, Mackiewicz-Pawlowska A et al, Microheterogeneity forms of alpha-1-acid glycoprotein as indicator of rheumatoid arthritis activity, *Clin Chim Acta* 1987; **163**:185–90.

29

Sex differences in the psychopharmacological treatment of depression

Olga Brawman-Mintzer and Kimberly A Yonkers

Introduction

Historically, psychopharmacological treatment was based on the assumption that women and men metabolize and respond to drugs in a like manner. There was little to refute this, since data collected during the initial stages of development depended upon the use of male subjects. Women of reproductive potential were restricted from participating in clinical trials until the compound was shown to be effective, since it was felt that the risk of exposing a fetus to a new drug in the case of unexpected and undetected pregnancy was too great. Empirical evidence illustrated how this led to decreased testing in young women.[1] This and other information led to reformulation of US Food and Drug Administration (FDA) policy and, in 1993, the FDA announced revised guidelines that encourage the inclusion of women with childbearing potential in clinical trials.[2] The National Institutes of Health introduced similar changes for government-sponsored studies around this time.[3]

Despite limitations on available data, there may be considerable sex differences in the pharmacokinetics (i.e. the absorption, distribution, biotransformation, and elimination of drugs) and the pharmacodynamics (i.e. the biochemical and physiological effects) of many pharmacological agents.[4-7] At minimum, certain sex-specific events such as the use of oral contraceptives (OCs), pregnancy, menstrual cycle phase and even end-organ receptor sensitivity can influence drug metabolism. Unfortunately, and despite the fact that women are prescribed psychotropic agents more often than are men, the available data on sex-related effects are limited.

This chapter will highlight recent data on sex differences in the pharmacokinetics and pharmacodynamics of drugs, and the effects of sex-specific events, such as menstrual cycle phase and the use of OCs, on the metabolism and clearance of agents used in the treatment of depression. We include benzodiazepine anxiolytics in this review because they are also commonly used in the treatment of depressed women. It should be noted that issues such as use of psychotropic agents during pregnancy and breast-feeding are important topics but covered elsewhere in this volume. This chapter has been informed by other work written by the authors.[8]

Sex differences in pharmacokinetics

Absorption and bioavailability

The amount of drug that is absorbed from the gastrointestinal tract depends on the acid–base and lipophilic properties of the medication and the physiology of the gastrointestinal tract. The degree of drug ionization will affect its solubility. Some work suggests that women may secrete less gastric acid than men, leading to potential gender differences in absorption.[9] A decrease in gastric acid secretion would lead to a decrease in the absorption of weak acids, but an increase in absorption of weak bases.

There are several studies which have found sex differences in gastric emptying and gastrointestinal transit time. For example, Wald et al[10] reported that gastrointestinal transit time was significantly prolonged in women during the premenstrual phase. Other researchers[11] have shown that women empty solids from their stomachs more slowly than do men. While the mechanism for these differences is unknown, researchers hypothesize that it may be due to the effects of progesterone and oestradiol on the musculature of the gastrointestinal tract. However, there are also studies that have failed to demonstrate significant effects of ovarian hormones on gastrointestinal transit time.[12] If there is slowing in transit time, particularly in the small intestine, a number of factors may be affected. Absorption could be increased secondary to increased time in the gastrointestinal tract or drug could be degraded to greater extent if the particular medication is

susceptible to metabolism by one of the enzymes found at the brush border (e.g. CYP3A4[13,14]). Notably, CYP3A4 is an important hepatic oxidative enzyme for psychotropics that appears to be more active in women than in men.[15] However, whether increased activity in women also holds for the gastrointestinal enzyme analogue or just the hepatic analogue is unknown.

It should be said that despite the potential differences in gastric acid secretion, gastrointestinal transit time, and differences in enzyme activity, only a few variations in the absorption and the bioavailability of specific agents have been observed. For example, Aarons et al[16] observed that, following oral administration, aspirin was absorbed more rapidly in women than in men, while other researchers[17] found higher parenteral bioavailability of aspirin in women than in men, indicating potentially clinically relevant sex differences in the enzyme activity of the gastrointestinal tract.

Distribution

A number of drug characteristics affect the distribution of the compound in the body, including acid–base properties, water and lipid solubility and the affinity of the drug for binding proteins.[18] Patient characteristics include differences in blood volume, cardiac output, percentage lean body mass and organ size.[19] In general, females have a lower ratio of lean body mass to adipose tissue.[20] Thus, drugs with high lipophilicity, a characteristic of many psychotropics, would be expected to demonstrate a greater volume of distribution in females. These drugs may also have more prolonged half-lives, and serum levels may be greater in patients with less lean body mass. This information may be critical to understanding patients' treatment responses and experience of side-effects. It is possible that female patients with a relatively higher percentage of adipose tissue may require higher initial doses, but maintenance over time of the same dose will cause drug accumulation, leading to potentially toxic effects. However, these effects have not been investigated in relation to patient sex.

Metabolism

Metabolic processes in the liver are conceptualized as phase I or phase II reactions. Phase I reactions include oxidation, hydroxylation, N-demethylation, reduction, and hydrolysis, and are mediated through cytochrome P450 (CYP450). Phase II reactions, which are very rapid and not usually rate-limiting, consist of synthetic reactions such as glucuronidation, sulphation, methylation and/or acetylation of parent molecules and/or phase I reaction products. Importantly, there are data indicating significant sex-related differences in hepatic enzyme activity.

Cytochromes P450

In 1971, O'Malley et al[21] reported that the metabolism of antipyrine differs by sex. At that time, antipyrine metabolism was thought to reflect total hepatic CYP450 activity. Since that time, many isoenzymes of CYP450 have been identified, and there are increasing data on potential sex differences in the activity of some but not all isoenzymes. Since the majority of antidepressants and antipsychotic drugs are either metabolized by, or inhibit to varying degrees, one or more CYP450 isoenzymes, the potential for sex differences may be of particular relevance to the clinician.

CYP3A3/4

CYP3A3/4 is an important CYP450 enzyme, since it constitutes as much as 60% of the total P450 content of in vitro liver specimens.[22] It is involved in the metabolism of a broad range of compounds, including alprazolam, midazolam, diazepam, terfenadine, astemizole, carbamazepine, sertraline, tricyclic antidepressants (TCAs), calcium channel blockers, erythromycin, steroids, quinidine, lidocaine and others.[23–26] There is in vitro evidence for varied inhibition of CYP3A3/4 by frequently prescribed antidepressants such as the selective serotonin inhibitors (SSRIs) fluvoxamine, fluoxetine and sertraline.[27] Consistent with this are in vivo data showing that plasma concentrations of some drugs metabolized by this CYP3A3/4 increase during concomitant therapy with fluvoxamine, nefazodone, fluoxetine and sertraline, but not paroxetine.[28] Thus, potential sex differences in the activity of this isoenzyme may be clinically important. Indeed, data indicate that young women have approximately 1.4 times the CYP3A3/4 activity of men. A study by Hunt et al used erythromycin as a CYP3A3/4 substrate. It was metabolized 25% more rapidly by microsomes made from the human female compared to human male liver.[15] A number of other drugs show a sex difference in clearance that is consistent with this finding, including diazepam,[29,30] verapamil[31] and midazolam.[32,33] Progesterone, which has been shown to activate CYP3A3/4 in vitro,[25,34] may be responsible for the observed sex differences in enzyme activity in vivo. However, other researchers have failed to find evidence for sex-related differences in CYP3A3/4-mediated drug metabolism, although these discrepancies may be due to interindividual variations in CYP3A3/4 activity.[35–40]

CYP2D6

CYP2D6 is the most extensively studied of the CYP450 isoenzymes and is also involved in the metabolism of a number of psychotropic medications.[41] Approximately 5–10% of Caucasians lack this isoenzyme and are designated 'poor metabolizers'. These individuals may exhibit greater bioavailability, higher plasma concentrations and prolonged elimination half-lives of, and possibly exaggerated pharmacological response to, standard doses of drugs that are metabolized by CYP2D6. Co-administration of drugs which inhibit CYP2D6 with drugs that are metabolized by this enzyme essentially converts individuals who are extensive metabolizers to poor metabolizers.

CYP2D6 metabolizes many different classes of drugs, including antidepressants, antipsychotics, beta-adrenergic blockers, type 1C antiarrhythmics, dextrometorphan and a number of chemotherapeutic agents. Codeine and venlafaxine are O-demethylated by this enzyme,[42,43] and nortriptyline, desipramine and imipramine are hydroxylated by CYP2D6. A number of different drugs potentially inhibit the CYP2D6 enzyme, including quinidine, fluphenazine, haloperidol, thioridazine, amitriptyline, desipramine, clomipramine, sertraline, fluoxetine and paroxetine.[23,41,44,45]

The influence of sex on CYP2D6-mediated metabolism has been examined in a few in vivo studies. Both the hydroxylation of clomipramine and oral clearance of desipramine are higher in men than in women,[46,47] although the authors of these articles did not account for differences in body weight. Similar results hold for propranolol[48–50] and ondansetron.[51]

CYP2C
Relevant isoenzymes in the CYP2C subfamily include 2C9, 2C10, 2C19 and others. Diazepam, clomipramine, amitriptyline and imipramine are demethylated by CYP2C enzymes, and it is believed that warfarin,[52] phenytoin,[53] tolbutamide[54] and certain non-steroidal anti-inflammatory agents[55] are also metabolized by CYP2C enzymes. Co-administration of fluoxetine, sertraline or fluvoxamine increases the plasma concentrations of a number of these drugs, and thus it is assumed that fluvoxamine, fluoxetine and sertraline may inhibit CYP2C isoenzymes.[56,57]

The activity of CYP2C19 may be higher in men than in women. Men clear methyl phenobarbital, a compound metabolized by CYP2C19, approximately 1.3 times faster than women,[58] and piroxicam exhibited similar sex effects.[33] However, adjusting for weight removed these differences.[59]

CYP1A2
The CYP1A2 isoenzyme is implicated in the metabolism of theophylline, caffeine,[60] TCAs[23,61] clozapine[62] and, possibly, thiothixene.[63] This enzyme is induced by cigarette smoke, charcoal-broiled foods, and cabbage,[23,61,64] and is inhibited by fluvoxamine in vitro.[61] Other SSRIs do not appear to inhibit this CYP1A2.

Data regarding sex-related differences in the activity of CYP1A2 are conflicting. Studies of caffeine and thiothixene metabolism suggest that CYP1A2 activity is higher in men than in women.[63,65] On the other hand, Nafziger and Bertino[66] report that theophylline is cleared significantly faster in young women than in men. Sex differences in theophylline metabolism are not present in elderly patients, suggesting that this difference could be hormone-dependent rather than resulting from genetic differences.[67] Further, data regarding clomipramine demethylation, a putative CYP1A2-dependent process, do not show an influence of sex.[46] In sum, given the available information, no definite conclusions on the effects of sex on CYP1A2 activity can be drawn at this point.

Conjugation
Many drugs are conjugated with sulphuric or glucuronic acid and excreted by the kidneys. Conjugation reactions are commonly a rapid, second metabolic step after the drug has been metabolized via relatively slower cytochrome-

mediated degradative reactions. Given that cytochrome-mediated metabolism is often the rate-limiting step, it may not be possible to detect any sex-related differences in conjugation reactions for drugs which have such differences.[7] However, a number of drugs are solely metabolized by conjugation and appear to display sex-related differences in their elimination. Two examples are the benzodiazepines temazepam and oxazepam, which are cleared faster by men than by women.[29,68] More rapid elimination in men is also observed for digoxin,[69] although the observed differences may be related to differences in renal function. The clearance of acetaminophen was also greater (22%) in young men than in young women.[70] However, not all compounds that are cleared by glucuronidation are influenced by the person's sex.[71]

The effects of menstrual cycle phase

The varying hormonal milieu may lead to possible menstrual phase-specific changes that can affect the metabolism of drugs in women. For example, gastrointestinal transit time is prolonged in the luteal phase,[72,73] which may increase absorption in the small intestine or increase exposure of a compound to metabolic enzymes.

Other potential menstrual phase-related changes that can affect drug metabolism include increases and decreases in the volume of distribution, although empirical data showing menstrual cycle-associated vascular fluid retention are lacking. However, an older study did find evidence of menstrual phase changes in transcapillary fluid dynamics, resulting in fluid shifts between intravascular and extravascular spaces.[74] If such changes were to occur,

increases in fluid retention could dilute the concentration of medications, resulting in lower drug plasma levels.

A small number of reports suggest a menstrual cycle effect on drug pharmacokinetics. Methylprednisolone elimination is more variable in premenopausal than in postmenopausal women or in men, suggesting a menstrual cycle effect.[75] However, there was no correlation between the magnitude of drug elimination and the phase of the menstrual cycle. Another drug whose clearance varied across the menstrual cycle was caffeine.[76] Clearance of caffeine was slower in the luteal phase than in the follicular phase of the menstrual cycle. In contrast, the elimination of phenytoin appears to be more rapid at the end of the luteal phase.[77] The menstrual cycle does not, however, appear to affect the metabolism of a number of other compounds studied, including alprazolam,[78] nitrazepam,[79] phenobarbital,[80] lithium[81] and fluoxetine.[82]

These data highlight the need to determine menstrual cycle phase when investigating pharmacodynamic as well as pharmacokinetic properties of psychotropic medications in women. It may also be useful to explore the potential effects of menstrual cycle phase when adverse effects of medications occur or when there are fluctuations in drug efficacy.

Oral contraception

OCs are among the most widely used medications in the world. In selected instances, OCs influence the pharmacokinetics and pharmacodynamics of other compounds.[6,7,83] For example, oestrogen stimulates protein synthesis, which in turn may affect the protein binding of various drugs. OCs may also influence the elimination of other drugs via inhibition of various cytochrome P450 isoenzymes.[6] The clearance of the benzodiazepines triazolam, alprazolam[84] and nitrazepam[79] was reduced when OCs were taken concomitantly. The TCA imipramine was also affected by the older, higher-dose OCs when administered intravenously.[85] This was not seen when imipramine was given orally, perhaps because this effect was counterbalanced by a change in oral availability and decreased apparent oral clearance. Clomipramine metabolism is not influenced by OCs, although its metabolic rate is enhanced by oestrogens and inhibited by progesterone in animal models.[86]

OCs may also affect conjugative reactions through enzyme induction. Benzodiazepines that undergo conjugation, such as temazepam, show higher clearance in the presence of OCs.[84] The interaction between psychotropics and OCs can be clinically significant.[87] In one study, diazepam-associated impairment in cognitive and psychomotor tasks was found in a simulated driving task. The performance of women who were chronically taking OCs showed greater impairment during the week off hormones, probably because benzodiazepine levels peaked more quickly during that interval. The authors postulated that OCs decrease the rate of absorption of diazepam, and during the week off hormones the plasma levels quickly rose to intoxicating levels. Contrasting results were reported by Kroboth et al,[88] who investigated different benzodiazepines (alprazolam, triazolam and lorazepam) and found that psychomotor changes were most marked in women who received OCs. However, in both cases plasma levels did not correlate with the observed clinical effect, and the specific benzodiazepines used in these reports differed, as did their metabolic pathways. Later investigation suggested that this pharmacodynamic effect may have been influenced by endogenous compounds such as the progesterone metabolites pregnanolone and allopregnanolone.[89]

In summary, given the potential interaction between exogenous hormones and various psychotropic medications, it may be important to inquire about the use of OCs prior to any psychopharmacological intervention.

Sex differences in psychotropic agents

Benzodiazepines

Relatively few studies have evaluated the therapeutic effects and side-effects of benzodiazepines in women; most available studies have focused primarily on potential sex-related differences in the pharmacokinetics of benzodiazepines. For example, in an older study, diazepam, which is oxidatively metabolized, had higher clearance in younger women than in younger men.[90] This difference disappeared in 62–84-year-old men and women. On the other hand, MacLeod et al[91] found that women metabolized diazepam more slowly than did men, regardless of age. Nitrazepam, a benzodiazepine metabolized by reduction, does not appear to have sex-related differences in clearance.[79] Similarly, the metabolism of alprazolam, a benzodiazepine that undergoes oxidation, is not influenced significantly by sex or menstrual cycle phase.[92] However, temazepam and oxazepam, which are conjugated and excreted, had slower clearance rates among female patients compared to males in several studies.[29,68,93] Age did not influence this effect.[93]

In sum, despite varied methodology in the available studies, current data suggest that there are sex-related differences in the metabolism of the various benzodiazepines.

Antidepressant agents

Although mood disorders are more prevalent in women than in men,[94] little attention has been devoted to the research of sex differences or specific antidepressant effects in women. This is not surprising in light of the historic exclusion of women from many pharmacological clinical treatment trials.

Despite the limited data, sex-related differences in the pharmacokinetics of antidepressants have been reported. For example, higher plasma levels of selected TCAs were observed in women compared to men. In an older study, women had higher plasma levels of imipramine than did men.[95] Similarly, Preskorn and Mac[96] found that women and older subjects had higher plasma levels of amitriptyline than did young male subjects. Hydroxylation clearance of clomipramine was found to be lower in women than in men,[46] while oral clearance of desipramine was shown to be greater in men than in women.[85] However, the authors of these articles did not normalize for body weight, and others have failed to find significant gender differences in plasma levels of amitriptyline and nortriptyline.[97] Finally, the volume of distribution of trazodone was shown to be greater in women and the elderly, but clearance was significantly reduced only in older men.[98]

In recent years, data have emerged on potential gender differences in the pharmacokinetics of newer antidepressants, including the SSRIs. Several research groups have observed that plasma concentrations of sertraline are approximately 35–40% lower in young men than in women and elderly men.[99] Similarly, plasma concentrations of fluvoxamine appear to be 40–50% lower in men than in women, with the magnitude of effect possibly greater at lower medication doses.[100] Of the other antidepressants, the levels of nefazodone are higher in

elderly women compared to younger subjects and elderly men,[101] but sex does not substantially alter the disposition or the tolerance of venlafaxine.[102]

Data regarding potential sex-related differences in treatment response to antidepressants are scarce. Several studies indicate that younger women may respond less well to TCAs compared to men, but may respond better to SSRIs and monoamine oxidase inhibitors (MAOIs). An older study which involved a database reanalysis evaluated the efficacy of TCAs and MAOIs by sex in atypical depression.[103] Results showed that depressed women with panic attacks had a more favourable response to MAOIs than to TCAs, whereas men who were depressed and had panic attacks responded more favourably to TCAs. Raskin[104] also conducted a database reanalysis and found that premenopausal women (younger than 40 years) responded less well to imipramine than did older women and men. These results are consistent with a meta-analysis of all published imipramine trials (35 studies incorporating outcome from 342 men and 711 women) that presented outcome by sex.[105] The analysis showed that 62% of men but only 51% of women ($P < 0.001$) were considered to be imipramine responders.

Steiner et al[106] presented results from a Smith-Kline Beecham database reanalysis of paroxetine, imipramine and placebo in outpatients with major depression. This analysis showed that women preferentially responded to the SSRI over the TCA or placebo. The superior response of women to the SSRI compared to imipramine was echoed in a subsequent study on dysthymic disorder which compared sertraline, imipramine and placebo.[107] No sex difference was found in treatment response to fluoxetine in another database reanalysis, although the authors did not include an imipramine cell for comparison.[108] Thus, in sum, it appears that there may be some clinically meaningful sex-specific differences in the pharmacokinetics, efficacy and tolerability of antidepressant medications.

Conclusions

In this chapter, the available literature regarding sex-related differences in the pharmacokinetics and pharmacodynamics of psychotropic medications is reviewed. The surprising outcome is the fact that there are significant gaps in the experimental data addressing these issues. None the less, there is evidence suggesting potentially meaningful sex-related varia-

tions in the pharmacokinetics and treatment response of various compounds. Further, the menstrual cycle phase and the use of OCs may influence the metabolism, distribution and clearance of certain drugs, although this effect is probably greatest for the older, higher-strength OCs. Selected benzodiazepines and antidepressants are influenced by sex, menstrual cycle phase and the concurrent use of OCs. Further, women may respond better to different classes of antidepressant agents than do men, specifically the SSRI and the MAOI agents. These data also indicate the need for further, well-controlled research in this field.

References

1. Kinney EL, Trautmann J, Gold JA et al, Underrepresentation of women in new drug trials. Ramifications and remedies, *Ann Intern Med* 1981; **95**:495–9.

2. Merkatz RB, Temple R, Subel S et al, The Working Group on Women in Clinical Trials, Women in clinical trials of new drugs: a change in Food and Drug Administration policy, *N Engl J Med* 1993; **329**:292–6.

3. Food and Drug Administration, Guideline for the study and evaluation of gender differences in the clinic evaluation of drugs, *Fed Register* 1993; **58**:39406–16.

4. Yonkers KA, Harrison W, The inclusion of women in psychopharmacologic trials, *J Clin Psychopharmacol* 1993; **13**:380–2.

5. Harris RZ, Benet LZ, Schwartz JB, Gender effects in pharmacokinetics and pharmacodynamics, *Drugs* 1995; **50**:222–39.

6. Yonkers KA, Kando JC, Hamilton J, Gender issues in psychopharmacologic treatment, *Directions in Psychiatry* 1995; **15**:1–8.

7. Kando JC, Yonkers KA, Relevant sex differences in the prescribing and monitoring of psychotropic medications. In: Dunner DL, Rosenbaum JF, eds, *The Psychiatric Clinics of North American Annual of Drug Therapy*, Vol. 4 (WB Saunders Company: Philadelphia, 1997) 1–20.

8. Stewart DE, Stotland NL, eds, *Psychological Aspects of Women's Health Care: The Interface between Psychiatry and Obstetrics and Gynecology*, 2nd edn (American Psychiatric Press: Washington, DC, 2000) in press.

9. Grossman MI, Kirsner JB, Gillespie IE, Basal and histalog-stimulated gastric secretion in control subjects and in patients with peptic ulcer or gastric cancer, *Gastroenterology* 1963; **45**:14–26.

10. Wald A, Van Thiel DH, Hoechstetter L et al, Gastrointestinal transit: the effect of the menstrual cycle, *Gastroenterology* 1981; **80**:1497–500.

11. Datz FL, Christian PE, Moore JG, Differences in gastric emptying rates between menstruating and postmenopausal women, *J Nuclear Med* 1987; **28**:1204–7.

12. Degen LP, Phillips SF, Variability of gastrointestinal transit in healthy women and men, *Gut* 1996; **39**:299–305.

13. Kolars JC, Awni WM, Merion RM, Watkins PB, First-pass metabolism of cyclosporin by the gut, *Lancet* 1991; **338**:1488–90.

14. Strobel HW, Hammond DK, White TB, White JW, Identification and localization of cytochromes P450 in gut, *Methods Enzymol* 1991; **206**:648–55.

15. Hunt CM, Westerkam WR, Stave GM, Effect of age and gender on the activity of human

hepatic CYP3A, *Biochem Pharmacol* 1992; **44**:275–83.

16. Aarons L, Hopkins K, Rowland M et al, Route of administration and sex differences in the pharmacokinetics of aspirin administered as its lysine salt, *Pharm Res* 1989; **6**:660–6.

17. Ho PC, Triggs EJ, Bourne DWA, Heazlewood VJ, The effects of age and sex on the disposition of acetylsalicyclic acid and its metabolites, *Br J Clin Pharmacol* 1985; **19**:675–84.

18. Riester EF, Pantuck EJ, Pantuck CB et al, Antipyrine metabolism during the menstrual cycle, *Clin Pharmacol Ther* 1980; **28**:384–91.

19. Gilman AG, Rall TW, Nies AS et al, *The Pharmacological Basis of Therapeutics* 8th edn (Pergamon Press: New York, 1990).

20. Seeman MV, Neuroleptic prescription for men and women, *Social Pharmacol* 1989; **3**:219–36.

21. O'Malley K, Crooks J, Duke E, Stevenson IH, Effects of age and sex on human drug metabolism, *Br Med J* 1971; **3**:607–9.

22. Guengerich FP, Mechanism-based inactivation of human liver microsomal cytochrome P450 IIIA4 by gestodene, *Chem Res Toxicol* 1990; **3**:363–71.

23. Pollock BG, Recent developments in drug metabolism of relevance to psychiatrists, *Harvard Rev Psychiatry* 1994; **2**:204–13.

24. Smith DA, Jones BC, Speculations on the substrate structure–activity relationship (SSAR) of cytochrome P450 enzymes, *Biochem Pharmacol* 1992; **44**:2089–98.

25. Kerr BM, Thummel KE, Wurden CJ et al, Human liver carbamazepine metabolism. Role of CYP3A4 and CYP2C8 in 10,11-epoxide formation, *Biochem Pharmacol* 1994; **47**:1969–79.

26. Murray M, P450 enzymes. Inhibition mechanisms, genetic regulation and effects of liver disease, *Clin Pharmacokinet* 1992; **23**:132–46.

27. von Moltke LL, Greenblatt DJ, Court MH et al, Inhibition of alprazolam and desipramine hydroxylation in vitro by paroxetine and fluvoxamine: comparison with other selective serotonin reuptake inhibitor antidepressants, *J Clin Psychopharmacol* 1995; **15**:125–31.

28. Andersen BB, Mikkelsen M, Vesterager A et al, No influence of the antidepressant paroxe-tine on carbamazepine, valproate, and phenytoin, *Epilepsy Res* 1991; **10**:201–4.

29. Greenblatt DJ, Divoll M, Harmatz JS, Shader RI, Oxazepam kinetics: effects of age and sex, *J Pharmacol Exp Ther* 1980; **215**:86–91.

30. Hulst LK, Fleishaker JC, Peters GR et al, Effect of age and gender on tirilazad pharmacokinetics in humans, *Clin Pharmacol Ther* 1994; **55**:378–84.

31. Schwartz JB, Capili H, Daugherty J, Aging of women alters S-verapamil pharmacokinetics and pharmacodynamics, *Clin Pharmacol Ther* 1994; **55**:509–17.

32. Gilmore DA, Gal J, Gerber JG, Nies AS, Age and gender influence the stereoselective pharmacokinetics of propranolol, *J Pharmacol Exp Ther* 1992; **261**:1181–6.

33. Rugstad HE, Hundal O, Home I et al, Piroxicam and naproxen plasma concentrations in patients with osteoarthritis. Relation to age, sex, efficacy and adverse events. *Clin Rheumatol* 1986; **5**:389–98.

34. Kerlan V, Dreano Y, Bercovici JP et al, Nature of cytochromes P450 involved in the 2-/4-hydroxylations of estradiol in human liver microsomes, *Biochem Pharmacol* 1992; **44**:1745–56.

35. May DG, Porter J, Wilkinson GR, Branch RA, Frequency distribution of dapsone N-hydroxylase, a putative probe for P4503A4 activity in a white population, *Clin Pharmacol Ther* 1994; **55**:492–500.

36. Schmucker DL, Woodhouse KW, Wang RK et al, Effects of age and gender on in vitro properties of human liver microsomal monooxygenases, *Clin Pharmacol Ther* 1990; **48**:365–74.

37. Lobo J, Jack DB, Kendall MJ, The intra- and inter-subject variability of nifedipine pharmacokinetics in young volunteers, *Eur J Clin Pharmacol* 1986; **30**:57–60.

38. Sitar DS, Duke PC, Benthuysen JL et al, Aging and alfentanil disposition in healthy volunteers and surgical patients, *Can J Anaesth* 1989; **36**:149–54.

39. Yee GC, Lennon TP, Gmur DJ et al, Age-dependent cyclosporine: pharmacokinetics in marrow transplant recipients, *Clin Pharmacol Ther* 1986; **40**:438–43.

40. Shimada T, Yamazaki H, Mimura M et al, Interindividual variations in human liver

cytochrome P-450 enzymes involved in the oxidation of drugs, carcinogens and toxic chemicals: studies with liver microsomes of 30 Japanese and 30 Caucasians, *J Pharmacol Exp Ther* 1994; **270**:414–23.

41. Brosen K, Recent developments in hepatic drug oxidation: implications for clinical pharmacokinetics, *Clin Pharmacokinet* 1990; **18**:220–39.

42. Brosen K, Gram LF, Clinical significance of the sparteine/debrisoquine oxidation polymorphism, *Eur J Clin Pharmacol* 1989; **36**: 537–47.

43. Otton SV, Ball SE, Chung SW et al, Comparative inhibition of the polymorphic enzyme CYP2D6 by venlafaxine (VF) and other 5HT uptake inhibitors, *Clin Pharmacol Ther* 1994; **55**:141.

44. Crewe HK, Lennard MS, Tucker GT et al, The effect of selective serotonin re-uptake inhibitors on cytochrome P4502D6 (CYP2D6) activity in human liver microsomes, *Br J Clin Pharmacol* 1992; **34**:262–5.

45. Otton SV, Wu D, Joffe RT et al, Inhibition by fluoxetine of cytochrome P4502D6 activity, *Clin Pharmacol Ther* 1993; **53**:401–9.

46. Gex-Fabry M, Balant-Gorgia AE, Balant LP, Garrone G, Clomipramine metabolism: model based analysis of variability factors from drug monitoring data, *Clin Pharmacokinet* 1990; **19**:241–55.

47. Abernethy DR, Greenblatt DJ, Shader RI, Imipramine and desipramine disposition in the elderly, *J Pharmacol Exp Ther* 1985; **232**: 183–8.

48. Walle T, Byington RP, Furberg CD et al, Biologic determinants of propranolol disposition: results from 1308 patients in the beta-blocker heart attack trial, *Clin Pharmacol Ther* 1985; **38**:509–18.

49. Walle T, Walle K, Mathur RS et al, Pharmacokinetics and drug disposition. Propranolol metabolism in normal subjects: association with sex steroid hormones, *Clin Pharmacol Ther* 1994; **56**:127–32.

50. Walle T, Walle UK, Cowart TD, Conradi EC, Pathway-selective sex differences in the metabolic clearance of propranolol in human subjects, *Clin Pharmacol Ther* 1989; **46**:257–63.

51. Pritchard JF, Bryston JC, Kernodle AE et al,

Age and gender effects on ondansetron pharmacokinetics: evaluation of healthy aged volunteers, *Clin Pharmacol Ther* 1992; **51**:51–5.

52. Rettie AE, Korzekwa KR, Kunze KL et al, Hydroxylation of warfarin by human cDNA-expressed cytochrome P450: a role for P4502C9 in the etiology of (S)-warfarin drug interactions, *Chem Res Toxicol* 1992; **5**:54–9.

53. Smith DA, Species differences in metabolism and pharmacokinetics: are we close to an understanding? *Drug Metab Rev* 1991; **23**:355–73.

54. Knodell RG, Hall SD, Wilkinson GR, Guengerich FP, Hepatic metabolism of tolbutamide: characterization of the form of cytochrome P450 involved in methyl hydroxylation and relationship to in vivo disposition, *J Pharmacol Exp Ther* 1987; **241**:1112–19.

55. Newlands AJ, Smith DA, Jones BC et al, Metabolism of nonsteroidal, anti-inflammatory drugs by cytochrome P450 2C, *Br J Clin Pharmacol* 1992; **34**:152P.

56. Jalil P, Toxic reaction following the combined administration of fluoxetine and phenytoin. Two case reports, *J Neurol Neurosurg Psychiatry* 1992; **55**:412–13.

57. Skjelbo E, Brosen K, Inhibitors of imipramine metabolism by human liver microsomes, *Br J Clin Pharmacol* 1992; **34**:256–61.

58. Hooper WD, Qing MS, The influence of age and gender on the stereoselective metabolism and pharmacokinetics of mephobarbital in humans, *Clin Pharmacol Ther* 1990; **48**:633–40.

59. Richardson CJ, Blocka KLN, Ross SG, Verbeeck RK, Effects of age and sex on piroxicam disposition, *Clin Pharmacol Ther* 1985; **37**:13–18.

60. Wrighton SA, Stevens JC, The human hepatic cytochromes P450 involved in drug metabolism, *Crit Rev Toxicol* 1992; **22**:1–21.

61. Brosen K, Skjelbo E, Rasmussen BB et al, Fluvoxamine is a potent inhibitor of cytochrome P4501A2, *Biochem Pharmacol* 1993; **45**:1211–14.

62. Jerling M, Lindstrom L, Bondesson U, Bertilsson L, Fluvoxamine inhibition and carbamazepine induction of the metabolism of clozapine: evidence from a therapeutic drug monitoring service, *Ther Drug Monit* 1994; **16**:368–74.

63. Ereshefsky L, Saklad SR, Watanabe MD et al, Thiothixene pharmacokinetic interactions: a study of hepatic enzyme inducers, clearance inhibitors, and demographic variables, *J Clin Psychopharmacol* 1991; **11**:296–301.

64. Guengerich FP, Human cytochrome P450 enzymes, *Life Sci* 1992; **50**:1471–8.

65. Relling MV, Lin JS, Ayers GD, Evans WE, Racial and gender differences in N-acetyl transferase, xanthine oxidase and CYP1A2 activities, *Clin Pharmacol Ther* 1992; **52**:643–58.

66. Nafziger AN, Bertino JS, Sex-related differences in theophylline pharmacokinetics, *Eur J Clin Pharmacol* 1989; **37**:97–100.

67. Cuzzolin L, Schinella M, Tellini U et al, The effect of sex and cardiac failure on the pharmacokinetics of a slow-release theophylline formulation in the elderly, *Pharm Res* 1990; **22**:137–8.

68. Divoll M, Greenblatt DJ, Harmatz JS, Shader RI, Effect of age and gender on disposition of temazepam, *J Pharmacol Sci* 1981; **70**:1104–7.

69. Yukawa E, Mine H, Higuchi S, Aoyama T, Digoxin population pharmacokinetics from routine clinical data: role of patient characteristics for estimating dosing regimes, *J Pharm Pharmacol* 1992; **44**:761–5.

70. Miners JO, Attwood J, Birkett DJ, Influence of sex and oral contraceptive steroids on paracetamol metabolism, *Br J Clin Pharmacol* 1983; **16**:503–9.

71. Greenblatt DJ, Abernethy DR, Matlis R et al, Absorption and disposition of ibuprofen in the elderly, *Arthritis Rheum* 1984; **27**:1066–9.

72. Sweeting J, Does the time of the month affect the function of the gut? *Gastroenterology* 1992; **102**:1084–5.

73. McBurney M, Starch malabsorption and stool excretion are influenced by the menstrual cycle in women consuming low fiber western diets, *Scand J Gastroenterol* 1991; **26**:880–6.

74. Pollan A, Oian P, Changes in transcapillary fluid dynamics—a possible explanation of the fluid retention in the premenstrual phase. In: Dennerstein L, Fraser I, eds, *Hormones and Behavior* (Elsevier: New York, 1986).

75. Lew KH, Ludwig EA, Milad MA et al, Gender-based effects on methylprednisolone

76. Lane JD, Steege JF, Rupp SL, Kuhn CM, Menstrual cycle effects on caffeine elimination in the human female, *Eur J Clin Pharmacol* 1992; **43**:543–6.

77. Shavit G, Lerman P, Korczyn AD et al, Phenytoin pharmacokinetics in catamenial epilepsy, *Neurology* 1984; **34**:959–61.

78. Kirkwood C, Moore A, Hayes P et al, Influence of menstrual cycle and gender on alprazolam pharmacokinetics, *Clin Pharmacol Ther* 1991; **50**:404–9.

79. Jochemsen R, van der Graaff M, Boeijinga JK, Breimer DD, Influence of sex, menstrual cycle and oral contraception on the disposition of nitrazepam, *Br J Clin Pharmacol* 1982; **13**:319–24.

80. Backstrom T, Jorpes P, Serum phenytoin, phenobarbital, carbamazepine, albumin; and plasma estradiol, progesterone concentrations during the menstrual cycle in women with epilepsy, *Acta Neurol Scand* 1979; **59**:63–71.

81. Chamberlain S, Hahn PM, Casson P, Reid RL, Effect of menstrual cycle phase and oral contraceptive use on serum lithium levels after a loading dose of lithium in normal women, *Am J Psychiatry* 1990; **147**:907–9.

82. Stewart DE, Fairman M, Barbadoro S et al, Follicular and late luteal phase serum fluoxetine levels in women suffering from late luteal phase dysphoric disorder, *Biol Psychiatry* 1994; **36**:201–2.

83. Yonkers KA, Kando JC, Cole JO, Blumenthal S, Gender differences in pharmacokinetics and pharmacodynamics of psychotropic medication, *Am J Psychiatry* 1992; **149**:587–95.

84. Stoehr GP, Kroboth PD, Juhl RP et al, Effect of oral contraceptives on triazolam, temazepam, alprazolam, and lorazepam kinetics, *Clin Pharmacol Ther* 1984; **36**:683–90.

85. Abernethy DR, Greenblatt DJ, Shader RI, Imipramine and desipramine disposition in the elderly, *J Pharmacol Exp Ther* 1984; **232**:183–8.

86. Fletcher HP, Miya TS, Bousquet WF, Influence of estradiol on the disposition of chlorpromazine in the rat, *J Pharmacol Sci* 1965; **54**:1007–9.

87. Ellinwood EH, Easier ME, Linnoila M et al,

Effects of oral contraceptives on diazepam-induced psychomotor impairment, *Clin Pharmacol Ther* 1983; **35**:360–6.

88. Kroboth PD, Smith RB, Stoehr GP, Juhl RP, Pharmacodynamic evaluation of the benzodiazepine–oral contraceptive interaction, *Clin Pharmacol Ther* 1985; **38**:525–32.

89. McAuley JW, Reynolds IJ, Kroboth FJ et al, Orally administered progesterone enhances sensitivity to triazolam in postmenopausal women, *J Clin Psychopharmacol* 1995; **15**: 3–11.

90. Greenblatt DJ, Allen MD, Harmatz JS, Shader RI, Diazepam disposition determinants, *Clin Pharmacol Ther* 1980; **27**:301–12.

91. MacLeod SM, Giles HG, Bengert B et al, Age- and gender-related differences in diazepam pharmacokinetics, *J Clin Pharmacol* 1979; **19**:15–19.

92. Greenblatt DJ, Wright CE, Clinical pharmacokinetics of alprazolam: therapeutic implications, *Clin Pharmacokinet* 1993; **24**:453–71.

93. Smith RB, Divoll M, Gillespie WR, Greenblatt DJ, Effect of subject age and gender on the pharmacokinetics of oral triazolam and temazepam, *J Clin Psychopharmacol* 1983; **3**:172–6.

94. Kessler RC, Nelson CB, McGonagle KA et al, Comorbidity of DSM-III-R major depressive disorder in the general population: results for the US National Comorbidity Survey, *Br J Psychiatry* 1996; **30** (suppl):17–30.

95. Moody JP, Tait AC, Todrick A, Plasma levels of imipramine and desmethylimipramine during therapy, *Br J Psychiatry* 1967; **113**: 183–93.

96. Preskorn SH, Mac DS, Plasma levels of amitriptyline: effects of age and sex, *J Clin Psychiatry* 1985; **46**:276–7.

97. Ziegler VE, Biggs JT, Tricyclic plasma levels: effect of age, race, sex, and smoking, *JAMA* 1977; **238**:2167–9.

98. Greenblatt DJ, Friedman H, Burstein ES et al, Trazodone kinetics: effect of age, gender, and obesity, *Clin Pharmacol Ther* 1987; **42**: 193–200.

99. Warrington SJ, Clinical implications of the pharmacology of sertraline, *Int Clin Psychopharmacol* 1991; **6**:11–21.

100. Hartter S, Wetzel H, Hammes E, Hiemke C, Inhibition of antidepressant demethylation and hydroxylation by fluvoxamine in depressed patients, *Psychopharmacology* 1993; **110**:302–8.

101. Barbhaiya RH, Buch AB, Greene DS, A study of the effect of age and gender on the pharmacokinetics of nefazodone after single and multiple doses, *J Clin Psychopharmacol* 1996; **16**:19–25.

102. Klamerus KJ, Parker VD, Rudulph RL et al, Effects of age and gender on venlafaxine and *O*-desmethylvenlafaxine pharmacokinetics, *Pharmacotherapy* 1996; **16**:915–23.

103. Davidson J, Pelton S, Forms of atypical depression and their response to antidepressant drugs, *Psychiatry Res* 1986; **17**:87–95.

104. Raskin A, Age–sex differences in response to antidepressant drugs, *J Nerv Ment Dis* 1974; **159**:120–30.

105. Hamilton JA, Grant M, Jensvold MF, Sex and treatment of depressions. When does it matter? In: Jensvold MF, Halbreich U, Hamilton JA, eds, *Psychopharmacology and Women. Sex, Gender, and Hormones* (American Psychiatric Press, Inc.: Washington DC, 1996) 241–60.

106. Steiner M, Wheadon D, Kreider M, Bushnell W, Antidepressant response to paroxetine by gender. Presented at the Annual Meeting of the American Psychiatric Association, San Francisco, CA, May 1993 (Abstract 462).

107. Yonkers KA, Kando JC, Gender differences in the pharmacotherapeutics of depression. Presented at the American Psychiatric Association Annual Meeting, New York, NY, 4–9 May 1996.

108. Lewis-Hall FC, Wilson MG, Tepner RG, Koke SC, Fluoxetine vs tricyclic antidepressants in women with major depressive disorder, *J Women's Health* 1997; **6**:337–43.

30

Psychosocial treatments for mood disorders in women
Scott Stuart and Michael W O'Hara

Introduction

Mood disorders have long been thought to have their origins in the endocrine and reproductive systems. The ancient Egyptians, for example, believed that mental disturbances were caused by dislocation of the uterus and other organs. The Greeks, including Hippocrates, also promoted the idea that a 'wandering' uterus was responsible for many physical and psychological maladies.[1] Even Freud and some subsequent psychoanalytic authors espoused the view that some manifestations of neuroticism and mood disorders were unique to women because of their peculiar negotiation of early childhood sexual experiences.[2]

The contemporary view of mood disorders is that their phenomenology is not significantly different between men and women. This is reflected in nearly all of the studies of psychosocial interventions for mood disorders, which typically involve the treatment of mood disorders that are not gender-specific (i.e. major depression and dysthymia). Though women are well represented in such studies, as

the rates of depression are higher in women and because women are more likely to seek treatment, very few studies have specifically examined the differential effects of psychotherapy on women and men.

The empirical research that has explored gender variations in response to psychotherapy has typically shown minimal differential effects. For example, a meta-analysis of 28 studies examining the efficacy of cognitive-behavioural therapy (CBT) for depression[3] did not reveal any effect for patient gender.[4] More recently, Thase et al[5] conducted a mega-analysis utilizing data from 595 depressed patients who had participated in six outpatient research protocols in which psychotherapy (CBT or Interpersonal Psychotherapy[6] (IPT)) or a combination of psychotherapy and tricyclic antidepressant medication was provided. In each of the protocols, therapy was administered for 16 weeks. The results of this mega-analysis suggested that older patients and women had somewhat slower recoveries than men. Additionally, relative to geriatric patients, mid-life patients (younger than 60 and, for women, perimenopausal) did well with combined treatments. The effect for gender, however, was rather weak and was noted by the authors to have little or no clinical significance. The findings of these analyses suggest that women of all ages benefit from psychotherapy for depression to about the same extent as men.

In contrast to these general psychotherapy studies, there are several areas in which psychosocial treatments for mood disorders specific to women have been more fully researched. These include treatments for women with depression during pregnancy, depression during the puerperium, and mood disorders associated with either the premenstrual period or the perimenopausal period. In this chapter, we review these studies in detail, and describe the issues common to these disorders which are often addressed in psychotherapeutic treatments.

Psychosocial treatment of mood disorders during pregnancy

Depression during pregnancy is quite common—estimates of the prevalence of antenatal depression in the community are in the range of 10%, a level which is similar to that of non-childbearing women.[7,8] There appears to be a very strong association between a history of psychiatric problems such as depression and a recurrence of these problems during pregnancy,[9] with estimates of risk of antenatal depression in women with a history of depression of about 25%.[8,10]

Antenatal depression is associated with a high degree of morbidity. Steer et al[11] reported that the relative risk of delivering a low-birthweight infant was 3.97 for women with Beck Depression Inventory[12] (BDI) scores of 21 or greater. There is also evidence which suggests that antenatal depression is associated with maladaptive behavioural change in the neonate.[13,14]

One of the most consistently replicated findings regarding antenatal depression is its association with poor social support.[15] Bernazzani et al[16] demonstrated that levels of antenatal depression are correlated with satisfaction with interpersonal relationships, and noted that the impact of poor interpersonal relationships was nearly as significant as that of previous psychiatric problems. Support from a woman's spouse or significant other[17] and the degree of intimacy in their relationship[18] appear to be particularly critical in this regard. The effects of poor social support on women from lower socio-economic classes are even more striking. Seguin et al[19] found that 47% of women of low socio-economic status had BDI scores of 10 or more during their second trimester of pregnancy, and that the BDI scores were closely tied to social support. Among low-income pregnant women, Collins et al[20] found that women with more social support had less complicated labours and deliveries and had newborns with higher Apgar scores. Poor social support has also been correlated with low-birthweight deliveries.[21] Given these factors, it is clear that antenatal depression requires treatment of some type. Further, the data suggest that an intervention aimed at improving social supports and interpersonal relationships may be of great benefit.

Current recommendations are that antidepressants be utilized for women with moderate to severe antenatal depression or in women with histories of severe depression and who are therefore at high risk for recurrence during pregnancy.[22] Most authors have suggested that antidepressant medication can be used relatively safely during pregnancy, and that the benefits of antidepressant usage outweigh the risks of treatment with medication. However, many pregnant women prefer psychological treatments during pregnancy, wishing to avoid medication if possible, often even in cases where it is warranted for severe depression. Consequently, psychotherapeutic treatments should be strongly considered for pregnant women suffering from mild to moderate levels of depression, or for those women who do not wish to take medication.[23]

Though there are many studies documenting the efficacy of psychotherapeutic treatments for depression in general,[24,25] there are at present only two empirical studies investigating the efficacy of specific psychological treatments for depression during pregnancy. Both involve modifications of IPT.[6] Stuart[26] has described the use of IPT for antepartum depression, and Spinelli[27] has published data from an open trial of IPT which suggest that it is helpful with depressed, pregnant women.

IPT is predicated on the premise that depression occurs in an interpersonal context, and that productive modification of patients' interpersonal relationships will result in a decrease in symptoms. IPT is a time-limited treatment, and is usually delivered over 12–16 sessions. Rather than focusing on past issues, IPT is designed to assist patients in dealing with 'here and now' problems in the service of symptom relief. Traditional IPT focuses on one or two of four interpersonal problem areas, which include grief issues, interpersonal disputes, role transitions, and interpersonal deficits. Stuart has suggested that the descriptor 'interpersonal sensitivity' is both more accurate and less pejorative than the term 'interpersonal deficits', and this nomenclature is used by some research groups.[28] Spinelli and Weissman[29] have described the addition of another IPT problem area specific to depression during pregnancy which they have labelled 'complicated pregnancy'. This problem area includes obstetrical difficulties, previous perinatal loss, or fetal anomaly. They describe a case of pregnancy induced by rape which is also subsumed under this category.

Stuart[26] has described a number of themes which are common during IPT for antenatal depression. Anticipated role transition is a frequent topic, as many pregnant women begin to plan for the changes created by the arrival of a newborn. Practical role transition issues, such as dividing time between work and child care, may be complicated by other issues such as finances and the desire to serve as the newborn's primary caregiver. Women may be ambivalent about giving up the social and emotional support they receive at work or in other relationships outside the home.

In addition, some women often experience ambivalence about their pregnancy. Pregnancy may occur unexpectedly, potentially interrupting other plans, or may occur at stressful points in a woman's relationship with her significant other. Women may also experience mixed feelings about the physical changes which occur during the pregnancy, particularly if their prenatal course is medically complicated.

Women who experience antenatal depression frequently voice concerns regarding the effect of the depression on their child, particularly if they are receiving antidepressant medication. Over and above these toxicity concerns, women may feel that there will be some unspecified harm to the baby in utero if they have ambivalent feelings about the pregnancy. Finally, many women, particularly those with a history of depression prior to pregnancy, also voice concern about continuing to be depressed postpartum, and are concerned about their ability to function as mothers.

A variety of other issues unique to pregnancy may be associated with depressive symptoms. These include pregnancies in which the father is absent or unknown, or in which the pregnancy leads to a significant change in the woman's relationship with the child's father.[26] Complicated prenatal courses and difficulty in conceiving are also common issues.[30] Women who have had to use artificial means to initiate a pregnancy may have difficulty with over-investment and over-idealization of the pregnancy. Finally, prenatal or perinatal loss of previous pregnancies may complicate the current pregnancy.

Spinelli[27] used IPT to treat 13 pregnant women who met DSM-III-R[31] criteria for major depression, and had Hamilton Rating Scale for Depression[32] (HRS-D) scores of 12 or more. The women were recruited and treated in a large metropolitan setting. After 16 weeks, the nine women who completed the IPT all met criteria for recovery—that is, a HRS-D score of less than 6. The study was limited to some degree because it was an open trial, because of the high rate of drop-out from treatment, and because all of the treatment was provided by a single therapist.

Stuart[26,33] has also described the use of IPT for antenatal women in a small pilot study involving three women. All were married, and two of the three were primiparous. At intake, all met criteria for a major depressive disorder according to DSM-IV.[34] None of the patients met criteria for major depression at the completion of treatment. BDI scores declined from 28.0 at intake to 9.0 at termination, and HRS-D scores declined from 25.0 to 9.3 at the end of therapy.

IPT appears to hold promise as a treatment for depressive symptoms during pregnancy, though a well-controlled treatment trial of IPT clearly needs to be conducted. The interpersonal and role transition themes which are the basis for IPT, and the time-limited nature of IPT (which fits well with the time-limited duration of pregnancy), render it an appropriate psychological treatment for depressed pregnant women. Though there has been no research regarding the use of other types of psychotherapies during pregnancy, it is likely that modifications of time-limited treatments such as CBT[3] will also prove to be effective for antenatal depression. Further research is clearly needed with both IPT and other forms of psychotherapy.

Psychosocial treatment of mood disorders during the puerperium

Several risk factors are associated with the development of postpartum depression. A prior psychiatric history, and a history of depression specifically, is clearly the greatest risk factor.[10] The presence of depressive symptoms during pregnancy is also a significant risk factor,[35] as is a family history of major depression.[36]

More importantly when psychosocial treatments are being considered, social factors have also been associated with increased risk for postpartum depression. Among these are being unmarried and having an unplanned pregnancy.[37] Women from lower social classes and with lower incomes are at higher risk, as are women with poor support from their spouses and with poor social support in general.[38] Preterm birth and difficulty with pregnancy and delivery may also be risk factors. These social factors may be focal points of psychotherapeutic interventions.

As with depression during pregnancy, most authors suggest that moderate to severe depression in breast-feeding mothers should be treated with medication (see Chapter 19). However, there are several caveats to treatment with antidepressants that should be noted. First, there are few prospective studies regarding the toxic effects of any of the anti-depressants on the neurodevelopment of breast-feeding infants. The data regarding safety have come primarily from retrospective examination of outcomes in exposed children, as well as case reports. Second, the number of exposures which have been examined in detail is quite limited, particularly with the newer antidepressants. Finally, the assessment of neurodevelopmental effects in breastfed children is based on examinations that are quite gross, and it is possible that more subtle effects of exposure may not have been noted.

Another issue highlighting the problems associated with the use of antidepressant medications is that many breast-feeding women do not wish to use medication of any type. This issue is compounded by a general lack of recognition of the severity of depression in many women. Whitton et al,[39] for example, investigated depressed women's perceptions of difficulties that they were experiencing during the postpartum period. They found that 97% of the women in their study felt there was 'something wrong', but only 32% believed they were suffering from depression. Many who did not believe they were depressed felt that their symptoms were either not severe enough to merit treatment or attributed them to family or child-care difficulties. Most strikingly, only 10% had discussed their symptoms with a health professional, and only 20% said that they would consider pharmacological treatment. Given the morbidity associated with postpartum depression, and the desire of many women to breast-feed while minimizing or avoiding any exposure of their child to psychotropic medication, it is clear that psychosocial interventions are paramount in the treatment of postpartum depression.

Psychosocial treatments for postpartum mood disorders can be categorized into two different types of intervention. The first involves prevention of depression, and involves treatment of either fairly large numbers of women from the general population, or involves prenatal or postpartum women who are at high risk for postpartum depression. These prevention trials may begin during pregnancy or early during the puerperium, and in either case are designed to prevent postpartum problems from occurring.

The second type of psychosocial intervention involves the treatment of women after they have already developed postpartum depression. Several different psychotherapy modalities have been used in this fashion, including individual therapy, group therapy, and marital therapy. Additionally, several novel approaches using in-home health-care visitors or telephone interventions have been described as tertiary treatments.

Preventive interventions

Preventive interventions for postpartum depression, with few exceptions, have been applied only to general populations. In other words, the women who receive preventive treatment have typically not been specifically selected because they are at high risk for postpartum depression, but rather are women selected from general obstetrical practices. Consequently, it is difficult to determine how effective these treatments are in preventing postpartum depression, as most of the women who are treated are not likely to develop postpartum depression even without treatment. None the less, the studies that have been published do illustrate a number of psychosocial issues common to postpartum women.

Halonen and Passman[40] conducted a prevention study in which pregnant women received relaxation therapy designed to alleviate postpartum distress. After participation in a class teaching relaxation for pain control during labour, women were assigned to one of four treatment conditions: discussion, exposure, relaxation training, or relaxation training and exposure combined. The authors based their work on the premise that relaxation has been found to be of benefit for decreasing the pain and anxiety of childbirth,[41] and might prove to be beneficial following childbirth as well. Forty-eight randomly selected women were treated in their homes by a trained therapist. The relaxation training took place in two sessions preceding childbirth, and during a 'refresher' session 2 days after birth.

From days 7 to 10 postpartum, women in the two relaxation groups reported significantly lower scores on the BDI than women in the other two groups. There were no differences between groups, however, when BDI scores at 1 month were compared. Moreover, the peak mean BDI score was only 11, indicating a very mild degree of depression. Though relaxation training appears to be of benefit to women, the treatment effect in this study was quite small, and it is not clear how well the intervention would fare with women either at risk for or diagnosed with postpartum depression.

Gordon and Gordon[42] conducted a prevention treatment trial using psychoeducational groups to prepare pregnant women for the emotional changes that frequently accompany childbirth. Women who attended antenatal classes at a community hospital were randomly assigned to participate in two additional psychoeducational classes during pregnancy. The experimental groups included women who participated in these groups by themselves, and those who participated in the groups with their husbands. Only 15% of the women who received additional classes experienced postpartum 'emotional upsets', as compared to 37% of the control women. At a 6-month follow-up, only 2% of the participant women were having

such upsets compared to 28% of controls. The authors noted that the women who attended the groups with their spouses had the best outcome, but provided no data supporting this conclusion.

As is true of most prevention trials, Gordon and Gordon did not specifically select women at risk for postpartum disorders. The authors also did not describe their assessment measures, and it is unclear what variables were used to assess outcome. In addition, they provided no definition for postpartum 'upset', and nor is its clinical relevance noted. The significance of their results is difficult to determine without this information.

Cowan and Cowan[43] conducted a prevention treatment trial using a psychoeducational group which met during both the prenatal and postpartum periods. Primiparous couples were enrolled in the group at about 3 months prior to delivery, and continued in the group until 3 months postpartum. Each group included both women and their partners, and was co-led by a male and a female therapist. The therapy focused primarily on the couples' marital relationships, particularly as they were affected by the anticipated and actual birth of their child. Normalization of stress during this transition period, and the 'joint' nature of the experience of childbirth and child-rearing, were emphasized. Each group met weekly for $2\frac{1}{2}$ h per session over the last 3 months of pregnancy and the first 3 months of the puerperium.

Forty-seven couples were split into two groups, one of which received the group intervention and one of which received no additional treatment. The presence of risk factors for depression was not used as a criterion for selection for the study. A comparison at 6 and 18 months postpartum did not demonstrate differences between the treatment and no-treatment groups in stressful life events. Additionally, 'satisfaction with self' measures did not differ between the mothers in either group. Although mothers who had participated in the treatment group reported more satisfaction with the couple's division of labour and household tasks, fathers in the treatment group reported less satisfaction. Couples in the treatment group reported fewer negative changes in their sexual relationship than did those in the no-treatment group, and the decline in marital satisfaction postpartum was less marked in the treatment group as well.

Unfortunately, though self-report measures of 'wellbeing' were used in the study, no measures of depressive symptoms were included. Moreover, the authors did not report any scores on the measures they did use at either intake or at the conclusion of treatment, so the degree of improvement that occurred is unclear. In conclusion, there are no data from this study which suggest that the intervention is effective in treating depression, or that the intensive time commitment from both patients and clinicians results in clinically significant benefit.

Elliott et al[44] reported on the use of group treatment for the prevention of postpartum depression. The intervention included both psychoeducational components and the opportunity for emotional processing. The authors described the psychoeducational component as 'anticipatory guidance', and aimed the therapy at helping women to anticipate changes that would occur both practically and emotionally after childbirth, as well as offering practical advice on how to avoid these potential pitfalls. Therapists provided specific information about postpartum depression and the need to establish adequate social supports. The authors also emphasized the need for continuity of psychological care, and provided the monthly group treatment to women from early in pregnancy to 6 months postpartum. Additionally, the authors specifically marketed the treatment as an 'educational programme' rather than as psychological counselling. They noted that women expect to receive prenatal classes, whereas there is often resistance to counselling, particularly as a preventive measure.

The groups met monthly beginning at about 4 months of pregnancy, and continued until 6 months postpartum. Each group had between 10 and 15 members and was led by a trained mental health professional. Early sessions were structured and psychoeducational, while the latter sessions had increased time for 'open discussion'. The last pregnancy meeting and all of the postpartum meetings had no formal agenda. In some cases, group treatment was supplemented by individual therapy. Both first- and second-time mothers were treated, though in separate groups. First-time mothers attended an average of 7 of 11 sessions, while second-time mothers attended an average of only 4 of 11 meetings.

The Elliott et al study is unique among prevention studies because the women selected for treatment were all identified as being at high risk for postpartum depression. Risk factors used to select subjects included: (1) previous psychiatric history; (2) high levels of anxiety; (3) poor marital relationship; and (4) lack of a confidant. Women were not interviewed for the presence of depression during the antepartum period, and mood symptoms were not assessed prior to beginning the treatment trial. During the postpartum period, women were interviewed with the Present State Exam[45] (PSE) and also completed the Edinburgh Postnatal Depression Scale[46] (EPDS). Women were considered 'depressed' if they indicated a depressed mood and one or more additional depressive symptoms on the PSE.

Significantly fewer women met this criteria for depression in the treatment group (12.5%) compared to the control group (33%) at 2 months postpartum. A non-significant trend in the same direction was noted at 3 months postpartum. EPDS scores averaged 6.9 for women in the treated group compared to 9.1 in the control group at 3 months postpartum, a difference which was significant.

The authors concluded that the programme was effective in reducing depression, and in engaging first-time mothers in the treatment. Although this treatment programme shows promise for the prevention of depression, it is not clear to what degree the depressive symptoms of the women were reduced from antenatal levels, as within-group comparisons were not conducted. Reliable pretreatment measures of depressive symptoms would also ensure that women in the two groups were distributed equally with respect to their depression severity.

Trotter et al[47] conducted a treatment trial in which the effect of social support during labour on the subsequent development of postpartum depression was assessed. In this South African study, women were randomly assigned to be accompanied by a 'doula' during their delivery, or to receive only standard medical care during delivery. In the South African system, a doula is a person 'specifically designated to provide emotional support rather than clinical care' to a woman during the labour process.

In this study, 63 women were randomly assigned to one of the two groups. All of the subjects were nulliparous, and were not assessed for the presence of depression or depressive symptoms prior to their delivery. The women in the study were not selected for the presence of risk factors for depression. Women were evaluated at 3 months postpartum using the Pitt Depression Questionnaire,[48] which is specifically designed to assess postpartum depression. Women in the group which received labour support from a doula had a mean depression score of 13.63 at 3 months, which was significantly better than those in the control group, who had a mean score of 18.29.

The results of the Trotter et al study are limited by several factors. From a research design standpoint, the authors did not assess depressive symptoms during pregnancy, so that the effects of the intervention on reducing depression are not clear. Additionally, women in the study continued to report moderate levels of depression even if they were assigned to the experimental group. It is also not clear how applicable this intervention would be across cultures, as the doula system is not common in many Western societies. None the less, the authors do present evidence which suggests that a relatively simple intervention may provide some benefit to women, and particularly strengthens the hypothesis that social support is essential in preventing postpartum depression.

Acute treatment trials

Acute interventions for postpartum depression have been designed to treat the symptoms of postpartum depression once they develop. Both group and individual tertiary treatments have been assessed. In contrast to preventive interventions, all of the women who receive acute treatment are specifically selected because they are experiencing postpartum depression. The criteria which define postpartum depression, however, vary among the studies. Outcome measures also vary among the interventions tested.

Morris[49] treated seven women with prolonged (greater than 1 year) postnatal depression for 11 months with group psychotherapy. The patients were described as having had significant reductions in their scores on the BDI[12] when pre- and posttreatment scores were compared. However, the means for the pre- and post-treatment scores were not reported, nor was information regarding the diagnoses of the patients involved in the trial.

Fleming et al[50] described the use of a social

support group for the treatment of women during the postpartum period. Women between 2 and 5 months postpartum were assigned to one of three treatment groups: a social support group which met weekly for 8 weeks, a no-intervention group in which no treatment was provided, and a group-by-mail group, in which women received a transcript of the group treatment sessions but did not participate in the group itself. The social support treatment was designed primarily to bring the depressed women into contact with other women experiencing similar problems, and was described by the authors as being 'relatively unstructured'.

Some of the women in the study were selected on the basis of having scored above the depression cut-off on the Current Experiences Scale (CES) and above a cut-off score on either the Multiple Affect Adjective Checklist[51] or the Edinburgh Postnatal Depression Scale[46] at 2 weeks postpartum. No mean scores for the depressed women were reported, and nor were psychiatric diagnoses. Interestingly, an equal number of non-depressed women were included in each of the experimental groups, and were treated concurrently in the same groups as the depressed subjects.

The results of the trial suggest that the treatment intervention was not particularly helpful to the depressed women. There was no difference between the depressed women receiving treatment and the women who received no treatment when CES scores were compared. In fact, depressed women in the social support group showed less improvement in their negative self-image than did the depressed women who received no treatment, perhaps because they had the opportunity to compare themselves to other non-depressed women who were included in the group. In addition, there were no differences related to either treatment or depression status with respect to women's attachment to their infants—the authors noted

that all women, regardless of mood state or treatment condition, maintained high levels of attachment to their infants. The authors concluded that their social support group treatment did not appear to be of benefit to depressed postpartum women.

Clark et al[52] investigated the effect of a programme utilizing group psychotherapy as treatment for postpartum depression. Their programme was described as being based loosely on a theoretical combination of psychodynamic, developmental, family systems, interpersonal and cognitive models of therapy, and utilized a 12-session programme in which a number of issues were addressed. These included psychoeducation regarding the birth of a child and its attendant consequences, self-observation of the relationship between mothers and their children, and use of the patients' own experiences of being parented as a context in which they could understand their feelings of being a parent.

The programme of Clark et al is unique in that it also included treatment for infants as well as mothers. One and one-half hours of each session were devoted to group therapy with mothers, while infants were simultaneously being treated in a developmental therapy group. The infant group was designed to assist the infants to become more regulated, more affectively attuned, and more socially engaged. The last 30 min of each session were then devoted to dyadic group activities with mothers and children which were monitored by a therapist. These activities were designed to foster more appropriate attachment between mother and child, and to enhance the mothers' feelings of competence in their parenting role. Fathers were also included in 2 of the 12 sessions, and were included primarily so that they could receive psychoeducational information.

Clark et al reported that significant reductions in patients' self-reported depression resulted from the treatment, with BDI scores decreasing from a mean of 18.9 at intake to 12.1 at termination ($P = 0.003$), and SCL-90-R[53] scores dropping from 1.68 at intake to 1.01 at termination ($P = 0.01$). In addition, some, but not all, of the subscale scores on the Parenting Stress Index[54] also improved significantly. Among those that improved were parental depression and sense of competence scores. Notably, scores regarding attachment with child, social isolation and relationship with spouse did not change significantly.

No information was given by the authors regarding the assessment of depression, or whether any or all of the patients met diagnostic criteria for depression. In addition, information is lacking regarding the use of concurrent medication. No information was given regarding the age of the patients, the time postpartum, parity, or previous psychiatric history. Additionally, the data regarding treatment changes are limited because no clinician ratings were reported. Moreover, the mean BDI scores at the conclusion of treatment would indicate that though improvement occurred, patients continued to remain at what would be considered mildly depressed levels.

Meager and Milgrom[55] also reported on the effects of group treatment for women with postpartum depression. Their treatment consisted of 10 weeks of group psychotherapy based loosely on the CBT of Beck et al.[3] There was no confirmation of a diagnosis of depression using a structured interview. Many of the subjects were already receiving antidepressant medication at the time of referral. Prior to treatment, the mean BDI score of the women was 30.7, indicative of the severe depression for which many of the women were already in treatment. The mean EPDS score was 27.7.

Four of the 10 women referred for group treatment dropped out of the study, and only 6 of 10 women in a no-treatment control group were available for posttreatment comparison. Women who completed the treatment had reductions in their average BDI scores from 29.7 to 16.8, compared to no change in the control group. EPDS scores dropped from 24.8 in the treated completers to 15.8 at 10 weeks, again compared to no change in the control group. Both within-group and between-group changes were significant. The authors note, however, that most of the women in both groups continued to have moderate depressive symptoms at treatment termination, and did not provide data regarding the women who dropped out of the trial.

Holden et al[56] conducted one of the most methodologically sound, controlled studies of acute treatment for postpartum depression. Fifty women from a well-described community-based population were divided into two groups—those who received psychological treatment, and a control group in which no postnatal counselling was provided. Women were selected for the study if they met Research Diagnostic Criteria[57] (RDC) for a diagnosis of either major or minor depression at about 12 weeks postpartum. The sample had a median score of 15.8 on the Edinburgh Postnatal Depression Scale[46] at intake (mean scores were not reported). The vast majority of women were multiparous, and about 40% had suffered a previous episode of depression.

The treatment programme consisted of eight weekly sessions of counselling provided by trained visiting nurses, most of whom had midwife experience and several of whom had additional psychiatric training. Patients in the treatment group received a mean of 8.8 sessions of therapy over about 13 weeks. The counselling was designed to be non-directive in orientation, and each session was to last at least 30 min. Twelve of the women in the study were receiving antidepressant medication in addition to the counselling.

The main finding of the study was that 18 of the 26 (69%) women in the treatment group who were depressed at intake no longer met criteria for either RDC major or minor depression at the conclusion of treatment, compared to 9 recovered women out of the 24 (38%) depressed women who were assigned to the control group. This difference was significant at the $P = 0.03$ level. Additionally, the median score on EPDS decreased from 15.5 to 12.0 in the control group as compared to 16.0 at intake and 10.5 posttreatment for those women who were in the group receiving counselling. There was no significant difference in the control group on pre- and post-scores, while the difference in the treatment group was significant at $P = 0.001$. Finally, blinded ratings based on the Goldberg Standardized Psychiatric Interview[58] demonstrated that observer ratings of depression decreased from a median score of 2.0 to 0.5 for the counselled group ($P = 0.001$) compared to pre- and post-evaluation scores of 2.0 in the control group.

This study is one of the most rigorous in defining an appropriate group for treatment intervention, as all of the patients met criteria for either major or minor depression at intake. Outcome was also clearly defined, with a clear advantage to the counselling treatment when posttreatment diagnoses were compared. However, the outcome data based on symptomatic scores are somewhat difficult to interpret. The use of median scores, rather than mean scores, may obscure the effect of variance of scores at intake and posttreatment. Thus, they may not accurately reflect the outcome of a majority of the women in the study, and may not reflect the outcome of the average woman. In addition, the outcome scores were compared only within each group, rather than between the two groups. In other words, there was no indication that there were significant differences in self-assessed and rater-assessed symptoms

between groups at the conclusion of treatment. Moreover, the median posttreatment EPDS scores of the two groups would suggest that even if the between-group difference was statistically significant, the between-group difference is probably not clinically distinguishable. Further, though there was some change in EPDS scores, both groups continued to be moderately depressed based on the EPDS even at the conclusion of treatment.

The results of this study suggest that non-directive counselling may be of help in promoting recovery from postpartum depression. The notion that psychiatric nurses can be adequately trained to deliver the treatment is also intriguing. However, though the data suggests that further study is warranted, there are limitations to the data analysis. The evidence suggests that though some women did improve, many continued to be mildly symptomatic after the conclusion of treatment.

In another study utilizing community screening to locate cases, Wickberg and Hwang[59] studied the effects of counselling visits by Swedish child health clinic nurses. The authors hypothesized that a non-directive and empathic approach to counselling would enable women to gain a more positive view of themselves and their lives, and would subsequently relieve their depression. The counselling in the study was provided by nurses who had received about 2 days of training in this method.

Women were recruited during routine visits to a child health care clinic and were entered into the study if they had scores of 12 or more on the EPDS at both 2 and 3 months postpartum. Women meeting this screening criterion were then interviewed using the Montgomery-Asberg Depression Rating Scale (MADRS)[60] and were enrolled in the randomized treatment phase of the project if they had MADRS scores of more than 10 and met DSM-III-R[31] criteria for major depression. The treated group received six weekly non-directive counselling sessions, and the control group received routine care.

Twelve of 15 women in the treatment group compared to 4 of 16 women in the control group no longer met criteria for DSM-III-R major depression at the completion of treatment. MADRS scores in the group receiving counselling decreased from 19.6 at intake to 10.9 at 6 weeks, whereas those of the control group began at 17.1 at intake and declined to 14.7 at 6 weeks. The between-group comparison of the MADRS scores was significant.

Given the duration of treatment in this study, the decline in MADRS scores is notable—conventional wisdom is that psychotherapeutic treatments for mild to moderate depression should be provided for at least 10–12 weeks. The authors noted that four severely ill women had to be dropped from the study, and this limits the findings to postpartum women with mild to moderate depression. Further, there were no self-report measures used in the study. Finally, even after the intervention was complete, women appeared to remain symptomatic to some degree—women in the treated group had posttreatment MADRS scores above the cut-off used for entry into the study.

Cooper and Murray[61] compared 8 weeks of non-directive counselling, CBT or psychodynamic psychotherapy to a no-treatment control group. One hundred and seventy primiparous women meeting DSM-III-R criteria for major depression at 6 weeks postpartum were enrolled. Women were screened from the community using the EPDS, and this was followed by interview with the Structured Clinical Interview for DSM-III-R.[62] Approximately 40 women were enrolled in each treatment cell.

The authors found that all of the treatments significantly advanced the remission of depression compared to the control group. Remission occurred in 75% of the women treated with non-directive counselling, 60% of the women in the CBT intervention, 50% of the women treated with psychodynamic psychotherapy, and 40% of the women in the control group. EPDS scores dropped from 14 to 10 in the non-directive counselling group, 13.5 to 9 in the CBT group, 12.7 to 8.8 in the psychodynamic group, and 12.4 to 11.3 in the control group. No information regarding the significance of these comparative scores is given by the authors.

The information provided by the authors regarding the makeup of the population, and concurrent psychopharmacological treatments, is limited, and the authors did not say who provided the counselling. Most of the studies conducted in the UK have utilized visiting nurses, most of whom have limited experience in providing counselling. This may explain the relatively poor results in the CBT and psychodynamic cells, as may the relatively short duration of treatment.

Appleby et al[63] reported on the treatment of postpartum depression using counselling based loosely on the CBT model. In this study, women from a community population were screened for depression and were selected if they scored above 10 on the EPDS and met RDC criteria for major or minor depressive disorder. A total of 87 women from 6 to 8 weeks postpartum were randomly assigned to one of four treatment cells: (1) treatment with fluoxetine and one session of counselling; (2) treatment with fluoxetine and six sessions of counselling; (3) treatment with placebo and one session of counselling; and (4) treatment with placebo and six sessions of counselling. The medication arm of the study was double-blinded, and the total duration of the study was 12 weeks. The counselling was described by the authors as being based on the CBT model of Beck et al,[3] but was designed to be delivered by non-specialists such as health visitors.

Highly significant improvements were seen in all four of the treatment groups, and fluoxetine was superior to placebo on all measures. Six sessions of counselling were superior to one session on the HRSD, but not on the EPDS. There were no interaction effects between medication and psychotherapeutic treatment.

The study was notable for a fairly high number of drop-outs in each cell—roughly 25–30% in each group. The average EPDS score of women completing the fluoxetine plus one session of counselling treatment declined from 16.4 to 5.4, while the average score of women in the fluoxetine plus six sessions of counselling group dropped from 16.9 to 5.3. The mean EPDS rating of women receiving placebo and one counselling session declined from 17.4 to 9.8, and that of women receiving placebo and six sessions of counselling from 16.8 to 9.9. On the HRSD, the mean score of the women in the fluoxetine plus one session group declined from 13.3 to 2.9, and the average rating of the women in the fluoxetine plus six sessions group declined from 13.2 to 2.8. The mean HRSD score of women receiving placebo and one session declined from 14.7 to 7.5, and that of women receiving placebo and six counselling sessions from 13.3 to 3.7.

The authors noted the 'unexpected' finding that many women improved greatly within 1 week after entering the treatment trial. They suggested that this may have been due either to a more rapid than anticipated response to fluoxetine, or to the benefits of women's expectations of entering into counselling. They specifically pointed out that their study was not designed to test the effectiveness of counselling, but was designed to reflect what might occur in clinical practice, in which a lengthy initial interview might be followed by counselling of a supportive nature. The study, according to the authors, was designed to assess the additional benefits of adding an antidepressant medication and of adding additional counselling sessions.

Stuart and O'Hara[64] reported on the use of IPT[6] for the treatment of postpartum depression. As noted above, IPT has been extensively evaluated for the treatment of depression in general. The IPT problem areas of role transition (from pregnancy to motherhood) and interpersonal disputes (typically conflict between the woman and her spouse) are particularly cogent for counselling with this population.

In the Stuart and O'Hara study, postpartum women meeting criteria for DSM-III-R[31] depression were treated over 12 consecutive weeks with IPT. Therapists providing treatment were highly experienced psychotherapists with PhD or MD degrees. Six women between 2 and 6 months postpartum (average 4.1 months) were enrolled in the open treatment trial, and women were evaluated both pre- and posttreatment with the BDI and the HRSD. BDI scores declined from 27.7 to 5.4 after 12 weeks, and the mean HRSD score declined from 18.2 to 5.2. Additionally, none of the women met criteria for major depression at the completion of treatment. Two of the patients received concurrent treatment with fluoxetine, while the other patients were medication-free. The difference in response between women receiving medication and those who did not was not significant.

The design of this trial and lack of a control group, as well as the limited number of women who were treated, clearly limit the conclusions that can be drawn. Additionally, the provision of treatment by experienced therapists is certainly more costly than treatment provided by visiting nurses or midwives, and could limit the applications of the treatment. Specific training is required to deliver IPT effectively[65] as opposed to 'supportive' or 'non-directive' counselling. None the less, this trial does suggest that IPT is of benefit to women with well-defined moderate to severe major depression. A large-scale controlled treatment trial in which depressed postpartum women receiving immediate treatment with IPT are compared to women placed on a 12-week waiting list is currently underway to test this hypothesis.

Telephone interventions for postpartum depression

One of the more novel psychosocial interventions for postpartum depression is the use of telephone interviews with women during the postpartum period. Stack and Shaver[66] described a programme in which women were contacted by phone at 2 weeks postpartum. The women in the study frequently raised concerns about their mental health, focusing specifically on symptoms of both depression and anxiety. No control group was present for comparison, however. Beech[67] and Bogie[68] also described telephone advisory services which, though designed primarily to assist with childcare issues, frequently picked up psychological complaints from the women who called for advice. In contrast, Donaldson[69] reported no differences in outcome at 8 weeks between a group of postpartum women who received weekly phone calls during the first 6 weeks postpartum and those in a control group who did not.

Self-help groups

Postpartum self-help support groups have also been advocated as a means of relieving postpartum depression.[70,71] Depression After Delivery, for example, is now established on an international basis as a self-help group for postnatal depression. These groups are typically led by laywomen who have had previous experience with postpartum depression. To date, no outcome studies regarding the effectiveness of self-help groups have been conducted.

Elliott et al[44] note that self-help groups for postpartum women have several marked differences from treatment groups. First, self-help groups consist of members who are self-referred for a previously existing and personally identified problem. Second, there is no leader or identified 'expert' to facilitate discussion. They note, however, that group leaders who have had children themselves may be perceived by group members as having more authority or expertise than those who have not had children.

Several authors have observed that there is little evidence supporting the efficacy of such self-help groups. There appear to be no differences in maternal adjustment when women who participate in support groups are compared to controls, and Lieberman[72] hypothesized that exploration of negative reactions to motherhood, and particularly to spousal support, may actually be associated with increased dissatisfaction. Wandersman[73] also noted that there was little evidence that support groups were effective in treating psychiatric symptoms. Limitations of the evaluation of support groups include a lack of objective data in almost all of the reports of such groups, and the fact that there have been no comparative trials conducted using control groups.

Conclusions

Despite the fact that postpartum depression is common, it remains an illness which is often unrecognized, both by postpartum women and by medical professionals. Those treatment trials which have incorporated community screening as a means of case finding have clearly demonstrated that women can be identified either through health clinics or by health visitors. Once identified as depressed, women appear to be willing to engage in treatment. Given the implications of untreated postpartum depression for both women and their children, it appears that community screening would be well worth the effort.

In contrast, the preventive measures which have been tested do not appear to be of particular benefit. This may be due in large part to the fact that, in most of the studies that have been conducted, women are not selected for treatment because they are at high risk for depression. Application of preventive measures to women who are not at high risk does not appear to be an effective utilization of resources. Further study is needed to determine whether preventive interventions are effective for high-risk women specifically, such as those with previous histories of postpartum depression.

Another issue that is yet to be resolved is the use of group treatment. While most of the studies which have yielded clinical improvement have used individual treatments, group treatments may be more appropriate as primary interventions for high-risk women. Additional research is also needed to determine the efficacy of postpartum self-help support groups in guiding clinicians in making appropriate referrals to these groups.

Acute psychotherapeutic treatment of postpartum depression also needs to be studied more. The psychotherapies to be tested in the future should be well defined, and should be modelled after therapies that have demonstrated effectiveness with non-postpartum depression, such as CBT or IPT. A reasonable rationale for use of the specific treatment should also be made. Finally, the need for highly trained versus 'lay' mental health professionals as therapists should also be more thoroughly investigated.

Psychosocial treatment of premenstrual dysphoria

A wide range of interventions have been used for premenstrual dysphoria.[74] Recently, there has been an intense focus on the efficacy of pharmacological interventions for well-defined 'premenstrual syndrome' or 'premenstrual dysphoric disorder'.[75] There is little question that antidepressant medications, particularly the selective serotonin reuptake inhibitors (SSRIs), are effective in reducing symptoms of premenstrual dysphoria.[75,76] However, despite the success of the newer antidepressants in reducing the debilitating symptomatology of more severe premenstrual dysphoria, most clinicians and researchers in this area recognize the need for comprehensive, multimodal treatment for most women experiencing severe premenstrual dysphoria (see Chapter 16).[74–77]

For many women, psychotherapy is an important component in the comprehensive treatment of premenstrual dysphoria. Some women have only a partial response to medical treatment, and require a psychological intervention to manage symptoms effectively. Other women may need counselling to manage the consequences of prolonged premenstrual dysphoria, which may include a diminished sense of self or disrupted interpersonal relationships. Successful management of premenstrual dysphoria with medication may also increase the salience of long-standing problems unrelated to the premenstrual dysphoria (e.g. personality disorder, marital distress, conflict with peers). Consistent with this perspective are the results of a survey of women seeking help in a premenstrual syndrome (PMS) clinic in London who indicated a preference for psychological treatments (e.g. learning coping skills, counselling).[78]

Among the few empirical studies of psychological interventions for premenstrual dysphoria[76,77] is a study by Morse et al,[79] who compared hormone therapy, coping skills training and relaxation in a study of 54 women with prospectively confirmed PMS. This study followed a reported case series of six women with a clear history of PMS who showed good response to rational-emotive group therapy.[80] Hormone therapy was provided for three cycles from day 17 to day 27, while coping skills training was provided in a group context over ten 90-minute sessions. Relaxation instructions were provided via audiotape. Several women in each condition failed to start therapy after assignment, and within the relaxation group there was significant attrition (only 4 of 16 completed the treatment through follow-up). Treatment continued over a period of 3 months and there was also a 6-month follow-up assessment. The results of the study indicated that there were significant symptom improvements for the hormone therapy and relaxation therapy groups in the first month. However, by the second month, the superior effects of the coping skills group were evident for both affective and cognitive symptoms. After the first cycle, the general trend was for the coping skills training group to improve, the hormone therapy group to deteriorate, and for women in the relaxation training group to discontinue. The coping skills group maintained their therapeutic gains through the 6-month follow-up. These findings are encouraging given the response of women with well-defined PMS to the coping skills training. Unfortunately, interpretation of the significance of the study findings is hampered by the treatment refusal and attrition rate.

Relaxation as a treatment fared much better in a study that compared 'relaxation response' techniques with daily charting alone, and with daily charting plus leisure reading over a 3-month period.[81] Relaxation response involves a meditation-like exercise in which attention is

focused on a single word while the subject sits in a relaxed state free from distraction for about 20 minutes twice a day.[82] Seventy-seven women with prospectively confirmed PMS entered the trial, and 46 women completed the 5-month protocol (including 2 months for confirmation of diagnosis). The authors found that overall physical symptoms were significantly more improved in the relaxation response group than in the other two groups. For women with more severe symptoms, the relaxation response group had significantly greater improvement of emotional symptoms and social withdrawal symptoms than the other two groups. The results of this study are promising; however, a 41% dropout rate clouds interpretation of the findings, particularly given the lack of specificity about attrition rates for each group.

Christensen and Oei[83] compared CBT to 'information-focused' therapy (IFT). IFT included a variety of interventions, such as relaxation training, nutritional education, and vitamin and lifestyle guidelines. Thirteen group sessions (2 hours per session) conducted on a weekly basis were provided in both groups to a total of 33 women (24 assigned to CBT and 9 assigned to IFT). There were no differences between groups on any outcome measures, although there were significant time effects for all variables. The findings of this study were inconclusive given the lack of group differences. One major problem with this study was the large imbalance in sample size in the two groups, almost guaranteeing that there would be no significant effects.

Cognitive-behavioural treatment has been evaluated in two treatment trials. In an Australian study,[84] women who described themselves on questionnaires as having relatively severe premenstrual symptoms were randomly assigned to CBT ($n = 13$), non-specific counselling ($n = 12$), and waiting list ($n = 12$) groups. The interventions were administered to groups of eight women each over a period of 6 weeks. Although the planned analyses revealed few significant effects, post hoc analyses did indicate that the cognitive-behavioural coping skills group reported significantly lower scores for premenstrual symptoms and irrational thinking. In a study of 37 women who met criteria for primary recurrent premenstrual tension syndrome, CBT was more effective than supportive group therapy or a waiting list condition in reducing intensity of negative events experienced during the premenstrual phase of the cycle.[85] CBT also was more effective in reducing 'mood swings' during the premenstrual phase than the waiting list condition.

Psychological interventions for premenstrual dysphoria have not been developed and evaluated with the same degree of rigour as pharmacological interventions. Most of the studies have involved relatively small samples. Also, because of the changing and disputed criteria for premenstrual dysphoria, there has been little homogeneity with respect to entry criteria for psychological studies. Moreover, the interventions themselves are diverse, as are the lengths of treatments provided in the various studies. As a consequence, it is difficult to make definitive statements about the role of psychological interventions, or more specifically psychotherapy, in the management of premenstrual dysphoria.

Despite the relatively undeveloped state of the literature on psychological interventions for premenstrual dysphoria, it is probably time to conduct larger trials of a well-defined cognitive-behavioural intervention. Ideally, such a study would include a factorial combination of a pharmacological intervention (active versus placebo) and psychotherapeutic intervention (active versus non/support). Certainly, given the similarity of effects of pharmacological and psychotherapeutic interventions for major depression, it is not unreasonable to expect

that competently provided psychotherapeutic interventions would be effective either on their own or in combination with pharmacotherapy.

Psychosocial treatment of mood disorders associated with menopause

There is very little evidence that menopause or the perimenopausal period are associated with increased risk for mood disorders.[86–88] Longitudinal studies following healthy women through the menopause have found little evidence of increased depressive symptomatology.[87,89,90] In fact, epidemiological research suggests that women of perimenopausal age are somewhat less likely than younger women to experience an affective disorder.[91] For those women who do experience depression, the clinical literature suggests that presentations of mood disorders during the perimenopausal years do not differ from presentations at other times.[86,92] In sum, there is little evidence supporting a discrete 'menopausal' depression.

Psychotherapy studies with depressed patients have almost always included women of perimenopausal age.[24,93–95] Typical psychotherapy studies include patients 18–60 years of age, and patients usually have a mean age of between 30 and 40. A majority of participants in most psychotherapy studies of depressed patients are usually women. In sum, women of perimenopausal age have been well represented in therapy trials with depressed patients, and psychotherapy appears to be quite effective with women in this age range.

Is there anything about menopause or the perimenopause that rates special consideration in psychotherapy? As a reproductive transition, menopause is gradual with no clear demarcation, unlike PMS, pregnancy, and childbirth.

Obviously, the cessation of regular menstruation and the impending loss of fertility may be greeted with mixed emotions, and may play a positive or negative role with respect to mood disorders. For some women, the loss of fertility may be added to other psychological losses and may increase the likelihood of a mood disorder, or increase the severity or duration of one that is ongoing. Alternatively, the cessation of regular menses and the reduction in the threat of unintended conception may reduce the burden for some women and decrease their risk for a mood disorder. In either case, the literature suggests that psychological functioning in the perimenopause is more likely to be determined by social and psychological factors than by the specific biological effects of menopause.

Although almost any issue could be addressed in psychotherapy with perimenopausal women, certain issues may be especially common with these women. For example, many women in mid-life are faced with parental care responsibilities. In the extreme, a woman may have a parent with physical or mental disabilities who is living with the family. She may be faced with managing the finances of elderly parents and providing much in the way of living assistance to them. At the same time, the perimenopausal woman may be coping with the turbulence of life with adolescent children, or, in contrast, with the prospect of children leaving home.[96] Chronic physical illnesses such as hypertension, cancer, arthritis and diabetes afflicting a woman or her partner are increasingly common in mid-life as well. Finally, marital problems may become apparent at this time, particularly if frequency of or satisfaction with sex is diminished for any reason. In sum, there are many psychological issues that may play a causal role in the onset of major depression during the perimenopausal years, and effective clinicians must be sensitive to these issues.

Conclusion

Psychosocial treatments are clearly needed for the spectrum of mood disorders experienced by women. The consequences of antenatal and postpartum depression in particular dictate that women be treated rapidly and aggressively. Many women do not wish to take medication, particularly during pregnancy or while breast-feeding, for fear that they will expose their children to what they perceive to be toxic medications. As both pregnancy and breast-feeding can be considered relative contraindications to the use of medications, it is reasonable practice to use effective psychotherapies as a first-line treatment for women with both antenatal and postpartum depression if their symptoms are mild to moderate. Psychotherapy is also likely to be a useful adjunct for women suffering from premenstrual mood symptoms.

The research regarding treatments for postpartum depression is clearly the most advanced at present, but much additional research is needed. The application of preventive interventions does not appear to be of benefit to general populations of women, but may hold great promise for women who are specifically at risk for depression during both pregnancy and the puerperium. Acute treatments for both antenatal and postpartum depressions need to be further evaluated. More work is also needed regarding the use of readily available resources for the treatment of depression during pregnancy and the postpartum period, such as nursing support and other interventions that could be provided by non-specialists. The efficacy and indications for referral to self-help groups also need to be investigated.

Our knowledge about the use of psychotherapeutic treatments for mood disorders specific to women is still in its infancy. There is great reason to be optimistic, however, as many of the psychotherapies that are effective with depression in general are likely to be helpful for depression associated with pregnancy and the postpartum.

References

1. Veith I, Four thousand years of hysteria. In: Horowitz MJ, ed., *Hysterical Personality* (Jason Aronson: New York, 1977) 9–93.
2. Freud S, *The Complete Psychological Works* (Hogarth Press: London, 1946).
3. Beck AT, Rush AJ, Shaw BF, Emery G, *Cognitive Therapy of Depression* (Guilford Press: New York, 1979).
4. Dobson KS, A meta-analysis of the efficacy of cognitive therapy for depression, *J Consult Clin Psychol* 1989; **57**:414–19.
5. Thase ME, Greenhouse JB, Frank E et al, Treatment of major depression with psychotherapy or psychotherapy–pharmacotherapy combinations, *Arch Gen Psychiatry* 1997; **54**:1009–1015.
6. Klerman GL, Weissman MM, Rounsaville BJ, Chevron ES, *Interpersonal Psychotherapy of Depression* (Basic Books: New York, 1984).
7. O'Hara MW, Social support, life events, and depression during pregnancy and the puerperium, *Arch Gen Psychiatry* 1986; **43**:569–73.
8. Gotlib IH, Whiffen VE, Mount JH et al, Prevalence rates and demographic characteristics associated with depression in pregnancy and the postpartum, *J Consult Clin Psychol* 1989; **57**:269–74.
9. Sharp D, Childbirth and mental health, *Practitioner* 1992; **236**:315–19.
10. O'Hara MW, *Postpartum Depression: Causes and Consequences* (Springer-Verlag: New York, 1995).
11. Steer RA, Scholl TO, Hediger ML, Fischer RL, Self-reported depression and negative pregnancy outcomes, *J Clin Epidemiol* 1992; **45**:1093–9.
12. Beck AT, Ward CH, Mendelson M et al, An inventory for measuring depression, *Arch Gen Psychiatry* 1961; **4**:561–71.
13. Zuckerman B, Bauchner H, Parker S, Cabral H, Maternal depressive symptoms during pregnancy, and newborn irritability, *J Dev Behav Pediatr* 1990; **11**:190–4.
14. Cutrona CE, Causal attributions and perinatal depression, *J Abnorm Psychol* 1983; **92**:161–72.
15. Paarlberg KM, Vingerhoets AJ, Passchier J et al, Psychosocial factors as predictors of maternal well-being and pregnancy-related complaints, *J Psychosom Obstet Gynecol* 1996; **17**:93–102.
16. Bernazzani O, Saucier JF, David H, Borgeat F, Psychosocial factors related to emotional disturbances during pregnancy, *J Psychosom Res* 1997; **42**:391–402.
17. Gjerdingen DK, Froberg DG, Fontaine P, The effects of social support on women's health during pregnancy, labor and delivery, and the postpartum period, *Fam Med* 1991; **23**:370–5.
18. Kitamura T, Shima S, Sugawara M, Toda MA, Clinical and psychosocial correlates of antenatal depression: a review, *Psychother Psychosom* 1996; **65**:117–23.
19. Seguin L, Potvin L, St Denis M, Loiselle J, Chronic stressors, social support, and depression during pregnancy, *Obstet Gynecol* 1995; **85**:583–9.
20. Collins NL, Dunkel-Schetter C, Lobel M, Scrimshaw SC, Social support in pregnancy: psychosocial correlates of birth outcomes and postpartum depression, *J Pers Social Psychol* 1993; **65**:1243–58.
21. Pittroff R, Social support in pregnancy can reduce the incidence of low birthweight deliveries, *Social Sci and Med* 1997; **45**:797–9.
22. Altshuler LL, Cohen L, Szuba MP et al, Pharmacologic management of psychiatric illness during pregnancy: dilemmas and guidelines, *Am J Psychiatry* 1996; **153**:592–606.
23. American Psychiatric Association, Practice Guideline for Major Depressive Disorder in Adults, *Am J Psychiatry* 1993; **150** (suppl): 1–26.
24. Elkin I, Shea MT, Watkins JT et al, National Institute of Mental Health Treatment of Depression Collaborative Research Program.

General effectiveness of treatments, *Arch Gen Psychiatry* 1989; **46**:971–82.

25. Robinson LA, Berman JS, Neimeyer RA, Psychotherapy for the treatment of depression: a comprehensive review of controlled outcome research, *Psychol Bull* 1990; **108**:30–49.

26. Stuart S, Use of interpersonal psychotherapy for other disorders, *Directions Clin Counseling Psychol* 1997; **7**:4–16.

27. Spinelli MG, Interpersonal psychotherapy for depressed antepartum women: a pilot study, *Am J Psychiatry* 1997; **154**:1028–30.

28. Stuart S, Use of interpersonal psychotherapy for depression. *Directions Psychiatry* 1997; **17**:263–74.

29. Spinelli MG, Weissman MM, The clinical application of interpersonal psychotherapy for depression during pregnancy, *Primary Psychiatry* 1997; **4**:50–7.

30. Carr ML, Normal and medically complicated pregnancies. In: Stewart DE, Stotland NL, eds, *Psychological Aspects of Women's Health Care: The Interface Between Psychiatry and Obstetrics and Gynecology* (American Psychiatric Press: Washington DC, 1993) 15–35.

31. American Psychiatric Association, *Diagnostic and Statistical Manual of Mental Disorders*, 3rd edn revised (American Psychiatric Association: Washington DC, 1987).

32. Hamilton M, Development of a rating scale for primary depressive illness, *Br J Social Clin Psychol* 1967; **6**:278–96.

33. Stuart S, Interpersonal psychotherapy for postpartum depression. In: Miller L, ed., *Postpartum Psychiatric Disorders* (American Psychiatric Press: Washington DC, 1999) 143–62.

34. American Psychiatric Association, *Diagnostic and Statistical Manual of Mental Disorders*, 4th edn (American Psychiatric Association: Washington DC, 1994).

35. Kendell RE, Rennie D, Clarke JA, Dean C, The social and obstetric correlates of psychiatric admission in the puerperium, *Psychol Med* 1981; **11**:341–50.

36. O'Hara MW, Postpartum mental disorders. In: Sciarra JJ, ed., *Gynecology and Obstetrics*, Vol. 6 (Harper and Row: Philadelphia, 1991) 1–17.

37. Cox JL, Connor YM, Henderson I et al, Prospective study of the psychiatric disorders of childbirth by self-report questionnaire, *J Affect Disord* 1983; **5**:1–7.

38. O'Hara MW, Swain AM, Rates and risk of postpartum depression: a meta-analysis, *Int Rev Psychiatry* 1996; **8**:37–54.

39. Whitton A, Appleby L, Warner R, Maternal thinking and the treatment of postnatal depression, *Int J Psychiatry* 1996; **8**:73–8.

40. Halonen JS, Passman RH, Relaxation training and expectation in the treatment of postpartum distress, *J Consult Clin Psychology* 1985; **53**:839–45.

41. Klusman LE, Reduction of pain in childbirth by alleviation of anxiety during pregnancy, *J Consult Clin Psychol* 1975; **43**:162–5.

42. Gordon RE, Gordon KK, Social factors in the prevention of postpartum emotional problems, *Obstet Gynecol* 1960; **15**:433–8.

43. Cowan CP, Cowan PA, A preventive intervention for couples becoming parents. In: Boukydis CF, ed., *Research Support for Parents and Infants in the Postnatal Period* (Ablex: New Jersey, 1987) 225–51.

44. Elliott SA, Sanjack M, Leverton TJ, Parent groups in pregnancy: a preventive intervention for postnatal depression. In: Gottlieb BH, ed., *Marshaling Social Support: Formats, Processes, and Effects* (Sage: Newbury Park, 1988) 87–110.

45. Finlay-Jones R, Brown GW, Duncan-Jones P et al, Depression and anxiety in the community: replicating the diagnosis of a case, *Psychol Med* 1980; **10**:445–54.

46. Cox JL, Holden JM, Sagovsky R, Detection of postnatal depression. Development of the 10-item Edinburgh Postnatal Depression Scale, *Br J Psychiatry* 1987; **150**:782–6.

47. Trotter C, Wolman WL, Hofmeyer J et al, The effect of social support during labor on postpartum depression, *South Afric J Psychol* 1992; **22**:134–9.

48. Pitt B, 'Atypical' depression following childbirth, *Br J Psychiatry* 1968; **114**:1325–35.

49. Morris JB, Group psychotherapy for prolonged postnatal depression, *Br J Med Psychol* 1987; **60**:279–81.

50. Fleming AS, Klein E, Corter C, The effects of a social support group on depression, maternal

attitudes and behavior in new mothers, *J Child Psychol Psychiatry* 1992; **33**:685–98.

51. Zuckerman M, Lubin B, *Manual for the Multiple Adjective Checklist* (Educational and Industrial Testing: San Diego, CA, 1985).

52. Clark R, Fedderly SS, Keller A, *Therapeutic Mother–Infant Groups for Postpartum Depression: Process and Outcome* (National Center for Clinical Infant Programs, Seventh Biennial National Training Institute: Washington DC, 1991).

53. Derogatis LR, Melisaratos N, The brief symptom inventory: an introductory report, *Psychol Med* 1983; **13**:595–605.

54. Abidin RR, *Parenting Stress Index* (Pediatric Psychology Press: Charlottesville, VA, 1983).

55. Meager I, Milgrom J, Group treatment for postpartum depression: a pilot study, *Aust NZ J Psychiatry* 1996; **30**:852–60.

56. Holden JM, Sagovsky R, Cox JL, Counseling in a general practice setting: controlled study of health visitor intervention in treatment of postnatal depression, *Br Med J* 1989; **298**:223–6.

57. Spitzer RL, Endicott J, Robins E, Research Diagnostic Criteria: rationale and reliability, *Arch Gen Psychiatry* 1978; **35**:773–82.

58. Goldberg DP, Cooper B, Eastwood MR et al, A standardized psychiatric interview for use in community surveys, *Br J Prevent Social Med* 1970; **24**:18–23.

59. Wickberg B, Hwang CP, Counseling of postnatal depression: a controlled study on a population based Swedish sample, *J Affect Disord* 1996; **39**:209–16.

60. Montgomery SA, Asberg M, A new depression scale designed to be sensitive to change, *Br J Psychiatry* 1979; **134**:382–9.

61. Cooper PJ, Murray L, Three psychological treatments for postnatal depression: a controlled comparison. Eighth International Conference of the Marcé Society, Cambridge, UK, 1994.

62. Spitzer RL, Williams JB, Gibbon M, First MB, The structured clinical interview for DSM-III-R (SCID). I. History, rationale, and description, *Arch Gen Psychiatry* 1992; **49**:624–9.

63. Appleby L, Warner R, Whitton A, Faragher B, A controlled study of fluoxetine and cognitive-behavioral counseling in the treatment of postnatal depression, *Br Med J* 1997; **314**:932–6.

64. Stuart S, O'Hara MW, Interpersonal psychotherapy for postpartum depression: a treatment program, *J Psychother Pract Res* 1995; **4**:18–29.

65. Rounsaville BJ, O'Malley S, Foley S, Weissman MM, Role of manual-guided training in the conduct and efficacy of interpersonal psychotherapy for depression, *J Consult Clin Psychol* 1988; **56**:681–8.

66. Stack JM, Shaver BJ, A postpartum telephone program of reassurance, information, and early intervention in a family practice, *Infant Ment Health J* 1985; **6**:98–106.

67. Beech CP, A new service for parents with crying babies, *Nursing Times* 1981; **77**:245–6.

68. Bogie A, A crying baby advisory service, *Health Visitor* 1981; **54**:535–7.

69. Donaldson N, *Effect of Telephone Postpartum Follow-up: a Clinical Trial* (University of California: San Francisco, 1987).

70. Mills JB, Kornblith PR, Fragile beginnings: identification and treatment of postpartum disorders, *Health Social Work* 1992; **17**:192–9.

71. Gruen DS, Postpartum depression: a debilitating yet often unassessed problem, *Health Social Work* 1990; **15**:261–70.

72. Lieberman MA, The effects of social support on responses to stress. In: Goldberger L, Breznitz S, eds, *Handbook of Stress: Theoretical and Clinical Aspects* (Free Press: New York, 1982).

73. Wandersman LP, An analysis of the effectiveness of parent–infant support groups, *J Primary Prevention* 1982; **3**:99–115.

74. Keye WR, Management of premenstrual syndrome: a biopsychosocial approach. In: Demers LM, McGuire JL, Phillips A, Rubinow DR, eds, *Premenstrual, Postpartum and Menopausal Mood Disorders* (Urban and Schwartzenberg Inc.: Baltimore, 1989) 81–128.

75. Freeman EW, Premenstrual syndrome: current perspectives on treatment and etiology, *Curr Opin Obstet Gynecol* 1997; **9**:147–53.

76. Steiner M, Premenstrual dysphoric disorder. An update, *Gen Hosp Psychiatry* 1996; **18**:244–50.

77. Pearlstein T, Nonpharmacologic treatment of premenstrual syndrome, *Psychiatr Ann* 1996; **26**:590–4.

78. Hunter MS, Swann C, Ussher JM, Seeking help for premenstrual syndrome: women's self-

reports and treatment preferences, *Sex Marital Ther* 1995; **10**:253–62.

79. Morse CA, Dennerstein L, Farrell E, Varnavides K, A comparison of hormone therapy, coping skills training, and relaxation for the relief of premenstrual syndrome, *J Behav Med* 1991; **14**:469–89.

80. Morse CA, Bernard ME, Dennerstein L, The effects of rational-emotive therapy and relaxation training on premenstrual syndrome: a preliminary study, *J Rational-Emotive Cognitive-Behavior Ther* 1989; **7**:98–110.

81. Goodale IL, Domar AD, Benson H, Alleviation of premenstrual syndrome symptoms with the relaxation response, *Obstet Gynecol* 1990; **75**:649–55.

82. Benson H, Beary JF, Carol MP, The relaxation response, *Psychiatry* 1974; **37**:37–46.

83. Christensen AP, Oei TP, The efficacy of cognitive behavior therapy in treating premenstrual dysphoric changes, *J Affect Disord* 1995; **33**:57–63.

84. Kirkby RJ, Changes in premenstrual symptoms and irrational thinking following cognitive-behavioral coping skills training, *J Consult Clin Psychol* 1994; **62**:1026–32.

85. Weiss CR, Cognitive-behavioral group therapy for the treatment of premenstrual distress, *Dissertation Abstracts Int* 1988; **49**:2389.

86. Dennerstein L, Psychiatric aspects of the climacteric. In: Studd JWW, Whitehead MI, eds, *The Menopause* (Blackwell Scientific Publications: Oxford, 1988) 43–54.

87. Matthews KA, Wing RR, Kuller LH et al, Influences of natural menopause on psychological characteristics and symptoms of middle-aged healthy women, *J Consult Clin Psychol* 1990; **58**:345–51.

88. Winokur G, The types of affective disorders, *J Nerv Ment Dis* 1973; **156**:82–96.

89. Busch CM, Zonderman AB, Costa PL, Menopause transition and psychological distress in a nationally representative sample: is menopause associated with psychological distress? *J Aging Health* 1994; **6**:209–28.

90. McKinlay JB, McKinlay SM, Brambilla DJ, Health status and utilization behavior associated with menopause, *Am J Epidemiol* 1987; **125**:110–21.

91. Myers JK, Weissman MM, Tischler GL et al, Six-month prevalence of psychiatric disorders in three communities, *Arch Gen Psychiatry* 1984; **41**:959–67.

92. Winokur G, Cadoret R, The irrelevance of the menopause to depressive disease. In: Sachar EJ, ed., *Topics in Psychoendocrinology* (Grune and Stratton, Inc.: New York, 1975) 59–66.

93. Shapiro DA, Barkham M, Rees A et al, Effects of treatment duration and severity of depression on the effectiveness of cognitive-behavioral and psychodynamic-interpersonal psychotherapy, *J Consult Clin Psychol* 1994; **62**:522–34.

94. Hollon SD, Najavitis L, Review of empirical studies on cognitive therapy. In: Frances AJ, Hales RE, eds, *American Psychiatric Press Review of Psychiatry* (American Psychiatric Press: Washington DC, 1988) 643–66.

95. Rehm LP, Kaslow NJ, Rabin AS, Cognitive and behavioral targets in a self-control therapy program for depression, *J Consult Clin Psychol* 1987; **55**:60–7.

96. McGrath E, Keita GP, Strickland BR, Russo NF, *Women and Depression: Risk Factors and Treatment Issues* (American Psychological Association: Washington DC, 1990).

31

Sociogeopolitical issues
Kelley Phillips

Contextual framework for the mental health care of women

Women are asking clinicians to reconceptualize their expertise to more accurately reflect gender-informed biological, psychological and social findings, so that their knowledge can be used more effectively by women to enhance the quality of their lives.

'Sociogeopolitical' is a term defined, for this discussion, as a woman's perspective and experience of her world. This context includes those factors in women's lives that create excess morbidity compared to men, owing to women's treatment in society because they are women. Issues include a woman's status as a person in her society and its political structure, her value as a member of her family, respect for her as an individual, her personal safety and security, and her access to education and to health care.[1,2] This social context interacts with women's biology and is mediated as feedback loops via biological, psychological and neuroendocrine systems, and is reflected in women's social and cultural settings.[3]

Women-focused care is described as a woman patient/client being the *subject* of her health consultation with her clinician. We are learning that the classification of women as objects using male-derived nomenclature is often quite inaccurate in developing appropriate treatments for women.[4] Rather than having something done to a woman, a test, an examination, a surgery, a procedure, a drug or a psychotherapy, she wishes to be a partner with her clinician in improving the quality of her health. Women's voices describing their health status and their life experiences and having these views of their world understood by their clinicians as real and meaningful and intrinsic to their health are essential for providing appropriate health and mental health care for women. This framework is extremely different from the prevalent male medical model describing scientific, social and clinical representations of women as an add-on to those findings for men.[5] A major problem with this male perspective is that it marginalizes women by explaining their context as abnormal because women's experiences, behaviours and biology are not the same as those of men.

Megatrends push science and medicine to shift from its 'androcentrism'

Medicine and health care are at a great crossroads. Major trends in science, health policies, clinical applications, funding and the level playing field of information technology are intersecting and profoundly changing the context of how research and its clinical applications are determined. The explosive rate of new health science makes it virtually impossible to inform clinicians in effective and timely ways using old models of training and continuing education. As the speed of acquisition of new knowledge increases, it becomes more difficult for clinicians to be relevant in providing health services. Kandel makes a plea for clinicians, health educators and translators of science and the social sciences to put science back into psychiatry. The current requirements for clinical psychiatrists demand a greater knowledge of the structure and functioning of the brain than is currently available in most training programmes. He also describes the unique domain that psychiatry occupies within academic medicine. Psychiatry's expertise is in the analysis of the interaction of social, psychological with biological determinants of behaviour. Feedback loops of social environment and brain exert actions on the brain to modify the expression of genes and thus the function of nerve cells. Learning produces alterations in gene expression. These findings do not seem to be reflected in current psychiatric practice.[3] This expertise by psychiatry can only be undertaken well by clinicians having a continuously updated understanding of the gender-specific biological, social and psychological components of behaviour.

Women's ways of accessing health care are also at a crossroads. How clinical services are delivered to women is being challenged. The traditional medical model has tremendous gaps in its framework to meet clinical needs. Women are flocking to alternative and collaborative health and medical services to better address their health care requirements.[6]

This chapter targets the *how* as well as the *what* of services offered to women that need changing. Understanding a women-centred perspective is especially relevant for clinicians, so that we do not contribute to the problems of devaluation and mistreatment of women. Women give meaning to their lives using a health context that is much broader than biology. The medical model focuses mostly on the male experience in the context of the biological sciences. Yet biology is only one dimension of gender difference in a world that is mostly defined by one gender's frame of reference. How research about women is designed and interpreted using male models is addressed, as well as how these flawed applications hinder the advancement of the health of women. The traditional models of health care developed around various body organs and systems—psychiatric, gastrointestinal, renal, cardiovascular, etc.—are not particularly meaningful to women who view this compartmentalization as not holistic, and therefore not very effective in assisting them with their health and wellbeing.[7] A women-centred model of care is outlined which every woman consumer, clinician and researcher can develop and refine. The focus is women consumers as experts in what they need and experts in knowing their bodies and their minds despite what others may describe for them. Attention is given to women's strengths, protective factors, and cultural beliefs regarding mental illness and treatment.

Making sense of psychiatric conceptualizations using a woman-centred lens involves having women as experts of their experiences, partnering with clinicians expert in specific clinical domains.[8] This view allows freedom to consider how different socio-cultural practices towards women impact adversely on their health status. It also encompasses how socio-cultural influences contribute to the greater rates of depression found in women.[9] These influences suggest that the rates of depression are affected by the meaning attached to the roles of gender, marital status, child care and work. Meaning is central for self-definition and is influenced by the value and status that dominant groups place on gender in different social roles. For example, in some Western countries such as the USA, young married women with preschool children are at particular risk for depression. However, this risk is low for married women from Mediterranean countries, where society highly values the home-making role.[9] Predominant political and socio-cultural realities for women contribute to their disproportion of mood disorders.[9] Specific gender trauma, from excising vulvas in the name of sexual control, to battering, rape, and incest, is predominantly experienced by women, especially those women interacting in the mental health arena.[10]

For clinicians who work with women, this means that 'women's position in society determines not only their health status but also the way in which health services are provided to them.'[11]

It is time to move on from an ability to *state* the need for a women-centred way of delivering services with and for women, to *understanding* the meaning of why this different way of working with women is so necessary for clinicians to be more effective in the healing process. This approach changes the content and context of health services and the way in which we research issues relevant for women. It is an evolution from a male perspective of women to a woman-centred perspective.

How do we get from here to there?

Women-centred health model: Equality, outreach, referral, education, advocacy, evaluation[12]

This model is a *strategic framework* developed for women consumers and clinicians to use as a change agent and resource to improve access to health services and treatment interventions at individual and systems levels. Different populations of women experience this framework as effective in improving their health.[13,14]

This woman-centred[15] approach to care for women is provided by men and women who are dedicated to advancing the art and science of women's health.

An *egalitarian* approach is used instead of a hierarchical one—woman is expert about her life, clinician is expert about some clinical domain in health care. Language is affirming, asserting, respecting and confident rather than lecturing or condemning. Ethical principles and practices that embody *how* we regard one another as gender, racially and culturally equal, and therefore relate to one another with mutual respect and trust, are incorporated in this model.[16,17]

Outreach includes reciprocity with women patient/clients as experts.

Education incorporates what health and illness means for a particular woman versus what disease means for a particular clinician.[14]

Advocacy includes respect for a woman client's autonomy and self-determination, a duty to do what is good for her, and consideration of her rights to be treated fairly and to receive a fair allocation of society's resources.[18]

This is an *integrative* approach to care. All the health and social services are coordinated and integrated with her, including complementary and alternative healing resources that are relevant to assist her with a particular health issue.

Clinician *skills* include listening to a woman's needs and providing gender-specific evidence-based assessments and technically appropriate interventions.

Evaluation of this model incorporates quality-of-life experiences and measures improvement in her health status.[19] Our clinical databases are skewed, based primarily on half our populations. It is essential that relevant information is elicited to be able to effect change. The *how* of eliciting this information is based on trust. Violence, AIDS, objectification, cardiovascular disease, malnutrition, depression, chronic pain, Alzheimer's disease, economics, coerced silence and stigma are key issues for women. Information systems are powerful tools in providing timely information for women clients and clinicians to use appropriate services and translate information into knowledge and action.

Incentives for clinicians focus on health improvements. Policy-makers and funders of health care are expecting clinicians to demonstrate how well they are contributing to the improvement of the health status of populations and groups and will pay for services based on the evidence that these services make a difference.

Orientation to care is a population-based perspective rather than a narrower disease-based focus. Public health perspectives of wellness, early intervention, health maintenance strategies, coordinated services, outreach and follow-up are essential components. Population-based models have the greatest effectiveness using the most efficient resources, yet enable individualized interventions to maximize women's health outcomes. For example, the personal context of a depressed woman with children whose husband assaults her is different from that of a single man with dual diagnoses of schizophrenia and drug dependence living in supported accommodation.

These personal contexts need to drive individual solutions to enhance positive health outcomes. Accessing and integrating relevant information (more than biology) to assist in appropriate treatment interventions is key.

The content—the *what* of this framework—will look different depending on each woman and/or family we relate to, but can be applied in all communities irrespective of region or country.[20]

This approach is a radical shift from the traditional medical model. It is one of a reciprocal arrangement, learning about a woman in the context of her current life experiences and relating to her as the primary partner and expert of her health-care team, for the purpose of contributing to her improved health outcomes. For example, rather than non-compliance to a clinician-directed plan being attributed to non-cooperation, a woman's response may be concern over side-effects that have not been taken seriously.[4] This perspective puts women in context, and broadens the focus to include the *psychosocial* component of the women-centred frame.[21]

Gender cross-cultural perspectives on women's mental health/violence[4]

Violence and control are the unwanted realities for women worldwide.[10] Women traumatized in their homes and/or communities have serious health consequences, such as mistrust that there is a safe personal world. They experience physical trauma, traumatic stress disorder, depression and diminished self-esteem. The prevalence rates for gender-based violence, including rape, domestic violence, mutilation, murder and sexual abuse, are high.[22] Up to 25% of American women experience physical and/or sexual assault by a current or former partner.[8,23] These rates are consistent with rates of abuse found in well-designed studies in

Canada, New Zealand, Belgium, Barbados, Norway, and India.[10] Countries such as Chile, Mexico, Sri Lanka, Korea, Malaysia, Kenya and Uganda report much higher rates of abuse: from one in three women to two in three women experience male partner abuse.[10]

The most prevalent abuse of women is by intimate male partners. The difference between violence against women versus violence against men is that the violence against women is done by those whom women trust, their partners, and these abusive experiences may continue or be repeated with coercion of silence. Violence against men is primarily by strangers or casual acquaintances.[10]

Violence towards women is not a new phenomenon but a historical legacy of how women are perceived in societies by dominant groups and treated as objects to be controlled.[24] Women have been treated as chattels and have been described as mad for challenging the status quo; laws have been written to sanction the status quo.[25]

It was not until 1994 that the United States Congress passed the *Violence against Women Act*, which addresses the issue of domestic violence.[25] This is the first time that American women have had their rights regarding domestic violence spelled out.

Consider gender-based violence, which spans the life cycle. American data show a one in three chance of molestation for girls. There is child physical and sexual abuse and rape, rape in adolescence and adulthood, one in four women battered during pregnancy, sexual harassment in the workplace, and sexual abuse by some health-care providers.[26] This is the contextual reality for many; the health sector needs to adapt and appropriately respond to this in order to better assist women.

These data are difficult for clinicians to relate to since violence is so emotionally charged. Gender trauma has not been part of the med-

ical model classification system until recently. There have been gaps in language, tools, training and integrated delivery systems to help clinicians assist women in an organized way.[27] Women choose a health setting for assistance with this issue, despite its current deficiencies, over police or crisis hot lines.[10] The health sector is the only public institution likely to interact with most women, and therefore it is essential that detection, support and treatments are developed from a public health perspective rather than treating the physical or emotional issues out of context with the social ones.

Consider also women's exposure to abuse not only from partners but also in shelters, in the workplace, in communities, and as immigrants or refugees, or against those with mental illness. Indeed, violence is considered to be one of the greatest health risk factors for women.[28]

Women with schizophrenia or mood disorders are very vulnerable to abuse, rape and the sequelae of unprotected sex, including AIDS. These women have cognitive impairment, affective instability, poor judgement and an environment of coercion and fear. Consider the prevalence rates: up to 70% of women in psychiatric inpatient settings have histories of physical or sexual abuse, 40% of women with pervasive mental disorders were incest victims, and 50% of women using mental health services have been sexually abused. These rates are at least twice those for men.[29]

Addressing this vast pervasive problem in a systemic way did not originate with the medical sector but rather from grass roots or consumer leadership. Nosology based on a biological model does not incorporate sociocultural values and aetiology in its framework, but rather is an add-on, which makes it difficult to scope out relevant issues surrounding aetiology, diagnoses, access to care and treatment strategies. Post-traumatic stress disorder, borderline personality disorder and eating disorders are diagnoses that are attempts by the medical sector to define illnesses that are responses to the environment.

Gender bias is illustrated by the Hindu practice in Bali, where women are considered to be unclean during menses. Public signs are posted stating that women who are menstruating are not allowed inside religious centres to pray.

New Zealanders have considered women's health status using a health services research perspective and have raised serious questions about the validity of policy decisions for the delivery of health services that serve women. Health data statistics have been developed independently of women's health issues and therefore there are gaps in the knowledge base. Kilgour has proposed a women's health model to sort out health-influencing variables that are *indicators* for health status and outcome variables that are *measures* of health status. Outcome measures include morbidity, mortality, disability and wellbeing. Their frame of reference incorporates a population perspective separating different groups within the population by age, gender and ethnicity. This is further refined by considering the political environment for women of funding, legislation, and treatment of native peoples. Health status is influenced by one's physical environment at home and at work, which may be the same place, experiences across the life and family cycle, adaptation and strengths, family, and religion. These are the health research issues that use a different lens than the traditional biomedical one. Although these policies and framework have been developed, there is concern that the political decisions about funding are still being made using the male perspective and that resources are not equitably distributed.[30]

Mental health is both an outcome of favourable circumstances and a necessary attribute of performing, achieving, creating, sharing and enjoying life. Mental health policy needs to address the educational needs of health-care workers for them to have a better understanding of power relations between men and women and the impact of these gender differences on the health of women.[4]

Clinical research practices

Rosser describes the androcentric bias in psychiatric diagnosis and clinical research.[5] A fundamental premise of scientists, that the scientific method is objective and has no bias, is challenged. The prevailing bias for women's health is one of male perspective. Since most scientists are men, values held by them as males are not distinguished as biasing, but rather are made congruent with the values of all scientists and thus become synonymous with the 'objective' view of the world.[31] Examples of this bias are pervasive. The physician's health study of 22 071 men looked at the effects of aspirin in decreasing the risk of myocardial infarction and generalized findings to men and women.[5] The definition of AIDS was not corrected by the Centers for Disease Control until 1993 to include women. Women may be the majority users of some medications, yet information gathered from clinical research may not have tested women, or the aetiology of the disease in women may not have been studied. The depressive effects of 'the pill' on women over several decades have not yet been fully addressed. Women matched with men on severity of cardiovascular illness receive much less than 'standard' care.[5] The choice and definition of problems for study reflect societal bias towards those who are powerful—white, middle–upper-class males.

Issues such as *the* scientific method become very polarized when the methodology is challenged as flawed.[31] Decades of research using quantitative analysis have been generalized for all women, when subjects have been primarily middle-class Caucasian men.[32] These gender, socio-cultural, political and economic biases raise serious questions about the validity and interpretation of findings, which then are translated into health policy for women, classifications of illness for women, and health services for women.[33] A research methodology that excludes women does not provide clinically relevant information for women.

Investigating gender differences in rates of depressive disorder, as well as sex differences within a particular depressive disorder, require different kinds of inquiry. Bebbington[9] points out that if there were a universal biological vulnerability in women for depression, then these rates should not be affected by sociodemographic attributes such as marital status or the effect of parenting small children, or a particular societal value attributed to the homemaking role. The qualitative research paradigm as compared with the quantitative one has different criteria and membership (consumers versus scientists) in identifying what science is and how it is used. In the qualitative model, those who use the information are those who live it. Therefore, access and dissemination of this information to women in an available form is critical.[34] Application of clinical research is shifted to women's worlds and experiences. Community surveys are the best sources for assessing sex differences in depressive disorders.[9]

Hamilton[1] describes profound barriers to change in the health research sector due to the conceptualization of modern medicine's theoretical framework as one of *biological primacy*. This occurs when a biological factor is assumed to be causal in describing a phenomenon and psychosocial factors are minimized. This reductionist approach to the complexity of human behaviour is described as a fundamental error

in thinking, 'attribution error'.[35] Thus the context (role) of situations as determinants of a person's behaviour is underestimated and devalued and the biological factors are overestimated. To correct this bias would involve several ways of assessing the relative importance of social, psychological and biological components for sex differences. Hormonal theories, life-cycle issues, coping styles and the impact of psychosocial adversity are a few lines of inquiry. A major political problem is that these research themes have not been appropriately or equitably integrated into the health funding umbrella, since there is male model bias about research funding and therefore bias in defining appropriate priorities for health research.[5]

A major rationale for excluding female animals or subjects, using the male model, was that the oestrous cycle complicated the interpretation of research findings. Over the last two decades in the USA, exclusionary policies for woman subjects in the three clinical phases of drug trials have been in effect. Women who menstruate were excluded in phase I and II studies because animal reproductive studies had not been completed and therefore fetal risk was the rationale for excluding this huge population of women. In phase III studies, which included larger controlled trials, non-pregnant women were included but the data were not evaluated to assess possible sex differences.[36] The issue that was not acknowledged for so long was that it is the oestrous cycle that creates so many of the different responses for women across all biological systems, such as immune, cardiovascular and neuroendocrine.

This underrepresentation of women and other subjugated groups was classic scientific practice in the USA in both the Food and Drug Administration (FDA), which evaluates the efficacy and safety of new drugs, and the National Institutes of Health, which fund clinical trials of marketed drugs to evaluate therapeutic utility or compare treatments for a particular disease.[36,37] It took until the 1990s, and after political pressure from women consumers, scientists, and politicians, for the United States' General Accounting Office (GAO) to review drugs approved by the FDA after a 1988 FDA guideline on inclusion of male and female subjects was issued. This guideline requested subset analyses to assess sex differences in response to the safety and effectiveness of new drugs. The GAO found that the guideline was not followed for two-thirds of the drugs, and that the proportion of women in the studies was not representative of the population of women with the illness studied. At last, this is the beginning of a new era for women, with the understanding that research using male subjects does not translate into practice very well for women.

A good example of missing important adverse events is the bupropion story. It is based on sex differences, testing a drug primarily on males, and then using it primarily on females.[38] Seizures were reported in women with bulimia who were treated with this antidepressant. After further study, the dosage for this drug was reduced. Hamilton and Yonkers[39] identified sex differences across the life cycle and menstrual cycle as they related to various psychopharmacological agents. Effects of oral contraceptives (decrease imipramine by one-third in women to reduce risk of toxicity), hormone replacement therapy, differences in smoking and alcohol intake between men and women on various psychotropic drugs, need to be incorporated into better designed studies to provide more appropriate guidelines for women. These guidelines will address sex differences and provide clinical decision analyses and act as powerful tools to assist clinicians in managing dosages, and medications along the menstrual and life cycle. Asking women whether the intensity of their symptoms change at certain times in their menstrual cycle helps

to stratify groups of women who need to titrate their medications based on the phase of their menstrual cycle. By not stratifying in this way, pooled data may not detect these differences.

This woman-centred model challenges how we collect data and research clinical areas that are relevant for women. It challenges how we traditionally define mental health and illness. It shifts from using a dominant group definition to describe *normal* behaviour and subjugated groups' different behaviour described as *abnormal* behaviour, to a model where a woman is considered in her sociogeopolitical frame of reference, and strategies are developed with her to more effectively enhance her health status.[40]

Labelling women with premenstrual syndrome as psychiatric rather than normalizing the experience as gynaecological is one example of a gender-different point of reference. Labelling women as having borderline personality disorders, which then gets translated by many clinicians as women who are difficult to treat, seductive, and bad, rather than addressing their real issues of incest, rape, physical and other sexual abuse, is another example of blame for difference from the predominant male group. Other examples of the late twentieth century description of women as bad, mad or inferior include the American Psychiatric nosology debates about premenstrual syndrome disorders, or self-defeating personality of women, where women are blamed for the circumstances in which they live.[41] Gender influences diagnosis, which currently may or may not be meaningful or accurate. Psychopathology refers to an actual disorder that may or may not be specified by diagnosis.[42] One major illness that has lacked a unique category is mood disorder in postpartum women. The prevalence was found to be 7.8% for postnatal depression in Maori and European women in New Zealand.[43] The treatment interventions are different, yet there is not a separate classification. Consequently it is difficult for this important group to be evaluated, since it is grouped together with other mood disorders. To teach and learn about postpartum women, there has to be a curriculum and a way of researching these issues to assist in intervention.

A women-centred approach does not mean that diagnoses are thrown out but rather are considered from a gender-meaningful perspective. Psychosocial realities are part of nosology.[21] By definition, this perspective causes us to consider our unconscious and conscious biases in attempting to be egalitarian and non-judgemental in working with the populations and individual women we serve.[44]

Psychiatric illness in women: implications for health-care clinicians

There are many differences for women as distinct from men that translate globally, socially, politically and culturally into how we view, experience, relate and contribute in each of our societies.[45] Similarly, it is difficult to understand what brown skin means if one has white skin, or understand a Hindu perspective if one has an Anglican experience, or what the meaning is of a different culture. These racial, cultural and gender experiences have tremendous impact on how women relate to traditional medical models of health care.

Why is this women-centred approach an important consideration in providing health services to women? It is critical to have a relationship that is grounded in mutual respect and regard for each other's human dignity if there is any expectation that an optimal health outcome will ensue.[46] This approach is based on research that demonstrates that women of all

colours, cultures, race and ethnic groups have been discriminated by psychiatric labelling, treatments and care developed based on male findings, because the dominant framework has been of white men.[4,47]

Women, if they have access to a formal health-care system, obtain most services, including mental health, from their primary care clinicians. A common example of a woman *experiencing* a male model approach is when she is told by her clinician that she is hypertensive, is prescribed medication and is told to lose weight and to stop smoking. Another example is when a woman is told that she is depressed, must take her antidepressant medication, since that intervention works best, and told to return in 1 month. The health status outcomes of these women have less than an optimal chance of improving, based on their interactions with their clinicians, lack of follow-up and lack of integration of other services to help them improve their health.

Innovative culturally sensitive and effective models of mental health delivery that recognize and tap into community resources for strengths and supports are available. These have been evaluated and demonstrate the efficacy and cost-benefits of cross-cultural training. Models building on family strengths and involving kinship networks are effective with women from traditional family-oriented cultures. Religion is an integral component for social interaction and spiritual wellbeing in African-American communities. The church is a strategic partner in developing culturally acceptable modes of treatment and assisting with the social–environmental issues/needs of African-American women who access treatment.[48] Evidence-based care uses clinical algorithms to demonstrate effective outcomes for women.[49] As clinical information is refined to be more specific for women, this new information can be integrated into these algorithms. Refined treatment strategies include assisting with and support for a safe place, appropriate interventions for women with post-traumatic stress disorders, therapy groups for battered women, individualized dosing schedules across menstrual cycles, and dosages not based on a 70-kg white male. Pharmacokinetics and pharmacodynamics are very different between men and women. Management of side-effects that are relevant to women, such as weight gain, is important in improving mood.

Women, who are viewed most differently from the dominant group due to differences of gender, culture, economics, or ethnicity, often *access* the dominant group health-care system, through an urgent or emergent venue in a crisis or in an unplanned way from the perspective of the clinician or health-care system. There are many reasons for this, but a major factor is the way in which the delivery system is configured. It is not particularly useful or meaningful for women. Her access is described as unplanned by clinicians and planners, but not by the person accessing these services, who is using them at the very time they are most needed.

A woman might describe her access through an urgent venue as the only reasonable way to use Western health services. Her purpose may be more than seeking treatment for physical trauma, but rather a search for a more holistic approach to her issues. She may be searching for assistance with her health and safety needs, and these may be best met 'after hours' from her perspective. A more successful model includes working with women and individualizing strategies that work for each woman to improve her health and safety.

If domestic violence is actively occurring, a primary treatment intervention is to assist a woman in her safety and welfare both physically and emotionally. Identifying that this woman is depressed or physically traumatized and treating her only for the *components* of her

reality does not meet quality standards of care.[27] If a clinician simply targets this woman's depression without other strategies and actions for her safety, she is often lost to follow-up, or dead. This approach is not comprehensive enough or collaborative enough to validate this woman's real life experience and to enable her to use the interventions effectively. Often there are other systems of care, links with community resources, that need to be integrated so that the services are coordinated with no gaps. It is the responsibility of the health team to assist a woman in the coordination of care. Woman-specific information, such as gender-specific and culturally appropriate evidence-based strategies for care, and communication tools that easily track interventions and time frames for appropriate service coordination, are key in assisting with effective treatment.[50,51]

The medical sector has recognized late domestic violence as a serious public health problem but has not really incorporated the issue into its clinical model, because the medical focus is response to *disease* rather than intervention and prevention of *illness*. The American Medical Association issued guidelines in 1992 that are followed by individual clinicians or organizations and therefore are implemented with great variance.[52] Clinicians need to be skilled in assisting women appropriately who are in violent situations. Recognition of this problem is necessary, and tools have been developed to assist clinicians in working with women in solving their safety and welfare issues.[27] This means that clinicians must be able to communicate with women consumers in emergency rooms or therapy sessions or primary care settings that they are there not only for treatment of physical injuries, but in order to assist them in maintaining their welfare.

Most treatment interventions for women have been tested and designed using a male biological model, and do not work as well for women.[53] Women experience twice as much major depression as men, more co-occurring depressions than men, and more atypical depressions than men. Postpartum depressions are prevalent and specific illnesses for women, but are not identified with a specific classification of diagnosis. Clinicians working with these women need to refine their treatment interventions and consider other ways of delivering them to effect better outcomes for women. Issues such as sex differences in presentation of depression, gaps in assessment, evaluation and treatment intervention skills, and sex differences in response to psychopharmacology, create vast areas for training, education, service delivery and research needs.

Many clinicians can recite the importance of cultural, gender, social class, racial and ethnic diversity, and sensitivity; we often feel that we do not know *what* and *how* to incorporate this information into our practices. What is meant by consumer focus? Clinical training schools are slow to change curricula, and those changes do not affect those clinicians who have completed their formal training. This is improving as some countries are developing women's health curricula, programmes and specialties that are about and for women rather than focused on their reproductive systems.[21] The old medical model focuses more on the biology of illnesses, minimizing the importance of the critical variables affecting the intensity and course of mood disorders. These include the meaning of the illness to a woman and its impact on her self-esteem.[48] Educational tools that include women-relevant assessment and evaluation screens and intervention techniques such as safety and violence issues, culturally sensitive approaches to care, and telecommunication consultation strategies and programmes are available to assist clinicians in incorporating this women-centred framework into their practices.[30,54] Those training programmes and service delivery systems that use gender-specific strategies will survive.

The good news is that there are gender-specific information and communication tools to assist us with bringing this specific knowledge to the place and time when a women works with her team. Clinical algorithms and evidence-based treatment interventions are available and need to be refined so that they are more specific for different populations of women. Those specialist clinicians who have expertise in assisting with improved outcomes for women need to consider working with other clinicians and community organizations using a consultation–liaison approach. Other systems of care have different names, such as shared care,[55] integrated care or strategic partnerships. This is one *how* of consumer focus delivery system.

Approaches for the promotion of women's mental health[56]

Strategies for clinicians using a woman's perspective and framework to promote women's mental health include:

- mental health definitions that are appropriate and within the context of a defined group of women
- development of aetiologies for mental illness that describe differences between groups at the socio-political level, rather than at an individual or family level, which attributes blame for rate differences
- evaluation of mental health status using appropriate contextual tools for assessment, diagnosis and treatment interventions
- access to gender and culturally appropriate services

- organizing and structuring mental health institutions and programmes so they are relevant and meaningful for women
- research that is gender and group specific with clinical application considerations
- training of mental health professionals using information technology tools to minimize the transition time from design to incorporating successful treatment interventions for women.

Undertreatment of depression

Primary care practitioners see more people with depression than do specialists, as do social workers compared with psychiatrists. Depressed women are underdetected and undertreated by their clinicians and many do not use their mental health system for treatment due to stigma and discrimination based on diagnosis and risk to security of paid employment. The point prevalence for women with major depression in Western nations is 4.5–9.3%, with 20–25% lifetime prevalence.[49] Untreated depression has great morbidity, with impaired social relationships, physical restriction, and diminished role functioning. Somatic complaints of pain or low energy, or vague complaints, may be the language used to convey distress. Women who present with these complaints are described by clinicians as very difficult. Doctors feel that they do not have the training, tools or skills to evaluate these ways of describing illness. There are difficulties in describing what is the meaning of symptoms, based on differences in power authority, gender, and culture. Clinicians skilled in assessment using a women's explanatory model[14] of a problem, working with women rather than a symptom, are effective. Using clinical guidelines for assessment and services for women, and revising them as new information is identified, is easier now that there are reliable and easy-to-use information systems to update clinicians at a time when the female consumer and the clinician need these resources. It is important that we use our information systems to access appropriate culturally sensitive clinical tools for training, evaluation, treatment, coordination and follow-up of services. Many women are lost to follow-up after the initial visit when depression is detected. Issues around supportive environment, education about side-effects, cost, stigma, and ease of follow-up are key for adherence.

The epidemiological catchment area (ECA) data demonstrate that black women have significantly greater rates of somatization disorders than any other group. Tools that are not refined to elicit appropriate ways of capturing depressive symptoms have been used by researchers to determine that black women have lower rates of depression than white women, but black women have more depressive symptoms. Generalized distress in black women has been ignored.[48] If assessment tools and research questions were framed from the perspectives of woman consumers, these findings would look very different and treatment strategies would follow.

Primary, secondary and tertiary prevention in models for the future

Information is powerful only if it is accessible and in a form that people can use. It is clear that health-care systems need to change. Clinical services need to be evaluated by outcome measures, by demonstrating improvement in the health status for a population of women. Instead, funders are currently measuring units of service rather than effective treatments. We need to identify that the *what* that is delivered is appropriate. Rather than conceptualize service delivery from the perspective of primary, secondary or tertiary intervention, it is more effective to consider integration of services to meet the woman consumer needs across the continuum of her *health and illness*.

This shift in focus is designed to empower individuals to direct and choose their own health options. This does not mean that clinicians are passive, but rather that a partnership is developed about wellness and health. How to implement these goals is key. If a woman is unsafe, or has no shelter, or no economic viability, as well as having a serious mood disorder, this is her reality. This context has tremendous impact on her mood disorder and quality of life. Strategies need to be worked out with her about what best meets her needs.

A health path to the future for women

As women embrace the dawning of a new millennium, we are told we have much to celebrate in the arena of women's health.

Some women's voices have been heard in the political and public policy arenas, which has made a difference in recognizing the different needs from men of women of different cultures, sexual orientation, religion and ages. For example, in the late 1980s the United States National Institutes of Health (NIH) allocated only 13.5% of its research budget to research illnesses of major consequence for women. In response, Congress in 1991 created an Office of Research on Women's Health to address specific issues for the health of women. Federal funding, which is so important in order for basic and clinical research to move forwards, has been mandated to reflect a more equitable gender and ethnic balance in research. In 1991, the NIH launched the Women's Health Initiative (WHI) to raise the priority of women's health and provide baseline data on understudied causes of death in women.[5]

The WHI, a 15-year clinical study, involving 160 000 postmenopausal women of all races and socio-economic status, is examining the major causes of death, disability and frailty in women. Now new women's programmes have been created in all the health institutes of the National Institutes of Health. No more, we hope, will we have study results generalized for both sexes with only males in the study.[57] Despite this current status of women's health research, women still reflect a cautionary note, given the pervasive male perspective of the power elites at the medical, political, scientific, educational and cultural levels in all societies. There is an urgent message for scientists, health policy makers and clinicians. The clinical applications of women's health policy and science must not fail women for yet one more generation.

The American College of Women's Health Physicians[21] has been created to address the holistic health needs of women by developing a relevant body of knowledge, research strategies and clinical practices that address these needs. This knowledge base is essential for clinicians to learn to meet required clinical and culturally sensitive competencies that serve different health service needs of all women.

Many women in the USA have turned to alternative medical approaches for their care, which exceeds their access to primary care. Examples include acupuncture, for chronic pain that has a high correlation with depression, biofeedback, which increases circulation for people with diabetes and greatly diminishes fecal incontinence, and chiropractic care for lower back pain. These are far more effective than other treatments.[58] Guided imagery is an important adjunctive to chemotherapy for treatment of cancer.[59] Women have sought out what works for them. Their clinicians need to help them match the best treatments for their individual needs. Clinicians can enhance the timeliness and effectiveness of response by being knowledgeable about other treatments and develop strategic partnerships with complementary health and medical services to serve women.

The lens through which to consider the health of women includes culture, life-cycle issues, ethnicity, class, sexual orientation, religion, and lifestyles. The appropriate health system uses different concepts, language and outcomes from the traditional male disease model. It is essential to translate these differences into one's clinical practice if one is providing health-care services for women. Public policy and funding agencies have refined priorities for health services. They include populations of people to treat, and have increased expectations that services provided will have positive impacts on the health status of treated individuals and groups. Health-care delivery has moved from the medical model of one-to-one treatments from a skilled practitioner with one patient or family, to a system of integrated

care that takes into consideration populations of people who desire interventions that will positively affect their health status. This is achieved using a team approach and a sex- and gender-specific lens.

Women view their health status within a context of the worlds in which they live. This social context perspective uses a macro lens rather than a micro diseased organ system. This big picture is political. There may be domestic violence in her home, or the societal rules of her culture may be oppressive and devalue her because of her gender, class, colour or religion. Clinicians need to meet women at their point of reference.

Acknowledgments

The author thanks Anne Kasper PhD and Eileen Hoffman MD for editorial comments.

References

1. Hamilton JA, Feminist theory and health psychology: tools for an egalitarian, woman-centered approach to women's health. In: Dan AJ, ed., *Reframing Woman's Health: Multidisciplinary Research and Practice* (Sage: Thousand Oaks, 1994) 56–66.
2. Miller JB, *Toward a New Psychology of Women* (Beacon Press: Boston, 1986).
3. Kandel ER, A new intellectual framework for psychiatry, *Am J Psychiatry* 1998; **155**:457–69.
4. Paltiel FL, Mental health of women in the Americas. In: Gomez EG, ed., *Gender, Women and Health in the Americas*, No. 541 (Pan American Health Organization, Scientific Publication: Washington, 1993) 131–48.
5. Rosser SV, *Women's Health—Missing from US Medicine*, 1st edn (Indiana University Press: Bloomington, IN, 1994).
6. VandeCreek L, Rogers E, Lester J, Use of alternative therapies among breast cancer outpa-

   tients compared with the general population, *Altern Ther Health Med* 1999; **5**:71–6.
7. Hoffman E, The malpractice of women's medicine. In: Hoffman E, ed., *Our Health, Our Lives, A Revolutionary Approach to Total Health Care for Women*, 1st edn (Pocket: New York, 1995) 1–17.
8. Warshaw C, Domestic violence: challenges to medical practice. In: Dan AJ, ed., *Reframing Women's Health: Multidisciplinary Research and Practice* (Sage: Thousand Oaks, 1994) 201–18.
9. Bebbington PE, Sex and depression, *Psychol Med* 1998; **28**:1–8.
10. Heise LL, Gender-based abuse: the global epidemic. In: Dan AJ, ed., *Reframing Women's Health: Multidisciplinary Research and Practice* (Sage: Thousand Oaks, 1994) 233–50.
11. Yew L, Need JA, Women's health needs, *Med J Aust* 1988; **148**:110–12.
12. Dan AJ, Introduction. In: Dan AJ, ed.,

Reframing Women's Health: Multidisciplinary Research and Practice (Sage: Thousand Oaks, 1994) ix–xxii.

13. Massion CT, Clancy CM, Maxell ME, Women's access to health care. In: Lemcke DP, Pattison J, Marshall LA, Cowley DS, eds, *Primary Care of Women*, 1st edn (Appleton and Lange: Norwalk, 1995) 1–6.

14. Brown KH, Corbett K, Sociocultural perspectives. In: Lemcke DP, Pattison J, Marshall LA, Cowley DS, eds, *Primary Care of Women*, 1st edn (Appleton and Lange: Norwalk, 1995) 7–14.

15. Johnson K, Women's health care: an innovative model, *Women Ther* 1987; **6**:305–11.

16. Oakley A, Class categories. In: Oakley A, ed., *Subject Women, Where Women Stand Today— Politically, Economically, Socially, Emotionally* (Pantheon: New York, 1981) 281–96.

17. Rieker PP, Jankowski MK, Sexism and women's psychological status. In: Willie CV, Rieker PP, Kramer BM, Brown BB, eds, *Mental Health, Racism, and Sexism*, 2nd edn (University of Pittsburgh Press: Pittsburgh, 1995) 27–50.

18. Marshall LA, Cain J, Ethical issues. In: Lemke DP, Pattison J, Marshall LA, Cowley DS, eds, *Primary Care of Women*, 1st edn (Appleton and Lange: Norwalk, 1995) 47–50.

19. Phillips KL, Preparing ourselves as behavioral health clinicians for the twenty-first century. In: Alperin RM, Phillips DG, eds, *The Impact of Managed Care on the Practice of Psychotherapy: Innovation, Implementation, and Controversy*, 1st edn (Brunner/Mazel: New York, 1997) 13–30.

20. Boyd JA, Ethnic and cultural diversity in feminist therapy: keys to power. In: White EC, ed., *The Black Women's Health Book: Speaking for Ourselves*, 2nd edn (Seal: Seattle, 1994) 226–34.

21. American College of Women's Health Physicians, *Guiding Principles Dedicated to the Art and Science of Women's Health* (ACWHP: Schaumburg, Illinois, 1996).

22. Koss MP, The negative impact of crime victimization on women's health and medical use. In: Dan AJ, ed., *Reframing Women's Health: Multidisciplinary Research and Practice* (Sage: Thousand Oaks, 1994) 189–200.

23. Straus MA, Gelles RJ, Societal change and change in family violence from 1975 to 1985 as revealed by two national surveys, *J Marriage Fam* 1986; **48**:465–79.

24. Brownmiller S, *Against Our Will, Men, Women, and Rape* (Simon and Schuster: New York, 1975).

25. Schornstein SL, Societal perspectives on domestic violence. In: Schornstein SL, ed., *Domestic Violence and Health Care, What Every Professional Needs to Know* (Sage: Thousand Oaks, 1997) 14–45.

26. Carmen E, Family violence and the victim-to-patient process. In: Dickstein LJ, Nadelson CC, eds, *Family Violence: Emerging Issues of a National Crisis* (American Psychiatric Press: Washington, 1989) 17–27.

27. Schornstein SL, The medical response. In: Schornstein SL, ed., *Domestic Violence and Health Care: What Every Professional Needs to Know* (Sage: Thousand Oaks, 1997) 70–97.

28. Winters M, Carbonell D, Glass L et al, Violence against women. In: *The Boston Women's Health Book: Our Bodies, Ourselves for the New Century* (Touchstone/Simon & Schuster: New York, 1998) 158–78.

29. Carmen E, Inner-city community mental health: the interplay of abuse and race in chronic mentally ill women. In: Willie CV, Rieker PP, Kramer BM, Brown BB, eds, *Mental Health, Racism, and Sexism*, 2nd edn (University of Pittsburgh Press: Pittsburgh, 1995) 217–36.

30. Kilgour R, *Exploring Women's Health Status, Data Requirements* (Discussion paper 10, Department of Health, Health Services Research: Wellington, 1991).

31. Rosser SV, Gender bias in clinical research: the difference it makes. In: Dan AJ, ed., *Reframing Women's Health: Multidisciplinary Research and Practice* (Sage: Thousand Oaks, 1994) 253–65.

32. Hamilton J, Parry B, Sex-related differences in clinical drug response: implications for women's health, *J Am Med Women's Assoc* 1983; **38**: 126–32.

33. Padgett DK, Women's mental health: some directions for research, *Am J Orthopsychiatry* 1997; **67**:522–34.

34. Hall JM, Stevens PE, Rigor in feminist research, *Adv Nurs Sci* 1991; **13**:16–29.

35. Fausto-Sterling A, *Myths of Gender: Biological Theories about Women and Men* (Basic Books: New York, 1985).

36. Harrison W, Brumfield MA, Psychopharma-

cological drug testing in women. In: Jensvold MF, Halbreich U, Hamilton JA, eds, *Psychopharmacology and Women: Sex, Gender and Hormones* (American Psychiatric Press: Washington, 1996) 371–91.

37. Bennett JC, Inclusion of women in clinical trials—policies for population subgroups, *N Engl J Med* 1993; 329:288–92.

38. Davidson J, Seizures and bupropion: a review, *J Clin Psychiatry* 1989; 50:256–61.

39. Hamilton JA, Yonkers KA, Sex differences in pharmacokinetics of psychotropic medications. In: Jensvold MF, Halbreich U, Hamilton JA, eds, *Psychopharmacology and Women: Sex, Gender and Hormones* (American Psychiatric Press: Washington, 1996) 11–71.

40. Townsend J, Racial, ethnic, and mental illness stereotypes: cognitive process and behavioral effects. In: Willie CV, Rieker PP, Kramer BM, Brown BB, eds, *Mental Health, Racism, and Sexism*, 2nd edn (University of Pittsburgh Press: Pittsburgh, 1995) 119–50.

41. Caplan PJ, The name game: psychiatry, misogyny and taxonomy, *Women Ther* 1987; 6:132–43.

42. Howell E, The influence of gender on diagnosis and psychopathology. In: Howell E, Bayes M, eds, *Women and Mental Health* (Basic Books: New York, 1981) 153–59.

43. Wilson DA, McKenzie JM, Mood disorders in postpartum women. In: Joyce PR, Romans SE, Ellis PM, Silverstone TS, eds, *Affective Disorders* (Department of Psychological Medicine: Christchurch, 1995) 241–56.

44. Lerner HG, *Women in Therapy* (J Aronson: Northvale, NJ, 1988).

45. Oakley A, Politics in a man's world. In: Oakley A, ed., *Subject Women, Where Women Stand Today—Politically, Economically, Socially, Emotionally* (Pantheon: New York, 1981) 297–315.

46. Chernomas W, Rainonen S, Research and therapy with women: a feminist perspective, *Can Ment Health* 1994; 42:2–6.

47. Levy L, ed., *Finding Our Own Solutions: Women's Experience of Mental Health Care* (National Association of Mental Health: London, 1986).

48. Lefley HP, Bestman EW, Training for culturally appropriate services. In: Willie CV, Rieker PP,

Kramer BM, Brown BB, eds, *Mental Health, Racism, and Sexism*, 2nd edn (University of Pittsburgh Press: Pittsburgh, 1995) 351–72.

49. Rush J, *Depression in Primary Care*, Vol. 1, *Detection and Diagnosis* (Clinical Practice Guideline 5, Agency for Health Care Policy and Research, United States Department of Health and Human Services: Washington, 1993).

50. Johnson K, Hoffman E, Women's health and curriculum transformation: the role of medical specialization. In: Dan AJ, ed., *Reframing Women's Health: Multidisciplinary Research and Practice*, 1st edn (Sage: Thousand Oaks, 1994) 27–39.

51. Johnson K, Hoffman E, Women's health, designing and implementing a new medical specialty, *J Women's Health* 1992; 1:95–9.

52. American Medial Association, *Diagnostic and Treatment Guidelines on Domestic Violence* (American Medical Association: Chicago, 1992).

53. Jensvold MF, Hamilton JA, Halbreich U, Future research directions: methodological considerations for advancing gender-sensitive pharmacology. In: Jensvold MF, Halbreich U, Hamilton JA, eds, *Psychopharmacology and Women, Sex, Gender, and Hormones* (American Psychiatric Press: Washington, 1996) 415–29.

54. Avery BY, Breathing life into ourselves: the evolution of the national black women's health project. In: White EC, ed., *The Black Women's Health Book: Speaking for Ourselves*, 2nd edn (Seal: Seattle, 1994) 4–10.

55. Turner T, de Sorkin A, Sharing psychiatric care with primary care physicians: the Toronto Doctors Hospital experience (1991–1995), *Can J Psychiatry* 1997; 42:950–4.

56. Turner CB, Kramer BM, Connections between racism and mental health. In: Willie CV, Rieker PP, Kramer BM, eds, *Mental Health, Racism, and Sexism*, 2nd edn (University of Pittsburgh Press: Pittsburgh, 1995) 3–25.

57. Blumenthal SJ, Toward a new prescription for women's mental and physical health: the US experience, *Bailliere's Clin Psychiatry* 2:593–618.

58. Fugh-Berman A, *Alternative Medicine: What Works* (Odonian Press: Tucson, 1996).

59. Naparstek B, *Staying Well with Guided Imagery* (Warner: New York, 1994).

INDEX